VETERINARY DERMATOPATHOLOGY

A macroscopic and microscopic evaluation of canine and feline skin disease

VETERINARY DERMATOPATHOLOGY

A macroscopic and microscopic
evaluation of canine and feline
skin disease

THELMA LEE GROSS, D.V.M.

Pathologist
California Dermatopathology Service;
Consulting Pathologist
California Veterinary Diagnostics
West Sacramento, California

PETER J. IHRKE, V.M.D.

Professor of Dermatology
School of Veterinary Medicine
University of California
Davis, California

EMILY J. WALDER, V.M.D.

Director, Histopathology Services
Veterinary Centers of America Laboratory
Los Angeles, California

with 727 illustrations

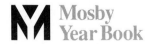
Mosby
Year Book

St. Louis   Baltimore   Boston   Chicago   London   Philadelphia   Sydney   Toronto

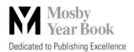
Mosby
Year Book
Dedicated to Publishing Excellence

Editor: Robert W. Reinhardt
Assistant Editor: Melba Steube
Project Manager: Gayle May Morris
Production Editor: Donna L. Walls
Designer: Liz Fett
Cover Art: Emily J. Walder

Printed in the United States of America

Mosby—Year Book, Inc.
11830 Westline Industrial Drive
St. Louis, Missouri 63146

Library of Congress Cataloging-in-Publication Data
Gross, Thelma Lee.
   Veterinary dermatopathology : a macroscopic and microscopic
evaluation of canine and feline skin disease / Thelma Lee Gross,
Peter J. Ihrke, Emily J. Walder.
      p.   cm.
   Includes index.
   ISBN 0-8016-5809-8
   1. Dogs—Diseases—Diagnosis. 2. Cats—Diseases—Diagnosis.
3. Veterinary dermatology. 4. Dogs—Histopathology. 5. Cats—
Histopathology. 6. Skin—Diseases—Diagnosis. I. Ihrke, Peter J.
II. Walder, Emily J. III. Title.
   SF992.S55G76   1992
   636.7'089'65—dc20
                                                        91-34242
                                                        CIP

92 93 94 95 96 GW/MV 9 8 7 6 5 4 3 2 1

To our Parents,

Seymour L. Gross, Elaine Linford Gross,
Jeannette P. Ihrke, *and* Louis Bernstein

with love and appreciation.

Preface

The correlation of the gross and microscopic features of skin disease is a pivotal focus of diagnostic dermatology. The philosophic goal of this book, which was conceived to fill a gap in the growing body of literature in veterinary dermatology, is to emphasize the benefit to be gained from the clinicopathologic method of diagnosis. Pathologists who desire to be proficient dermatopathologists should increase their knowledge of the clinical aspects of skin disease by working closely with clinicians, reading clinically oriented literature, and following cases to determine outcome. The clinical description submitted with the biopsy specimen thus becomes a critical tool of the dermatopathologist as it provides the gross features of the disease under investigation. For what is clinical dermatology if not "gross pathology" of the skin? Similarly, those who engage in clinical practice should become familiar with the basic microscopic lesions of skin diseases and how these relate to etiopathogenesis, severity of the clinical signs, and prognosis. A clinician can then interpret the biopsy report more effectively and develop a list of clinical differential diagnoses that are derived in part from the histopathologic description and morphologic diagnosis of the skin biopsy. Hopefully, this book will facilitate such a cooperative approach to the diagnosis of skin diseases in dogs and cats.

Pattern analysis of inflammatory skin disease was first developed by A. Bernard Ackerman, a physician dermatopathologist, and has been adapted in these pages to veterinary dermatopathology. Section One, which describes inflammatory, dysplastic, and degenerative skin diseases of dogs and cats, is organized by histopathologic patterns. Section Two, which describes cutaneous neoplasms of dogs and cats, is organized by tissue of origin. In general, the pattern selected to characterize an individual disease was considered the most typical and therefore the most diagnostic. Some diseases were considered to have two patterns of equal diagnostic importance and were described in separate chapters. The system of pattern diagnosis outlined in these pages may differ from other methods of pattern analysis devised for veterinary dermatopathology. Such a system is inherently subjective; the particular method chosen is not as critical as selecting a system and adhering to it, making alterations as new knowledge dictates.

This book is not intended to replace or compete with textbooks of clinical veterinary dermatology, and it places its emphasis on the morphologic aspects, or gross and microscopic appearance, of skin diseases of dogs and cats. The reader is referred to *Small Animal Dermatology,* 4th edition, by Drs. George Muller, Robert Kirk, and Danny Scott, and other clinical references for details on clinical aspects of skin diseases, such as therapy and prognosis, not covered in this book.

Veterinary dermatopathology is still a young and rapidly growing field. This book contains descriptions of some diseases which are newly recognized or previously unreported. Because of the current rapid generation of knowledge in this field, mistakes are anticipated. Rather than exclude some entities that are still imperfectly understood, the authors have chosen to describe them to the best of their abilities and/or according to the reports currently available, being aware that interpretation of some of these fledgling diseases may change radically over the next few years. It is our intention that this book not only provide information, but also stimulate argument and investigation.

The authors would like to thank Drs. James Conroy, Valerie Fadok, Richard Halliwell, Tony Stannard, and Ronald Barr for setting us on our course. We thank the current and past clinical dermatology residents at the University of California, School of Veterinary Medicine who have participated over the years in the genesis of the clinical portion of this book through questioning dogma, seeking answers, and providing the continuous impetus to keep up with the expotentially expanding information in veterinary dermatology.

We are grateful to Lorna McAdam for help in the preparation of this manuscript; to Bruce Mackie of McBain Instruments, and to Andrew and Tom DeLucia of Infinity Photographics for photographic assistance and support; and to Penny Atkinson, Susan Ann Barker, and Linda Hall for histotechnical excellence in the preparation of slides for photomicrography. We thank Dr. Ralf Mueller for his able assistance as proofreader. Sincere appreciation is also given to Dr. William Spangler as this project would not have been possible without his understanding and support of the time demands for its completion.

Special thanks is extended to Dr. M. Donald McGavin, who guided the photomicrographic technique of the illustrations. We are deeply in his debt.

Thelma Lee Gross
Peter J. Ihrke
Emily J. Walder

Contents

INTRODUCTION **The Skin Biopsy,** 1

SECTION ONE
INFLAMMATORY, DYSPLASTIC, AND DEGENERATIVE DISEASES
Thelma Lee Gross and Peter J. Ihrke

PART I **DISEASES OF THE EPIDERMIS,** 9

1 **Superficial Pustular Diseases of the Epidermis,** 10
Impetigo, 10
Superficial spreading pyoderma, 12
Mucocutaneous candidiasis, 14
Pemphigus foliaceus, 16
Pemphigus erythematosus, 18
Subcorneal pustular dermatosis, 20

2 **Bullous and Vesicular Diseases of the Epidermis and the Dermal-Epidermal Junction,** 22
Discoid lupus erythematosus, 22
Systemic lupus erythematosus, 24
Hereditary lupoid dermatosis of the German Shorthaired
Pointer, 26
Bullous pemphigoid, 28
Pemphigus vulgaris, 31
Pemphigus vegetans, 33
Canine familial dermatomyositis, 34
Ulcerative dermatosis of Shetland Sheepdog and Collie, 36
Epidermolysis bullosa, 38

3 **Necrotizing Diseases of the Epidermis,** 41
Erythema multiforme, 41
Toxic epidermal necrolysis, 44
Superficial necrolytic dermatitis, 46
Chemical and thermal burns, 48

4 **Spongiotic Diseases of the Epidermis,** 51
Allergic contact dermatitis, 51
Irritant contact dermatitis, 52
Feline eosinophilic plaque, 55

ix

5 Exudative and Ulcerative Diseases of the Epidermis, 58
Pyotraumatic dermatitis, 58
Feline allergic miliary dermatitis, 59
Feline indolent ulcer, 63
Feline idiopathic ulcerative dermatosis, 65

6 Hyperplastic Diseases of the Epidermis, 68
Chronic hyperplastic dermatitis, 68
Fibropruritic nodules, 70
Acral lick dermatitis, 71
Hypothyroidism, 74
Canine Sertoli cell tumor, 75
Actinic keratosis, 76
Acanthosis nigricans of Dachshunds, 79
Hyperplastic dermatosis of the West Highland White Terrier, 81
Psoriasiform-lichenoid dermatosis of the Springer Spaniel, 83
Lichenoid keratosis, 85

7 Hyperkeratotic Diseases of the Epidermis, 88
Primary seborrhea, 88
Seborrheic dermatitis, 90
Seborrheic dermatitis and *Malassezia pachydermatis* infection, 92
Vitamin A–responsive dermatosis, 94
Canine ear margin seborrhea, 95
Schnauzer comedo syndrome, 96
Ichthyosis, 98
Sebaceous adenitis, 100
Zinc-responsive dermatosis, 102
Generic dog food dermatosis, 104
Acrodermatitis of Bull Terriers, 106

PART II DISEASES OF THE DERMIS, 111

8 Perivascular Diseases of the Dermis, 112
Superficial spreading pyoderma, 112
Atopy, 114
Food allergy, 117
Canine flea allergy dermatitis, 119
Feline allergic miliary dermatitis, 122
Canine sarcoptic acariasis, 123
Feline notoedric acariasis, 125
Cheyletiellosis, 126
Cutaneous dirofilariasis, 128
Hookworm dermatitis, 130
Allergic contact dermatitis, 131

9 Vascular Diseases of the Dermis, 135
Urticaria and angioedema, 135
Immune-mediated vasculitis, 138
Septic vasculitis, 139

10 Lichenoid (Interface) Diseases of the Dermis, 141
Mucocutaneous pyoderma, 141
Discoid lupus erythematosus, 143
Systemic lupus erythematosus, 145
Pemphigus erythematosus, 147

Vogt-Koyanagi-Harada—like syndrome, 148
Vitiligo, 150
Erythema multiforme, 153
Actinic keratosis, 155
Psoriasiform-lichenoid dermatosis of the Springer Spaniel, 156
Lichenoid keratosis, 157
Mycosis fungoides, 158

11 **Infectious Nodular and Diffuse Granulomatous and Pyogranulomatous Diseases of the Dermis, 163**
Actinomycosis and nocardiosis, 163
Feline leprosy, 166
Opportunistic mycobacterial infection, 169
Feline dermatophytic mycetoma, 172
Cutaneous infections of systemic fungi, 174
Cutaneous cryptococcosis, 177
Cutaneous infections of other opportunistic fungi and algae, 179
Sporotrichosis, 181
Cutaneous pythiosis, 184
Cutaneous leishmaniasis, 186

12 **Noninfectious Nodular and Diffuse Granulomatous and Pyogranulomatous Diseases of the Dermis, 190**
Foreign body reactions, 190
Cutaneous xanthoma, 193
Sterile granuloma and pyogranuloma syndrome, 194
Cutaneous histiocytosis, 198
Systemic histiocytosis of the Bernese Mountain Dog, 201
Juvenile sterile granulomatous dermatitis and lymphadenitis, 203

13 **Nodular and Diffuse Diseases of the Dermis with Prominent Eosinophils or Plasma Cells, 207**
Arthropod-bite granuloma, 207
Feline mosquito-bite hypersensitivity, 210
Spider bites, 212
Feline eosinophilic plaque, 213
Feline eosinophilic granuloma, 215
Canine eosinophilic granuloma, 218
Feline plasma cell pododermatitis, 220

14 **Dysplastic and Depositional Diseases of Dermal Connective Tissue, 223**
Calcinosis cutis, 223
Calcinosis circumscripta, 226
Cutaneous mucinosis/myxedema, 228
Cutaneous amyloidosis, 229
Cutaneous asthenia, 232
Feline skin fragility syndrome, 234

PART III **DISEASES OF THE HAIR FOLLICLES, 237**

15 **Pustular and Nodular Diseases without Follicular Destruction, 238**
Superficial bacterial folliculitis, 238
Feline dermatophytosis, 241
Canine dermatophytosis, 243

Pemphigus foliaceus, 245
Sebaceous adenitis, 247
Sterile eosinophilic pustulosis, 250

16   **Pustular and Nodular Diseases with Follicular Destruction, 252**
Deep bacterial folliculitis and furunculosis, 252
Canine callus and callus pyoderma, 255
Canine acne, 257
Feline acne, 258
Kerion, 261
Demodicosis, 262
Rhabditic dermatitis, 266
Eosinophilic furunculosis of the face, 269
Actinic comedones, 270

17   **Atrophic Diseases of the Hair Follicle, 273**
Hypothyroidism, 273
Canine hyperadrenocorticism, 275
Canine Sertoli cell tumor, 278
Canine female hyperestrogenism, 280
Growth hormone/castration-responsive dermatosis, 281
Post-clipping alopecia, 285
Telogen effluvium, 286
Post-rabies vaccination alopecia, 287
Canine familial dermatomyositis, 289
Alopecia areata, 291
Cicatricial alopecia, 292
Canine traction alopecia, 294
Feline psychogenic alopecia, 295

18   **Dysplastic Diseases of the Hair Follicle, 298**
Color mutant alopecia, 298
Black hair follicular dysplasia, 301
Canine follicular dysplasia, 302
Acquired pattern alopecia, 306
Congenital hypotrichosis, 307

PART IV   **DISEASES OF THE PANNICULUS, 311**

19   **An Overview of Panniculitis, 312**
Panniculitis, 312

20   **Diseases of the Panniculus, 316**
Post-rabies vaccination alopecia, 316
Post-injection panniculitis, 316
Traumatic panniculitis, 319
Idiopathic sterile nodular panniculitis, 321
Erythema nodosum–like panniculitis, 323
Feline pansteatitis, 323
Sterile pedal panniculitis of the German Shepherd Dog, 324

SECTION TWO
NEOPLASTIC DISEASES OF THE SKIN
Emily J. Walder and Thelma Lee Gross

INTRODUCTION, 327

PART V EPITHELIAL TUMORS, 329

    21 **Epidermal Tumors,** 330
        Actinic keratosis, 330
        Pigmented epidermal nevus, 331
        Cutaneous horn of feline footpad, 331
        Viral squamous papilloma, 334
         Exophytic papilloma, 334
         Verruca plana, 335
         Inverted papilloma, 335
        Idiopathic squamous papilloma, 336
        Squamous cell carcinoma, 336
         Well-differentiated squamous cell carcinoma, 337
         Poorly differentiated squamous cell carcinoma, 338
         Acantholytic squamous cell carcinoma, 338
         Spindle-celled squamous cell carcinoma, 339
        Multicentric squamous cell carcinoma in situ, 340
        Benign feline basal cell tumor, 341
        Basal cell carcinoma, 343
         Solid basal cell carcinoma, 344
         Keratinizing basal cell carcinoma, 347
         Clear-cell basal cell carcinoma, 348

    22 **Follicular Tumors,** 351
        Follicular cyst, 351
         Infundibular cyst, 352
         Isthmus-catagen cyst, 353
         Proliferating isthmus-catagen cyst, 353
         Matrical cyst, 354
         Hybrid cyst, 354
        Dermoid cyst, 355
        Dilated pore, 356
        Follicular hamartoma, 357
        Focal adnexal dysplasia, 358
        Trichofolliculoma, 359
        Trichoepithelioma, 360
        Infundibular keratinizing acanthoma, 361
        Tricholemmoma, 364
         Bulb type, 364
         Isthmus-catagen type, 365
        Pilomatricoma, 365
        Trichoblastoma, 367
         Ribbon type, 367
         Trabecular type, 369
         Granular cell type, 370
        Matrical carcinoma, 371

    23 **Sebaceous Tumors,** 374
        Sebaceous duct cyst, 374

Nodular sebaceous hyperplasia, 374
Sebaceous nevus, 376
Sebaceous adenoma, 376
  Simple sebaceous adenoma, 377
  Compound ductular and glandular adenoma, 377
Sebaceous epithelioma, 377
Sebaceous carcinoma, 380
Nodular perianal (hepatoid) gland hyperplasia and perianal (hepatoid)
    gland adenoma, 381
  Nodular perianal gland hyperplasia, 382
  Perianal gland adenoma, 382
Perianal (hepatoid) gland carcinoma, 384

24 Sweat Gland Tumors, 386
Apocrine cyst, 386
Apocrine cystomatosis, 386
Apocrine cystadenoma, 387
Apocrine adenoma, 389
  Apocrine glandular adenoma, 389
  Mixed (compound) apocrine adenoma, 390
  Canine ductular (basaloid) apocrine adenoma, 390
  Feline ductular (basaloid) apocrine adenoma, 391
Apocrine carcinoma, 392
  Apocrine cystadenocarcinoma, 392
  Well-differentiated apocrine adenocarcinoma, 393
  Poorly differentiated apocrine carcinoma, 393
  Mixed (compound) apocrine adenocarcinoma, 394
  Ductular apocrine adenocarcinoma, 394
Eccrine carcinoma, 396

25 Nailbed Epithelial Tumors, 398
Nailbed epithelial inclusion cyst, 398
Nailbed inverted squamous papilloma, 399
Nailbed keratoacanthoma, 400
Nailbed squamous cell carcinoma, 403

PART VI MESENCHYMAL TUMORS, 406

26 Fibrocytic Tumors, 407
Collagenous nevus, 407
Nodular dermatofibrosis, 408
Skin tag, 409
Dermatofibroma, 410
Fibroma, 411
Fibrosarcoma, 413
Myxoma, 415
Myxosarcoma, 416

27 Vascular Tumors, 419
Scrotal vascular hamartoma, 419
Hemangioma, 419
Hemangiosarcoma, 422
Lymphangioma, 426
Lymphangiosarcoma, 427

28 Other Mesenchymal Tumors, 430
Lipomatosis, 430
Lipoma, 430
Fibrolipoma, 431
Infiltrative lipoma, 432
Liposarcoma, 433
  Well-differentiated liposarcoma, 434
  Myxoid liposarcoma, 435
  Pleomorphic liposarcoma, 435
Hemangiopericytoma, 436
Tail dock neuroma, 438
Schwannoma, 438
Malignant schwannoma, 441
Leiomyoma, 443
Leiomyosarcoma, 444
Benign fibrous histiocytoma, 445
Malignant fibrous histiocytoma, 446
  Giant cell type (giant cell tumor of soft parts), 447
  Storiform-pleomorphic type (fibroblastic-pleomorphic type), 447
  Dermatofibrosarcoma type (dermatofibrosarcoma protuberans), 448

29 Melanocytic Tumors, 451
Melanocytoma, 451
  Compound melanocytoma, 452
  Dermal melanocytoma, 454
  Balloon-cell melanocytoma, 456
Lentigo, 456
Melanoma-acanthoma, 458
Malignant melanoma, 459

30 Histiocytic and Mast Cell Tumors, 465
Canine cutaneous histiocytoma, 465
Feline mast cell tumor, 468
  Well-differentiated type, 468
  Poorly differentiated type, 469
  Histiocytic type, 470
Canine mast cell tumor, 470
  Grade 1, 471
  Grade 2, 471
  Grade 3, 471

31 Lymphocytic Tumors, 474
Cutaneous extramedullary plasmacytoma, 474
Malignant lymphoma, 476
  Nonepitheliotropic, 478
  Epitheliotropic, 481
Lymphomatoid granulomatosis, 482

INFLAMMATORY, DYSPLASTIC, AND DEGENERATIVE DISEASES

THELMA LEE GROSS
PETER J. IHRKE

Introduction

THE SKIN BIOPSY

The skin biopsy is one of the most valuable diagnostic tools in dermatology. Diagnosis of many skin diseases evolves from and is supported by results of the skin biopsy. Proper technique in obtaining the skin specimen is only one feature of the effective skin biopsy. Recognizing the indications, proper timing, careful site selection, and preparation for submission of the specimens to a laboratory are all critical supporting factors.

The skin biopsy may have benefits other than offering a diagnosis. Ruling out serious diseases such as neoplasia may be just as significant for the animal and owner. Confirmation of the tentative clinical diagnosis through histopathologic evaluation of the skin reinforces clinical diagnostic techniques employed by the clinician, thus providing a method of self-assessment. When the histopathologic findings suggest a disease that is different from the clinical diagnosis, or when they lead to investigation of a potentially new or previously unrecognized disease, then the skin biopsy becomes a source of continuing education for both the clinician and the pathologist. The skin biopsy also may be used to predict prognosis during the course of therapy; however, for financial reasons the prognostic skin biopsy has been underused in veterinary medicine.

Indications for the skin biopsy

The skin biopsy usually is employed in an attempt to establish a definitive diagnosis. Diseases which are subtle or unusual clinically, or those which have not responded as expected to therapy, are prime candidates for biopsy. Specimens for biopsy always should be obtained from skin disease that is devastating physically (e.g., bullous and ulcerative lesions in widespread distribution), or from lesions that are suspected to be neoplastic.

The diagnostic specificity of the skin biopsy should not be overrated: many skin diseases, particularly those of allergic etiology, are similar histopathologically. Although suspected allergic diseases are not prime candidates for biopsy, histopathologic examination of the skin may help to rule out complicating or coexisting problems such as pyoderma or endocrinopathy. Thus the skin biopsy can be as valuable for what it does not reveal as for what it does. "Chronic superficial hyperplastic dermatitis" is not a specific diagnosis, but it can help to prioritize a list of clinical differential diagnoses because it suggests investigation of an allergic cause.

Selection of the specimen for skin biopsy

The critical goal of selection is to obtain primary lesions and avoid secondary lesions. Primary lesions are those which are the result of the principal pathogenic process and thus will be most diagnostic. Primary lesions include papules, pustules, bullae, nodules, scaling, erythema, alopecia, or depigmentation. Secondary lesions evolve from primary lesions and represent aged and therefore less diagnostic changes. As pustules eventuate in crusts and bullae become ulcers, these secondary changes will obscure the diagnostic features of the disease. Secondary lesions also can result from superimposed processes, such as self-trauma leading to erosion, ulceration, or lichenification of the skin, or from secondary superficial bacterial infection leading to exudation and crusting. Secondary lesions follow primary lesions temporally; thus lesions should be selected that are most recent in onset. In cases where primary lesions are not obvious, careful questioning of the owner or observation of a hospitalized animal often will indicate which lesions are the youngest. Smaller primary lesions should be removed in their entirety, or the advancing edge of a larger lesion should be selected. Areas immediately adjacent to ulcers rather than ulcers should be sampled, since ulcerated skin will provide the pathologist only with dermal tissue.

Multiple specimens always should be obtained unless only solitary lesions are present. Care should be taken to sample lesions that are most representative of the entire disease process. Procuring multiple specimens will increase the chances of obtaining diagnostic lesions and is vital when the disease is characterized by a variable appearance grossly, or when clinical lesions are subtle. Diagnostic pathology laboratories generally charge no additional fee for the evaluation of two or three specimens from the same disease process.

In general, the biopsy site should include abnormal skin only, particularly when punch technique is used (see below). Normally, identification of histopathologic lesions does not require comparison with normal skin. If clinical lesions are subtle (e.g., mild erythema or scaling), or if alopecia is the primary clinical sign, a separate specimen of normal skin should be sampled and identified for the dermatopathologist. In this way, changes that might not be obvious in an isolated abnormal specimen may be illuminated by comparison with a normal specimen.

Specimen selection for direct immunofluorescent testing or immunohistochemical testing is slightly different since areas *directly adjacent* to well-developed primary lesions (bullae or vesicles) should be sampled. The erythematous zone surrounding a bulla or ulcer should be obtained for direct immunofluorescent testing or immunohistochemical testing if a bullous autoimmune disease is suspected. Lesional skin may yield false negative results since deposited immunoglobulins and complement may be swept away by secondary inflammation.

Dermatopathologists usually are experienced in biopsy site selection and often can provide information about sampling confusing cases. The pathologist should be contacted prior to biopsy if there are questions about the site of biopsy, number of biopsy specimens required, or method of submission.

Methods of skin biopsy

Elliptical wedge biopsy using a scalpel is a common method of skin biopsy. This technique has the advantage of producing a larger specimen which can be oriented easily by the laboratory technician for sectioning. Solitary lesions are often best removed using this technique. Wedge biopsy is preferred if neoplasia is suspected since the biopsy procedure will have the added benefit of surgical removal. Wedge biopsy is required for diseases involving the panniculus since this deep tissue is usually underrepresented in most punch biopsy specimens. Fragile lesions such as bullae or large pustules may be ruptured by the shearing and torque applied during punch technique; wedge resection will allow removal of these lesions without damage. Since wedge biopsy requires substantial time, multiple sutures, and frequently general anaesthesia, this technique is employed less frequently than warranted in many veterinary hospitals.

Punch biopsy has the substantial advantage of ease of specimen procurement under local anesthesia and results in a minimal surgical wound. Consequently, the procedure is more acceptable to many owners and thus encourages permission for skin biopsy. Punch technique facilitates the taking of multiple specimens for biopsy, which optimizes the diagnostic benefit of the procedure.

The site of sample selection will differ between wedge and punch techniques. It is acceptable to include a transitional zone and normal tissue at one end or pole of the elliptical wedge specimen since the technician can easily orient the tissue and commonly is trained to transect the specimen through its long axis. However, punch specimens *always* should include only abnormal tissue. If normal tissue is included, routine processing by bisection of the specimen and imbedment of one-half may eliminate most or all of the lesional tissue. If normal tissue is being submitted for comparison, a separate punch specimen must be obtained.

Size of the specimen for skin biopsy

Wedge biopsy specimens should never be more than 2 cm in width and length regardless of the size of the lesion sampled. Adequate fixation of excessively large specimens may not occur in formalin.

Disposable biopsy punches of 4-mm, 6-mm, and

8-mm diameter are used most commonly. Six-mm punch specimens are generally the minimal acceptable size, since specimens obtained from larger punches have proportionately less procurement artifact and are more likely to yield diagnostic lesions. Four-mm biopsy punches generally are reserved for difficult sites such as the planum nasale and skin near the eye.

Michel's fixative and transport media does not penetrate tissue as readily as formalin. Consequently, specimens for direct immunofluorescent testing should not be thicker than 4 mm in diameter. The clinician can either use a 4-mm punch or halve a larger specimen.

Instrumentation for the skin biopsy

A skin biopsy will be performed more frequently if the procedure is facilitated by having all necessary instrumentation readily available. Ideally, a separate cold sterilization tray containing the required instruments should be utilized. Since delicate handling of fragile tissue is imperative, a pair of small curved iris scissors and several pairs of fine eye forceps should be included. Small curved hemostats, a small needleholder, suture scissors, and a small scalpel handle also are needed. Disposable 6-mm, 8-mm, and 4-mm punches are the only specialized instruments required. Most disposable punches may be placed in the cold sterilization tray after initial use and reused three or four times.

Skin biopsy technique

Most canine skin biopsy specimens may be obtained using only local anesthesia and physical restraint. Occasionally, general anesthesia or tranquilization is indicated for a fractious animal, or for animals which have lesions localized to the muzzle, periorbital region, or footpads. General or dissociative anesthesia is required more often for feline skin biopsy. Prospective sites are clipped carefully with the goal of removing hair without creating inflammation. Skin biopsy sites should *not* be scrubbed, cleansed, or prepared in any way since surface material is an important part of the specimen.

After the hair is clipped, an indelible marker pen is used to indicate the location of the biopsy. Four dots are placed equidistant from the exact center of the proposed site. Two percent lidocaine is used for routine local anaesthesia. The barrel of the syringe may be rinsed with epinephrine before withdrawing the lidocaine. Epinephrine will aid in hemostasis and restrict the spread of the local anaesthetic. One cc of lidocaine generally is sufficient for each skin biopsy site. The lidocaine is introduced sublesionally in the subcutaneous tissue directly under the lesion using a 25- or 26-gauge needle. Proper blockage is enhanced by gently repositioning the needle several times and depositing the anaesthetic in a fan-like pattern. Since sensory nerves radiate peripherally from the spine, the recommended site of injection is the side of the biopsy site which is closest to the spinal column so that needle repositioning will not cause further discomfort in the patient.

Skin biopsy is performed between 5 and 10 minutes after the injection of the local anaesthetic. The indelible ink dots prevent the inadvertent sampling of nonblocked regions since the bleb of local anaesthetic may no longer be visible.

Local anaesthesia using subcutaneous lidocaine should not be used if a disease of the subcutaneous fat (panniculitis) is suspected. Ring block, regional anaesthesia, or general anaesthesia is recommended to obtain subcutaneous tissue without artifact.

Skin biopsy is accomplished by using a disposable punch or a scalpel. If a disposable biopsy punch is used, the punch is rotated gently in one direction until the blade has entered the subcutaneous tissue. The punch is rotated in one direction because back-and-forth rotation increases the likelihood of specimen damage from shearing forces. With practice, the clinician will note a sudden easing of pressure when the punch has successfully entered the subcutaneous tissue.

Remembering the delicacy of fresh, nonfixed tissue, the specimen should be removed gently with a pair of fine eye forceps and curved iris scissors. Care must be taken to grasp the specimen only by hair stubble, subcutaneous fat, or the edge of the dermal-epidermal junction. If excess blood is present on the specimen, it may be blotted by gently rolling the specimen on absorbent paper toweling. The specimen may be gently placed with the subcutaneous side of the specimen on a small piece of wooden tongue depressor or cardboard. The splint with the attached specimen is then floated specimen side down or emersed in the fixative. The use of a splint encourages proper anatomic orientation of the specimen during fixation. The timely placement of the specimen in the fixative is critical since artifactual changes begin to occur within one minute after sample procurement.

Suturing of the biopsy site, if indicated, is performed. Four-mm punch sites do not require suturing. Six- and eight-mm punch sites require either a purse string suture or several simple interrupted sutures.

Handling of the specimen for skin biopsy

Fresh biopsy specimens must be handled with the utmost care since artifacts are induced easily and may render a specimen useless. Minimal manipulation should occur before the specimen is placed in fixative. Compression and tears will result from the improper use of surgical instruments.

Ten percent neutral phosphate-buffered formalin is the fixative of choice for routine histopathological evaluation. The volume of fixative always should be at least 10 times the volume of the specimen. Fixation in formalin requires at least 12 hours before processing for histopathology. In colder climates, improperly fixed specimens may freeze during transport. Formalin freezes at −11 degrees Centigrade (−24 degrees Fahrenheit). To prevent this problem, specimens must remain at room temperature in formalin for at least 6 hours before exposure to extreme cold.

Michel's transport media and fixative is required for specimens which will be processed for immunofluorescent studies. Michel's media-fixed specimens cannot be used for histopathology. Michel's media maintains its preservative properties over long periods of time if kept from air. Specimens placed in tightly sealed vials of properly buffered Michel's media may be maintained for several years before processing.

Submission of the skin biopsy specimen

Specimens should be submitted to a dermatopathologist, if possible, since most pathologists specializing in skin have experience in clinical dermatology or have a collegial affiliation with a veterinary dermatologist. It is vital to the diagnostic outcome of the biopsy to include signalment (breed, age, and sex) and a detailed description of the clinical lesions. Clinical findings, including type of lesions present and their distribution on the animal, essentially represent the "gross pathology" of the case and are thus fundamental requirements. A dermatopathologist cannot perform optimally if this information is withheld, no matter how perfectly the specimen was obtained.

Specimens for immunofluorescent testing or immunohistochemical testing generally should be submitted at the same time as specimens for routine histopathology. The pathologist should be requested to hold the specimen and to process it only if necessary for the diagnosis. In this way, time is saved in cases where immunologic studies are indicated, and money is saved in circumstances where these tests are not required for the diagnosis.

Mailers frequently are provided by the pathology laboratory. Formalin-filled containers should be sealed tightly and then wrapped with tape to prevent leakage during transit. The history should be written on the form with an indelible ballpoint pen because formalin can dissolve water soluble ink if leakage occurs. Shipment of specimens for biopsy in the same container with other samples stored on ice is not recommended since freezing artifact may result.

General approach to the histopathologic interpretation of the skin biopsy

Specimens are generally bissected, retaining half of the specimen in fixative for potential further study. The laboratory technician should orient the specimens similarly during sectioning, ideally with the epidermis downward, so that optical inversion by the microscope lenses results in a "natural" orientation with the epidermis at the top of the field.

The principle diagnostic pattern or patterns must first be determined when interpreting a skin biopsy using pattern analysis. Low-power magnification (4 ×) is used to scan the specimen and the principal features are determined with reference to a list of previously recognized patterns. A proposed system of patterns is presented in the accompanying box. These patterns are not defined exclusively by location and type of inflammation, but pertain also to hyperplastic, atrophic, or dysplastic changes, or deposition of abnormal products in the skin. Several patterns may be coexistent in a given biopsy specimen; some patterns may not be as prominent or as consistent throughout the specimen. With practice, and as familiarity with the principal diagnostic patterns is gained, the most significant pattern or patterns will be identified preferentially.

When an overall pattern (or patterns) is selected, higher power examination is required to determine more subtle features of the histopathologic changes, such as type of cellular infiltrate present, or presence of infectious organisms. These secondary features are critical to pattern diagnosis since they allow division into smaller subcategories (e.g., granulomatous diseases of the dermis with infectious organisms).

Once the pattern is identified, the presumptive diagnosis usually is within a list of known differential diagnoses, all of which are characterized by the specific pattern. At this stage, specific diagnosis often involves correlation with the clinical features or gross appearance of the case under diagnosis. For this purpose, review of the clinical history is critical, and the ultimate diagnosis may depend on the accuracy of the clinical data submitted with the biopsy specimen.

Some patterns are not as diagnostically useful as others. For example, in many cases of perivascular dermatitis, the best that can be offered (particularly if the gross pathology is not known) is a diagnosis of possible allergic dermatitis. This limitation may be reduced in the future as subtle histopathologic differences among individual diseases which share a common pattern are revealed through clinicopathologic correlation.

Pattern diagnosis is a useful tool of diagnostic dermatopathology, and one which ultimately strengthens the selective observation of the pathologist, which is the basis of all tissue diagnosis. Microscopic findings alone are not patterns; it is only when characteristic changes are identified consistently with specific diseases that patterns emerge. With practice and experience, the pathologist may develop variations of the system outlined in this book which have individual application and usefulness (see the accompanying box). Systems of pattern diagnosis should not be rigid; they are subjective tools only, and it is the consistent application of the technique which is more important that the actual pattern system utilized.

SUGGESTED READINGS

Hargis AM: Integumentary system. In Thompson RG, editor: Special veterinary pathology, Toronto, 1988, BC Decker, pp 1-68.

Yager JA and Scott DW: The skin and its appendages. In Jubb KVF, Kennedy PC and Palmer N, editors: Pathology of domestic animals, ed 3, Orlando, 1985, Academic Press, vol 1, pp 407-549.

Histopathologic patterns of skin disease

Diseases of the epidermis
Superficial pustular
Bullous and vesicular (dermal-epidermal junction)
Necrotizing
Spongiotic
Exudative and ulcerative
Hyperplastic
Hyperkeratotic

Diseases of the dermis
Perivascular
Vascular
Lichenoid (interface)
Nodular and diffuse pyogranulomatous and granulomatous (with and without infectious organisms)
Nodular and diffuse with eosinophils or plasma cells
Dysplastic and depositional

Diseases of the hair follicle
Pustular and nodular (with and without follicular destruction)
Atrophic
Dysplastic

Diseases of the panniculus

Diseases of the epidermis

Superficial pustular diseases of the epidermis

Superficial pustular disease are characterized by the formation of pustules in the superficial epidermis. Lesions result from breakdown in the integrity of the keratinocytes by spongiosis or acantholysis, as well as from the accumulation of inflammatory cells, which migrate from the underlying dermal vasculature in response to superficial infectious agents or ongoing epidermal damage. Pustules may be subcorneal, intragranular, or loosely organized in the upper layers of the epidermis. Pustules may be discrete or poorly defined and may contain neutrophils, eosinophils, and acantholytic cells.

IMPETIGO (Synonym: puppy pyoderma)
Clinical features (Figures 1-1 and 1-2)

Impetigo is a common bacterial skin disease in dogs, characterized by superficial nonfollicular pustules. As in other types of canine pyoderma, *Staphylococcus intermedius* is the primary pathogen. Underlying causes are not known, although inflammation secondary to fecal debris or urine scalding in the perineal region and groin has been suggested.

Crusted papules are more common than are intact pustules since pustules are fragile and rupture easily. Intact pustules are creamy white or yellow. Yellow crusts and sparse, mildly erythematous papules may be the predominant clinical feature. A hand lens is useful for determining that pustules are interfollicular rather than follicular since follicular pustules will have central protruding hairs. This determination is important clinically since impetigo responds more readily to therapy than does folliculitis. Lesions are seen primarily in the glabrous inguinal and axillary regions. Pruritus is absent or mild.

Occasionally, a bullous form of impetigo may be seen in adult dogs in conjunction with immune suppression. Pustules are large and may span several follicles. This phenomenon is seen most frequently with naturally occurring or iatrogenic hyperglucocorticoidism.

Impetigo is seen most commonly in prepubescent and pubescent dogs. Breed or sex predilections have not been noted. Mild flea allergy dermatitis is the major clinical differential diagnosis if pustules are not intact.

Biopsy site selection

Skin biopsy specimens should be obtained from intact pustules if available. Crusted papules are not ideal as they represent pustules in advanced stages of degeneration.

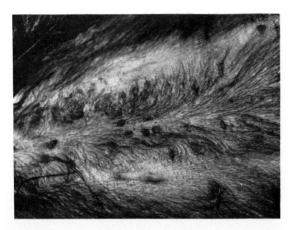

FIGURE 1-1. Impetigo on the ventral abdomen of a pubescent dog. Note the multiple crusted papules and the sparse intact pustules.

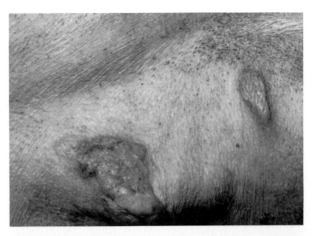

FIGURE 1-2. Bullous impetigo of the ventral abdomen of an 11-year-old Boxer dog with hyperadrenocorticism. A single large, intact, asymmetric pustule is surrounded by an erythematous halo (*at right*). The nipple exhibits calcinosis cutis.

Histopathology (Figure 1-3)

The typical microscopic lesion is a discrete subcorneal pustule that is composed predominantly of neutrophils. Generally, pustules are elevated above the epidermal surface and are located between hair follicles. In bullous impetigo, broader pustules span one or two hair follicles. Spongiosis often occurs beneath pustules; very rarely mild separation of keratinocytes (acantholysis) is seen. Pustules become crusts as neutrophils degenerate, and new stratum corneum often develops at the base of these older lesions. The epidermis is mildly to moderately acanthotic.

A bacterial stain often reveals gram-positive cocci within pustules. Stains are useful diagnostically only if the pustule is intact, as any ruptured pustule may develop secondary bacterial colonization.

The dermis has superficial perivascular to interstitial, mixed inflammation with neutrophils predominating. Mild to moderate dermal edema is common.

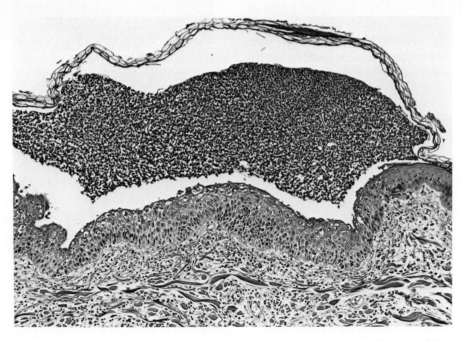

FIGURE 1-3. Impetigo in a dog. Note the large, discrete subcorneal pustule with subjacent mild spongiosis. (×90.)

The principal differential diagnosis is pemphigus foliaceus, particularly in the case of bullous impetigo. Acantholysis is absent or minimal in impetigo, and intact pustules reveal bacteria, in contrast to the sterile intact pustules of pemphigus foliaceus.

SUPERFICIAL SPREADING PYODERMA
Clinical features (Figures 1-4 and 1-5)

Superficial spreading pyoderma is a common canine bacterial skin disease. *Staphylococcus intermedius* is the primary pathogen, as in other types of canine pyoderma. Superficial spreading pyoderma may be seen alone or more commonly in conjunction with superficial bacterial folliculitis. Predisposing factors are not known but the frequent initiation of lesions in the glabrous intertriginous regions of the groin and axillae suggests that moisture and heat retention, coupled with frictional microtrauma associated with movement, may play a role in the development of superficial spreading pyoderma.

Erythematous macules spread from transient tiny pustules as point sources and enlarge peripherally to create coalescing arciform lesions. The superficial keratin layer lifts and peels peripherally, forming a collarette at the margin of the expanding macule. Central as well as subtle peripheral crusting may be present. Hyperpigmentation is a frequent sequela. Substantial alopecia, frequently in ringlike patterns, may be seen with superficial spreading pyoderma.

Lesions often are confined to the glabrous skin of the ventrum but may be more generalized on the trunk. In haired regions, alopecia may occur within the confines of the erythematous macules. Pruritus is variable and may not correlate with the degree of erythema.

Age, breed, or sex predilections have not been reported. Clinical differential diagnoses are legion since lesions at different stages of development may be nondescript, especially if pruritus and self-trauma are present. Superficial spreading pyoderma may resemble flea allergy dermatitis, superficial bacterial folliculitis, dermatophytosis, pemphigus foliaceus, sterile eosinophilic pustulosis, and subcorneal pustular dermatosis. Differentiation is aided by clinical signs, distribution, and histopathology.

Biopsy site selection

Specimens for skin biopsy should be obtained from the advancing edge of circular, scaling, and erythematous lesions. The central alopecic area that is sometimes hyperpigmented is older and less likely to yield diagnostic results. Care should be taken to ensure that scales or crusts remain intact on the specimen. If present, pustules also should be sampled.

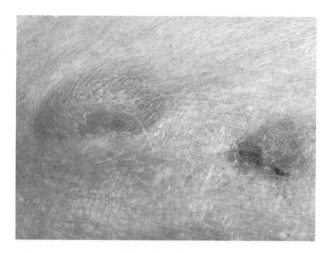

FIGURE 1-4. Superficial spreading pyoderma in a dog. Two asymmetric erythematous macules have slight peripheral scaling.

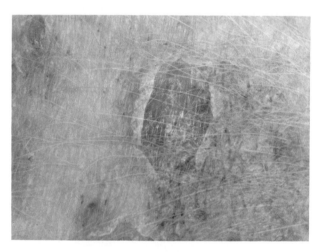

FIGURE 1-5. Superficial spreading pyoderma in the glabrous skin of the ventral abdomen of a dog. A large collarette peels peripherally from the border of the erythematous macule.

Histopathology (Figures 1-6 and 1-7)

Microscopic appearance is variable and is highly dependent on the stage and site of lesions obtained for biopsy. Because lesions evolve rapidly in an outward direction, it may be difficult to obtain a diagnostic biopsy.

The most characteristic epidermal lesions consist of small, loosely organized and spongiotic, superficial epidermal pustules that rapidly form crusts. Rarely, superficial folliculitis is observed, characterized by accumulations of neutrophils in follicular infundibula.

Gram-positive cocci may be seen within superficial layers of keratin and may be accompanied by granular basophilic cellular debris, recently referred to as the

FIGURE 1-6. Superficial
spreading pyoderma in a dog.
A large spongiotic pustule is
loosely organized in the superficial epidermis. (×90.)

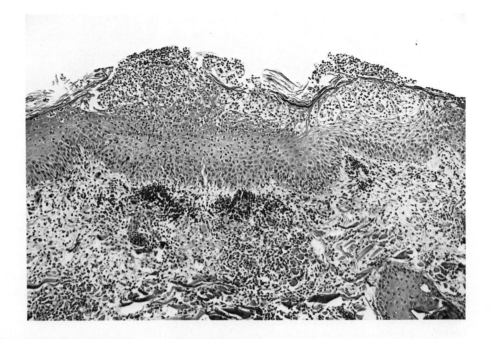

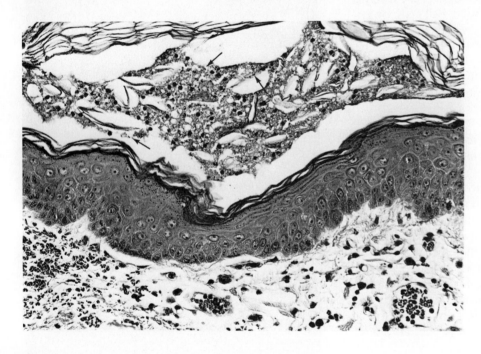

FIGURE 1-7. Dunstan's blue
line. Degenerating nuclear debris, fragments of keratin, and
numerous small cocci *(arrows)*
are intermingled at the advancing edge of a pustule. Note elevated stratum corneum at top.
(×220.)

"blue line."* On occasion, lifting of keratin is evident
above or adjacent to the blue line, and this may correspond to the peripheral scaling, or epidermal collarette,
seen clinically. In this respect, lesions of superficial
spreading pyoderma resemble those of very early exudative epidermitis, a *Staphylococcus hyicus* infection seen
in pigs. Early macroscopic skin lesions of scaling in
gnotobiotic pigs correspond to microscopic splitting of
the keratin layer and superficial colonization by

staphylococci.* Dermal inflammation, predominantly
neutrophilic, is superficial and perivascular to interstitial in orientation (see Chapter 8). In less optimal specimens, epidermal lesions may be absent and dermal
lesions may predominate, making differentiation from
chronic dermatitis difficult.

Differential diagnoses include impetigo and impetiginization due to self-trauma from pruritus. Pustules

---

* From Dunstan RW: Personal communication, 1989.

* From Lloyd DH, Allaker RA, and Gross TL: Unpublished data,
May 1986.

of superficial spreading pyoderma are rarely as discrete as those of impetigo and do not confine themselves neatly to the subcorneal space. Lesions of impetiginization found in chronic hyperplastic dermatitis due to allergy are compact neutrophilic crusts, often admixed with parakeratosis or hyperkeratosis, and sometimes accompanied by erosion; frank pustules usually are not seen.

MUCOCUTANEOUS CANDIDIASIS
Clinical features (Figures 1-8 and 1-9)

Mucocutaneous candidiasis is a very rare fungal disease seen in dogs, caused by the yeast *Candida* species. Mucocutaneous candidiasis usually is seen secondary to underlying immunosuppressive or debilitating systemic disease.

Ulcers and erosions are coated with adherent, tenacious, foul-smelling exudate. The oral mucosa and mucocutaneous junction are the most frequently involved sites. Lesions also may be seen in the external ear, perineum, nares, vulva, scrotum, nail beds, or glabrous skin. Secondary bacterial invasion contributes to morbidity, and pain may be severe. Candidiasis may complicate superficial necrolytic dermatitis (see Chapter 3); review of a case previously published by Pichler and one author* indicates histopathologic features compatible with superficial necrolytic dermatitis.

Sex or breed predilections have not been noted. Candidiasis may be seen more frequently in older animals since immunosuppression and debilitation can be contributing factors.

Clinical differential diagnoses should include chronic diseases causing mucocutaneous and mucous-membrane ulceration and exudation. Uremic stomatitis, pemphigus vulgaris, bullous pemphigoid, systemic lupus erythematosus, erythema multiforme, superficial necrolytic dermatitis, and epitheliotropic malignant lymphoma (mycosis fungoides) should be considered. Stained smears from the exudate are a diagnostic aid if blastoconidia and pseudohyphae are demonstrated, but a definitive diagnosis cannot be made without biopsy and culture.

Biopsy site selection

Intact, crusted lesions should be selected. Care should be taken to leave crusts attached to the specimens. The pathology service should be instructed to include any separated crusts in the slide preparation. Ulcers should not be sampled since an intact epidermis or mucosa is essential to the identification of organisms in tissue.

* Thelma Lee Gross.

Histopathology (Figures 1-10 and 1-11)

Microscopic findings consist of moderate to severe, superficial epidermal pustulation, generally composed of neutrophils. Large areas of surface pustulation and serocellular crusting with parakeratosis may be present; discrete small pustules generally are not seen. Subjacent spongiosis is often prominent. Secondary erosion and ulceration are common. Intact epidermis is moderately acanthotic.

Discovery of yeast and pseudohyphae of *Candida* species in superficial crusts or pustules is diagnostic. Yeast may be found on routine examination with hematoxylin and eosin stain, but are more obvious with the use of periodic acid-Schiff stain, which reveals brilliant magenta, oval-shaped, budding yeast, measuring 3 to 4 μ in diameter, as well as tangled pseudohyphae.

Dermal inflammation is superficial perivascular to interstitial, and includes a prominent component of

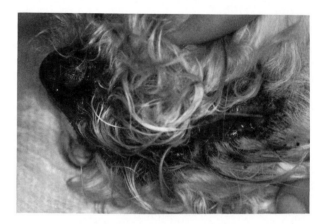

FIGURE 1-8. Perioral mucocutaneous candidiasis in an elderly Poodle with superficial necrolytic dermatitis.

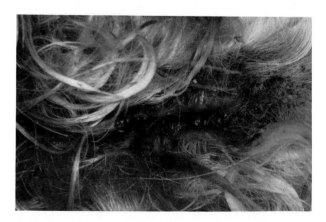

FIGURE 1-9. Closer view of the dog in Fig. 1-8. Dark crusts and tenacious mucoid deposits adhere to erosions and mat the surrounding hair.

neutrophils, mixed with lymphocytes, plasma cells, and macrophages. Dermal edema is variable, but usually is mild to moderate.

The pustular inflammation of mucocutaneous candidiasis is reminiscent of that of superficial spreading pyoderma but is generally more severe. Discovery of yeast is required for definitive diagnosis. Candidiasis can complicate superficial necrolytic dermatitis; lesions compatible with superficial necrolytic dermatitis (laminar epidermal edema and degeneration) should be searched for in specimens with superficial yeast colonization.

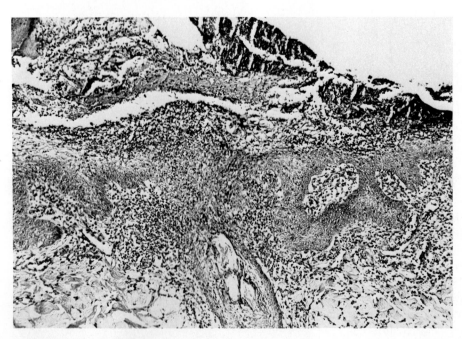

FIGURE 1-10. Mucocutaneous candidiasis in a dog. A large superficial pustule is accompanied by marked epidermal edema. (×90.)

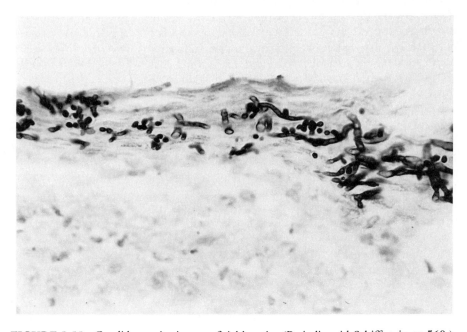

FIGURE 1-11. *Candida* species in superficial keratin. (Periodic acid-Schiff stain × 560.)

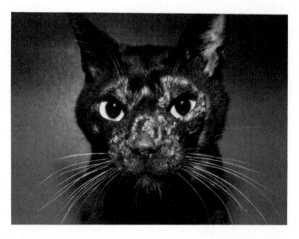

FIGURE 1-12. Pemphigus foliaceus in a cat. Note symmetric crusting and alopecia. (*Courtesy AC Mundell, Seattle, Washington; case material from the University of California, Davis.*)

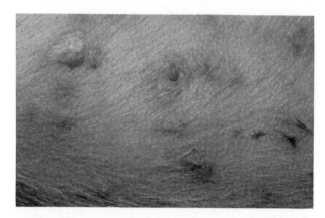

FIGURE 1-13. Pemphigus foliaceus in a dog. Multiple, intact, and recently ruptured vesicopustules are not circular, in contrast with most pustules caused by bacterial pyoderma.

PEMPHIGUS FOLIACEUS
Clinical features (Figures 1-12 through 1-14)

Pemphigus foliaceus is an uncommon bullous autoimmune skin disease seen in the dog and cat. In this type V hypersensitivity reaction, autoantibody in the superficial layers of the epidermis binds to components of the desmosome, which are then internalized by phagocytosis, leading to the conversion of plasminogen to plasmin by plasminogen activators. Acantholysis results, creating superficial vesicles and bullae.

Transient superficial pustules (or vesicopustules) develop in waves. Individual pustules may be large (2 to 6 mm in diameter) and irregular in shape and vary in color from translucent, to gray-white, to yellow. Animals may progress from absence of lesions to sudden development of dozens of pustules. Pustules quickly eventuate in thick, adherent crusts with marked exfoliation. These exfoliative crusts are the most common clinical lesions of pemphigus foliaceus. Alopecia is variable. Characteristic footpad lesions in dogs consist of erythematous swelling at the pad margins and cracking and villous hypertrophy of the pads.

The most common sites of involvement in the dog are the dorsal muzzle, planum nasale, pinnae, periorbital skin, and footpads. Truncal lesions are variable but may be diffuse. Bilateral symmetry is a common feature. Occasionally, the disease may be predominantly confined to the face or footpads. Chronic facial pemphigus foliaceus is often characterized by severe crusting and thickening of the skin. Mucocutaneous and mucous membrane lesions are rare. Pruritus is noted in less than one-half of affected dogs. In cats, lesions are often restricted to the face, ears, interdigital webs, and nipples.

The Bearded Collie, Akita, Chow Chow, Newfoundland, Schipperke, and Doberman Pinscher are

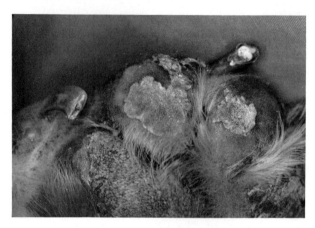

FIGURE 1-14. Canine pemphigus foliaceus restricted to the paw pads. Keratinous crusts peel away from intact, normal-appearing pad material, demonstrating the wavelike progression of the disease. A positive Tzanck preparation was made from a soft, necrotic focus in the central pad.

genetically predisposed. Predominantly facial pemphigus foliaceus is seen more commonly in the Chow Chow and Akita. Canine pemphigus foliaceus usually is a disease of middle age. There is no sex predilection in the dog. Predilections have not been reported for the cat.

Superficial bacterial folliculitis is the major clinical differential diagnosis. Pustules seen with pemphigus foliaceus usually are larger and more irregular in contour than the pustules seen with superficial bacterial folliculitis. Pemphigus foliaceus can appear visually similar to other crusting, pustular and exfoliative skin diseases such as dermatophytosis, lupus erythematosus, demodicosis, zinc-responsive dermatosis, sebaceous adenitis, and mycosis fungoides. However, the symmetry and periodic "waves" of pustules observed in pemphigus foliaceus are important differentiating features.

FIGURE 1-15. Canine pemphigus foliaceus. A subcorneal pustule contains acantholytic cells. (×90.)

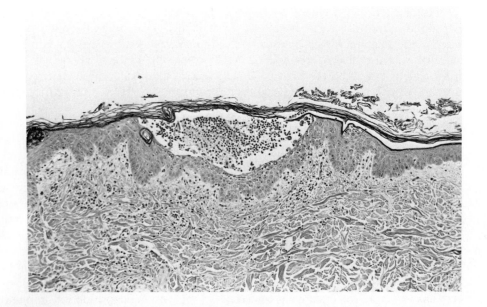

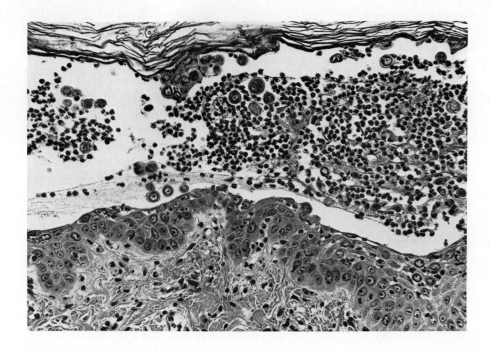

FIGURE 1-16. Higher magnification of subcorneal pustule from a dog with pemphigus foliaceus. Prominent acantholytic cells are free floating; partially acantholytic cells adhere to the roof of the pustule. (×220.)

Biopsy site selection

Because of the fragile and transient nature of primary lesions in pemphigus foliaceus, early lesions (pustules and vesicopustules) should be obtained promptly. Diagnostic histopathology may not be forthcoming from older crusted lesions. If only crusted lesions are available, these should be procurred carefully and the pathology service should be instructed to include any dissociated crusts in the slide preparation. Sites directly adjacent to early pustules should be sampled for direct immunofluorescent or immunohistochemical testing.

Histopathology (Figures 1-15 and 1-16)

Broad, discrete, subcorneal, or intragranular pustules within a variably acanthotic epidermis are the typical histopathologic lesions of pemphigus foliaceus. Pustules often span several follicles and may extend into the follicular infundibula. Deeper follicular inflammation occurs occasionally (see Chapter 15). Deeper forms of pemphigus foliaceus are associated with more pronounced epidermal hyperplasia; chronic facial pemphigus foliaceus is often of this histopathologic appearance.

Pustules are composed of neutrophils and often eosinophils. Individualized, rounded, eosinophilic, acantholytic keratinocytes are present in small to large numbers within pustules. Free-floating "rafts" of partially adherent acantholytic cells, and adherence of acantholytic cells to the overlying stratum corneum, are both characteristic histopathologic features of pemphigus foliaceus. Spongiosis or active acantholysis, characterized by rounding up of keratinocytes that appear to be "springing" from the underlying epidermis, are found beneath pustules. Because pustules are transient, active acantholysis often is not present and the diagnosis may then depend on demonstration of degenerated free keratinocytes in crusts. Some caution is warranted in relying on free keratinocytes alone to make the diagnosis of pemphigus foliaceus, since spongiosis, as seen in superficial pyoderma and other inflammatory diseases of the epidermis, can also result in separation of keratinocytes from the underlying epidermis.

Rarely, acantholysis without pustule formation may be seen in the superficial epidermis. Affected keratinocytes are hypereosinophilic and slightly rounded and are separated from the underlying epidermis.

Pemphigus foliaceus of the footpads often shows degenerating pustules and crusts entrapped in thick layers of dense hyperkeratosis or focal parakeratosis. Early pustules demonstrating active acantholysis at the base are rarely seen in randomly obtained specimens, but free acantholytic keratinocytes are easily demonstrated within pustules or crusts that are entrapped in the keratin layer.

A rare variant of pemphigus foliaceus is characterized by prominent spongiotic eosinophilic pustulation of the epidermis or superficial hair follicles. Acantholysis is not a feature. Affected animals develop typical histopathologic lesions of pemphigus foliaceus in later stages of the disease. Interestingly, eosinophilic spongiosis most commonly precedes pemphigus vulgaris rather than pemphigus foliaceus in humans.

Dermal inflammation is superficial, mixed, and perivascular to interstitial and is accompanied by edema, vascular ectasia, and congestion. Neutrophils and eosinophils usually are prominent and are intermingled with macrophages, lymphocytes, and plasma cells. In some cases of pemphigus foliaceus, particularly those which are principally confined to the dorsal muzzle and planum nasale, there may be band-like or lichenoid dermal inflammation that includes macrophages, lymphocytes, plasma cells, and neutrophils. Pigmentary incontinence, or the accumulation of melanophages in the superficial dermis, may be prominent.

Immunoglobulin (Ig) G or IgM, and frequently C_3, are found in the intercellular spaces of the epidermis with immunofluorescent or immunohistochemical testing. In contrast to that seen in pemphigus vulgaris, immunoglobulin deposition may be confined to the superficial epidermis. Only 40% to 50% of random biopsy specimens are positive for immunoglobulin deposition, but sequential biopsy specimens from affected animals may increase the likelihood of a positive result.

The principal histopathologic differential diagnosis is bullous impetigo. Intact pustules of impetigo may contain cocci and occasional free keratinocytes. However, active acantholysis is absent. Pemphigus erythematosus, a rare variant of pemphigus foliaceus (see below), is characterized by combined lichenoid dermal inflammation and superficial pustules, as observed in facially predominant pemphigus foliaceus. The principal method of differentiating these two diseases is through immunofluorescent or immunohistochemical testing; pemphigus erythematosus exhibits deposition of immunoglobulin along the basement membrane in addition to the intercellular spaces of the epidermis.

PEMPHIGUS ERYTHEMATOSUS
Clinical features (Figures 1-17 and 1-18)

Pemphigus erythematosus is a rare variant of pemphigus foliaceus and has been reported in the dog and cat. This disease has been characterized as either a benign form of pemphigus foliaceus or a crossover syndrome between pemphigus and lupus erythematosus.

Clinical signs are very similar to those of pemphigus foliaceus. The lesions of pemphigus erythematosus are confined to the face. Symmetric crusting, exudation, and alopecia of the face are as seen with pemphigus foliaceus. Depigmentation of the dorsal muzzle and planum nasale coupled with attendant photoaggravation are common distinguishing features of pemphigus erythematosus. Clinical appearance coupled with a positive antinuclear antibody (ANA) test suggest a diagnosis of pemphigus erythematosus.

The Collie and the German Shepherd Dog may be at increased risk. Canine age or sex predilections have not been noted. Statistical predilections have not been reported for the cat.

Clinical differential diagnoses should include pemphigus foliaceus with predominantly facial lesions, discoid lupus erythematosus, mycosis fungoides, and Vogt-Koyanagi-Harada-like disease. Careful examination of dogs with predominantly facial pemphigus foliaceus generally reveals lesions at other sites. A positive antinuclear antibody (ANA) test and direct immunofluorescent or immunohistochemical testing results are prerequisites for a confirmatory diagnosis of pemphigus erythematosus in the dog.

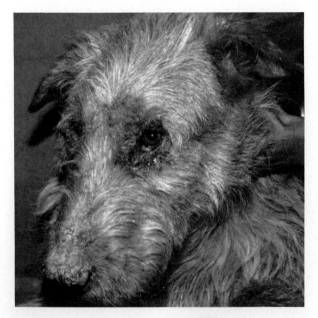

FIGURE 1-17. Pemphigus erythematosus in an Airedale Terrier. Lesions are confined to the dorsal muzzle, planum nasale, periorbital region, and the pinnae. *(From Ihrke PJ and others: Pemphigus foliaceus in dogs: 37 cases, J Am Vet Med Assoc 186:61, 1985. Reprinted with permission.)*

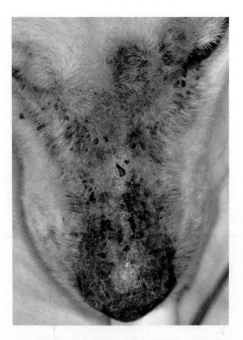

FIGURE 1-18. Pemphigus erythematosus in a Spitz cross-breed. Adherent, thick crusts symmetrically cover the dorsal muzzle and planum nasale.

Biopsy site selection

See previous discussion of Pemphigus Foliaceus.

Histopathology (Figures 1-19)

Superficial (subcorneal) pustulation and acantholysis are as described previously for pemphigus foliaceus.

Although in man pemphigus erythematosus is indistinguishable from pemphigus foliaceus, in dogs dermal inflammation may be lichenoid, closely resembling that of discoid lupus erythematosus (see Chapter 10).

Immunofluorescent or immunohistochemical testing should demonstrate deposition of immunoglobulin in the intercellular spaces of the epidermis as well as at

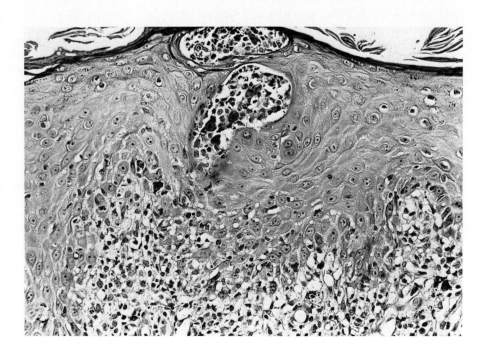

FIGURE 1-19. Canine pemphigus erythematosus. Two small intraepidermal pustules contain acantholytic cells. Note the lichenoid infiltrate with basal cell vacuolation.(×220.)

the basement membrane zone. This represents a combination of the patterns of immunoglobulin deposition seen in both pemphigus and lupus erythematosus.

Pemphigus erythematosus histopathologically resembles lesions of facially predominant pemphigus foliaceus that have lichenoid dermal inflammation. Without confirmatory immunologic findings, assignment of a diagnosis of pemphigus erythematosus to pemphigus foliaceus with lichenoid inflammation is speculative. Adherence to the immunologic criteria of pemphigus erythematosus requires that the diagnosis be made only when immunohistochemical or immunofluorescent testing is compatible.

SUBCORNEAL PUSTULAR DERMATOSIS
Clinical features

Subcorneal pustular dermatosis is a very rare, controversial superficial pustular skin disease in the dog. It is the authors' belief that this syndrome has been greatly overdiagnosed in the past. The etiology of the disease is unknown.

Affected dogs are reported to have a generalized or multifocal, pustular, and exfoliative dermatitis. The face and ears are commonly involved. The pustules may be green or yellow. Pustules are transient and are accompanied by crusting, scaling, alopecia, erythema, and epidermal collarettes. Pruritus is variable but may be extreme.

Miniature Schnauzers are reported as a breed at high risk. Age or sex predilections have not been noted.

Major clinical differential diagnoses include superficial bacterial folliculitis, pemphigus foliaceus, dermatophytosis, or pruritic skin disease with secondary superficial bacterial folliculitis. Repeated bacterial cultures of intact pustules and dermatophyte cultures of crusts are negative in subcorneal pustular dermatosis.

Biopsy site selection

Care should be taken to biopsy new, intact pustules since the differentiating features of the subcorneal pustular diseases cannot be distinguished in disrupted or aged lesions.

Histopathology

Subcorneal pustules without bacterial colonization or acantholysis are the principal histopathologic prerequisites for the diagnosis. Pustules may be accompanied by spongiosis of the underlying epidermis. Additionally, immunofluorescent or immunohistochemical testing must be negative. In general, subcorneal pustular dermatosis has been diagnosed histopathologically by exclusion; results of clinical response to therapy have been as important as histopathologic findings in obtaining a diagnosis.

Canine cases of subcorneal pustular dermatosis differ from human cases of subcorneal pustular dermatosis, inasmuch as pustules from canine lesions are generally not sharply elevated with a flat, nonspongiotic base. Delineation of this disease, or group of diseases, awaits further investigation. Differential diagnoses include impetigo and pemphigus foliaceus, both of which are considerably more common than subcorneal pustular dermatosis. Pustules of pemphigus foliaceus demonstrate prominent acantholysis; intact pustules of impetigo should contain bacteria.

SUGGESTED READINGS

Impetigo

Fourrier P, Carlotti D, and Magnol J-P: Les pyodermites superficielles, Pratique Medicale et Chirurgicale de l'Animal de Compagnie 23:473-484, 1988.

Ihrke PJ: Bacterial infections of the skin. In Greene CE, editor: Infectious diseases of the dog and cat, Philadelphia, 1990, WB Saunders, pp 72-79.

Ihrke PJ: The management of canine pyodermas. In Kirk RW, editor: Current veterinary therapy VIII, Philadelphia, 1983, WB Saunders, pp 505-517.

White SD and Ihrke PJ: Pyoderma. In Nesbitt GH, editor: Dermatology: contemporary issues in small animal practice, New York, 1987, Churchill Livingstone, pp 95-122.

Superficial spreading pyoderma

Fourrier P, Carlotti D, and Magnol J-P: Les pyodermites superficielles, Pratique Medicale et Chirurgicale de l'Animal de Compagnie 23:473-474, 1988.

Ihrke PJ: The management of canine pyoderma. In Kirk RW, editor: Current veterinary therapy VIII, Philadelphia, 1983, WB Saunders, pp 505-517.

Mucocutaneous candidiasis

Foil CS: Cutaneous fungal diseases. In Nesbitt GH, editor: Dermatology: contemporary issues in small animal practice, New York, 1987, Churchill Livingstone, pp 123-158.

Pichler ME, Gross TL, and Kroll W: Cutaneous and mucocutaneous candidiasis in a dog, Comp Cont Educ 7:225-230, 1985.

Pemphigus foliaceus

Caciolo PL, Nesbitt GH, and Hurvitz AI: Pemphigus foliaceus in eight cats and results of induction therapy using azathioprine, J Amer Anim Hosp Assoc 20:571-577, 1984.

Halliwell REW: Pemphigus foliaceus in the canine: a case report and discussion, J Amer Anim Hosp Assoc 13:431-436, 1977.

Ihrke PJ and others: Pemphigus foliaceus in dogs: a review of 37 cases, J Am Vet Med Assoc 186:59-66, 1985.

Ihrke PJ and others: Pemphigus foliaceus of the footpads in three dogs, J Am Vet Med Assoc 186:67-69, 1985.

Manning TO and others: Pemphigus diseases in the feline: seven case reports and discussion, J Amer Anim Hosp Assoc 18:433-443, 1982.

Robledo MA and Diaz LA: Pathophysiology of pemphigus. In Soter NA and Baden HP, editors: Pathophysiology of dermatologic diseases, New York, 1991, McGraw-Hill, pp 179-191.

Scott DW and others: Immune-mediated dermatoses in domestic animals: ten years after—part I, Comp Cont Educ 9:425-435, 1987.

Pemphigus erythematosus

Robledo MA and Diaz LA: Pathophysiology of pemphigus. In Soter NA and Baden HP, editors: Pathophysiology of dermatologic diseases, New York, 1991, McGraw-Hill, pp 179-191.

Scott DW and others: Immune-mediated dermatoses in domestic animals: ten years after—part I, Comp Cont Educ 9:425-435, 1987.

Scott DW and others: Unusual findings in canine pemphigus erythematosus and discoid lupus erythematosus, J Am Anim Hosp Assoc 20:579-584, 1984.

Scott DW and others: Pemphigus erythematosus in the dog and cat, J Am Anim Hosp Assoc 16:815-823, 1980.

Subcorneal pustular dermatosis

McKeever PJ and Dahl MV: A disease in dogs resembling human subcorneal pustular dermatosis, J Am Vet Med Assoc 170:704-708, 1977.

Muller GH, Kirk RW, and Scott DW: Small animal dermatology, ed 4, Philadelphia, 1989, WB Saunders, pp 828-831.

Bullous and vesicular diseases of the epidermis and dermal-epidermal junction

Bullous and vesicular diseases are characterized by the formation of clefts, leading to vesicles or bullae. Separation most commonly occurs between the dermis and epidermis and results from either basal cell degeneration or loss of structural integrity of the basement membrane zone. Diseases that produce suprabasilar clefting due to acantholysis also are included. Some diseases in this group may not be characterized by clinical vesiculation; for simplicity and clarity, diseases that show degeneration of the suprabasilar or basilar epidermis, or of the basement membrane zone, are included regardless of clinical manifestation of dermal-epidermal separation. Bullous and vesicular diseases frequently are the result of autoimmune processes that deposit autoantibodies that damage the basement membrane zone, basal cells, or the intracellular cement substance of the epidermis. Genetic defects in the structural integrity of the basal cell layer or basement membrane zone also may lead to the formation of dermal-epidermal clefts, vesicles, or bullae.

DISCOID LUPUS ERYTHEMATOSUS
Clinical features (Figures 2-1 through 2-3)

Discoid lupus erythematosus is a relatively common autoimmune skin disease of the dog. Cases previously diagnosed as nasal solar dermatitis, or "Collie nose," were likely discoid lupus erythematosus. In humans, actinic radiation is postulated to be instrumental in altering the antigenic nature of keratinocytes, thus inducing an autoimmune response. Since canine discoid lupus erythematosus is at least photo-aggravated if not photo-induced, lesions often are more severe in the summer and in parts of the world with high solar intensity.

Lesions are commonly restricted to the face. Early lesions, characterized by depigmentation, erythema, and scaling, frequently are confined to the planum nasale and occur in a symmetric pattern. The planum often exhibits a loss of the normal "cobblestone" architecture. Alopecia, crusting, erosion, ulceration, and scarring occur in more severe cases. Chronic, scarred, atrophic lesions are fragile and may be abraded easily, resulting in hemorrhage. Lesions may be present on the dorsum of the muzzle, lips, periorbitally, and on the ears. Rarely, focal oral ulcers and lesions on the genitals and distal extremities have been reported.

The Collie, Shetland Sheepdog, German Shepherd Dog, and Siberian Husky exhibit a breed predilection for discoid lupus erythematosus. As a subgroup, white

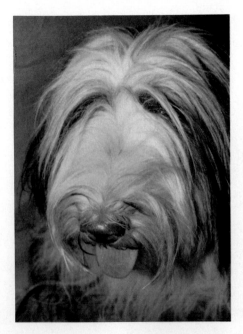

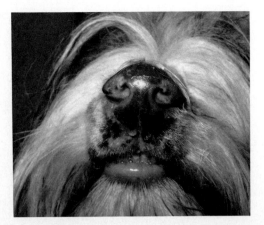

FIGURE 2-2. Closer view of the dog in Figure 2-1. Note the depigmentation and erosion of the planum nasale.

FIGURE 2-1. Mild canine discoid lupus erythematosus in a Bearded Collie. The dorsal planum is mildly depigmented.

German Shepherd Dogs are at greater risk. Affected siblings and mother-daughter cohorts have been recognized. A slight female sex bias has been noted. Age predilection has not been reported.

Major clinical differential diagnoses include systemic lupus erythematosus, dermatophytosis, pemphigus foliaceus, nasal pyoderma, and Vogt-Koyanagi-Harada-like syndrome. An ANA test and a chemistry screening profile should be performed to aid in differentiation from systemic lupus erythematosus. The ANA test should be negative in discoid lupus erythematosus. Lesions do not violate the planum nasale in dermatophytosis, and fistulation is seen in nasal pyoderma. Poliosis and uveitis usually are prominent coexistant features of Vogt-Koyanagi-Harada-like syndrome. Histopathology also is useful in differentiating all of the diseases mentioned above except for systemic lupus erythematosus.

Biopsy site selection

Recent sites of depigmentation, characterized by graying or partial loss of pigment, are optimal sites for skin biopsy. Traumatized lesions or lesions with severe crusting, ulceration, or scarring should be avoided. Lesions of the lip and dorsal muzzle are more likely to yield diagnostic results. Potential difficulties with hemostasis and scarring are additional reasons to avoid the planum nasale or pinnae unless other more suitable sites for biopsy are not affected.

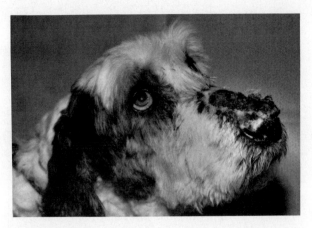

FIGURE 2-3. Severe canine discoid lupus erythematosus in an Old English Sheepdog. Ulceration and scarring deface the entire dorsal muzzle.

Histopathology (Figure 2-4)

Patchy, mild-to-moderate vacuolar degeneration of the basal cell layer is a characteristic epidermal feature of discoid lupus erythematosus. Colloid or Civatte body formation is a consistent finding but may be rare within a given specimen. Colloid or Civatte bodies (first described in lichen planus and lupus erythematosus of humans) are degenerated basal cells, which are generally rounded, individualized, and brightly eosinophilic; these may represent a type of apoptotic cell, as seen in erythema multiforme (see Chapter 3). Small vesicles at the dermal-epidermal junction, secondary to basal cell damage, are seen rarely. Artifactual dermal-epidermal separation at the margin of a specimen may be observed more commonly. Only tissue weakened through the dermal-epidermal junction will

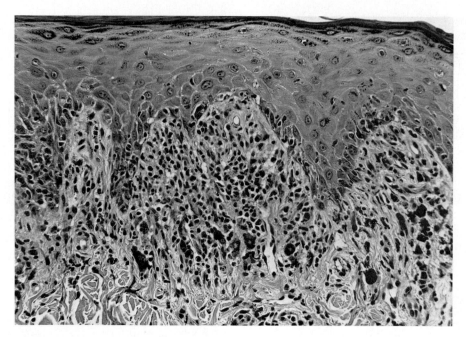

FIGURE 2-4. Canine discoid lupus erythematosus. Vacuolar degeneration of the basal cell layer has resulted in a moth-eaten appearance of the dermal-epidermal junction. Note the lichenoid infiltrate and pigmentary incontinence. (×220.)

separate in this manner during processing, and consequently this "usable artifact" is valid evidence of basal cell or basement membrane damage.*

Secondary erosion or ulceration, and superficial pustulation and crusting are observed in severe cases. Moderate acanthosis usually occurs; epidermal atrophy occasionally is present. The basement membrane may be markedly thickened in some cases; this is a nonspecific finding, however, and can be observed in other chronic inflammatory dermatoses.

The dermis has a lichenoid mixed inflammatory infiltrate (see Chapter 10), which may extend around adnexal appendages. Inflammation is usually moderate but can be mild. Pigmentary incontinence usually is present and reflects loss of melanin by damaged basal cells and its incorporation into macrophages in the superficial dermis.

Immunofluorescent or immunohistochemical testing may show deposition of granular deposits of immunoglobulin, usually IgG, (occasionally IgM) and complement at the dermal-epidermal junction. Positive results are not automatically forthcoming in random biopsy specimens, and a negative result should not exclude the diagnosis if histopathology is characteristic.

Systemic lupus erythematosus and canine familial dermatomyositis are the principal histopathologic dif-

* From Stannard AA: Personal communication, August 1986.

ferential diagnoses. Discoid lupus erythematosus may have a more intense, band-like dermal infiltrate than has systemic lupus erythematosus (see Chapter 10) and less severe basal cell degeneration; however, these two diseases can be indistinguishable histopathologically, and clinical differentiation is required. Dermatomyositis is characterized by patchy basal cell necrosis and/or vacuolation, but differs from discoid lupus erythematosus by the presence of follicular atrophy and the absence of a lichenoid dermal infiltrate. Cases of discoid lupus erythematosus with prominent basal cell degeneration must also be differentiated from ulcerative dermatosis of the Shetland Sheepdog and Collie, hereditary lupoid dermatosis of the German Shorthaired Pointer, and erythema multiforme. Knowledge of breed affected is helpful in differentiating the first two diseases. Erythema multiforme shows individual keratinocyte necrosis at all levels of the epidermis, in addition to basal cell degeneration.

SYSTEMIC LUPUS ERYTHEMATOSUS
Clinical features (Figures 2-5 and 2-6)

Systemic lupus erythematosus is a rare, multisystemic autoimmune disease reported in the dog and cat. Both organ-specific and non–organ-specific circulating autoantibodies are directed against a wide variety of tissue antigens. The ANA test should be positive. Tissue damage may be due to immune complex deposition (Gell and Combs Type III), direct cytotoxic action (Type II), or even cell-mediated immunity (Type IV), as in lupus-induced autoimmune thyroiditis. A wide spectrum of disease is associated with multifactorial immunologic injury to a variety of organ systems. Reported abnormalities in the dog include fever of unknown origin, polyarthritis, glomerulonephritis, anemia, thrombocytopenia, skin disease, neutropenia, and central nervous system disease. The frequency of lupus-related skin disease in the dog is controversial. The opinion of the authors is that skin disease is seen in less than 20% of dogs with systemic lupus erythematosus. Fever of unknown origin, weight loss, glomerulonephritis, hemolytic anemia, and skin disease are signs of systemic lupus erythematosus in the cat.

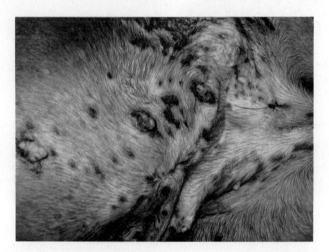

FIGURE 2-5. Canine systemic lupus erythematosus. Widespread erosions and ulcerations of the ventral abdomen have erythematous, thickened margins and necrotic crusts.

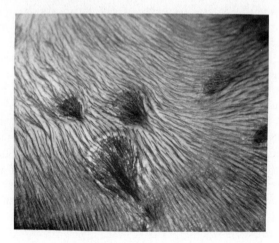

FIGURE 2-6. Closer view of the dog in Fig. 2-5. Adherent crusts entrap the remaining hair within the lesions.

Clinically, the dermatologic signs of systemic lupus erythematosus are pleomorphic. Erythema, scaling, crusting, depigmentation, and alopecia may be seen. Ulcers may eventuate from bullae in the skin, mucocutaneous junctions, and oral mucous membranes. Generalized exfoliative dermatitis, ulcers of the footpads, panniculitis, and lesions closely mimicking discoid lupus erythematosus have been noted. The face, ears, and distal extremities are common sites of involvement. Partial symmetry, especially facial, is an important diagnostic clue. Photo-aggravation may be seen. Lymphadenopathy is common. A rare variant, similar to subacute or chronic cutaneous lupus erythematosus in humans, has been seen in the dog. Lesions were widespread and polycyclic, psoriasiform, and ulcerative.

The Spitz, Collie, Shetland Sheepdog, German Shepherd Dog, and Poodle are at increased risk. Purebred cats in general, and Siamese cats specifically, are overrepresented.* Age or sex predilection has not been reported in the dog or cat.

Clinical differential diagnoses are legion, based on the pleomorphic nature of the disease. Discoid lupus erythematosus, other bullous autoimmune diseases, keratinization disorders, vasculitis, and idiopathic sterile nodular panniculitis are the more important differential diagnoses. Evidence of involvement of multiple organ systems should increase the clinician's suspicion for systemic lupus erythematosus.

Biopsy site selection

Care should be taken to avoid ulcers or erosions, since an intact epidermis is necessary to substantiate the diagnosis. Erythematous areas adjacent to ulcers may yield diagnostic results. If panniculitis is suspected, full-thickness wedge technique is recommended to ensure that subcutaneous fat is included in the specimen. Oral specimens rarely are beneficial, since ulcers, which are inherently not diagnostic, are common in this location. In addition, the mucosa may be disrupted easily from the submucosa in apparently intact lesions.

Histopathology (Figure 2-7)

The histopathologic findings of systemic lupus erythematosus may be nondiagnostic, a dilemma that also is encountered in human medicine. Classically, histopathologic and immunofluorescent or immunohistochemical findings are similar to those of discoid lupus erythematosus (see above). Basal cell vacuolation, and necrosis of basal cells with formation of colloid or Civatte bodies, may be more severe in systemic lupus erythematosus and may lead to marked vesicula-

---

* From Pedersen NC: Personal communication, March 1990.

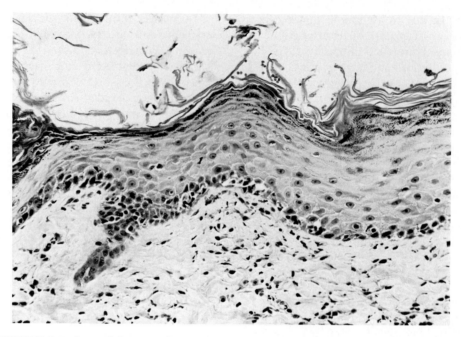

FIGURE 2-7. Systemic lupus erythematosus in a cat. Prominent vacuolar degeneration of the basal cell layer; note the mild interface dermatitis. (×20.)*(Case material from WS Rosenkrantz, Garden Grove, California.)*

tion and ulceration. Superficial hair follicles may be similarly affected. Lichenoid or interface inflammation of the dermis is present but may not be as intense as that of discoid lupus erythematosus (see Chapter 10).

Differential diagnoses to consider for systemic lupus erythematosus (in addition to discoid lupus erythematosus) include ulcerative dermatosis of the Shetland Sheepdog and Collie, hereditary lupoid dermatosis of the German Shorthaired Pointer, and erythema multiforme. If the breed affected is not known, differentiation of systemic lupus erythematosus from the first two diseases may be problematic, as all may be characterized by significant basal cell damage. Lupoid dermatosis is generally not ulcerative, in contrast to the other two diseases. Erythema multiforme shows individual keratinocyte necrosis at all levels of the epidermis, in addition to basal cell degeneration. Systemic lupus erythematosus should be characterized by deposition of immunoglobulin at the basement membrane zone.

HEREDITARY LUPOID DERMATOSIS OF THE GERMAN SHORTHAIRED POINTER
Clinical features (Figures 2-8 and 2-9)

Hereditary lupoid dermatosis as named by White is a scaling, exfoliative skin disease seen in the German Shorthaired Pointer. Recognition of this disease ex-

clusively in this breed to date suggests a hereditary origin. White has observed a case for which 3 of 10 siblings, as well as 1 half-sibling, were reputedly also affected.* Although similar histopathologically, the disease does not share the immunologic features of systemic or discoid lupus erythematosus and is distinct clinically.

Scale and variable crusting are the most prominent clinical features. White observed fronds of keratin surrounding hair shafts.* Thickening of the skin may be evident. Lesions may begin on the head and back but usually generalize. The dog observed by White had most severe involvement of the head, hocks, and scrotum.* Pruritus and pain are variable. Pyrexia and peripheral lymphadenopathy may be observed.

The syndrome has been seen only in the German Shorthaired Pointer. Age of onset has been between 5 and 7 months. Sex predilection has not been noted, but few cases have been observed.

Clinical differential diagnoses should include primary keratinization disorders such as primary seborrhea and ichthyosis, and sebaceous adenitis. The young age of onset would be atypical for sebaceous adenitis. Occurrence exclusively to date in the German Shorthaired Pointer and the distinct histopathologic appearance will allow differentiation from primary keratinization disorders.

* From White SD: Personal communication, June 1990.

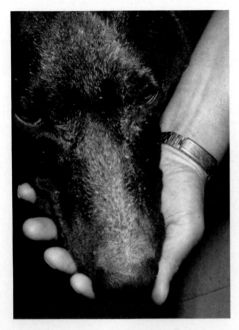

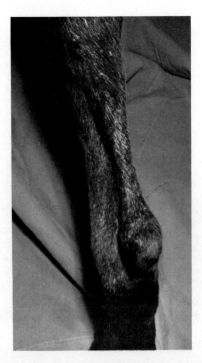

FIGURE 2-8. Hereditary lupoid dermatosis of the German Shorthaired Pointer. Somewhat symmetric scaling is present on the dorsal muzzle. *(Courtesy SD White, Fort Collins, Colorado.)*

FIGURE 2-9. Hereditary lupoid dermatosis in dog of Fig. 2-8. Note scaling involving the caudal lower limb. *(Courtesy SD White, Fort Collins, Colorado.)*

Biopsy site selection

Multiple specimens should be selected from lesions of varying stages. If early lesions can be identified, these may more reliably reveal typical basal cell damage.

Histopathology (Figures 2-10 and 2-11)

The epidermis is mild to moderately acanthotic and may have multifocal parakeratosis and crusting and moderate hyperkeratosis. There may be mild spongiosis with exocytosis of neutrophils and lymphocytes.

FIGURE 2-10. Hereditary lupoid dermatosis of the German Shorthaired Pointer. Note patchy basal cell vacuolation and hyperkeratosis (×90.)

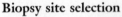

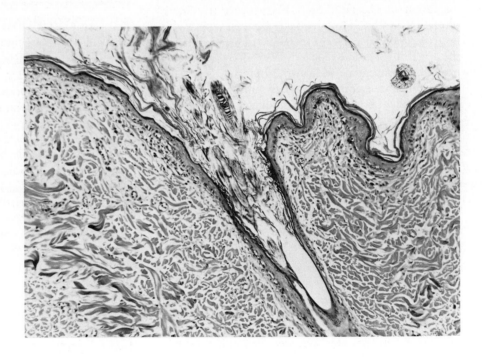

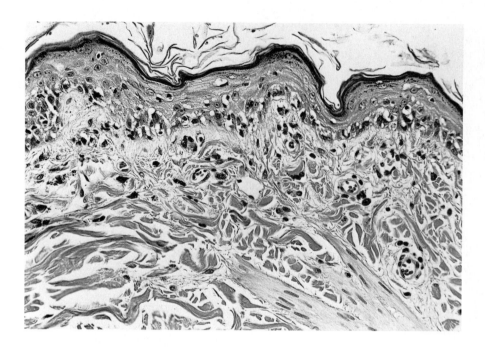

FIGURE 2-11. Higher magnification of hereditary lupoid dermatosis demonstrating lupus-like basal cell vacuolation and degeneration. (×220.)

The most characteristic lesions are severe vacuolar degeneration of the basal cell layer of the epidermis, accompanied by individual cell necrosis. These changes are striking similar to those of lupus erythematosus, particularly the systemic form, and it is from this similarity that the name *lupoid* is derived. Necrotic cells are shrunken and rounded or angular; nuclei are pyknotic. Occasionally, individual keratinocyte necrosis may extend mildly throughout the epidermis. Mild dermal-epidermal separation is present and is often seen at the margins of specimens as useable artifact (see earlier discussion in Discoid Lupus Erythematosus). Frank ulceration also has been observed. Similar vacuolar and necrotic lesions also affect the superficial hair follicles to the level of the adnexal glands. Occasionally there is marked accompanying follicular atrophy.

Pigmentary incontinence is often prominent in the superficial dermis, and is the result of basal cell damage. Lymphocytes, macrophages, mast cells, neutrophils, and plasma cells accumulate in mild or moderate numbers around superficial vessels or interstitially in close approximation to the overlying epidermis.

Histopathologic differential diagnoses include systemic lupus erythematosus, discoid lupus erythematosus, canine familial dermatomyositis, ulcerative dermatosis of the Shetland Sheepdog and Collie, and erythema multiforme. Knowledge of breed affected and young age of onset may be most helpful in differentiating lupoid dermatosis. Systemic lupus erythematosus and discoid lupus erythematosus are strikingly similar histopathologically to lupoid dermatosis; however, immunoglobulin deposition at the basement membrane zone has not been identified in lupoid dermatosis. Basal cell damage is generally much milder in dermatomyositis than in lupoid dermatosis. Although the degree of basal cell degeneration is similar between lupoid dermatosis and ulcerative dermatosis; frank ulceration is generally not a feature of lupoid dermatosis. Erythema multiforme will closely mimic those cases of lupoid dermatosis in which necrosis is seen at all levels of the epidermis. Clinical differentiation may be required; erythema multiforme generally does not occur in dogs less than 1 year of age.

BULLOUS PEMPHIGOID
Clinical features (Figures 2-12 and 2-13)

Bullous pemphigoid is a rare, vesiculobullous autoimmune skin disease of the dog. Autoantibodies are directed against bullous pemphigoid antigen, a biosynthetic product of keratinocytes and a normal constituent of the dermal-epidermal junction. Cleavage occurs within the lamina lucida. Since the lesion is subepidermal, intact vesicles or bullae are seen more commonly than with other bullous autoimmune skin diseases, such as pemphigus, in which lesions form intraepidermally. The wide variation in clinical presentation suggests that more than one entity may be currently grouped as bullous pemphigoid in the dog. Cases with predominantly periorbital and oral involvement exhibit features more similar to cicatricial pemphigoid in humans.

Turgid bullae with irregular borders develop rapidly. Smaller satellite vesicles and bullae form in the vicinity of the initial lesions. Commonly, the bullae rupture, leading to multifocal ulceration as the most

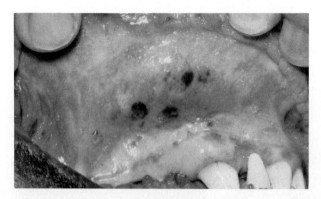

FIGURE 2-12. Bullous pemphigoid affecting the buccal mucosa of a Doberman Pinscher. Multiple intact bullae are present amid well-demarcated ulcers resulting from ruptured bullae. *(Courtesy LP Schmeitzel, Knoxville, Tennessee; case material from the University of California, Davis.)*

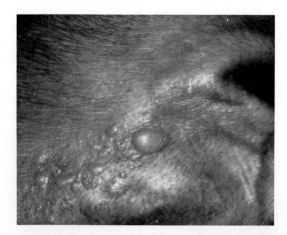

FIGURE 2-13. Bullous pemphigoid of the inner pinnae surface of the dog in Figure 2-12. Note the centrally located, large, intact bulla and multiple smaller bullae. *(Courtesy LP Schmeitzel, Knoxville, Tennessee; case material from the University of California, Davis.)*

common clinical sign. Generally, the ulcers do not coalesce and tend to remain the same size as the previously existent bullae. Bullae are more likely to remain intact in comparatively protected sites such as the buccal gingiva, pinnae, and axillae. Secondary bacterial involvement may occur. Scarring is common but variable in severity. Most dogs have oral, perioral, and periorbital involvement, but lesions are almost always present at other locations such as the intertriginous zones of the axillae and groin. Other sites include mucocutaneous junctions of the anus, vulva, and prepuce, as well as skin of the nailbeds and inner surface of the pinnae. Acute and chronic forms of canine bullous pemphigoid have been recognized. Dogs severely affected with the acute form of the disease may be systemically ill.

The Doberman Pinscher and Collie are reported to be at increased risk. However, at least some of the Collies reported as having bullous pemphigoid may have had a different subepidermal vesiculobullous disease, ulcerative dermatosis of the Shetland Sheepdog and Collie (see below). The Dachshund also may be at increased risk. Bullous pemphigoid may be more common in older dogs. Sex predilections are not reported.

Major clinical differential diagnoses include pemphigus vulgaris, systemic lupus erythematosus, ulcerative dermatosis of the Shetland Sheepdog and Collie, erythema multiforme, toxic epidermal necrolysis, and other bullous drug eruptions. Histopathology and immunohistochemical or immunofluorescent testing are generally required for differentiation.

Biopsy site selection

If present, an intact bulla or vesicle should be removed in its entirety, preferably by excisional biopsy. Sheering forces created during punch biopsy may rup-

ture fragile lesions. Biopsy should be performed as soon as possible since intact lesions may be transient and ruptured lesions are less likely to yield diagnostic specimens. If an intact lesion is not available, tissue from the immediate margin of a recent bulla may be adequate for histopathologic interpretation. Alternatively, the dog may be hospitalized for a "vesicle watch."

Histopathology (Figures 2-14 and 2-15)

There may exist several diseases in the dog characterized by subepidermal bullae and vesicles. These may have variable clinical presentation and differences in histologic characteristics, including shape of bullae, degree and type of accompanying dermal inflammation, and presence or absence of immunoglobulin or complement at the basement membrane zone. Only a small percentage share all the features of bullous pemphigoid in man. Further investigation is needed to subdivide this group.

Classically, as in bullous pemphigoid in humans, a large vesicle or bulla develops at the dermal-epidermal junction as a result of immune-mediated injury. Thus, in early lesions there is intact epidermis above a clean separation between dermis and epidermis. Variation in shape and contents of bulla occurs. Some bullae are turgid with serum, whereas others are flat and enclose small amounts of fibrin. Bulla may contain variable numbers of eosinophils or neutrophils. As the lesion ages, the epidermal roof of the bulla may be spongiotic; degeneration eventuates in ulceration.

The dermis is generally only minimally inflamed beneath early bullae. Small numbers of eosinophils or neutrophils and a few mixed mononuclear cells may be

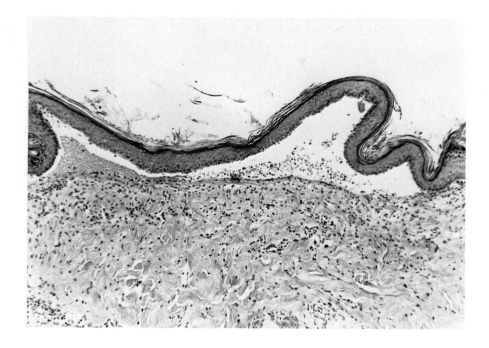

found superficially in a perivascular and interstitial pattern. Edema may be seen. Secondary ulceration results in severe dermatitis.

In ideal cases, immunofluorescent or immunohistochemical testing reveals deposition of immunoglobulin, usually IgG or IgM, and complement at the basement membrane zone. The pattern is usually thin and smooth, in contrast to the granular or clumped pattern more characteristic of lupus erythematosus. Failure to demonstrate antibody does not exclude the diagnosis in typical cases.

The major differential diagnosis is epidermolysis bullosa. Epidermolysis bullosa may be identical histopathologically but is negative for deposition of immunoglobulin and can be differentiated based on clinical features.

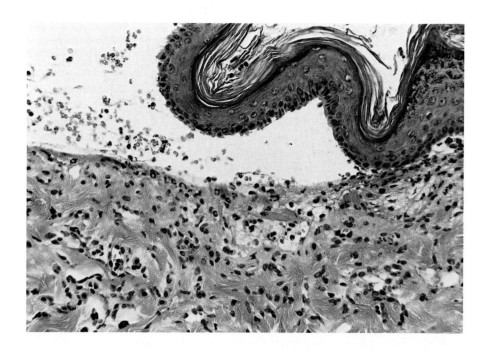

FIGURE 2-15. Higher magnification of the bulla in Figure 2-14. Note the red blood cells and small numbers of neutrophils and eosinophils in the bulla. (×235.)

PEMPHIGUS VULGARIS
Clinical features (Figures 2-16 and 2-17)

Pemphigus vulgaris is a rare bullous autoimmune skin disease reported in the dog and cat. In this type V hypersensitivity reaction, autoantibody binds to components of the desmosome, which are then internalized by phagocytosis leading to the conversion of plasminogen to plasmin by plasminogen activators. Acantholysis results, creating suprabasilar vesicles and bullae.

Fragile, irregularly shaped vesicles and bullae develop in groups. Dissolution of these vesicles and bullae rapidly leads to erosions that are substantially larger than previously existent intact bullae. Secondary surface bacterial infection results in widespread ulceration. The resultant ulcers are irregularly shaped and may coalesce. A positive Nikolsky sign (the artificial extension of a blister or ulcer induced by digital pressure to adjacent mucous membrane or skin) may be elicited.

The oral cavity and mucocutaneous junctions of the lips, eyelids, nostrils, anus, prepuce, and vulva are the most common sites. Corneal ulcers may be present. Stannard reported esophageal involvement. Partial bilateral symmetry may be noted. At least 90% of affected animals have oral involvement, and oral ulceration is often the initial clinical sign. Coalescing ulcers on the tongue, palate, and gingiva that are not contiguous with the teeth should increase clinical suspicion for pemphigus vulgaris. Lip involvement usually is seen with extensive oral disease. Thick, ropey, tenacious, odorous saliva is an additional feature. Less commonly, skin distant from mucocutaneous junctions may also be affected; rarely, pemphigus vulgaris of the haired skin alone has been reported. Onychomadesis may be seen. Anorexia and depression are common.

Age, breed, or sex predilections have not been noted for either the cat or dog. Little data is available since pemphigus vulgaris is considerably less common than most other autoimmune skin diseases.

Major clinical differential diagnoses include bullous pemphigoid, erythema multiforme, systemic lupus erythematosus, toxic epidermal necrolysis, and mycosis fungoides, all of which may cause oral ulcers. Histopathology may allow differentiation, and the intercellular deposition of immunoglobulin should be demonstrable in pemphigus vulgaris. In addition, superficial necrolytic dermatitis and mucocutaneous candidiasis can present with perioral skin disease; however, frank oral ulceration is not a feature of these diseases. If lesions are limited to the oral cavity, the many causes of feline and canine ulcerative stomatitis must also be considered.

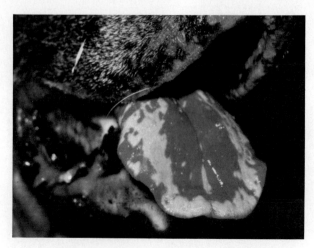

FIGURE 2-16. Pemphigus vulgaris in an adult Great Dane. Extensive erosion and secondary ulceration are present on the tongue, oral mucous membranes, and muzzle.

Biopsy site selection

Intact vesicles or margins of recent ulcers should be removed for biopsy. In general, specimens from the lips or other cutaneous sites are more likely to yield diagnostic results than are specimens from the oral mucosa, which are extremely fragile. Rapid natural degradation of vesicles or bullae also makes sampling difficult. Due to the frailty of the lesions, wedge biopsy technique more commonly yields diagnostic specimens than does punch biopsy.

Histopathology (Figures 2-18 and 2-19)

The typical lesion of pemphigus vulgaris is a suprabasilar cleft or separation due to acantholysis, leading

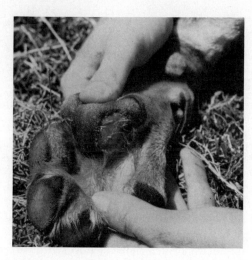

FIGURE 2-17. Pemphigus vulgaris involving the footpad of the dog in Figure 2-16. The pad epithelium has been shed, exposing the dermal tissue.

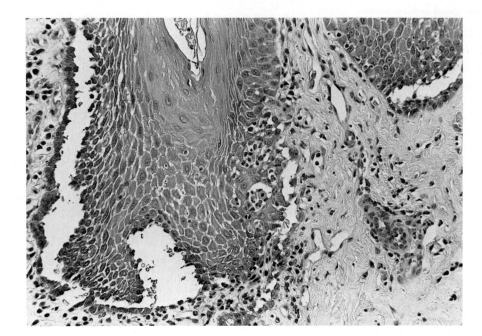

FIGURE 2-18. Suprabasilar cleft in canine pemphigus vulgaris. Note involvement of the superficial hair follicle. (×220.) *(Case material from MB Calderwood Mays, Gainesville, Florida.)*

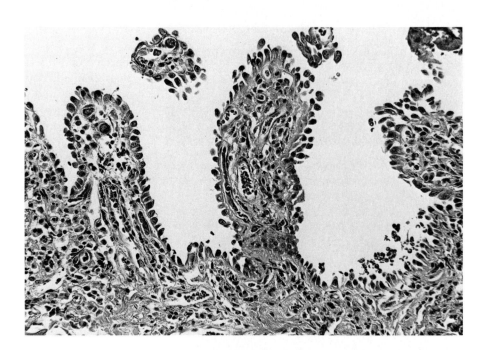

FIGURE 2-19. Canine pemphigus vulgaris. Residual basal cells are in tombstone-like configuration along the base of the cleft. (×220.)

to formation of a bulla. Lesions involve the mucosa or epidermis and frequently extend to superficial hair follicles. Acantholysis of the salivary ducts has been reported by Stannard. A row of plump or rounded basal cells, commonly called "tombstone" cells, remain at the base of the cleft. Active acantholysis may be seen above the cleft. Inflammation is absent from intact bullae. Often the roof of the bulla is absent in specimens, leaving a row of basal cells still attached to the basement membrane. Secondary ulceration and superficial inflammation and exudation (crusting) are common sequelae.

Superficial dermal inflammation (lymphocytes, plasma cells, and neutrophils) is variable, and severity is contingent partly upon the presence of ulceration. Pigmentary incontinence may be present.

Immunofluorescent or immunohistochemical findings are similar to those of pemphigus foliaceus. There is transepidermal intercellular deposition of immunoglobulin, usually IgG, and occasionally complement. As in pemphigus foliaceus, a positive result does not always result from random biopsy. Obtaining multiple sequential specimens for immunohistologic evaluation may increase the chances for a positive result.

If the classic histopathologic features are present, there are no known differential diagnoses for pemphigus vulgaris. Theoretically, drug eruption could mimic pemphigus vulgaris. Pemphigus vegetans, a variant of pemphigus vulgaris, is also typified by suprabasilar clefting and acantholysis, but is additionally characterized by severe hyperplasia and pustulation of the epidermis.

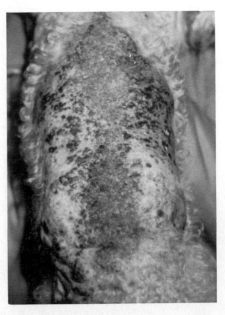

PEMPHIGUS VEGETANS

Clinical features (Figure 2-20)

Pemphigus vegetans is an extremely rare autoimmune skin disease reported in the dog. It is considered to be a benign variant of pemphigus vulgaris. Host resistance factors have been implicated in humans.

Pemphigus vegetans has been described as a chronic "vesiculopustular disorder that evolves into verrucous vegetations and papillomatous proliferations, which ooze and are studded with pustules."* Lesions have been primarily truncal in a very limited case sampling. Pruritus and pain may be noted, but otherwise, other signs are not present.

Age, breed, or sex predilections have not been established. Clinically, deep pyoderma and deep follicular pemphigus foliaceus should be considered as differential diagnoses. Histopathology allows differentiation.

Biopsy site selection

Vegetative erythematous plaques, papillomatous lesions, or intact pustular lesions should be selected for

FIGURE 2-20. Pemphigus vegetans in a dog. Note the proliferative, verrucous character of the lesions. *(From Scott DW: Pemphigus vegetans in a dog, Cornell Vet 67:380, 1977. Reprinted by permission.)*

biopsy. Wedge technique is advisable since the lesions may be fragile.

Histopathology (Figures 2-21 and 2-22)

Pemphigus vegetans is characterized by suprabasilar clefting due to acantholysis, similar to pemphigus vulgaris. Clefting often involves superficial hair follicles as well as the overlying epidermis. Pemphigus vegetans

---

* From Scott DW. In Muller GH, Kirk RW, and Scott, DW, eds: Small animal dermatology, ed 4, Philadelphia, 1989, WB Saunders, p 502.

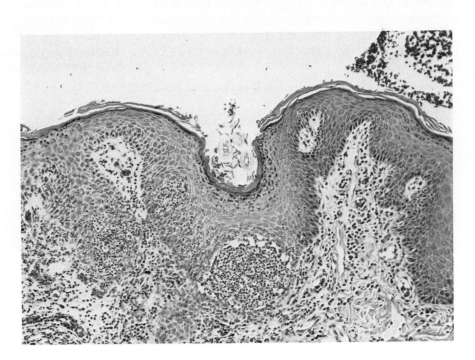

FIGURE 2-21. Canine pemphigus vegetans. Suprabasilar pustules are forming within the hyperplastic epidermis and superficial hair follicles. (×120.)

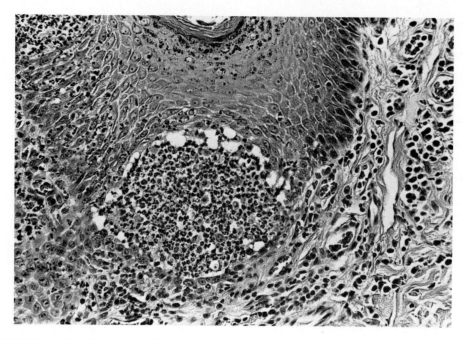

FIGURE 2-22. Higher magnification of the suprabasilar pustule shown in Figure 2-21. Note the free acantholytic cells. (×220.)

is also pustular (like pemphigus foliaceus) and is characterized by papillomatous hyperplasia of the epidermis and superficial follicular epithelium. Suprabasilar pustules often extend through the entire thickened epidermis or wall of the hair follicle and contain prominent eosinophils, fewer neutrophils, and variable numbers of acantholytic cells. Dermal inflammation is superficial and mixed and includes eosinophils, neutrophils, lymphocytes, macrophages, and plasma cells.

There are no histopathologic differential diagnoses for pemphigus vegetans, as long as suprabasilar clefting is recognized. Care should be taken not to confuse deep follicular pemphigus foliaceus, which does not demonstrate suprabasilar clefting, with pemphigus vegetans.

CANINE FAMILIAL DERMATOMYOSITIS
Clinical features (Figures 2-23 and 2-24)

Canine familial dermatomyositis is a heritable inflammatory disease of muscle and skin. The etiopathogenesis is unknown. Autoimmune and viral etiologies have been postulated for a similar disease in humans. Lesions of skin and muscle vary markedly in severity. Spontaneous regression is common. Severely affected dogs exhibit lifelong disease with cyclic recrudescence.

Transient papules, pustules, and vesicles eventuating in crusted erosions, ulcers, and alopecia may be seen early in the disease. Scarring is a feature of severe,

chronic lesions. Pigmentary aberrations give rise to poikilodermatous change.

Initial lesions usually occur over bony prominences, especially on the muzzle, and in periorbital and perioral locations. Later, similar lesions are seen on the pinnae (especially the tips of the ears), nail folds, tip of the tail, and over bony prominences of the distal extremities and other pressure points. Pain and pruritus are not common unless ulceration or secondary pyoderma are present. Photo-aggravation occurs, and trauma or estrus may trigger relapse.

Muscle involvement is often subtle and may be limited to temporal and masseter muscle atrophy. Difficulties with mastication and swallowing may occur. Severely affected dogs show growth retardation,

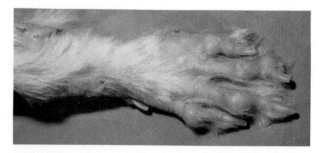

FIGURE 2-23. Canine familial dermatomyositis in a Shetland Sheepdog puppy. Extensive alopecia is present on the forelimb. Pale crusts adhere to erosions over bony prominences.

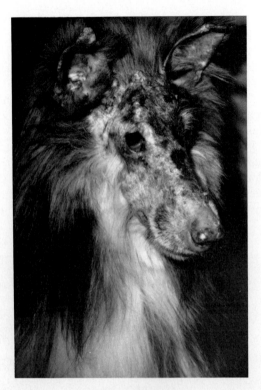

FIGURE 2-24. Chronic canine familial dermatomyositis in an adult Shetland Sheepdog. Extensive alopecia and crusting are present on the face and pinnae.

megaesophagus, lameness, and widespread muscle atrophy. Infertility is an additional feature of severe dermatomyositis.

Familial canine dermatomyositis is seen almost exclusively in Shetland Sheepdogs, Collies, and their related crossbreeds. Rarely, dermatomyositis has also been documented in the Chow Chow, German Shepherd Dog,* and Kuvasz, as well as in other purebred dogs. Initial lesions usually occur by 6 months of age. Sex predilection has not been noted.

Demodicosis, dermatophytosis, facial pyoderma, and discoid lupus erythematosus are the major clinical differential diagnoses. Concurrent clinical, electromyographic, or histopathologic evidence of muscle disease is indicative of dermatomyositis.

Biopsy site selection

Lesions showing erythema and alopecia are preferred sites for biopsy. Secondarily infected or scarred lesions are not optimal for demonstration of typical histopathology. Vesicular lesions are excellent specimens for biopsy but rarely are observed clinically.

Histopathology (Figure 2-25)

Scattered degeneration of individual basal cells is the typical epidermal feature of dermatomyositis but may not be present in individual biopsy specimens. Affected basal cells may be either vacuolated or necrotic. Necrotic basal cells are shrunken and brightly eosinophilic (colloid bodies). Secondary vesiculation is present occasionally, or there may be diagnostically

* From Miller WH, Jr: Personal communication, 1990.

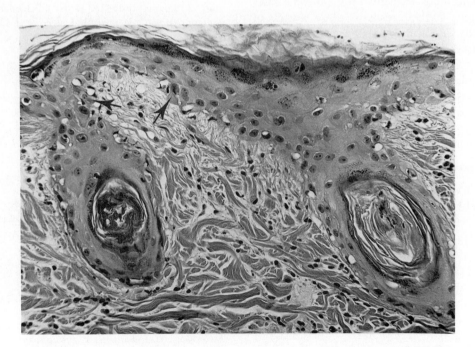

FIGURE 2-25. Canine familial dermatomyositis. Basal cells are mildly vacuolated and occasionally shrunken and necrotic *(arrows)*; outer hair follicles also are affected. (×220.)

useful, artifactual dermal-epidermal separation at the margins of the specimen (see earlier discussion in discoid lupus erythematosus). Vesicles often contain small numbers of red blood cells. Secondary ulceration is uncommon but may occur if vesicular lesions are extensive. Superficial crusting is variable.

Dermal inflammation is generally superficially diffuse and mild and often loosely encircles follicles. Lymphocytes and histiocytes predominate; mast cells and neutrophils may also be observed. Intense inflammation, which includes prominent neutrophils, may be seen accompanying ulceration in severe lesions. Dermal scarring is rare but can occur in the wake of severe ulceration and inflammation. Follicular basal cell degeneration and resultant follicular atrophy usually are observed and may be more consistently observed than basal cell lesions of the epidermis (see Chapter 17).

Deeper biopsies, particularly in periocular location, occasionally will show inflammation of skeletal muscle. Myositis is characterized by mixed inflammation, including lymphocytes, macrophages, plasma cells, and sparse neutrophils, myofiber degeneration (fragmentation, vacuolation, increased eosinophilia), regeneration, fibrosis, and atrophy. In general, random biopsy of clinically affected muscle groups, such as the temporal or masseter muscles, may not show lesions. Electromyography is a more reliable method of documenting muscle disease and locating appropriate sites for muscle biopsy.

Lupus erythematosus is the principal differential diagnosis. Prominent lichenoid dermal inflammation, as seen in discoid lupus erythematosus and some cases of systemic lupus erythematosus, is not a feature of dermatomyositis. Follicular atrophy usually is not present in lupus erythematosus. Hereditary lupoid dermatosis of the German Shorthaired Pointer may be similar, particularly if follicular atrophy is present. Basal cell degeneration is generally more severe in lupoid dermatosis and can assist in differentiation when knowledge of the breed affected is not available to the pathologist.

ULCERATIVE DERMATOSIS OF THE SHETLAND SHEEPDOG AND COLLIE

Clinical features (Figures 2-26 and 2-27)

Ulcerative dermatosis of the Shetland Sheepdog and Collie is a newly recognized, poorly understood syndrome that may represent a subgroup of canine familial dermatomyositis. Transient vesiculobullous eruptions lead to coalescing ulcerations with an undulating serpiginous border. The intertriginous areas of the groin and axillae are most often affected. Lesions may involve the mucocutaneous junctions of the eyes,

mouth, genitals, and anus. Partial bilateral symmetry may be seen. Pain may be evident if secondary pyoderma is present. A concomitant myositis has been documented by electromyography in some affected dogs.

This syndrome has been recognized, to our knowledge, only in the adult Shetland Sheepdog and Collie. Sex predilection has not been noted.

In the past, this syndrome was probably misdiagnosed as hidradenitis suppurativa, or, more recently, as bullous pemphigoid. Other clinical differential diagnoses should include erythema multiforme, systemic lupus erythematosus, and pemphigus vulgaris. ANA

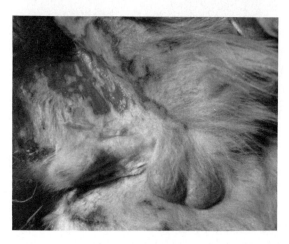

FIGURE 2-26. Ulcerative dermatosis in an adult Shetland Sheepdog. Ulcers on the ventral abdomen exhibit undulating, serpiginous borders. *(Courtesy AC Mundell, Seattle, Washington; case material from the University of California, Davis.)*

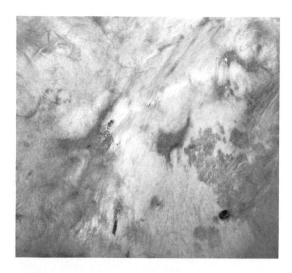

FIGURE 2-27. Ulcerative dermatosis in an adult Shetland Sheepdog. Well-demarcated serpiginous ulcers are present amid chronic scarring on the ventral abdomen. Note striae from older, healed lesions located centrally.

testing has been consistently negative in ulcerative dermatosis. Histopathology and immunofluorescent or immunohistochemical testing will allow separation in most cases.

Biopsy site selection

Foci of erythema at the margins of crusting or ulcerated lesions are preferred sites for the demonstration of characteristic histopathologic lesions. Due to fragility of the dermal-epidermal junction in lesions of

ulcerative dermatosis, wedge technique is recommended.

Histopathology (Figures 2-28 and 2-29)

The histopathologic lesions of ulcerative dermatosis are qualitatively similar to but much more severe than those of canine familial dermatomyositis. Shrunken, brightly eosinophilic, necrotic basal keratinocytes (colloid bodies) may be numerous. Occasionally, necrosis of scattered keratinocytes of the spinous

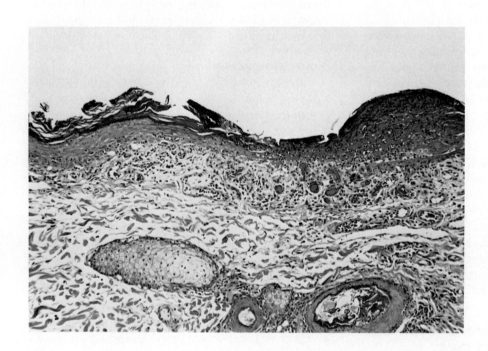

FIGURE 2-28. Ulcerative dermatosis in a Shetland Sheepdog. The ulcer is covered by a serocellular crust; intact epidermis shows basilar vacuolation. (×95.)

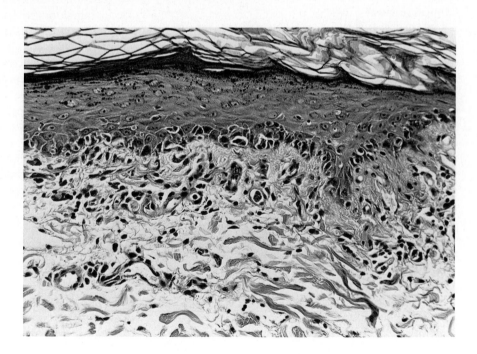

FIGURE 2-29. Ulcerative dermatosis in a Shetland Sheepdog. Basal cells are shrunken and necrotic. (×220.)

layer may also be observed. Vacuolation of basal cells is mild to moderate. Dermal-epidermal vesiculation is common and leads to ulceration and exudation. Damage to basal cells allows weakening of the dermal-epidermal junction, and the "usable artifact" of dermal-epidermal separation may be seen at the margins of specimens (see Discoid Lupus Erythematosus, above). Although outer cells of superficial hair follicles also are frequently necrotic or vacuolated, follicular atrophy as seen in dermatomyositis is not observed. Lesions of ulcerative dermatosis may be more fulminating than those of dermatomyositis and thus do not allow the more chronic process of follicular atrophy to occur. The superficial dermis contains a mixed mononuclear infiltrate. Inflammation may be perivascular to mildly lichenoid as lymphocytes migrate into the overlying basal cell layer and obscure the dermal-epidermal junction. Neutrophils are prominent in ulcerated lesions.

The principal differential diagnoses include erythema multiforme, systemic and discoid lupus erythematosus, and hereditary lupoid dermatosis of the German Shorthaired Pointer. Individual keratinocyte necrosis is prominent at all levels of the epidermis in erythema multiforme and is not principally confined to the basal cell layer as it is in ulcerative dermatosis. Lupus erythematosus may closely resemble ulcerative dermatosis; however, immunofluorescent and immunohistochemical testing have been negative in ulcerative dermatosis. Lupoid dermatosis has significant basal cell damage but is not generally ulcerative; knowledge of breed affected also will allow differentiation.

EPIDERMOLYSIS BULLOSA
Clinical features

Epidermolysis bullosa is a term used in human medicine to describe a group of hereditary mechanobullous diseases of unknown etiology. Structural defects occur at various levels of the basement membrane zone, resulting in fragility of the dermal-epidermal junction. Congenital and acquired forms have been described in humans. Cases with clinical and histopathologic features similar to congenital epidermolysis bullosa of man have been observed by the authors and others in young dogs, and a recent case report by Dunstan convincingly documented junctional epidermolysis bullosa in a Toy Poodle.

Affected animals develop multiple oral and cutaneous vesicles and bullae leading to ulceration. Footpads, intertriginous skin, and other frictional sites may be preferentially affected. Lesions may be produced iatrogenically with friction.

Collies previously reported as having epidermolysis bullosa simplex most likely had canine familial dermatomyositis. Currently, breed or sex predilections have not been identified. Affected animals with congenital epidermolysis bullosa usually develop lesions shortly after birth.

Clinical differential diagnoses include bullous autoimmune skin diseases, toxic epidermal necrolysis, and chemical or thermal burns. Differentiation usually should not be problematic. A history of probable exposure generally accompanies chemical or thermal burns. Autoimmune diseases commonly occur in middle-aged or older animals, and toxic epidermal necrolysis usually is associated with a drug history. Autoimmune skin disease or toxic epidermal necrolysis should not be localized to frictional skin. Histopathology should confirm the diagnosis.

Biopsy site selection

Bullae or vesicles should be obtained carefully by wedge technique to preserve the integrity of these fragile lesions. Margins of early ulcers may show diagnostic changes at the dermal-epidermal junction.

Histopathology (Figures 2-30 and 2-31)

Three principal forms of epidermolysis bullosa have been identified in humans. Epidermal or epidermolytic epidermolysis bullosa involves basal cell degeneration; junctional epidermolysis bullosa is characterized by fragility of the basement membrane; and dystrophic or collagenolytic epidermolysis bullosa affects anchoring fibrils or other structures of the superficial dermis.

In junctional epidermolysis bullosa, the epidermis is cleanly separated from the underlying dermis to form a bulla or vesicle. Dunstan described the earliest lesions of junctional epidermolysis in a poodle as vacuoles occurring along the basement membrane. Mature vesicles contained occasional red blood cells or hair fragments. Inflammation was sparse in early lesions. As the bullae evolved to ulcers, there was secondary superficial dermal influx of neutrophils and mixed mononuclear cells.

Histopathologically, bullous pemphigoid may closely resemble junctional epidermolysis bullosa. Since not all random biopsy specimens obtained from dogs with bullous pemphigoid will have positive immunofluorescence at the basement membrane, ultimate differentiation from epidermolysis bullosa may require knowledge of signalment and clinical signs.

SUGGESTED READINGS

Discoid lupus erythematosus

Griffin CE and others: Canine discoid lupus erythematosus, Vet Immunol Immunopathol 1:79-87, 1979.

Olivry T and others: Le lupus erythemateux discoide du chien a propos de 22 observations, Pratique Medicale Chirurgicale de L'Animal de Compagnie 3:205-214, 1987.

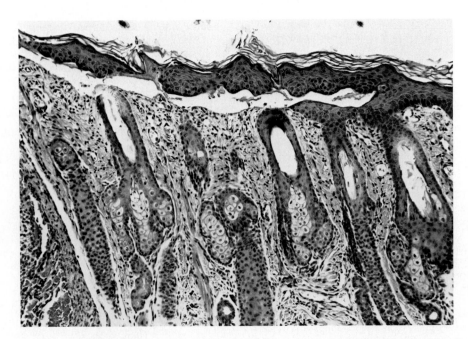

FIGURE 2-30. Canine junctional epidermolysis bullosa. Note the large subepidermal bulla. (×105.) *(Case material from RW Dunstan, East Lansing, Michigan.)*

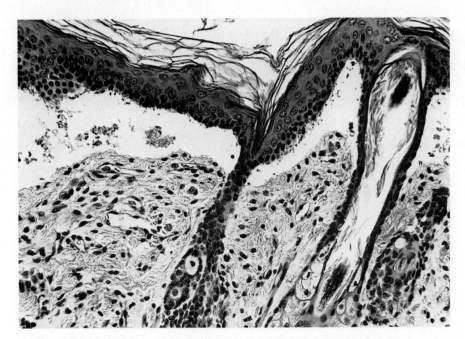

FIGURE 2-31. Higher magnification of the bulla in Fig. 2-30. Basal cells remain intact in the roof of the bulla. (×220.)

Scott DW and others: Immune-mediated dermatoses in domestic animals: ten years after. Part II, Comp Cont Educ 9:539-553, 1987.

Sontheimer RD and Fine J-D: Biology of the dermal-epidermal interface and the pathophysiology of bullous pemphigoid, epidermolysis bullosa acquisita, and lupus erythematosus. In Soter NA and Baden HP, editors: Pathophysiology of dermatologic diseases, New York, 1991, McGraw-Hill, pp 303-325.

Systemic lupus erythematosus

Halliwell REW and Gorman NT: Veterinary clinical immunology, ed 1, Philadelphia, 1989, WB Saunders, pp 324-333.

Pedersen NC and Barlough JE: Systemic lupus erythematosus in the cat, J Am Anim Hosp Assoc 19:5-13, 1991.

Scott DW and Anderson WI: Panniculitis in dogs and cats: a retrospective analysis of 78 cases, J Am Anim Hosp Assoc 24:551-559, 1988.

Sontheimer RD and Fine J-D: Biology of the dermal-epidermal interface and the pathophysiology of bullous pemphigoid, epidermolysis bullosa acquisita, and lupus erythematosus. In Soter NA and Baden HP, editors: Pathophysiology of dermatologic diseases, New York, 1991, McGraw-Hill, pp 303-325.

Zamansky GB: Sunlight-induced pathogenesis in systemic lupus erythematosus, J Invest Dermatol 85:179-180, 1985.

Hereditary lupoid dermatosis of the German Shorthaired Pointer

References not available.

Bullous pemphigoid

Ackerman LJ: Pemphigus and pemphigoid in the dog and cat. Part II. Pemphigoid, Comp Cont Educ Pract Vet 7:281-286, 1985.

Kunkle GA and others: Bullous pemphigoid in a dog: a case report with immunofluorescent findings, J Am Anim Hosp Assoc 14:52-57, 1978.

Scott DW: Pemphigoid in domestic animals, Clin Dermatol 5:155-163, 1987.

Scott DW and others: Immune-mediated dermatoses in domestic animals: ten years after. Part I, Comp Cont Educ 9:423-435, 1987.

Sontheimer RD and Fine J-D: Biology of the dermal-epidermal interface and the pathophysiology of bullous pemphigoid, epidermolysis bullosa acquisita, and lupus erythematosus. In Soter NA and Baden HP, editors: Pathophysiology of dermatologic diseases, New York, 1991, McGraw-Hill, pp 303-325.

Pemphigus vulgaris

Manning and others: Pemphigus diseases in the feline: seven case reports and discussion, J Am Anim Hosp Assoc 18:433-443, 1982.

Robledo MA and Diaz LA: Pathophysiology of pemphigus. In Soter NA and Baden HP, editors: Pathophysiology of dermatologic diseases, New York, 1991, McGraw-Hill, pp 179-191.

Scott DW and others: Immune-mediated dermatoses in domestic animals: ten years after. Part I, Comp Cont Educ 9:423-435, 1987.

Scott DW and others: Pemphigus vulgaris without mucosal or mucocutaneous involvement in two dogs, J Am Anim Hosp Assoc 18:401-404, 1982.

Stannard AA and others: A mucocutaneous disease in the dog, resembling pemphigus vulgaris in man, J Am Vet Med Assoc 166:575-582, 1975.

Suter MM and others: Ultrastructural localization of pemphigus vulgaris antigen on canine keratinocytes in vivo and in vitro, Am J Vet Res 51:507-511, 1990.

Pemphigus vegetans

Scott DW: Pemphigus vegetans in a dog, Cornell Vet 67:374-384, 1977.

Scott DW and others: Immune-mediated dermatoses in domestic animals: ten years after. Part I, Comp Cont Educ 9:423-435, 1987.

Canine familial dermatomyositis

Gross TL and Kunkle GA: The cutaneous histology of dermatomyositis in Collie Dogs, Vet Pathol 24:11-15, 1987.

Hargis AM and others: A skin disorder in three Shetland Sheepdogs: comparison with familial canine dermatomyositis of collies, Comp Cont Educ 7:306-315, 1985.

Hargis AM and others: Familial canine dermatomyositis. Initial characterization of the cutaneous and muscular lesions, Am J Pathol 116:234-244, 1984.

Haupt KH and Hargis AM: Familial canine dermatomyositis. In Kirk RW, editor: Current veterinary therapy X. Philadelphia, 1989, WB Saunders, pp 606-609.

Kunkle GA and others: Dermatomyositis in Collies, Comp Cont Educ 7:185-192, 1985.

Ulcerative dermatosis of the Shetland Sheepdog and Collie

References not available

Epidermolysis bullosa

Dunstan RW and others: A disease resembling junctional epidermolysis bullosa in a toy poodle, Am J Dermatopathol 10:442-447, 1988.

Lever WF and Schaumburg-Lever G: Histopathology of the skin, ed 7, Philadelphia, 1990, JB Lippincott, pp 77-79.

Necrotizing diseases of the epidermis

This group of epidermal diseases is characterized by necrosis of keratinocytes and may be the result of external trauma or internal metabolic or immune-mediated alteration of the epidermis. Superficial hair follicles are often affected. Necrosis may be diffuse and superficial, or it may affect individual cells throughout the epidermis or superficial hair follicles. Necrotizing diseases will have prominent associated ulceration as devitalized keratinocytes are sloughed.

ERYTHEMA MULTIFORME
Clinical features (Figures 3-1 and 3-2)

Erythema multiforme is a cutaneous reaction pattern of multifactorial etiology seen uncommonly in the dog and rarely in the cat. An immunologic basis for the syndrome has been hypothesized for both humans and domestic animals. It is currently believed that the process of cell death occurring in erythema multiforme, also called *apoptosis,* is the result of initiation of a "death program" through cell-mediated or unknown factors.* Most documented cases of erythema multiforme in small animals are associated with drug hypersensitivity. Neoplasia and infection are less common initiators. Erythema multiforme is characterized clinically by a remarkably pleomorphic eruption considering the commonality of the histopathologic changes.

Typically, the onset is acute, as erythematous macules and papules develop rapidly in partially symmetric patterns. The lesions may appear urticarial. Crusting commonly occurs as the lesions spread peripherally and form arciform patterns. Epidermal collarettes may be present. Annular target lesions with central clearing are visually striking at some stages of the syndrome. In the less common severe form of erythema multiforme, widespread ulcers may eventuate from the urticarial or plaquelike lesions. Although lesions may be seen anywhere, truncal lesions are more frequent and especially involve the glabrous skin of the groin. Other common sites of involvement include the mucocutaneous junctions, oral mucosa, ears, and axillae. Pain or pruritus may be present.

A subgroup of idiopathic erythema multiforme has been seen in older dogs without a history compatible with drug hypersensitivity or without other concurrent disease. Lesions are more exudative and proliferative and often predominantly involve the face and ears. The authors have identified occult leukemia, pancreatic endocrine tumor, and *Pneumocystis* pneumonia (probably indicating immune dysfunction) as sub-

* From Fadok VA: Personal communication, 1990.

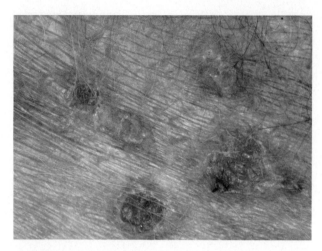

FIGURE 3-1. Erythema multiforme in a dog caused by a drug reaction to trimethoprim-sulfa. Coalescing erythematous target lesions are present on the ventral abdomen.

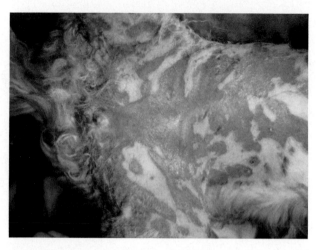

FIGURE 3-2. Severe erythema multiforme in a dog caused by a drug reaction to ampicillin. Widespread coalescing erosions and ulcers with serpiginous borders involve most of the ventral abdomen. *(From Ihrke PJ: Topical therapy: use, principals and vehicles, dermatologic therapy, Part I, Comp Cont Ed 1:30, 1980. Reprinted by permission.)*

sequent findings in several of these dogs. Breed or sex predilections have not been noted for any of the forms of erythema multiforme.

Clinical differential diagnoses are legion because of the pleomorphic nature of erythema multiforme. Milder more common manifestations may resemble urticaria, superficial spreading pyoderma, bacterial folliculitis, and early lesions of bullous autoimmune skin diseases. Rarely, erythema multiforme may be so severe that it must be differentiated from necrotizing syndromes such as toxic epidermal necrolysis, burns, systemic lupus erythematosus, and vasculitis or other causes of ischemic necrosis. Rarely, erythema multiforme and toxic epidermal necrolysis may coexist in the same patient. Superficial necrolytic dermatitis, zinc-responsive dermatosis, and generic dog food dermatosis are additional differential diagnoses for erythema multiforme seen in older dogs because of the proliferative and exudative nature of these lesions. Histopathology usually will allow differentiation of erythema multiforme from the diseases mentioned above.

Biopsy site selection

Areas of erythema without crusting or ulceration are ideal sites for skin biopsy. An intact epidermis is crucial for the diagnosis of this syndrome.

Histopathology (Figures 3-3 and 3-4)

Individual cell necrosis of keratinocytes, or apoptosis, is the most characteristic histologic lesion of erythema multiforme. Solitary or grouped, brightly eosinophilic cells are present at all levels of the epidermis. Lymphocytes migrate into the affected epidermis and may closely surround the apoptotic keratinocytes, a

process termed *satellitosis*. Progression of keratinocyte necrosis usually leads to ulceration. Secondary neutrophilic infiltration and crusting are then observed. Variable vacuolar degeneration of the basal cell layer also is present. Superficial perivascular to interface, lymphocytic and histiocytic dermal inflammation is present (see Chapter 10), but neutrophils and plasma cells may predominate in cases with severe erosion or ulceration.

Idiopathic erythema multiforme seen in older dogs is histopathologically similar. Acanthosis and lymphocytic satellitosis may be more pronounced. Striking superficial follicular apoptosis, as seen in experimental graft-versus-host disease of dogs,* may be more prominent in this form of erythema multiforme; however, this finding is not diagnostic, since some dogs with drug-induced erythema multiforme also may have follicular lesions. In erythema multiforme of older dogs, the epidermis may have numerous brightly eosinophilic keratinocytes that appear dyskeratotic, since they are unassociated with lymphocytic satellitosis and eventuate in superficial hyperkeratosis rather than erosion or ulceration. Since the generation of the individual necrotic keratinocyte (or apoptotic keratinocyte) and the dyskeratotic cell involve similar ultrastructural changes (and may represent a final common pathway to keratinocyte self-destruction), the visual similarity between apoptosis and dyskeratosis of the keratinocyte is not surprising.

---

* From Sale GE: In vitro and in vivo animal models of graft versus host disease. In Sale GE and Shulman HM: The pathology of bone marrow transplantation, 1984, Masson Publishing, Inc, pp 19-30.

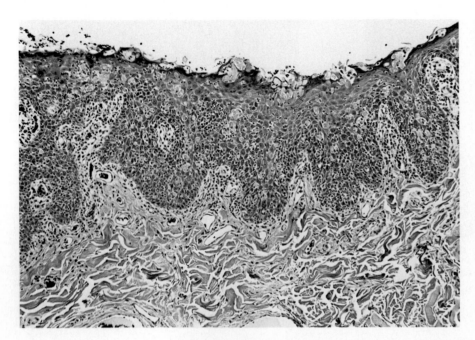

FIGURE 3-3. Erythema multiforme in a dog. Widespread individual keratinocyte necrosis; confluence of necrotic cells is apparent superficially. (×90.)

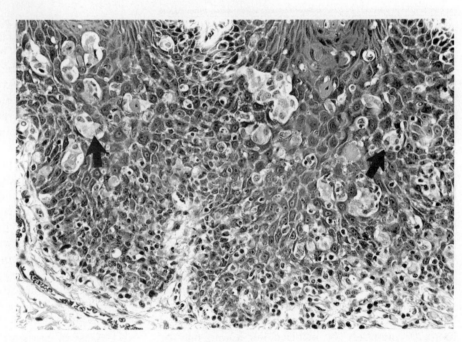

FIGURE 3-4. Erythema multiforme in a dog. Note pale necrotic keratinocytes and occasional lymphocytic satellitosis *(arrows).* (×220.)

Confluent areas of necrosis derived from severe individual cell necrosis in lesions of erythema multiforme may resemble toxic epidermal necrolysis (see subsequent discussion). Although the two diseases may be etiopathogenically related, severely necrotic erythema multiforme is clinically and histopathologically distinct from toxic epidermal necrolysis. Confluent necrosis in erythema multiforme always is associated with dermal and often epidermal inflammation; lesions of toxic epidermal necrolysis consist of diffuse epidermal necrosis without associated inflammation, at least in the earliest lesions.

Differentiation of erythema multiforme from systemic and discoid lupus erythematosus, as well as ulcerative dermatosis of the Shetland Sheepdog and Collie, is required because these diseases all may show degeneration of basal cells and an interface or lichenoid dermal inflammatory infiltrate. In erythema multiforme, individual necrosis of keratinocytes is more prominent and is seen at all levels of the epidermis; lupus erythematosus and ulcerative dermatosis have necrosis that is principally confined to the basal cell layer.

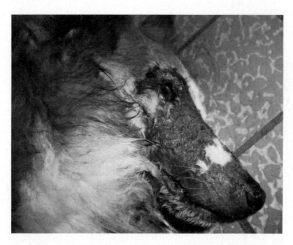

FIGURE 3-5. Toxic epidermal necrolysis in a Collie associated with a splenic fibrosarcoma. Note the confluent ulcers covering most of the face. *(Case material from REW Halliwell, Edinburgh.)*

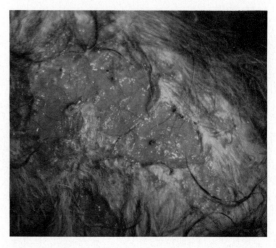

FIGURE 3-6. Toxic epidermal necrolysis in a mixed-breed dog. The dog had received multiple drugs prior to the development of the skin disease. Large confluent areas of ulceration and new smaller ulcers are present on the lateral thorax.

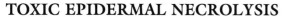

TOXIC EPIDERMAL NECROLYSIS

(Synonym: TEN)

Clinical features (Figures 3-5 and 3-6)

Toxic epidermal necrolysis is a rare, severe, life-threatening, ulcerative disorder of the oral mucosa and skin that has been seen in the dog and cat. Lymphocyte- and macrophage-mediated immunologic injury is a proposed mechanism. Drug hypersensitivity is the most commonly implicated underlying cause, although visceral neoplasia and infections also have been documented.

Initially, widespread macular erythema progresses to confluent erythema. The animal may be tender to palpation. Full-thickness confluent epidermal necrosis results in ulceration as the necrotic epidermis is shed. A positive Nikolsky's sign usually is present. The epidermis may be shed in translucent sheets resembling moist tissue paper. Sloughing may result from contact during handling. Facial skin, mucocutaneous junctions, and footpads commonly are involved but lesions may be widespread. The pharynx, esophagus, trachea, and mainstem bronchus may be affected. Concurrent hemorrhagic diarrhea in some cases suggests that gastrointestinal mucosa also may be affected.

Age, breed, or sex predilections have not been noted with drug-associated toxic epidermal necrolysis. Toxic epidermal necrolysis secondary to visceral neoplasia would be expected to occur more frequently in older animals.

Major clinical differential diagnoses include thermal burns, severe erythema multiforme, pemphigus vulgaris, bullous pemphigoid, systemic lupus erythematosus, and vasculitis or other causes of ischemic necrosis. The rapid spread and dramatic severity of toxic epidermal necrolysis aid in differentiating this syndrome from erythema multiforme. Controversy exists as to whether toxic epidermal necrolysis represents a pathophysiologically similar but more severe and fulminating form of erythema multiforme. Irrespective of this controversy, it is of clinical importance to separate erythema multiforme and toxic epidermal necrolysis because the biologic behavior of these two disorders is dissimilar. Toxic epidermal necrolysis is always a potentially life-threatening disease, whereas erythema multiforme most often follows a relatively benign, although occasionally chronic, course. On rare occasion, dogs may present with erythema multiforme that progresses to toxic epidermal necrolysis, or they may present with erythema multiforme and toxic epidermal necrolysis simultaneously.

Biopsy site selection

Areas of erythema without evidence of ulceration should be selected. Intact epidermis is vital to the histopathologic diagnosis of this disease.

Histopathology (Figures 3-7 and 3-8)

Lesions of toxic epidermal necrolysis are striking and consist of acute coagulation necrosis of the epidermis. The nuclei of affected keratinocytes lose detail and are pale or hyperchromatic; the cytoplasm is hypereosinophilic. In early lesions, keratinocytes retain their normal configuration and the overall architecture of the epidermis is intact. In older lesions, the devitalized epidermis separates from the subjacent dermis to form

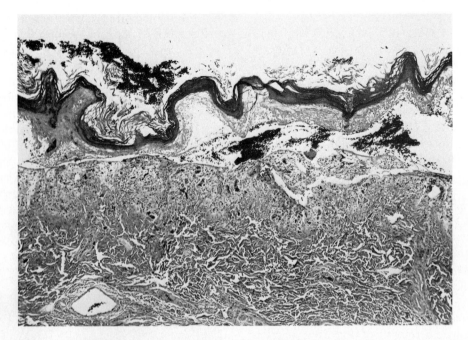

FIGURE 3-7. Toxic epidermal necrolysis in a dog. Diffusely necrotic epidermis is separating from underlying dermis to form a large bulla. (×35.)

large bullae. Bullae rupture, which results in ulceration. After separation from the dermis, the epidermis may lose all architectural detail and severe ballooning degeneration may occur.

Inflammation is not observed until the epidermis begins to separate from the dermis. Ulceration leads to severe secondary dermatitis that includes prominent neutrophils. Because of the potentially fatal nature of this disease, it is vital that the pathologist immediately alert the clinician as to the likelihood of toxic epidermal

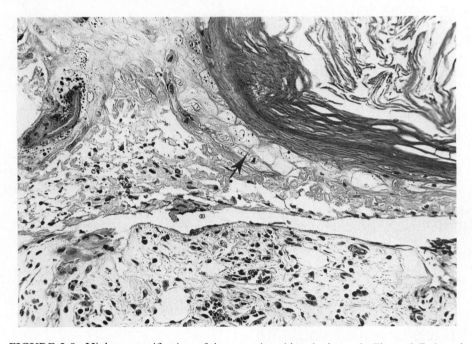

FIGURE 3-8. Higher magnification of the necrotic epidermis shown in Figure 3-7. Acutely necrotic keratinocytes are beneath the stratum corneum. Note the ballooning degeneration *(arrow)*. (×235.)

necrolysis so that any potentially causative drugs may be stopped.

Toxic epidermal necrolysis and severe erythema multiforme are distinct morphologically. Primary lesions of erythema multiforme include individual keratinocyte necrosis and inflammation; early toxic epidermal necrolysis has confluent epidermal necrosis and no inflammation. Histologically, toxic epidermal necrolysis may be similar to acute superficial burn, which also is manifested as coagulation necrosis of the epidermis.

SUPERFICIAL NECROLYTIC DERMATITIS (Synonyms: SND, diabetic
dermatopathy, hepatocutaneous syndrome, necrolytic migratory erythema)

Clinical features (Figures 3-9 through 3-11)

Superficial necrolytic dermatitis is an uncommon, necrotizing skin disorder of dogs associated with incompletely characterized internal metabolic disease. Superficial necrolytic dermatitis of dogs is most often associated with severe vacuolar hepatopathy and diabetes mellitus. This syndrome bears some resemblance to necrolytic migratory erythema (glucagonoma syndrome) of humans, which commonly is associated with a pancreatic endocrine tumor that secretes glucagon (glucagonoma) as well as high levels of plasma glucagon. Glucagon-producing pancreatic endocrine tumors have been identified in a minority of canine cases. Hyperglucagonemia may still be implicated in the pathogenesis of canine superficial necrolytic dermatitis as low level increases in plasma glucagon have been found by the authors and others in dogs with superficial necrolytic dermatitis but without apparent pancreatic endocrine tumors. Plasma levels of glucagon were not as-

sayed in two reported canine cases of glucagon-producing pancreatic endocrine tumors. Skin lesions appear to be the direct result of depressed plasma amino acid levels, as in humans. Plasma amino acid profiles show marked reduction in concentration of most amino acids with percentage reductions of up to 80%.

Erosions and ulcerations, with alopecia, exudation, and thick, adherent crusts are seen on the footpads and around the mucocutaneous junctions of the lips, eyes, anus, and vulva. Lesions also may be seen on the ears; pressure points, including the elbows and hocks; ventral thorax; and scrotum. Facial and pedal lesions have a striking bilateral symmetry. Secondary infection with dermatophytes or bacteria or colonization by yeast is common. Pruritus and pain frequently are evident.

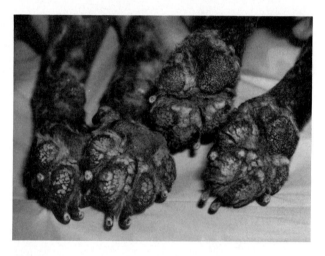

FIGURE 3-10. Superficial necrolytic dermatitis in an aged mixed-breed dog. The footpads of all four feet are heavily crusted. Fissures with exudation are evident on the footpads and at the margins of the pads.

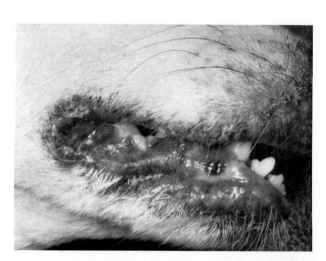

FIGURE 3-9. Superficial necrolytic dermatitis in an aged mixed-breed dog. Perioral and mucocutaneous erosions, ulcers, and crusts are present. *(Courtesy IJ Ameti, Orange, California.)*

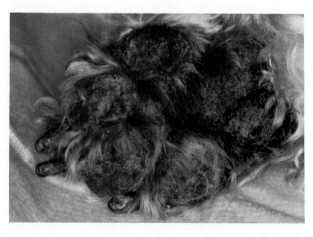

FIGURE 3-11. Closer view of footpad from aged poodle with superficial necrolytic dermatitis. Note the deeply fissured carpal pad.

Superficial necrolytic dermatitis is seen primarily in older dogs. Current data indicate that females are over-represented. Breed predilections have not been noted.

Clinical differential diagnoses include idiopathic erythema multiforme in older dogs, drug eruption, pemphigus foliaceus, systemic lupus erythematosus, zinc-responsive dermatosis, and generic dog food dermatosis. The presence of associated metabolic internal disease is a prime distinguishing clinical feature. Histopathology is useful in the differentiation of these diseases.

Biopsy site selection

Erythematous plaques with mild to moderate adherent crusts are ideal sites. Care should be taken not to disturb the crusts when taking the biopsy. Footpads may be less likely to yield diagnostic results because of the difficulty in obtaining a representative specimen, but pad margins may be suitable. Areas of ulceration should be avoided.

Histopathology (Figures 3-12 and 3-13)

On low power, the distinctive epidermal feature of superficial necrolytic dermatitis is the "pink, white, and

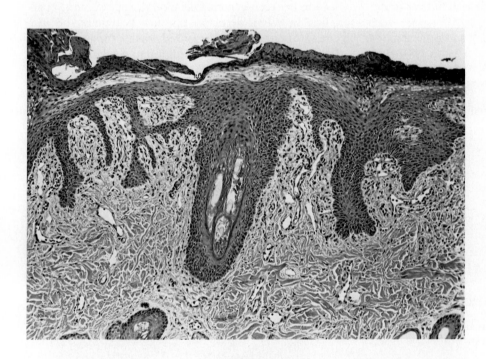

FIGURE 3-12. Superficial necrolytic dermatitis. Note layering of the superficial parakeratotic crust, subadjacent edema, and deep hyperplastic keratinocytes in the affected epidermis. (×95.)

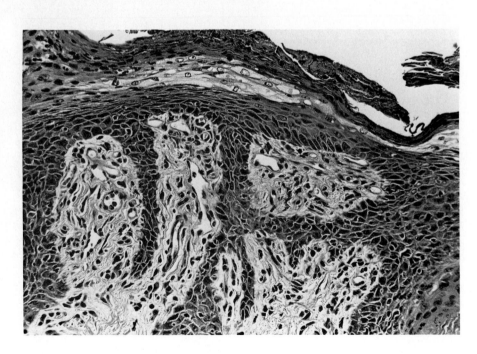

FIGURE 3-13. Higher magnificaton of the epidermis in Figure 3-12. The middle layer of the epidermis shows prominent edema and degeneration of keratinocytes. (×220.)

blue sandwich." Parakeratosis and crusting make up the top eosinophilic layer, edema and necrolysis of keratinocytes form the pale middle layer, and hyperplastic basal cells compose the deepest basophilic layer. Superficial pustulation may be seen. Bacteria, dermatophytes, or yeast may be present in the superficial layer. Devitalized cells of the middle layer lack discrete borders and pallor is due to diffuse intracellular and intercellular edema. Secondary clefting through this devitalized layer occasionally is observed and may lead to erosion or ulceration. The subjacent layers of the epidermis are hyperplastic and thus have increased basophilic staining because of the increased nuclear to cytoplasmic ratio.

Dermal inflammation is mixed and is generally superficial and perivascular to interstitial. Neutrophils may be prominent, depending on the degree and stage of overlying epidermal degeneration. Macrophages, lymphocytes and plasma cells may be observed.

Differential diagnoses include zinc-responsive dermatosis, generic dog food dermatosis, and mucocutaneous candidiasis. Zinc-responsive dermatosis is differentiated from superficial necrolytic dermatitis by the lack of laminar epidermal edema and degeneration. If this histopathologic feature is absent, as occurs in chronic lesions of superficial necrolytic dermatitis, clinical differentiation may be required. Clinical differentiation between generic dog food dermatosis and superficial necrolytic dermatitis also may be required because both diseases are characterized by superficial epidermal necrolysis and edema, in addition to parakeratosis. Mucocutaneous candidiasis is histopathologically very similar; superficial necrolytic dermatitis with secondary yeast colonization may be indistinguishable from mucocutaneous candidiasis and may represent a partially overlapping syndrome (see Chapter 1).

CHEMICAL AND THERMAL BURNS
Clinical features (Figures 3-14 through 3-16)

Thermal and chemical burns are relatively common injuries in the dog and cat. Burns may be due to either thermal injury or the direct toxic action of a noxious substance on the skin or mucous membranes. Burns in domestic animals are categorized as partial thickness or full thickness based on the depth of involvement. Ther-

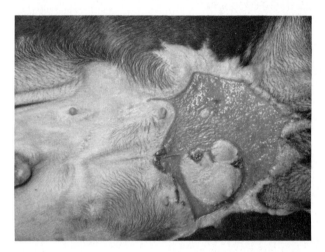

FIGURE 3-14. Thermal burn in a Doberman Pinscher puppy. Islands of less affected tissue are surrounded by ulceration.

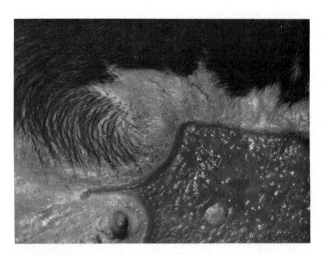

FIGURE 3-15. Closer view of puppy in Figure 3-14. Wound contraction is evident at the margins of the ulcer.

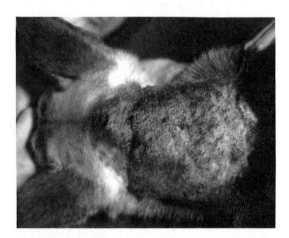

FIGURE 3-16. Chemical burn in a German Shepherd Dog caused by application of a nondiluted flea and tick dip. Punctate areas of ulceration are present on the swollen, erythematous affected area. The haircoat has been clipped from the lesion. *(From Ihrke PJ: Topical therapy: use, principals and vehicles, dermatologic therapy, Part I, Comp Cont Ed 1:31, 1980. Reprinted by permission.)*

mal burns are seen more frequently than chemical burns and often cause deeper injury. Partial-thickness thermal and chemical burns may be clinically indistinguishable unless residue of the chemical agent is present on the haircoat or underlying skin. Boiling water, electric heating pads, dog drying cages, and fires are the most common causes of thermal burns.

Since lesions may be hidden by the haircoat, burns may be more obvious in nonhaired areas. Progression of the burn beyond the initially observed site of damage may occur for several days after the presenting signs are noted. Well-demarcated erythema is the earliest clinical sign of a burn. Erosion and ulceration vary depending on the depth of injury. In full-thickness burns, the damaged skin becomes firm and dry because of avascular necrosis and eventually may slough. Bacterial infection from necrosis of tissue and impairment of local defense mechanisms is common. Life-threatening sepsis may be seen. Pain may be the initial presenting complaint. As expected, age, breed, or sex predilections have not been noted.

Clinical differential diagnoses include toxic epidermal necrolysis, erythema multiforme, pemphigus vulgaris, bullous pemphigoid, and vasculitis or other causes of ischemic necrosis, including physical trauma. Lack of progression of lesions after the initial 5 days is an important differentiating feature of burns, unless the insult is repetitive. Biologically abnormal patterns such as straight or angular borders, "drip" configura-tions, or unusual symmetry may increase the suspicion of burn.

Biopsy site selection

Areas of erythema without ulceration are preferred for skin biopsy, since they may be more diagnostic for burn trauma. Chronic or severe changes such as ulceration, deep necrosis, secondary inflammation, and scarring rarely yield a definitive diagnosis.

Histopathology (Figures 3-17 and 3-18)

Acute coagulation necrosis of the epidermis is present in mild early lesions. Milder trauma may be confined to the outer edges of a more severe burn. Spongiosis may be severe and leads to vesiculation. Erosion and ulceration are common in advanced lesions and are accompanied by crusts composed of exuded serum and neutrophils.

Thermal burns of partial thickness often produce necrosis of superficial follicular and adnexal epithelium and superficial dermal collagen. Dermal-epidermal separation may occur as cohesion is lost between nonviable tissues. Severe dermal inflammation, including large numbers of neutrophils, is the result of tissue damage and secondary bacterial infection. Subcutaneous vasculitis with thrombosis may be a sequela of burn trauma. Full-thickness burns, which are less common, result in complete dermal destruction and necrosis of the superficial panniculus.

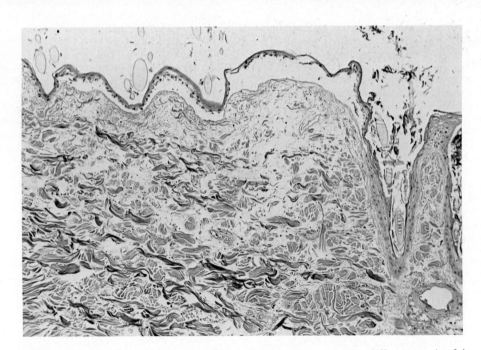

FIGURE 3-17. Partial-thickness thermal burn in a dog, demonstrating diffuse necrosis of the epidermis and superficial dermis. Note elevation of devitalized epidermis to form a subepidermal bulla. (×90.)

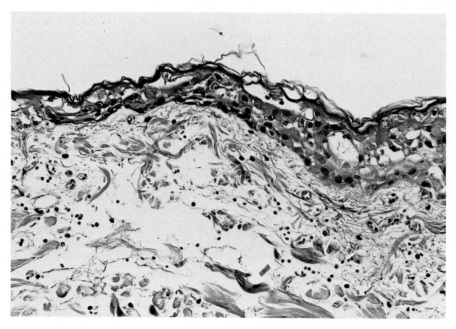

FIGURE 3-18. Diffuse necrosis and ballooning degeneration of the epidermis in a partial-thickness thermal burn from a dog. (×220.)

Toxic epidermal necrolysis is an important differential diagnosis if the burn is epidermally confined. Vasculitis is considered a differential diagnosis for deeper thermal burns that have vascular damage and inflammation. Historical and clinical information may be required to differentiate vasculitis from thermal burns.

SUGGESTED READINGS

Erythema multiforme

Elias PM and Fritsch PO: Erythema multiforme. In Fitzpatrick TB, Eisen AZ, Wolf K, and others, editors: Dermatology in general medicine, ed 3, New York, 1987, McGraw-Hill, pp 555-563.

Halliwell REW and Gorman NT: Veterinary clinical immunology, Philadelphia, 1989, WB Saunders, pp 378-382.

Hees J and others: Levamisole-induced drug eruptions in the dog, J Am Anim Hosp Assoc 21:255-260, 1985.

Lever WF and Schaumburg-Lever G: Histopathology of the skin, ed 7, Philadelphia, 1990, JB Lippincott, pp 135-138.

Mason KV: Fixed drug eruption in two dogs caused by diethylcarbamazine, J Am Anim Hosp Assoc 24:301-303, 1988.

McMurdy MA: A case resembling erythema multiforme major (Stevens-Johnson syndrome) in a dog, J Am Anim Hosp Assoc 26:297-300, 1990.

Medleau L and others: Trimethoprim-sulfonamide-associated drug eruptions in dogs, J Am Anim Hosp Assoc 26:305-311, 1990.

Scott DW, Miller WH, and Goldschmidt MH: Erythema multiforme in the dog, J Am Anim Hosp Assoc 19:453-459, 1983.

Toxic epidermal necrolysis

Fritsch PO and Elias PM: Toxic epidermal necrolysis. In Fitzpatrick TB, Eisen AZ, Wolf K, and others, editors: Dermatology in general medicine, ed 3, New York, 1987, McGraw-Hill, pp 563-567.

Lever WF and Schaumburg-Lever G: Histopathology of the skin, ed 7, Philadelphia, 1990, JB Lippincott, pp 135-138.

Scott DW and others: Toxic epidermal necrolysis in two dogs and a cat, J Am Anim Hosp Assoc 15:271-279, 1979.

Superficial necrolytic dermatitis

Gross TL and others: Glucagon-producing pancreatic endocrine tumors in two dogs with superficial necrolytic dermatitis. J Am Vet Med Assoc 197:1619-1622, 1990.

Lever WF and Schaumburg-Lever G: Histopathology of the skin, ed 7, Philadelphia, 1990, JB Lippincott, pp 211-212.

Miller WH and others: Necrolytic migratory erythema in dogs: a hepatocutaneous syndrome, J Am Anim Hosp Assoc 26:573-581, 1990.

Muller GH, Kirk RW, and Scott DW: Small animal dermatology, ed 4, Philadelphia, 1989, WB Saunders, pp 639-641.

Turnwald GH and others: Failure to document hyperglucagonemia in a dog with diabetic dermatopathy resembling necrolytic migratory erythema, J Am Anim Hosp Assoc 25:363-369, 1989.

Walton DK and others: Ulcerative dermatosis associated with diabetes mellitus in the dog: a report of four cases, J Am Anim Hosp Assoc 22:79-88, 1986.

Chemical and thermal burns

Fox SM: Management of thermal burns. I, Comp Cont Ed 7:631-632, 1985.

McKeever PJ: Thermal injuries. In Kirk RW, editor: Current veterinary therapy VII, Philadelphia, 1980, WB Saunders, pp 191-194.

Swaim SF and others: Heating pads and thermal burns in small animals, J Am Anim Hosp Assoc 25:156-162, 1989.

Spongiotic diseases of the epidermis

Spongiotic dermatitis is characterized by the accumulation of edema in the intercellular spaces of the epidermis. Severe spongiosis may lead to breakdown in the integrity of the epidermal architecture, resulting in vesiculation. Generally, inflammatory cell influx accompanies the spongiotic changes. Spongiotic foci usually eventuate in focal parakeratosis.

Many diseases, not described in this chapter, are characterized by mild spongiosis. Allergic skin diseases, for example, produce multifocal spongiosis. The diseases included in this chapter are those in which spongiosis is characteristically a significant and predominant feature. Not all stages of these diseases will show spongiosis; obtaining the earliest lesions possible is critical to the diagnosis.

ALLERGIC CONTACT DERMATITIS
Clinical features (Figures 4-1 and 4-2)

Allergic contact dermatitis is an uncommon skin disease seen in dogs and cats caused by a type IV, or delayed, hypersensitivity reaction. The syndrome occurs in previously sensitized dogs or cats and is initiated by a nonirritating concentration of the offending substance. Historically, offending substances often have been present in the environment for greater than 2 years! Conversely, sensitization may occur in as short a period as 1 month.

Erythema, papules, and vesicles, sometimes with exudation, rapidly eventuate in crusted lesions. If exposure is limited, healing occurs. Lichenification, hyperpigmentation, alopecia, and gradual expansion of the lesions result from chronic exposure. Lesions are seen primarily in hairless or relatively hairless body regions, since the haircoat is normally protective against most contactants (except liquids and aerosols). The most commonly involved sites include the ventral interdigital webs, groin, axillae, genitalia, muzzle, ears, and perineum. Pruritus is variable in intensity but usually is present. Positive patch tests may be more papular and vesicular than typical clinical lesions, since very early lesions are rarely seen in clinical cases.

In a Danish study, Thomsen (1986) reported that the German Shepherd Dog is at increased risk. Walton has reported that the yellow Labrador Retriever is at increased risk in the United Kingdom. Allergic contact dermatitis usually is seen in adult animals. Sex predilection has not been noted.

Irritant contact dermatitis is the primary clinical differential diagnosis for allergic contact dermatitis. Clinical signs compatible with contact dermatitis in a single animal within a multiple animal household favor allergic over irritant contact dermatitis.

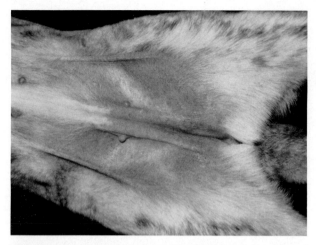

FIGURE 4-1. Allergic contact dermatitis in a mixed-breed dog caused by cedar chip bedding. The nonhaired area of the ventral abdomen is diffusely erythematous. Lesions do not extend into haired areas. *(From Ihrke PJ: Topical therapy, use, principals and vehicles, dermatologic therapy, Part I, Comp Cont Ed 1:33, 1980. Reprinted by permission.)*

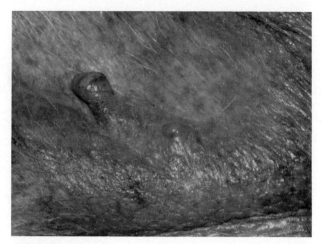

FIGURE 4-2. Closer view of the dog in Fig. 4-1. Small papules are seen against a background of diffusely erythematous, exudative skin.

Allergic contact dermatitis frequently is more papular than irritant contact dermatitis and is more likely to be chronic. Atopy and food allergy also may resemble allergic contact dermatitis clinically. Lesions of contact dermatitis in glabrous skin may subside strikingly at the junction with haired skin, in contrast to other allergic diseases.

Biopsy site selection

Erythematous macules or papules represent early stages of the disease, and if present, they should be sampled for biopsy. These early or acute lesions should be chosen over chronic lesions, characterized by hyperpigmentation and lichenification, which are not diagnostic histopathologically. Lesions with severe self-trauma also should be avoided. The most diagnostic specimens for histopathology may be obtained from positive patch tests at 24 to 48 hours.

Histopathology (Figures 4-3 and 4-4)

Acute lesions are best exemplified by biopsy from positive patch tests at 24 to 48 hours. Multifocal spongiosis may progress to vesiculation and is usually accompanied by exocytosis of inflammatory cells. Lymphocytic exocytosis was reported by Kunkle in a patch test reaction from a dog with allergic contact dermatitis to *Tradescantia fluminensis*. Thomsen (1989) reported epidermal necrosis and neutrophilic exocytosis in patch test reactions in dogs using a standardized series of European contact allergens, mostly inorganic in nature. Spongiosis and intraepidermal inflammation evolve to superficial crusts with parakeratosis.

Most biopsy specimens are obtained from areas of chronic inflammation and self-trauma. In these cases, the epidermis is characterized by acanthosis with usually mild spongiosis and secondary impetiginization caused by self-trauma, as seen in chronic hyperplastic dermatitis caused by allergic skin diseases (see Chapter 6). Dermal inflammation consists of superficial perivascular lymphocytic and histiocytic infiltrates with variable, usually minimal, eosinophils (see Chapter 8).

Histopathologic lesions of allergic contact dermatitis may be indistinguishable from those of irritant contact dermatitis, particularly in more advanced lesions. Lymphocytic exocytosis may be a more prominent feature of allergic contact dermatitis, especially in early lesions, compared to prominent neutrophilic infiltration in early irritant contact dermatitis. Necrosis of the epidermis is generally not a feature of allergic contact dermatitis, but may be found in severe cases of acute irritant contact dermatitis. Chronic allergic contact dermatitis mimics chronic dermatitis of any cause.

IRRITANT CONTACT DERMATITIS
Clinical features (Figures 4-5 and 4-6)

Irritant contact dermatitis is an uncommon inflammatory skin disease seen in dogs and cats caused by direct contact with an irritating concentration of an offending substance. Immune mechanisms are not involved. The irritating substance damages the skin by direct toxic action. Causes include corrosive substances such as strong acids and alkalis, as well as less potent irritants such as soaps, detergents, solvents, and various other chemicals. Moisture, which decreases the normal skin barrier function and increases the effective contact area by allowing diffusion of the irritant, will predispose to irritant-induced skin damage. Previously exist-

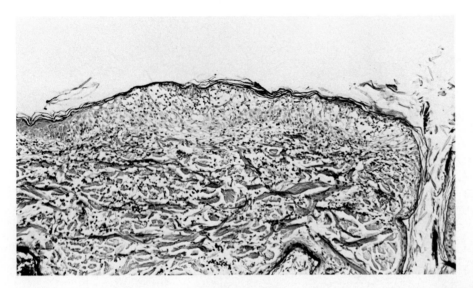

FIGURE 4-3. Allergic contact dermatitis in a dog (positive patch test at 48 hours). Locally extensive spongiosis is accompanied by exocytosis of mononuclear cells. (×105.)

FIGURE 4-4. Higher magnification of the epidermis shown in Fig. 4-3. Severe spongiosis is progressing to vesiculation. Note the exocytosis of mononuclear cells. (×250.)

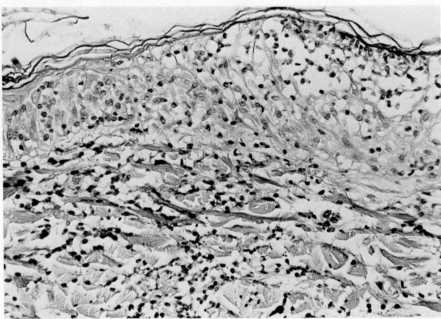

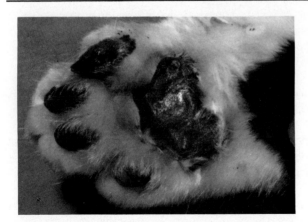

FIGURE 4-5. Irritant contact dermatitis on the footpad of a cat. The pads are diffusely swollen and multifocally eroded.

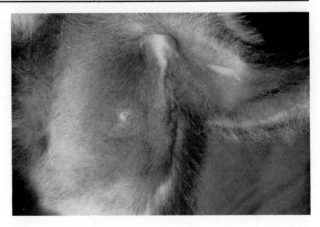

FIGURE 4-6. Irritant contact dermatitis in a Siamese cat after accidental emersion in motor oil. The affected axilla is alopecic, hyperpigmented, and lichenified.

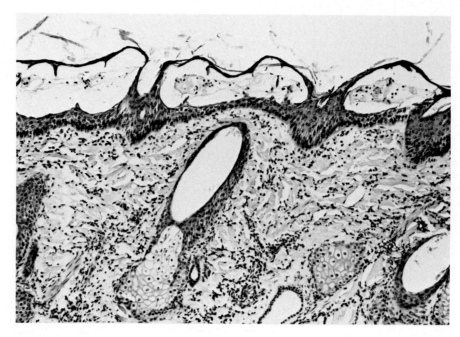

FIGURE 4-7. Irritant contact dermatitis in a dog. Acute vesiculation of the superficial epidermis. (×90.)

ing inflammatory skin diseases will increase susceptibility to irritant contact dermatitis. Contact time, concentration, and the total dose of the agent are additional determinative factors.

Clinical signs and affected sites are virtually identical to allergic contact dermatitis (see preceding discussion). Acute irritant contact dermatitis may be less vesicular and papular than allergic contact dermatitis. Pain may be more common and pruritus may be less common with irritant contact dermatitis. Irritant contact dermatitis is less likely to be chronic, since identification and elimination of the offending substance may be accomplished more readily. Breed, age, or sex predilections have not been noted and would not be expected.

Allergic contact dermatitis is the primary clinical differential diagnosis. In most circumstances, the lesions of irritant contact dermatitis are clinically indistinguishable from allergic contact dermatitis. Single episodes are more common with irritant contact dermatitis, since the cause is more readily determined than in allergic contact dermatitis. Clinical signs compatible with contact dermatitis in multiple animals in the same environment favor irritant rather than allergic contact dermatitis. Chronic irritant contact dermatitis also can mimic many other chronic dermatoses, since the grossly visible chronic reaction patterns of the skin are limited.

Biopsy site selection

See the preceding discussion on allergic contact dermatitis.

Histopathology (Figure 4-7)

Acute irritant contact dermatitis rarely is seen histopathologically and has not been well documented in dogs and cats. In humans, acute epidermal lesions of irritant contact dermatitis consist of spongiosis and intracellular edema, leading to spongiotic vesiculation and reticular degeneration. Epidermal necrosis may develop. Neutrophils may be prominent in lesions of acute irritant contact dermatitis and may accumulate in the damaged epidermis. Thomsen (1989) described a similar histopathologic appearance for allergic contact dermatitis in dogs (see preceding discussion).

Acute irritant contact dermatitis is transient. Consequently, lesions of chronic irritant contact dermatitis may be more commonly presented to the pathologist. Unfortunately, these lesions are not specifically diagnostic and consist of acanthosis, parakeratosis, and crusting. Mild superficial perivascular infiltrations of lymphocytes and macrophages are seen.

Histopathologically, lesions may be indistinguishable from allergic contact dermatitis, particularly in more advanced lesions. Neutrophils may be more prominent in early lesions of irritant contact dermatitis, compared to lymphocytes in allergic contact dermatitis.

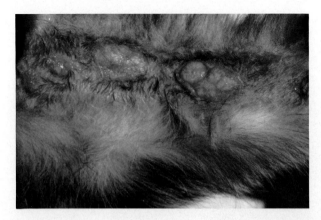

FIGURE 4-8. Feline eosinophilic plaques on the hindlimb of a cat. Individual plaques are raised, well-demarcated, alopecic, eroded, and intensely erythematous. Larger plaques show the partial contours of lesions that have coalesced.

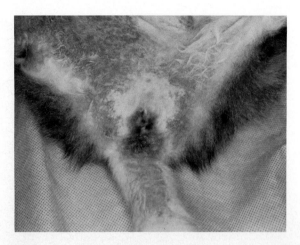

FIGURE 4-9. Multiple eosinophilic plaques on the ventral abdomen and tail of a cat. (*Courtesy BA Atlee, Davis, California; case material from the University of California, Davis.*)

Epidermal necrosis may be a feature of severe irritant reactions, but is rarely seen in allergic contact dermatitis. Chronic irritant contact dermatitis mimics chronic dermatitis of any cause.

FELINE EOSINOPHILIC PLAQUE
Clinical features (Figures 4-8 and 4-9)

Feline eosinophilic plaque is a common, highly pruritic skin disorder of cats. An underlying allergic hypersensitivity is suspected frequently but less commonly documented. Flea allergy dermatitis, atopy, and food allergy have all been seen in conjunction with eosinophilic plaques. In addition, feline eosinophilic plaques have responded to flea control, hyposensitization, and elimination diets.

Raised, well-demarcated, intensely erythematous, round to oval, eroded or ulcerated, oozing, alopecic plaques are noted most commonly on the abdomen and medial thighs. Plaques vary between 0.5 and 5 cm in diameter, may be single or multiple, and may coalesce. Constant licking of the affected area is a common feature and indicates the severity of pruritus. Regional lymphadenopathy usually is present.

Age or breed predilections have not been reported. According to Scott, females may be at increased risk.

Clinical differential diagnoses should include neoplasms such as mast cell tumor, metastatic mammary adenocarcinoma, and malignant lymphoma. Since malignant tumors may closely mimic eosinophilic plaques, skin biopsy is always indicated.

Biopsy site selection

Ulcers and severely crusted lesions should be avoided. Erythematous plaques with minimal erosive or exudative changes are ideal specimens for biopsy. If multiple lesions are present, the clinician should select a site that may be less readily traumatized by the cat after surgery.

Histopathology (Figures 4-10 and 4-11)

Epidermal changes consist of severe acanthosis and variable spongiosis with eosinophilic exocytosis. Spongiosis may be mild to severe, is diffuse in distribution, and often involves follicular infundibula. An unusual and striking variation is the presence of severe epidermal and follicular mucinosis. Spaces between epidermal and follicular epithelial cells become widened by deposition of pale gray or gray-blue mucin, often to the point of vesiculation. Severe secondary erosion or ulceration may be found in advanced lesions. Dermal inflammation consists of variably intense, usually diffuse, infiltrations of eosinophils that extend to the middle (follicular) dermis, but also may reach the superficial panniculus (see Chapter 13).

Overall, the histopathologic features of eosinophilic plaque are qualitatively similar to those of allergic miliary dermatitis, but are more dramatic and less focal. Since eosinophilic plaque and miliary dermatitis both may be manifestations of allergic skin disease in the cat (and can exist concurrently), histopathologic separation of severe lesions of miliary dermatitis from lesions of eosinophilic plaque may not be critical diagnostically. The depth of eosinophilic inflammation seen in some eosinophilic plaques may resemble nonmiliary lesions of feline food allergy, as well as lesions of feline mosquito bite hypersensitivity; however, the diffuse spongiosis of typical eosinophilic plaque is not observed. In addition, foci of collagen degeneration, not seen in eosinophilic plaque, may be present in lesions of mosquito bite hypersensitivity (see Chapter 13).

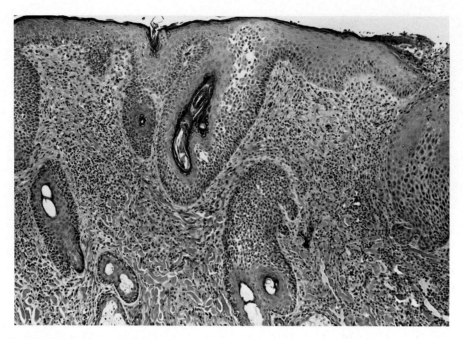

FIGURE 4-10. Feline eosinophilic plaque. Marked acanthosis is accompanied by spongiosis; superficial hair follicles also are affected. (×90.)

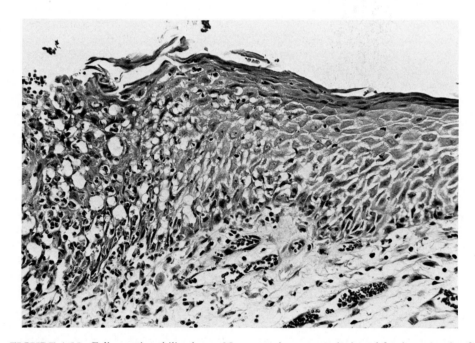

FIGURE 4-11. Feline eosinophilic plaque. Note prominent spongiosis and focal exocytosis of eosinophils. (×220.)

SUGGESTED READINGS

Allergic contact dermatitis

Belsito DV: Pathophysiology of allergic contact dermatitis. In Soter NA and Baden HP, editors: Pathophysiology of dermatologic diseases, New York, 1991, McGraw-Hill, pp 159-168.

Grant DI and Thoday KL: Canine allergic contact dermatitis: a clinical review, J Small Anim Pract 21:17-27, 1980.

Kunkle GA and Gross TL: Allergic contact dermatitis to *Tradescantia fluminensis* (wandering Jew) in a dog, Comp Cont Ed 5:925-930, 1983.

Krawiec DR and Gaafar SM: A comparative study of allergic and primary irritant contact dermatitis with DNCB in dogs, J Invest Dermatol 65:248-251, 1975.

Lever WF and Schaumburg-Lever G: Histopathology of the skin, ed 7, Philadelphia, 1990, JB Lippincott, pp 106-110.

Muller GH: Contact dermatitis in animals, Arch Dermatol 96:425-432, 1967.

Muller GH, Kirk RW, and Scott DW: Small animal dermatology, ed 4, Philadelphia, 1989, WB Saunders, pp 464-470.

Reedy LM and Miller WH: Allergic skin diseases of dogs and cats, Philadelphia, 1989, WB Saunders, pp 159-169.

Thomsen MK and Kristensen F: Contact dermatitis in the dog, Nord Vet Med 38:129-147, 1986.

Thomsen MK and Thomsen HK: Histopathological changes in canine allergic contact dermatitis patch test reaction, Acta Vet Scand 30:379-384, 1989.

Walton GS: Allergic contact dermatitis. In Kirk RW, editor: Current veterinary therapy VI, Philadelphia, 1977, WB Saunders, pp 571-575.

Irritant contact dermatitis

Fadok VA: Irritant contact dermatitis. In Kirk RW, editor: Current veterinary therapy VIII, Philadelphia, 1983, WB Saunders, pp 476-480.

Krawiec DR and Gaafar SM: A comparative study of allergic and primary irritant contact dermatitis with DNCB in dogs, J Invest Dermatol 65:248-251, 1975.

Lever WF and Schaumburg-Lever G: Histopathology of the skin, ed 7, Philadelphia, 1990, JB Lippincott, pp 106-110.

Muller GH, Kirk RW, and Scott DW: Small animal dermatology, ed 4, Philadelphia, 1989, WB Saunders, pp 771-774.

Feline eosinophilic plaque

Gross TL, Kwochka KW, and Kunkle GA: Correlation of histologic and immunologic findings in cats with miliary dermatitis, J Am Vet Med Assoc 189:1322-1325, 1986.

Muller GH, Kirk RW, and Scott DW: Small animal dermatology, ed 4, Philadelphia, 1989, WB Saunders, 563.

Scott DW: Observations on the eosinophilic granuloma complex in cats, J Am Anim Hosp Assoc 11:261-270, 1975.

CHAPTER 5

Exudative and ulcerative diseases of the epidermis

Exudative dermatitis is characterized by the accumulation of inflammatory cells on the surface of the epidermis, leading to the formation of crusts (inflammatory exudate). Crusting may be primary, as in nontraumatized lesions of miliary dermatitis in which allergy-induced migration of neutrophils and eosinophils results in their accumulation and degeneration on the epidermal surface. Ulcerative dermatitis is a primary feature of skin diseases characterized by prominent self-trauma, such as pyotraumatic dermatitis. These ulcerative diseases also are exudative; self-trauma leads to erosion or ulceration, which induces subsequent surface migration of inflammatory cells, usually neutrophils.

Many skin diseases are characterized by some crusting and epidermal damage, particularly allergic skin diseases that may produce erosion and crusting through self-trauma from pruritus. Any disease characterized by surface pustulation, such as superficial pyoderma or pemphigus foliaceus, also can lead to crusting as pustules degenerate. The diseases in this chapter include those for which epidermal exudation and crusting are considered primary events; this chapter also include diseases in which self-traumatic ulceration and exudation are the predominant pathologic processes occurring in the skin.

PYOTRAUMATIC DERMATITIS (Synonyms: acute moist dermatitis, "hot spot")

Clinical features (Figures 5-1 and 5-2)

Pyotraumatic dermatitis is a self-induced traumatic skin disease that is seen commonly in the dog and rarely in the cat. It is believed to be initiated by a vicious itch-scratch cycle secondary to underlying pruritic (especially allergic) skin disease. The characteristic lesions appear to result from licking, chewing, and scratching. Confusingly, extreme self-trauma in some dogs will not initiate pyotraumatic dermatitis, whereas surprisingly minimal self-trauma will cause this condition in other dogs. Most canine pyotraumatic dermatitis is seen secondary to flea allergy dermatitis. In cats, lesions similar to the canine disease clinically and histopathologically have been seen secondary to flea allergy dermatitis, especially in the dorsal lumbosacral region. Other allergic skin diseases, otitis externa, and anal sacculitis occasionally have been implicated in dogs. Pyotraumatic dermatitis also may be seen secondary to deep pyoderma in some breeds. (See deep bacterial folliculitis and furunculosis in Chapter 16.)

The clinically characteristic lesion is a rapidly developing, self-traumatized, erythematous, exudative, alopecic, sharply demarcated, slightly elevated plaque. Erosion and ulceration occur, and adherent, viscid debris mats the surrounding hair. Lesions are

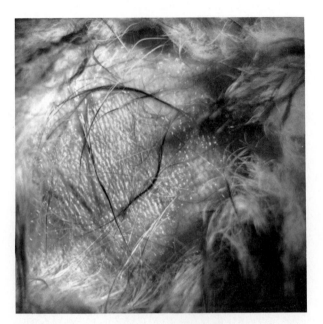

FIGURE 5-1. Pyotraumatic dermatitis in a German Shepherd Dog secondary to flea allergy dermatitis. The well-demarcated lesion is erythematous, swollen, and alopecic.

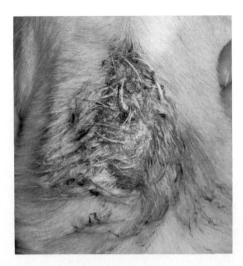

FIGURE 5-2. Pyotraumatic dermatitis on the ventral neck of a German Shepherd Dog. Hair from the periphery is matted in the dried exudate.

rapidly progressive and may coalesce. Since the lesions of pyotraumatic dermatitis usually are associated with flea allergy dermatitis, most lesions are seen primarily in the dorsal lumbosacral region and on the lateral thighs. Lesions also may be seen near the ears or anal sacs. Pain or pruritus is a consistent feature.

Canine breed predilections have been noted for large, dense-coated breeds such as the German Shepherd Dog, Golden Retriever, Labrador Retriever, Collie, and the Saint Bernard. Pyotraumatic dermatitis also is seen secondary to focal deep pyoderma in breeds such as the Golden Retriever and the Saint Bernard. Age or sex predilections have not been noted. A marked seasonality is recognized; pyotraumatic dermatitis is seen most frequently in warm, humid weather.

Pyotraumatic dermatitis is visually distinctive and differential diagnoses are few. The clinician may need to search carefully for underlying diseases, since early neoplasms (sweat gland adenocarcinoma) or bacterial infections may resemble or initiate pyotraumatic dermatitis.

Biopsy site selection

Skin biopsy commonly is not employed to obtain a diagnosis. However, skin biopsy should be performed in recurrent or chronic cases or when neoplasia or underlying deep pyoderma is suspected. Newer lesions, preferably with intact epithelium, should be sampled in these cases. If deep pyoderma is suspected, then periph-

eral, small, exudative lesions are most likely to yield diagnostic results.

Histopathology (Figures 5-3 and 5-4)

Epidermal lesions predominate and consist of severe erosion to ulceration and exudation. Superficial crusts contain degenerating neutrophils and serum, in addition to necrotic epidermal debris. Colonization of crusts by gram-positive cocci is common. Lesions are usually sharply demarcated from the adjacent epidermis, which may be spongiotic. Epidermal borders may have mild to moderate acanthosis in chronic lesions.

Necrosis may extend into the superficial dermis in severe cases. The dermis often contains mild to moderate neutrophilic inflammation and edema confined to the base of the erosion or ulcer. Pyotraumatic dermatitis occurring in conjunction with deep follicular inflammation will have evidence of folliculitis or furunculosis (see Chapter 16).

Differential diagnoses are few because the lesions are distinctive. In cats, idiopathic ulcerative dermatosis may appear similar histopathologically.

FELINE ALLERGIC MILIARY DERMATITIS (Synonym: miliary dermatitis)
Clinical features (Figures 5-5 and 5-6)

Miliary dermatitis is a multifactorial clinical cutaneous reaction pattern seen in cats. Most miliary dermatitis is due to cutaneous hypersensitivity and therefore may be termed *allergic miliary dermatitis*. Ectoparasitic, inhalant, food, and drug hypersensitivities have been documented. In locales where fleas are common, miliary

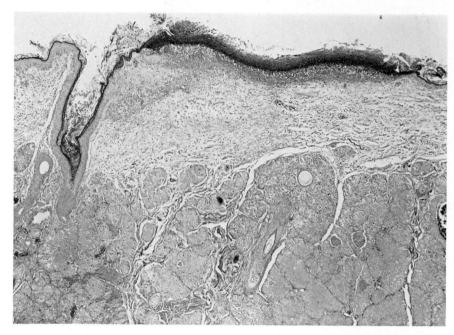

FIGURE 5-3. Pyotraumatic dermatitis in perianal skin of a dog. A large discrete ulcer is covered by a prominent serocellular crust. Note subjacent large perianal glands. (×40.)

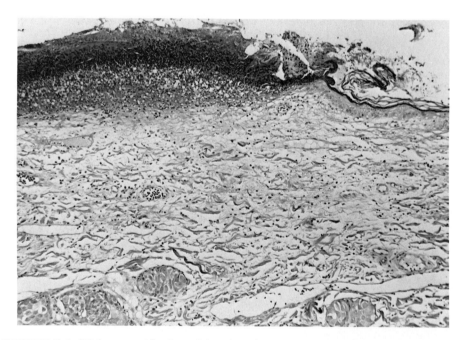

FIGURE 5-4. Higher magnification of the ulcer shown in Fig. 5-3. Note the sharp line of demarcation from the intact epidermis. (×90.)

dermatitis should be considered the result of hypersensitivity to fleas until proven otherwise. Other parasitic infestations inducing allergic miliary dermatitis include cheyletiellosis, otodectic acariasis, trombiculidiasis, and pediculosis. Visually similar skin lesions are seen uncommonly in conjunction with dermatophytosis or staphylococcal folliculitis.

Feline allergic miliary dermatitis is more often palpable rather than visible in cats with intact haircoats. Multiple, discrete, erythematous papules with adherent

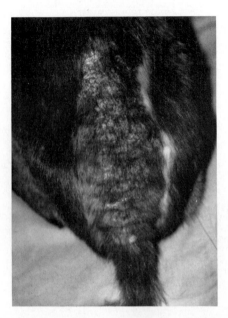

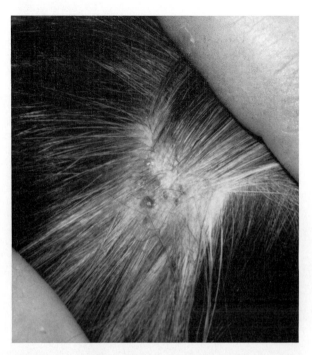

FIGURE 5-5. Severe feline allergic miliary dermatitis. Hair has been clipped from the dorsal lumbar sacral area to show multiple, confluent erythematous crusted papules.

FIGURE 5-6. Feline allergic miliary dermatitis. Grouped, erythematous, crusted papules on the back of the neck.

brownish crust are present. The crusted papule seen in feline allergic miliary dermatitis is a primary lesion and not the result of self-trauma. Pruritus is variable but usually present in all but the mildest cases. Pruritus with attendant self-trauma leads to excoriation, and increased erythema and crusting. Self-traumatic alopecia is seen in severe cases and results in increased visibility of miliary lesions.

Localization of lesions to the neck, dorsum, or tail base is noted in cats with flea allergy dermatitis. Lesions may be generalized in severe cases. Facial miliary dermatitis may be the initial or only sign of food hypersensitivity.

Breed, age, or sex predilections have not been noted. Clinical differential diagnoses include the rare, nonallergic causes of miliary dermatitis such as dermatophyte and bacterial infections.

Biopsy site selection

Nontraumatized, recently erupted, crusted papules are ideal for biopsy. If pruritus is extreme, special care should be taken to avoid traumatized lesions. If lesions are present between the shoulder blades, this site is recommended for biopsy, since self-trauma is not readily accomplished in this location.

Histopathology (Figures 5-7 through 5-9)

Primary epidermal lesions consist of discrete foci of superficial serocellular crusting, accompanied by focal spongiosis. Small accumulations of neutrophils and eosinophils are seen within the epidermis beneath the crusts. The affected epidermis may be focally necrotic underneath the crust and have a brightly eosinophilic, coagulated appearance. Occasionally, marked epidermal vesiculation with eosinophilic exocytosis (eosinophilic vesiculopustulation) is seen. Mild to moderate acanthosis and mild spongiosis of the adjacent epidermis and hair follicles may be present. Secondary focal erosion or ulceration is seen and presumptively is due to self-trauma. More severe lesions may exhibit extensive spongiosis and broader foci of erosion and ulceration. Dermal inflammation is superficial to middermal and perivascular to interstitial and consists predominantly of eosinophils and mast cells (see Chapter 8).

Severely spongiotic and eroded or ulcerated lesions of allergic miliary dermatitis may resemble those of eosinophilic plaque. Since eosinophilic plaque and miliary dermatitis both may be manifestations of allergic skin disease in the cat (and can exist concurrently), histopathologic separation of severe lesions of miliary dermatitis from lesions of eosinophilic plaque may not be critical diagnostically. Pemphigus foliaceus also may have prominent crusting, but free keratinocytes (acantholytic cells) should be visible in crusts and are absent in lesions of miliary dermatitis.

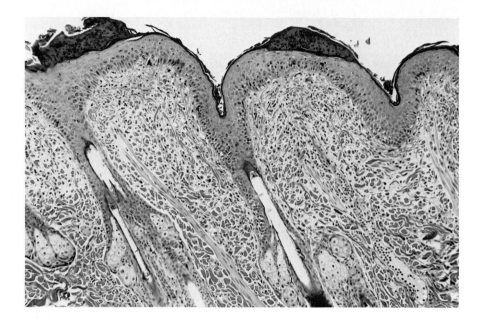

FIGURE 5-7. Feline allergic miliary dermatitis. Moderately acanthotic epidermis is covered by discrete serocellular crusts. (×90.)

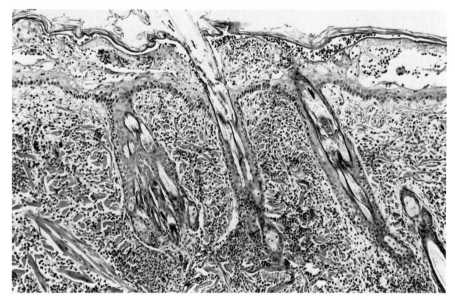

FIGURE 5-8. Marked eosinophilic vesicopustulation in a severe lesion of allergic miliary dermatitis. (×90.)

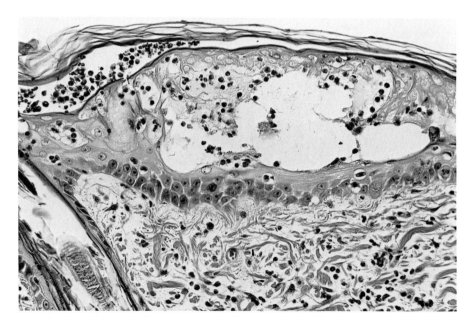

FIGURE 5-9. Higher magnification of eosinophilic vesicopustule in Figure 5-8. (×220.)

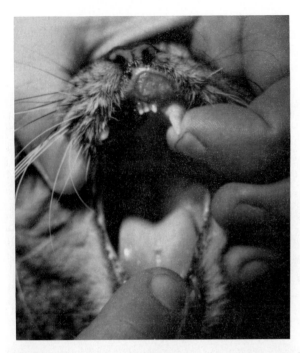

FIGURE 5-10. Feline indolent ulcer. A well-demarcated, dish-like ulcer with an elevated margin is present at the mucocutaneous junction of the upper lip just lateral to the philtrum.

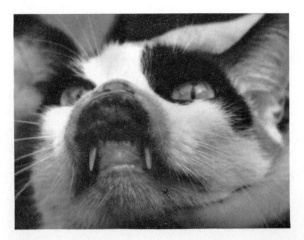

FIGURE 5-11. Severe feline indolent ulcer. The lesion resulted from bilateral indolent ulcers becoming confluent to involve most of the upper lip.

FELINE INDOLENT ULCER (Synonyms: feline eosinophilic ulcer, rodent ulcer)

Clinical features (Figures 5-10 and 5-11)

Feline indolent ulcer is a common feline syndrome or reaction pattern of uncertain etiology. An underlying allergic hypersensitivity is suspected frequently but less commonly documented. Flea allergy dermatitis, atopy, and food allergy have been seen in conjunction with feline indolent ulcer. Furthermore, feline indolent ulcers have responded to flea control, hyposensitization, and elimination diets. Feline indolent ulcers have been shown to commonly coexist with feline eosinophilic granuloma in a closed, inbred colony of cats studied by Power. These cats had not had exposure to fleas or other ectoparasites and could not be documented as having atopy or food allergy as determined by intradermal skin testing and elimination diets.

Well-demarcated dishlike ulcers with an elevated margin develop from focal areas of intense erythema. The elevated margins are firm and have an orange-tan color, whereas the central ulcerated area is granular and whitish-yellow. Lesions vary in size from 2 mm to 5 cm. The most common site is the juncture of the skin and mucous membrane of the upper lip apposing the lower canine tooth, just lateral to the philtrum. Lesions usually are solitary and unilateral, but may be bilateral and occasionally become confluent to involve most of the upper lip. Rarely, similar lesions may develop at other sites. The lesions are asymptomatic, although regional lymphadenopathy may be present. Malignant transformation to squamous cell carcinoma has been noted by Muller, Kirk, and Scott, but the authors have not observed this phenomenon.

Breed or age predilections have not been reported. Scott reports that females may be at increased risk.

Although indolent ulcers are visually distinctive, clinical differential diagnoses should include neoplasms such as squamous cell carcinoma or mast cell tumor, as well as ulcers associated with underlying infectious granulomas. Since malignant tumors or infectious granulomas may mimic indolent ulcers, skin biopsy always is indicated.

Biopsy site selection

Wedge biopsy or deep punch biopsy is recommended so that the specimen will include deeper dermal tissue beneath the ulcer. General anesthesia usually is advisable, since hemostasis may be a problem.

Histopathology (Figures 5-12 and 5-13)

Sequential sampling of feline indolent ulcers* shows variation in the histopathologic appearance over time. Acute lesions (48 to 96 hours) show moderate to severe ulceration with minimal underlying necrosis. Chronic lesions exhibit severe ulceration of the epidermis or mucosa, as well as deep and cavitating necrosis

* Case material from Power HT: Santa Cruz, California, 1990.

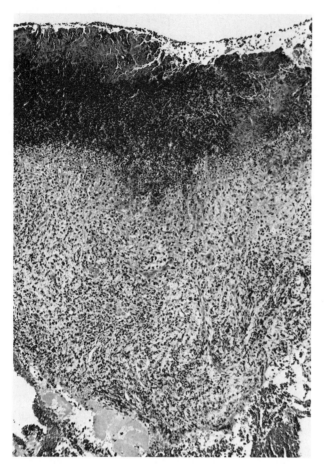

FIGURE 5-12. Feline indolent ulcer. Severe exudation, ulceration, and necrosis overlie deep inflammation. (×90.)

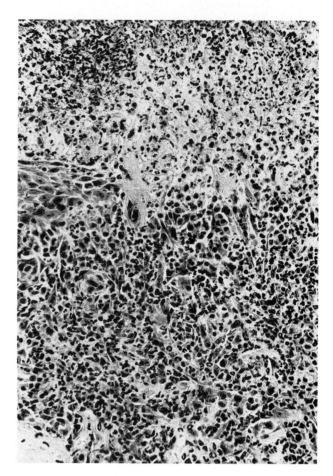

FIGURE 5-13. Higher magnification of indolent ulcer demonstrating prominent eosinophilic inflammation. (×220.)

of the underlying tissue. These deep foci of necrosis contain masses of degenerating eosinophils and neutrophils and are embedded superficially with colonies of bacteria. The intact epidermis is hyperplastic at all stages and may be spongiotic.

Acute indolent ulcer contains predominantly eosinophils, mast cells, and macrophages. Neutrophils are seen acutely and remain at all stages in concert with ulceration. Eosinophils and macrophages persist as the lesion ages, and plasma cells and lymphocytes, frequently in nodular clusters, first become evident at 5 to 7 days. Lesions of several months' duration may contain predominantly eosinophils and macrophages; plasma cells and lymphocytes are variable. Fibrovascular tissue proliferates as the lesion ages, and capillaries are prominent among inflammatory cells. Mature fibrous connective tissue is conspicuous in lesions of 4 to 6 months' duration. Inflammation extends deeply at all stages of indolent ulcer and often involves the muscle of the lip. Acutely affected muscle fibers may be swollen and nuclei pyknotic or fragmented.

Eosinophil degranulation and collagen degeneration may be a feature of indolent ulcer, similar to eosinophilic granuloma. This change is most prominent in early lesions and is generally mild and focal. Multinucleated giant cells may direct the eye to small foci of collagen degeneration not detected at first perusal. According to Power, clinically typical indolent ulcers (ulcers that affect the lip just lateral to the philtrum) do not show prominent eosinophilic degranulation and collagen degeneration; this is in contrast to lesions from the commissural area of the lip or lower lip (sites of eosinophilic granuloma). The significance of this variation is not known; both eosinophilic granuloma and indolent ulcer may represent variation of a common eosinophilic disorder in cats.

Other differential diagnoses to consider include mosquito bite hypersensitivity, deeply inflamed lesions of food allergy, or deeply inflamed eosinophilic plaque. Knowledge of localization to the upper lip allows differentiation; indolent ulcer also will have more severe ulceration and necrosis of the underlying dermis.

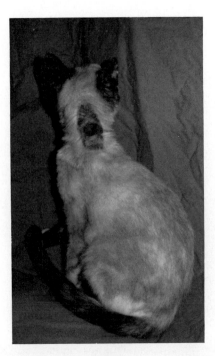

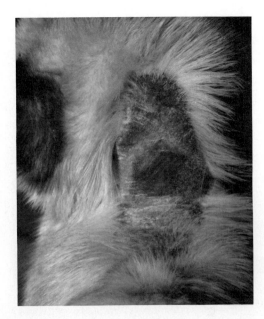

FIGURE 5-15. Closer view of the cat in Fig. 5-14. The lesion is alopecic, erythematous, and crusted.

FIGURE 5-14. Feline idiopathic ulcerative dermatosis in a kitten. An oval, well-demarcated ulcer developed rapidly between the shoulder blades.

FELINE IDIOPATHIC ULCERATIVE DERMATOSIS (Synonym: chronic ulcerative dermatosis with linear subepidermal fibrosis)

Clinical features (Figures 5-14 and 5-15)

Feline idiopathic ulcerative dermatosis is an uncommon syndrome of unknown etiology. A hypersensitivity reaction to subcutaneously injected vaccines or medications has been a proposed cause because of the frequent localization of the lesion between the scapulae or on the caudal neck (popular injection sites in the cat). However, the syndrome has been seen in cats that apparently have never received injections at these sites. Future investigation may reveal multiple causes.

A focal, alopecic, well-demarcated ulcer develops. Adherent necrotic debris covers the ulcer and mats remaining or adjacent hair. Peripheral swelling or erythema is mild. Chronic lesions may have a firm and elevated border. Lesions usually are solitary. The site is highly characteristic; the lesions are seen almost exclusively on the thoracic midline between the scapulae or on the caudal neck. The lesion may be painful. Regional lymphadenopathy is noted occasionally, but systemic signs are not present.

Breed or sex predilections have not been noted. According to Scott, the syndrome may be more common in cats less than 1 year of age.

Clinical differential diagnoses for idiopathic ulcerative dermatosis are few, since this syndrome is visually distinctive. A thermal or chemical burn at this site might appear similar. Because the etiology of this syndrome has not been demonstrated conclusively, the clinician and pathologist should investigate cases of this syndrome further in an attempt to elucidate the underlying cause or causes.

Biopsy site selection

Wedge biopsy is preferred over punch biopsy, since specimens obtained from the margins of ulcers will include both the ulcer and adjacent skin. Subcutaneous tissue should be included, since a reaction to vaccine or other subcutaneously injected medications has been hypothesized.

Histopathology (Figures 5-16 and 5-17)

The epidermis is extensively ulcerated and necrosis of the superficial dermis is seen. The intact epidermis at the borders of the ulcer is acanthotic. The necrotic dermis may have a coagulated appearance and the ulcer bed often contains a layer of devitalized epidermal or superficial dermal tissue embedded with degenerating neutrophils. Characteristically, the adjacent and subjacent viable dermis is uninflamed. Mild numbers of neutrophils, occasional eosinophils, and a few mixed mononuclear cells may be present. According to Scott, older lesions (of at least 6 months' duration) have variable and occasionally severe superficial laminar dermal

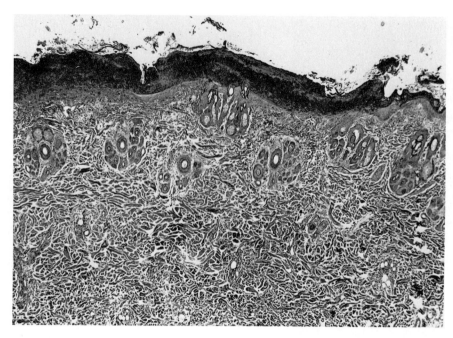

FIGURE 5-16. Feline idiopathic ulcerative dermatosis. Extensive ulceration is accompanied by prominent superficial exudate (crust). (×40.)

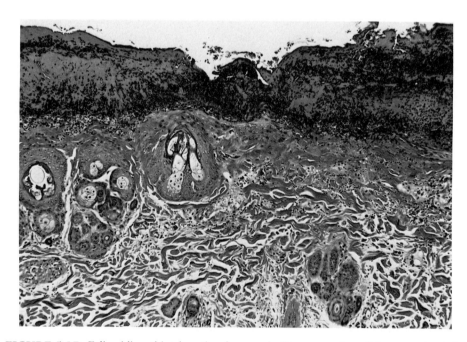

FIGURE 5-17. Feline idiopathic ulcerative dermatosis. Note extension of the necrosis to the level of the isthmus of hair follicles. (×90.)

fibrosis, which extends as a band beneath the adjacent acanthotic epidermis. Fibrosis of this type has not been observed by the authors in lesions of 4 to 6 weeks' duration.

Lesions of idiopathic ulcerative dermatosis should be differentiated from those of persistent self-trauma as a result of allergic skin disease, for example, a severely ulcerated eosinophilic plaque, or pyotraumatic dermatitis (very rare in cats). In general, eosinophils are a prominent feature of allergic ulcers; eosinophils are scant or absent in idiopathic ulcerative dermatosis.

SUGGESTED READINGS

Pyotraumatic dermatitis

Reinke SI and others: Histopathologic features of pyotraumatic dermatitis. J Am Vet Med Assoc 190:57-60, 1987.

Feline allergic miliary dermatitis

Gross TL, Kwochka KW, and Kunkle GA: Correlation of histologic and immunologic findings in cats with miliary dermatitis, J Am Vet Med Assoc 189:1322-1325, 1986.

Kunkle GA: Miliary dermatitis, eosinophilic granuloma complex, and symmetric hypotrichosis as manifestations of feline allergy. In Kirk, RW, editor: Current veterinary therapy X, Philadelphia, 1989, WB Saunders, pp 583-586.

Feline Indolent Ulcer

Muller GH, Kirk RW, and Scott DW: Small animal dermatology, ed 4, Philadelphia, 1989, WB Saunders, pp 561-563.

Power HT: Eosinophilic granuloma in a family of specific pathogen-free cats. Proceedings of the American Academy of Veterinary Dermatology/American College of Veterinary Dermatology, San Francisco 6:45, 1990.

Feline idiopathic ulcerative dermatosis

Mason K and Rosser EJ: Cutaneous drug eruptions. In Von Tscharner C and Halliwell REW, editors: Advances in veterinary dermatology, volume 1, London, 1990, Bailliere Tindall, pp 426-433.

Scott DW: An unusual ulcerative dermatitis with linear subepidermal fibrosis in cats. Proceedings of the American Academy of Veterinary Dermatology/American College of Veterinary Dermatology, San Francisco, 6:60, 1990.

CHAPTER 6

Hyperplastic diseases of the epidermis

Hyperplastic skin diseases are characterized by the proliferation of epidermal keratinocytes. Follicular infundibular epithelium frequently also is affected. Epidermal hyperplasia (acanthosis) may be due to internal factors (metabolic, hereditary) or external factors (self-traumatic). Changes in the surface keratin may accompany hyperplasia and principally consist of densification of the keratin layer, as in chronic self-trauma, or an increase in the normal basket-weave keratin, as in endocrine disease.

Many chronic diseases may feature epidermal hyperplasia, for example, those of infectious or autoimmune origin. The diseases of this chapter include those in which hyperplasia is a primary pathologic feature.

CHRONIC HYPERPLASTIC DERMATITIS
Clinical features (Figures 6-1 and 6-2)

Chronic hyperplastic dermatitis is a commonly encountered histopathologic reaction pattern in veterinary dermatopathology. Chronic hyperplastic dermatitis is seen primarily in the dog; chronic allergy is the most common cause. Pruritus with attendant self-trauma is the unifying feature of the diseases characterized by chronic hyperplastic dermatitis. The most beneficial reason for skin biopsy of suspected chronic hyperplastic dermatitis may be to rule out other diseases with a more specific histopathologic appearance, such as occult neoplasia or an endocrinopathy. Other pruritic skin diseases, such as pyoderma and keratinization disorders, may have histopathologic features of hyperplastic dermatitis in chronic stages.

Clinical changes in response to chronic self-trauma include alopecia, lichenification, and hyperpigmentation. Crusting is a common additional feature. Secondary pyoderma often may complicate chronic hyperplastic dermatitis; however, intact pustules rarely are evident, since they are effaced rapidly by self-trauma.

The clinical history and distribution pattern often are helpful in differentiating the allergic skin diseases. Flea allergy dermatitis may be the most likely consideration if the dorsal lumbosacral area, groin, and caudal thighs are most severely affected. If chronic hyperplastic skin disease is most conspicuous on the head and paws, underlying atopy or food allergy should be suspected. Chronic allergic contact dermatitis, a rare disease, tends to involve the glabrous, exposed areas such as the muzzle, groin, axilla, ventral interdigital webs, and the perineum. The clinical differences between allergic skin diseases blur in chronic cases, since the distribution pattern may become generalized.

Breed and age predilections may aid in the clinical differentiation of chronic hyperplastic dermatitis caused by allergy. The reader is referred to the specific sections detailing allergic skin diseases in Chapters 4 and 8.

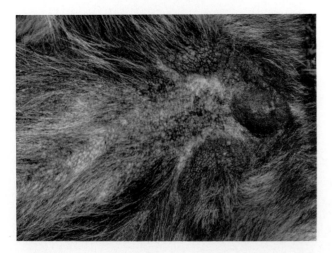

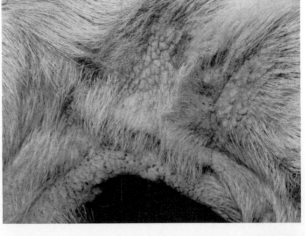

FIGURE 6-1. Chronic hyperplastic dermatitis in a dog with flea allergy dermatitis. Lichenification and hyperpigmentation are present in the perivulvar region and the adjacent ventral abdomen. Note the cobblestone appearance of the lichenified, chronically traumatized lesions.

FIGURE 6-2. Chronic hyperplastic dermatitis in the axilla of a dog with atopy. Alopecia and lichenification are indicative of chronicity.

Biopsy site selection

Biopsy site selection is not critical, since clinical features of this histopathologic reaction pattern are uniform. Since primary lesions are not present in most cases of chronic hyperplastic dermatitis, skin biopsy often will not be rewarding. If primary lesions also are present, they should be sampled in the hope of obtaining a more specific diagnosis.

Histopathology (Figure 6-3)

Chronic allergic skin disease is the most commonly encountered underlying cause of chronic hyperplastic dermatitis. Epidermal lesions include moderate to severe irregular acanthosis, as well as thickening of the follicular infundibulum. In some cases of hyperplastic dermatitis caused by allergy, there may be patchy spongiosis and exocytosis of lymphocytes or, rarely, eosinophils. Variable erosion, as well as discrete foci of superficial epidermal pustulation and crusting, also termed

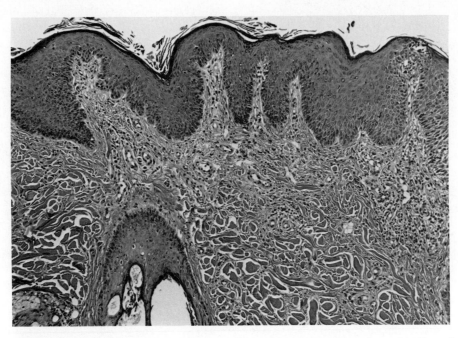

FIGURE 6-3. Chronic hyperplastic dermatitis in a dog with flea allergy dermatitis. Irregular hyperplasia of the epidermis is accompanied by focal mild spongiosis *(at right)*. (×90.)

impetiginization, probably result from self-trauma.

Dermal inflammation is superficial and perivascular to interstitial in most cases of chronic hyperplastic dermatitis. The inflammatory infiltrate is highly variable, both in cell type and severity. Sebaceous gland hyperplasia may be a feature of chronic pruritic hyperplastic dermatitis. In chronic hyperplastic dermatitis of allergic origin, suggestion of the specific allergic disease can sometimes be made based on the predominant types of inflammatory cells observed (see Chapter 8).

Many other dermatoses in chronic stages may have some of the histopathologic features of chronic hyperplastic dermatitis. For example, a similar histopathologic pattern may be seen with keratinization defects and chronic superficial spreading pyoderma; however, additional features not present in chronic allergic skin disease may aid in characterization of these disorders (see Chapters 1 and 7).

FIBROPRURITIC NODULES
Clinical features (Figures 6-4 and 6-5)

Fibropruritic nodules as named by Walder, are uncommon lesions seen in conjunction with the chronic self-trauma of canine flea allergy dermatitis. These lesions appear to be specific for flea allergy dermatitis and have not been seen in conjunction with any other allergic skin diseases of dogs.

Multiple, firm, sessile or pedunculated, alopecic

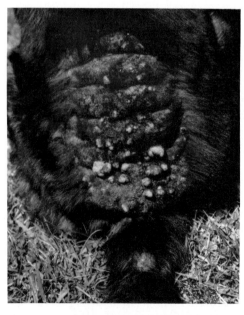

FIGURE 6-4. Multiple fibropruritic nodules in the dorsal lumbosacral area of a dog with chronic flea allergy dermatitis. The affected area is partially clipped to enhance the visibility of the lesions.

nodules develop, which vary in size from 0.5 to 2 cm in diameter. Individual nodules may be nonpigmented and erythematous or hyperpigmented. Hyperpigmented nodules may be visually striking if the surrounding skin remains normally pigmented. Erosions and ulcers may be present in larger lesions. As many as 50 nodules may be seen in long-standing cases. Fibropruritic nodules are located predominately in the bilaterally symmetric, alopecic wedge seen in the dorsal lumbosacral area of dogs with long-standing flea allergy dermatitis.

The syndrome may be more common in German Shepherd Dogs and their related crossbreeds. Fibropruritic nodules are seen most commonly in dogs greater than 8 years of age. Sex predilections have not been noted.

Differential diagnoses are few, since lesions are visually characteristic. Cutaneous neoplasms should be considered, particularly in dogs of advancing age.

Biopsy site selection

Sample selection is not critical as long as lesions are not severely ulcerated. Usually, wedge resection biopsy of an entire nodule is performed for cosmetic purposes.

Histopathology (Figures 6-6 and 6-7)

The overall configuration of the lesion is nodular as fibropruritic nodules protrude in a tumor-like fashion above the surface of the skin. The epidermis is severely hyperplastic and the keratin layer is dense, as seen in other lesions of chronic, severe self-trauma such as acral lick dermatitis. Ulceration and crusting may be present.

Dermal fibrosis is variable and may create obliteration of adnexa. In general, coarse, thick bundles of colla-

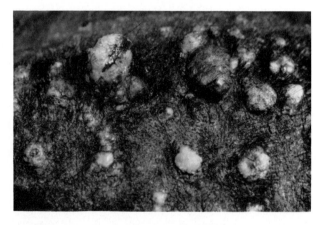

FIGURE 6-5. Closer view of the dog in Figure 6-4. Some of the nodules are hyperpigmented and others are nonpigmented. The largest nodule is ulcerated from self-trauma. The skin surrounding nodules is uniformly hyperpigmented and lichenified.

FIGURE 6-6. Fibropruritic nodule in a dog with flea allergy dermatitis. Note the irregular epidermal hyperplasia and subjacent fibrosis. (×22.)

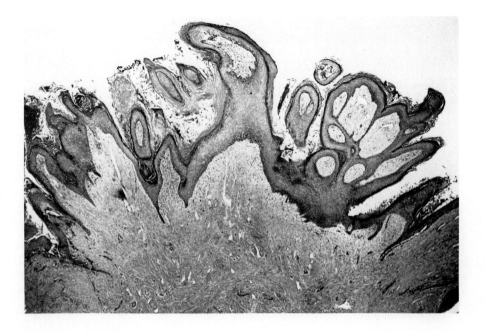

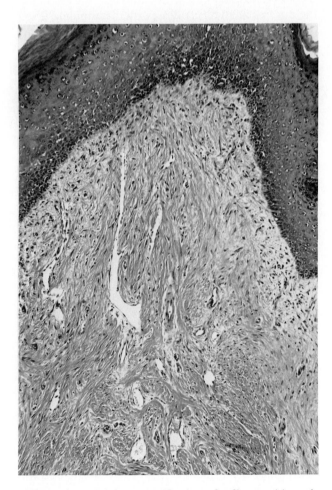

FIGURE 6-7. Higher magnification of a fibropruritic nodule demonstrating dense fibrosis beneath a hyperplastic epidermis. (×90.)

gen proliferate haphazardly in the dermis, creating a fibroma-like mass. Inflammation within the collagenous tissue is usually scant, but may include prominent neutrophils if there is ulceration. Mild accumulations of lymphocytes, macrophages, and plasma cells may be present just beneath the epidermis, and mild pigmentary incontinence may be evident. The adjacent intact (nonfibrotic) dermis may have perivascular accumulations of eosinophils, mast cells, lymphocytes, and macrophages, as seen in flea allergy dermatitis (see Chapter 8).

The principal differential diagnosis is dermal fibroma (see Chapter 26). A fibropruritic nodule tends to be less discrete than a fibroma; the epidermis is generally more hyperplastic. Inflammation is not a feature of a nonulcerated fibroma but is typical for a fibropruritic nodule.

ACRAL LICK DERMATITIS (Synonyms: lick granuloma, acral pruritic nodule)
Clinical features (Figures 6-8 and 6-9)

Acral lick dermatitis is a relatively common syndrome in the dog characterized by self-trauma to a focal area, usually a distal extremity, resulting in an alopecic, firm, oval plaque. Boredom is incriminated in the genesis of a vicious itch-lick cycle. Less commonly, a preexisting focal stimulus (infection, trauma, prior surgery, neoplasm) acts as an inflammatory or psychic nidus leading to the initiation of an itch-lick cycle. The recent success of endorphin blockers in the treatment of this syndrome indicates that endogenous opiate release may encourage habituation. Self-mutilation may

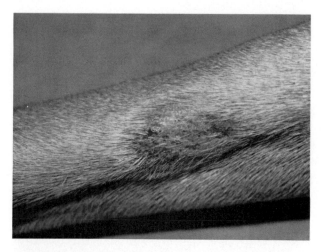

FIGURE 6-8. Early acral lick dermatitis on the forelimb of a Doberman Pinscher. The lesion is well demarcated and alopecic and has small, multifocal ulcers.

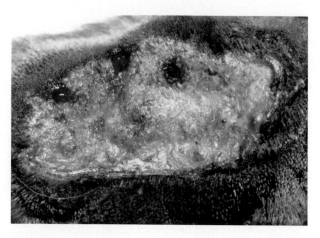

FIGURE 6-9. Severe acral lick dermatitis on the forelimb of a Golden Retriever. The crateriform ulcer has peripheral hyperpigmentation and thickening. *(Courtesy HT Power, Santa Cruz, California; case material from the University of California, Davis.)*

be performed in private. Frequently, the owner is unaware of any self-traumatic component to the syndrome and often resists this suggestion.

Typical lesions are well-circumscribed, firm, alopecic plaques. Lesions usually are solitary, oval, and vary in length between 2 and 6 cm. Coexisting lesions may merge to form larger foci with an irregular outer contour. A central irregular ulcer with a scalloped border, surrounded by a characteristic hyperpigmented halo, is present in active lesions. Surface exudate rarely is seen since licking removes any debris. In dogs with light-colored coats, peripheral salivary staining may be seen. A hand lens is useful in identifying fistulous tracts indicative of secondary bacterial infection. It is the opinion of the authors that secondary deep pyoderma in acral lick dermatitis is the direct result of self-trauma, which leads to follicular rupture and hair displacement into the deep dermis.

The anterior carpal and metacarpal areas are the most common sites. Other sites include the anterior radial, metatarsal, and tibial regions. Rarely, similar lesions may be created on the tail, stifle, or hip.

Large, active, attention-demanding breeds such as the Doberman Pinscher, Great Dane, German Shepherd Dog, Labrador Retriever, and Irish Setter are at increased risk. However, acral lick dermatitis may be seen in any breed or in mixed breed dogs. Adult dogs over 3 years of age are most commonly affected. The syndrome may be more common in male dogs.

Clinical differential diagnoses include focal neoplasms, kerion dermatophytosis, focal areas of bacterial furunculosis, and fungal granulomas. Location of the lesion, breed, history of persistent licking, and the characteristic ulceration surrounded by hyperpigmentation assist in differentiation. Histopathology will aid in ruling out visually similar diseases and determining if secondary pyoderma is present.

Biopsy site selection

Punch biopsy specimens should be obtained from nonulcerated areas. Care must be taken to obtain deep dermal tissue (to investigate the possibility of secondary pyoderma) without damaging delicate underlying structures of the distal extremities, such as flexor tendons, blood vessels, or nerves.

Histopathology (Figures 6-10 through 6-12)

Severe thickening of epidermal and superficial follicular epithelium is accompanied by compact hyperkeratosis and multifocal parakeratosis. Small neutrophilic serocellular crusts often are trapped in the keratin layer. Erosion or focal to extensive ulceration with exudation is often seen. The degree of epithelial hyperplasia is marked, but in the majority of cases cannot be termed pseudoepitheliomatous hyperplasia. Keratin horns, increased mitotic activity, and irregular, deeply projecting cords of hyperplastic epithelium, often to levels below the adnexa (appearing as islands in cross section), are observed in pseudoepitheliomatous hyperplasia, but are rare in acral lick dermatitis.

Superficial dermal fibrosis, often in a vertical streaking pattern, is seen between intact hair follicles. Mixed dermal inflammation is perivascular, perifollicular, or diffuse and includes lymphocytes, neutrophils, macrophages, and plasma cells. There is often prominent and distinctive plasmacytic inflammation around distended apocrine sweat glands. Deep folliculitis and furunculosis may be accompanied by rupture of hair

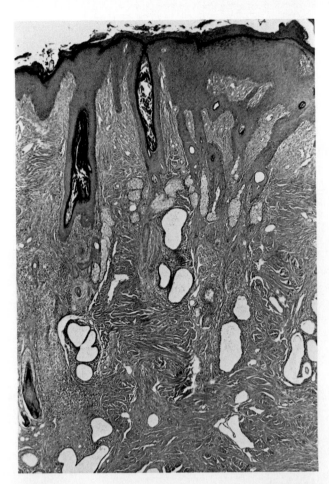

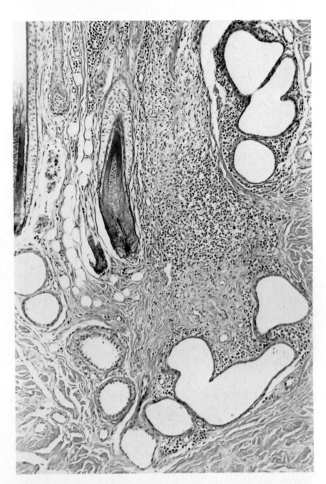

FIGURE 6-10. Acral lick dermatitis in a dog. Irregular hyperplasia of the epidermis and follicular infundibular epithelium is accompanied by dermal fibrosis, dilation of apocrine sweat glands, and periglandular inflammation. (×35.)

FIGURE 6-11. Higher magnification of dilated apocrine sweat glands and periglandular inflammation in Fig. 6-10. (×90.)

FIGURE 6-12. Epidermal hyperplasia, compact hyperkeratosis, and vertical streaking fibrosis of acral lick dermatitis. (×90.)

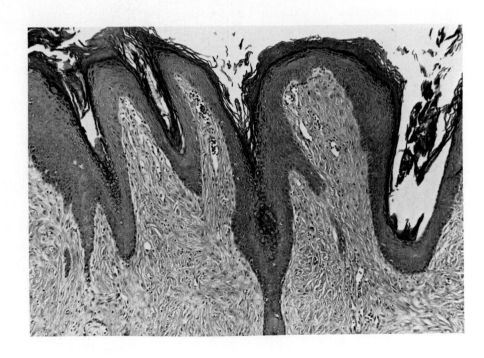

follicles and displacement of hairs into the deep dermis or panniculus. This displacement may be the direct result of licking, which pushes a stiff hair shaft through the follicular wall.

Acral lick dermatitis is histopathologically distinctive if typical features of plasmacytic periadnexal inflammation and vertical streaking fibrosis are observed. Lesions are similar to those of persistently traumatized skin of any cause; knowledge of the location of the lesion is often helpful in differentiation.

HYPOTHYROIDISM
Clinical features (Figures 6-13 and 6-14)

Hypothyroidism is the most common endocrinologic skin disease of the dog. Most documented cases of canine hypothyroidism are caused by either lymphocytic thyroiditis or idiopathic thyroid atrophy. Lymphocytic thyroiditis is thought to be due to a complex autoimmune process involving derangements in both cellular and humoral immunity. Idiopathic atrophy of the thyroid most likely is a primary degenerative disorder of the thyroid gland.

Thyroid hormone is necessary for normal cellular metabolic functions in all organ systems. Major mechanisms of action include stimulation of amino acid transport, mitochondrial oxygen consumption, and protein synthesis. Deficiency of thyroid hormone affects metabolic processes throughout the body. Consequently, symptoms are so variable that even a listing of all possible other dermatologic and nondermatologic signs is beyond the scope of this book. Conversely, hypothyroidism as a cause of skin disease probably is greatly overdiagnosed. Other alopecic skin diseases

may be partially thyroid hormone-responsive, since thyroid hormone promotes cycling into the active anagen phase of hair growth.

Bilaterally symmetric truncal alopecia, poor coat quality, coat color change, hyperpigmentation, and lichenification are the most common clinical signs. Retarded regrowth of hair after clipping may be noted. Secondary seborrhea, characterized by scaling and crusting, and secondary pyoderma also are common. These signs may be present in any combination and may be subtle. Lesions are most commonly truncal but may involve the distal extremities or head.

Breeds at reported increased risk include the Chow Chow, Great Dane, Irish Wolfhound, Boxer, English Bulldog, Dachshund, Afghan Hound, Newfoundland, Alaskan Malamute, Doberman Pinscher, Brittany, Poodle, Golden Retriever, Miniature Schnauzer, Airedale Terrier, and Irish Setter. However, hypothyroidism may be seen in any breed. Most affected dogs are over 6 years of age, but dogs of any age may be affected. Sex predilection has not been noted.

Clinical differential diagnoses include other endocrinopathies, follicular dysplasia, and primary seborrhea. Differentiation among these diseases is based on laboratory evaluation of thyroid function, and histopathology.

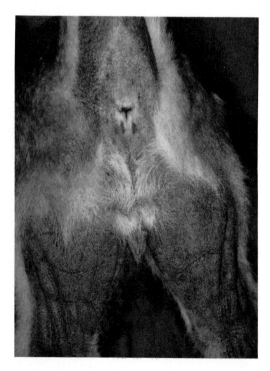

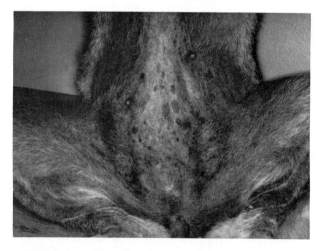

FIGURE 6-13. Hypothyroidism in an adult dog. Hyperpigmentation, lichenification, and alopecia are noted symmetrically in the ventral abdomen.

FIGURE 6-14. Hypothyroidism in the dog shown in Fig. 6-13. Severe symmetric lichenification and hyperpigmentation with alopecia are present on the caudal hindlimbs and the ventrum of the tail.

Biopsy site selection

Biopsies should be obtained from older sites of involvement demonstrating maximum alopecia and minimum inflammation. Lesions with obvious secondary pyoderma should be avoided.

Histopathology (Figure 6-15)

The epidermis and follicular infundibula usually are moderately hyperplastic, and there is mild to moderate hyperkeratosis. Hyperplasia can be present without inflammation; however, secondary pyoderma may contribute to the degree of epidermal and follicular infundibular hyperplasia observed. Epidermal hyperpigmentation may be present and is characterized by increased melanin at all levels of the epidermis.

The dermis may be variably inflamed, depending on the presence of secondary pyoderma, and is commonly characterized by superficial perivascular to interstitial and periadnexal mixed inflammation, consisting of lymphocytes, macrophages, plasma cells, and neutrophils. Folliculitis, or superficial epidermal pustulation as seen in superficial spreading pyoderma (see Chapter 1), may be seen. In sharp contrast to the hyperplastic follicular infundibulum, the deeper portion of the hair follicle is atrophic and generally in the telogen phase (see Chapter 17).

Epidermal lesions may be similar to those of other chronic hyperplastic skin diseases discussed in this chapter. The presence of follicular atrophy is a distin-guishing feature of hypothyroidism, as well as other endocrinopathies. Hypothyroidism may be histopathologically indistinguishable from skin disease caused by Sertoli cell tumor (see below) and clinical differentiation usually is required.

CANINE SERTOLI CELL TUMOR
Clinical features (Figures 6-16 and 6-17)

Functional Sertoli cell tumors leading to hyperestrogenism and feminization cause an uncommon canine endocrinopathy with characteristic dermatologic signs. The syndrome usually is associated with cryptorchidism.

Subtle symmetric alopecia or coat color change in the flank folds may be the earliest presenting sign. Bilaterally symmetric alopecia characteristically begins in the perineal and genital region and may progress with chronicity to the abdomen, chest, flanks, and neck. Hyperpigmentation is uncommon in early cases, but macular hyperpigmentation, especially on the neck, or diffuse hyperpigmentation in areas of alopecia may be seen in advanced cases. Lichenification, always in conjunction with hyperpigmentation and alopecia, may be seen in chronic and severe cases and may be accompanied by greasy keratinous deposits. Gynecomastia, a pendulous prepuce, and attraction to other male dogs commonly occur. Linear preputial erythema, described by Griffin as a well-demarcated linear band of macular

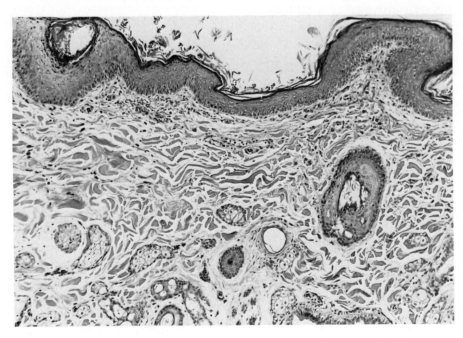

FIGURE 6-15. Hypothyroidism in a dog. The epidermis and follicular infundibular epithelium are irregularly hyperplastic. ($\times$90.)

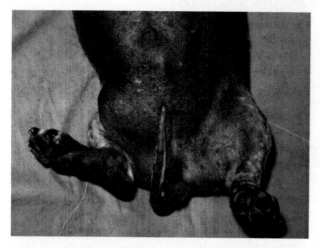

FIGURE 6-16. Skin disease in an adult Dachshund with a Sertoli cell tumor. Lichenification, hyperpigmentation, and alopecia are present diffusely on the ventral abdomen. The large Sertoli cell tumor in the abdominal cavity protrudes in the right inguinal region.

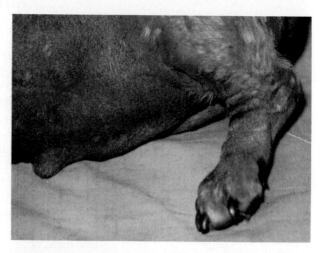

FIGURE 6-17. Closer view of the dog in Fig. 6-16. Diffuse hyperpigmentation and lichenification are present on the abdomen and prepuce.

erythema with mottled hyperpigmentation on the ventral prepuce, is an important cutaneous marker of Sertoli cell tumors. Tumor size and duration often correlate with the severity of clinical signs. Less than 10% of Sertoli cell tumors are malignant; metastasis is seen occasionally.

Boxers, Shetland Sheepdogs, Pekingese, Weimaraners, and Cairn Terriers are predisposed. Middle-aged or older male dogs most commonly are affected.

Clinical differential diagnoses include other endocrinopathies and follicular dysplasia, particularly those manifested as flank alopecia (see Chapter 18). Histopathologic confirmation of a Sertoli cell tumor and subsequent reversal of cutaneous signs following castration are diagnostic.

Biopsy site selection

Multiple biopsy specimens should be obtained from areas of maximum alopecia. If lichenified and hyperpigmented areas are present, they should be sampled in addition to areas of maximum alopecia.

Histopathology (Figure 6-18)

The epidermis may demonstrate variable acanthosis and the follicular infundibula also may be hyperplastic. Not all specimens will show acanthosis; random biopsy may reveal a normal epidermal thickness. Increased melanin pigmentation of the epidermis is often observed and is characterized by deposition of pigment at all viable levels of the epidermis. Mild to moderate hyperkeratosis is often present.

The dermis shows variable inflammation, including mild to moderate, superficial, perivascular to inter-stitial accumulations of lymphocytes, macrophages, plasma cells, and neutrophils. Inflammation may also extend around adnexal appendages. Inflammation may reflect the presence of secondary pyoderma. Follicular atrophy is present (see Chapter 17).

Epidermal lesions in the skin disease caused by Sertoli cell tumors resemble those of other chronic dermatoses discussed in this chapter; follicular atrophy is a differentiating feature. The skin disease caused by Sertoli cell tumors and hypothyroidism may be histopathologically identical (see preceding discussion) and clinical differentiation is required.

ACTINIC KERATOSIS (Synonyms: solar keratosis, squamous cell carcinoma in situ)
Clinical features (Figures 6-19 and 6-20)

Actinic keratoses are solar-induced preneoplastic lesions which are seen in the dog and cat. Lesions occur in nonpigmented and lightly haired skin exposed to excessive ultraviolet light. Many affected dogs are known sunbathers. Ample epidemiologic and experimental evidence exists that solar irradiation induces a continuum of changes in keratinocytes, ranging from dysplasia to carcinoma in situ to invasive squamous cell carcinoma; however, the precise mechanisms are not known. The central pathogenic mechanism is probably monoclonal malignant transformation of keratinocytes. Actinic keratoses of both dogs and cats may progress to invasive squamous cell carcinoma if exposure to solar irradiation continues. (See Chapter 21 for further discussion of actinic keratoses in dogs and cats.)

The clinical appearance in dogs is highly variable. Lesions range from scaly red to reddish-brown, ill-defined macules and papules to darkly crusted, indu-

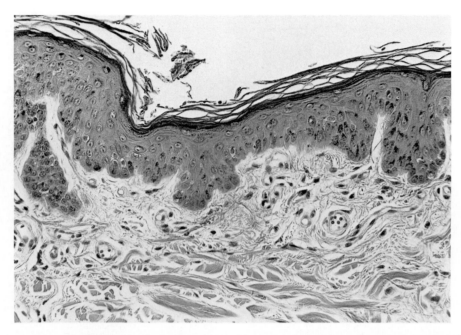

FIGURE 6-18. Skin from a dog with a Sertoli cell tumor. Irregular acanthosis is accompanied by epidermal hypermelanosis. (×220.)

rated, keratotic plaques and nodules. Actinic comedones may be present (see Chapter 16). Larger, ulcerated nodular lesions are most indicative of squamous cell carcinoma. Palpation of visually normal skin may detect irregular firmness and thickening, suggesting that preneoplastic change is more widespread than is visually apparent. The glabrous skin of the ventral and lateral abdomen and inner thighs is most frequently affected. One side of the abdomen and the opposite inner thigh may be more prominently affected, as described by Mason and observed by the authors, indicating favoring of one side during recumbency in sunbathing. Secondary pyoderma with follicular rupture is a common sequela; the lesions of pyoderma most commonly generate from actinic comedones (see Chapter 16).

In cats, lesions consist of erosions, ulcers, or erythematous, slightly elevated plaques. Hemorrhagic crusts may overlie ulcers or erosions. Severe ulceration

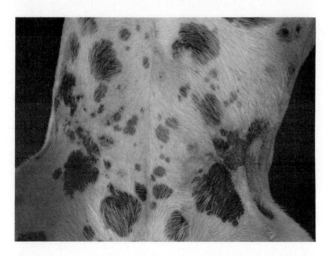

FIGURE 6-19. Actinic keratoses in an adult Dalmatian with a history of sunbathing. Mottled erythema, scaling, and crusting are present diffusely on the ventral abdomen. Note the focal erosions and ulcers with markedly erythematous borders. *(Courtesy LG Morehouse.)*

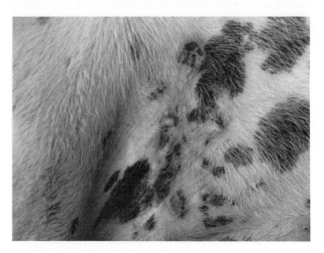

FIGURE 6-20. Closer view of the actinic keratoses shown in Fig. 6-19. Irregular crusted ulcers are present in the lateral flank fold. *(Courtesy LG Morehouse.)*

FIGURE 6-21. Feline actinic keratosis. Note that hyperplasia and dysplasia also affect the follicular infundibula. (×90.)

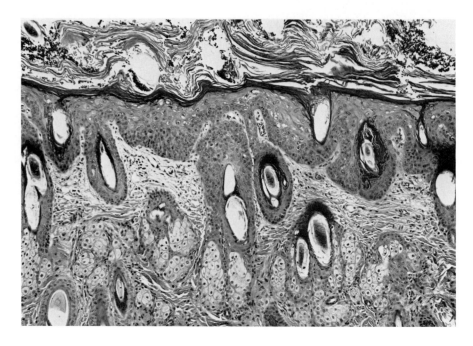

may be indicative of squamous cell carcinoma; however, ulceration cannot be used as a marker of occult squamous cell carcinoma, since pruritus may initiate self-trauma in preneoplastic actinic keratoses. Actinic keratoses of cats are seen most commonly on the margins of the pinna, planum nasale, and dorsal muzzle. Symmetry may be marked.

Lightly pigmented Dalmatians, Whippets, American Staffordshire Terriers, and Beagles are at increased risk for malignant and premalignant solar-induced lesions. Most feline actinic keratoses are seen in white cats. Lesions occur most commonly in older animals. Animals spending substantial time outdoors in areas of the world with increased solar exposure are at greater risk. Many affected dogs are reported to be sunbathers and spend long periods of time in dorsal or lateral recumbency in direct sunlight.

In the dog, solar-induced squamous cell carcinomas and hemangiomas and superficial and deep bacterial folliculitis and furunculosis are the major differential diagnoses for actinic keratoses. In the cat, clinical differential diagnoses include solar-induced squamous cell carcinoma and autoimmune diseases such as pemphigus foliaceus and discoid lupus erythematosus. Since it is impossible clinically to differentiate premalignant actinic keratosis from solar-induced malignancies, biopsy of suspected actinic keratosis is mandatory.

Biopsy site selection

Specimens for biopsy should be obtained from different stages of the disease. If present, samples should include discolored macules, areas of erythema, crusted plaques, nodules, and margins of ulcers in order to reveal the full spectrum of disease present and to un-

cover possible neoplasia. If possible, solitary lesions should be resected in their entirety to prevent possible progression to overt neoplasia.

Histopathology (Figures 6-21 and 6-22)

Epidermal changes vary in severity, depending on the stage of the disease. The principal diagnostic feature of actinic keratosis is epidermal hyperplasia with dysplasia. Dysplastic epithelial changes may extend down superficial hair follicles to the level of the isthmus, particularly in the cat. Advanced lesions may be markedly proliferative and have a papillomatous configuration. Hyperplasia and dysplasia without invasion through the basement membrane indicate actinic keratosis (carcinoma in situ); penetration into the underlying dermis signifies squamous cell carcinoma and may occur in advanced lesions (see Chapter 21).

Dysplasia is manifested by loss of normal stratification and is characterized by the absence of distinct basal and spinous layers, as well as the lack of an orderly maturation process. There is an increased nuclear-to-cytoplasmic ratio among dysplastic keratinocytes, particularly in the deeper layers of the epidermis. An increased mitotic index at all levels of the epidermis is present and dyskeratosis, or premature keratinization of keratinocytes, is often prominent. Vacuolated cells containing glycogen may be seen.

Acantholysis may be observed within an actinic keratosis, particularly when there is severe dyskeratosis. Acantholysis occurs as widespread dyskeratosis results in loss of cohesion among keratinocytes. Parakeratosis in parallel layers, so-called stacked parakeratosis, is observed most commonly in the dog.

Dermal inflammation may be prominently li-

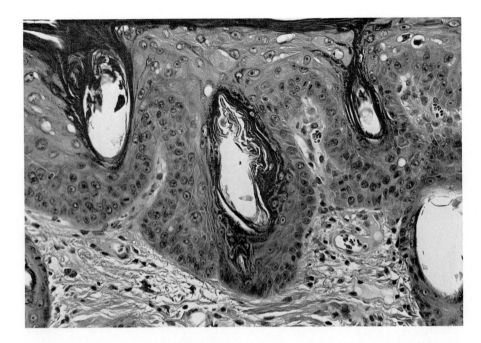

FIGURE 6-22. Higher magnification of the actinic keratosis shown in Fig. 6-21 demonstrates uneven nuclear size, increased nuclear-to-cytoplasmic ratio, and lack of orderly maturation of keratinocytes. (×220.)

chenoid in the dog and may be accompanied by solar elastosis and laminar fibrosis leading to scarring alopecia (see Chapter 10). Solar elastosis is also observed in the cat. Follicular keratosis (actinic comedones) with ensuing rupture and furunculosis, may accompany actinic keratoses in dogs and may be the sole feature of chronic sun exposure in some animals (see Chapter 16).

Because epidermal lesions are characteristic, differential diagnoses are few. Lichenoid keratoses may have a similar low-power appearance but are not characterized by epidermal dysplasia. Some actinic keratoses, particularly those with prominent glycogenation of dysplastic cells or with extension of dysplastic epithelium to superficial follicles, may be identical histopathologically to lesions of Bowen's disease (multicentric squamous cell carcinoma in situ; see Chapter 21), and are referred to as "bowenoid" actinic keratoses. The epidermis and superficial hair follicles of these lesions may have a more strikingly disorganized or "windblown" appearance than actinic keratoses, and the dysplastic keratinocytes may be more vacuolated. Clinical differentiation may be required; lesions of Bowen's disease are generally widespread and located in non–sun-exposed sites.

ACANTHOSIS NIGRICANS OF DACHSHUNDS
Clinical features (Figures 6-23 and 6-24)

Acanthosis nigricans is most specifically a rare, idiopathic primary genodermatosis seen exclusively in Dachshunds. The disease is characterized by symmetric hyperpigmentation, lichenification, and alopecia of the

axillae. Unfortunately, the term acanthosis nigricans also has been used generically to describe a multifactorial, clinical cutaneous reaction pattern, characterized by similar lesions and seen in a variety of different breeds.

Acanthosis nigricans of Dachshunds begins with subtle, bilaterally symmetric axillary hyperpigmentation. Lesions progress slowly to lichenification and alopecia. Accumulation of greasy, odoriferous, keratinous debris is common in severely affected dogs. In advanced cases, the abdomen, groin, perineum, chest, neck, forelimbs, and hocks may be involved. Pyoderma is a common sequela to severe disease. Pruritus is variable and can be absent in early stages.

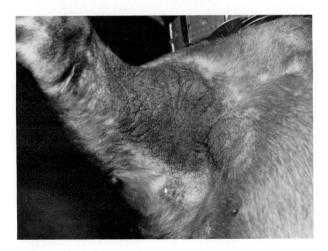

FIGURE 6-23. Acanthosis nigricans in a Dachshund. Affected axilla and ventral neck are alopecic, hyperpigmented, and lichenified.

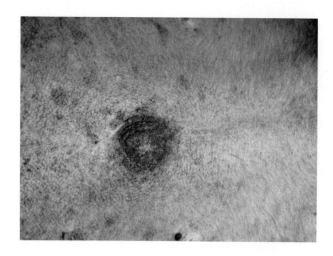

FIGURE 6-24. Acanthosis nigricans in a Dachshund. Early lichenification and hyperpigmentation seen in the umbilical region were preceded by axillary lesions.

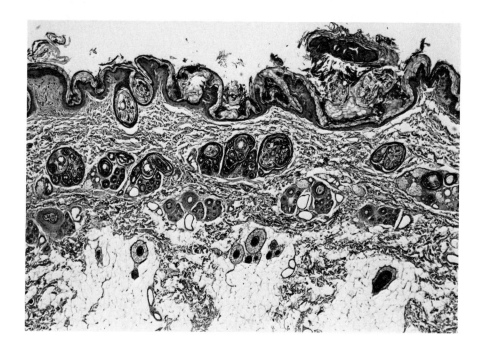

FIGURE 6-25. Acanthosis nigricans in a Dachshund. Irregular acanthosis is accompanied by mild hyperkeratosis. (×35.)

Acanthosis nigricans of Dachshunds commonly develops initially in dogs less than 2 years of age. Sex predilection has not been reported.

Even in the Dachshund breed, acanthosis nigricans should be a diagnosis of exclusion. Superficial bacterial folliculitis and superficial spreading pyoderma, as well as the numerous other causes of axillary pruritus, including atopy and food allergy, must be investigated and ruled out before acanthosis nigricans is diagnosed. Allergic skin diseases usually involve sites in addition to the axillae and groin, but chronic and severe cases of acanthosis nigricans may be very similar. Unlike cases of pyoderma, acanthosis nigricans should not have an excessively erythematous exfoliative margin with papules or collarettes.

Biopsy site selection

Multiple samples should be taken from both hyperpigmented and lichenified central lesions, as well as from the advancing border. Marginal specimens are most useful in ruling out other visually similar diseases.

Histopathology (Figures 6-25 and 6-26)

The epidermis is irregularly and often severely acanthotic. There may be mild to moderate hyperkeratosis and focal parakeratosis often is observed. Keratinocytes, especially those in the basal cell layer, are heavily pigmented. The dermis has a mild to moderate, superficial perivascular to interstitial infiltrate of lymphocytes, macrophages, and a few neutrophils or plasma cells. Pigmentary incontinence sometimes is

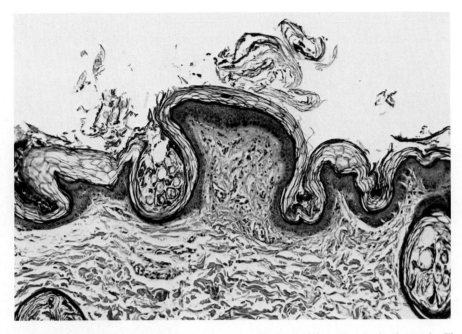

FIGURE 6-26. Higher magnification of the acanthosis and hyperkeratosis shown in Fig. 6-25. (×90.)

prominent. Follicular keratosis may be striking in some cases.

Histopathologically, the lesions of acanthosis nigricans are nondiagnostic and are essentially identical to those of chronic hyperplastic dermatitis. Correlation with the breed affected and the clinical distribution of lesions, in addition to systematic clinical exclusion of other possible causes, are required for the definitive diagnosis of acanthosis nigricans.

HYPERPLASTIC DERMATOSIS OF THE WEST HIGHLAND WHITE TERRIER (Synonym: epidermal dysplasia and *Malassezia pachydermatis* infection in West Highland White Terriers, "Westie seborrhea")
Clinical features (Figures 6-27 and 6-28)

Hyperplastic dermatosis of the West Highland White Terrier is an uncommon, severe, chronic skin disease with clinical features similar to primary seborrhea and seborrheic dermatitis. The restriction of this syndrome to the West Highland White Terrier, coupled with evidence of familial involvement, indicates the probability of a hereditary disease. Previously, diseases of abnormal keratinization, including primary seborrhea and ichthyosis, have been reported in West Highland White Terriers. However, in contrast to Cocker Spaniels, West Highland White Terriers with clinical evidence of chronic seborrhea often do not have

histopathologic evidence of a keratinization disorder. Therefore, it cannot be assumed that a true keratinization defect exists in this breed until studies of epidermal maturation have been performed.

Recently, epidermal dysplasia with secondary *Malassezia pachydermatis* infection has been described by Scott in West Highland White Terriers. The authors have not noted histopathologic features compatible with epidermal dysplasia in West Highland White Terriers. Because of this difficulty, the term hyperplastic dermatosis has been chosen until more data are available. Secondary infection with *Malassezia pachydermatis* has not been a consistent feature of clinically similar skin disease in West Highland White Terriers seen in California. This difference could be associated with an overall decreased frequency of both fungal and yeast infections in an environment with less humidity.

This confusing syndrome is complicated further by the frequent coexistence in the West Highland White Terrier of allergic skin diseases such as flea allergy dermatitis, atopy, and food allergy. Thus, differentiation of hyperplastic dermatosis of the West Highland White Terrier from chronic allergic dermatoses may be challenging, since the severely affected dog is often the end product of multiple coexistent skin diseases.

An authoritative chronology of the development of clinical signs is not available from firsthand clinical experience. Most cases seen by the authors have be-

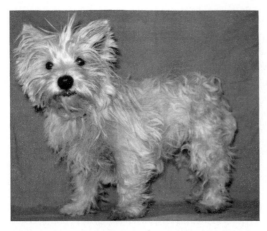

FIGURE 6-27. Hyperplastic dermatosis of the West Highland White Terrier. Partial alopecia of the chest and a generally disheveled coat are present.

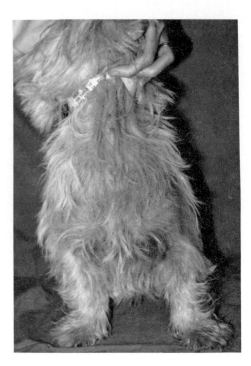

FIGURE 6-28. Closer view of the dog in Fig. 6-27. Alopecia, erythema, lichenification, and hyperpigmentation are present on the ventral neck and chest. Note the thickened skin folds.

come chronic before presentation to a referral center. Affected dogs have generalized erythema with alopecia, lichenification, and hyperpigmentation. Thickened skin folds develop on the legs and occasionally on the trunk. The skin is often malodorous and may have adherent, brownish-gray, greasy debris. Crusting may be present. Pruritus and accompanying self-trauma vary in intensity but are noted frequently. Secondary superficial pyoderma is common and intertrigo may be present in thickened folds of skin. Owners report that lesions often begin on the trunk but rapidly generalize. In advanced cases, lesions may involve virtually all haired body surfaces. Regional or generalized lymphadenopathy is a consistent feature.

The syndrome, as described here, is seen only in West Highland White Terriers. The age of onset may be from less than 1 year of age to middle age. Clinical signs commonly commence at less than 1 year of age in severely affected dogs. Sex predilections have not been noted.

Clinical differential diagnoses should include generalized demodicosis, atopy, food allergy, and flea allergy dermatitis; however, the documentation of any of these diseases should not preclude the coexistence of hyperplastic dermatosis of the West Highland White Terrier. Impression smears and fungal cultures should be performed to determine if secondary yeast infection is present.

Biopsy site selection

Multiple biopsy specimens should be taken from affected areas showing minimal self-trauma. Sites that have no evidence of secondary pyoderma are preferred.

Histopathology (Figures 6-29 and 6-30)

Epidermal features principally consist of severe acanthosis with mild hyperkeratosis. There is patchy or diffuse mild spongiosis with lymphocytic exocytosis. Parakeratosis often is mildly present as multifocal mounds accompanied by serocellular crusting. Hyperplasia may be accompanied by a scalloped or rounded lower border of the epidermis and basal cells may appear crowded; however, features compatible with epidermal dysplasia, such as uneven nuclear size, an increased mitotic index, or premature keratinization, have not been recognized by the authors. Colonization of the keratin layer by *Malassezia pachydermatis* has been an occasional feature of the cases observed by the authors.

Perivascular to interstitial inflammation is seen in the superficial dermis. Neutrophils, macrophages, plasma cells, and lymphocytes are present in varying proportions. Sebaceous glands are often markedly hyperplastic and may be distributed loosely throughout the middle dermis. Squamous metaplasia of sebaceous glands may be present.

Histopathologically, lesions resemble seborrheic dermatitis of other breeds. However, parakeratotic mounds at the edges of follicles, as seen in seborrheic dermatitis, are usually absent, and there are no coexist-

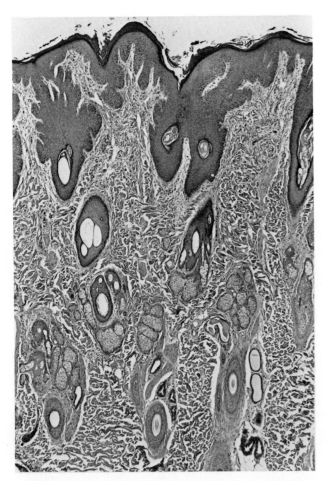

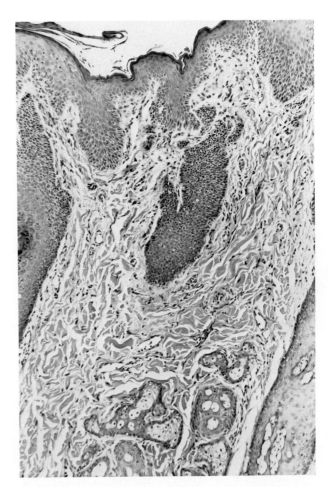

FIGURE 6-29. Hyperplastic dermatosis of the West Highland White Terrier. Severe irregular hyperplasia of the epidermis and follicular infundibular epithelium is accompanied by compact parakeratosis. (×40.)

FIGURE 6-30. Hyperplastic dermatosis of the West Highland White Terrier, demonstrating irregular acanthosis and mild spongiosis, mild superficial dermal inflammation, and prominent sebaceous glands. (×90.)

ent features of primary seborrhea, notably prominent epidermal and follicular hyperkeratosis. Lesions also are similar to chronic dermatitis of allergic causes. A scallop-bordered acanthotic epidermis and sebaceous gland hyperplasia have both been seen in lesions of chronic allergic dermatitis and are believed to be the direct result of chronic, pruritus-associated self-trauma; these lesions are not specifically diagnostic for hyperplastic dermatosis of the West Highland White Terrier.

PSORIASIFORM-LICHENOID DERMATOSIS OF THE SPRINGER SPANIEL (Synonym: lichenoid-psoriasiform dermatosis of the Springer Spaniel)

Clinical features (Figures 6-31 and 6-32)

Psoriasiform-lichenoid dermatosis is an uncommon, asymptomatic skin disease seen in the English

Springer Spaniel. The etiology is unknown but the strong breed predilection suggests heritability.

The syndrome is characterized clinically by erythematous to yellow, waxy, crusted papules that coalesce to form plaques. Lesions are found on the medial surface of the pinnae, external ear canal, prepuce, and the ventral abdomen. Pruritus is not noted. Affected dogs also may have generalized scaling, as in primary seborrhea.

Although psoriasiform-lichenoid dermatosis is reported as a disease of English Springer Spaniels, on rare occasion, clinically and histopathologically indistinguishable lesions have been seen in other breeds. Initial lesions occur during the first 1½ years of life. Sex predilection has not been noted.

Clinical differential diagnoses should include lichenoid keratoses (see subsequent discussion). Psoriasiform-lichenoid dermatosis occurs in the English

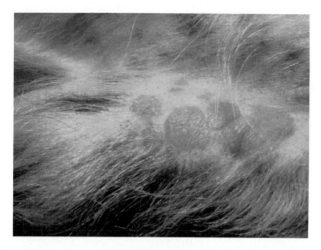

FIGURE 6-31. Psoriasiform-lichenoid dermatosis in an English Springer Spaniel. Erythematous papules and coalescing plaques are present in the groin. *(Courtesy of MP Schick, Atlanta, Georgia.)*

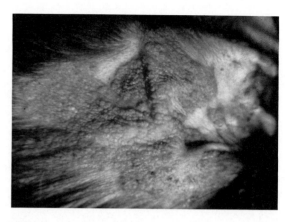

FIGURE 6-32. Psoriasiform-lichenoid dermatosis in an English Springer Spaniel. Waxy, erythematous, coalescing plaques and papules are seen on the medial surface of the pinna. *(Courtesy of WS Rosenkrantz, Garden Grove, California.)*

Springer Spaniel, and lesions commonly are multicentric. Lichenoid keratoses are found in any breed and are most often solitary.

Biopsy site selection

Solitary plaques with minimal crusting and erosion are preferred sites for biopsy. Multiple specimens from lesions in varying stages of development are ideal. Care must be taken during pinnal biopsy procedures not to damage the fragile underlying cartilage.

Histopathology (Figures 6-33 and 6-34)

The name psoriasiform-lichenoid dermatosis is preferred to lichenoid-psoriasiform dermatosis, since epidermal features are more distinctive than dermal features of the disease. The epidermis is irregularly acanthotic, often with deep projections into the dermis. This form of epidermal hyperplasia is similar to "psoriasiform" hyperplasia, which is described in humans with hyperplastic diseases that resemble psoriasis. Mild hyperkeratosis with focal parakeratosis is present. Characteristically, there are discrete, often round, in-

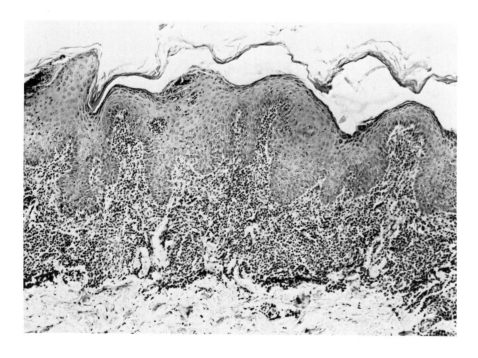

FIGURE 6-33. Psoriasiform-lichenoid dermatosis of an English Springer Spaniel. Irregular acanthosis is accompanied by discrete, round intraepidermal pustules. Note the lichenoid dermatitis. (×90.)

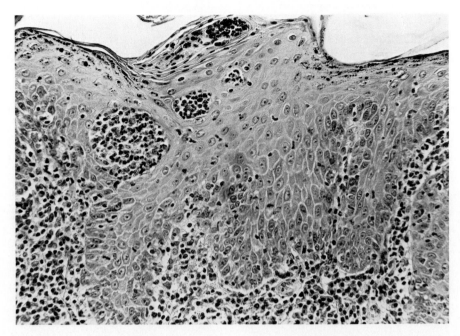

FIGURE 6-34. Higher magnification of the epidermis in Fig. 6-33, demonstrating intraepidermal pustules. Mound-shaped superficial parakeratosis contains a degenerating pustule (Munro's microabscess). (×220.)

traepidermal pustules that contain eosinophils, neutrophils, or a mixture of both. Pustules progress to well-demarcated, mound-shaped parakeratotic crusts, which resemble Munro's microabscesses, as described for psoriasis in humans. Necrosis of individual basal keratinocytes is seen rarely. Specimens from areas of generalized scaling show hyperkeratosis and follicular keratosis, similar to primary seborrhea (see Chapter 7). Dermal inflammation is lichenoid and predominantly plasmacellular (see Chapter 10).

Psoriasiform-lichenoid dermatosis histopathologically parallels lichenoid keratosis (see below), and differentiating clinical features are required for a definitive diagnosis.

LICHENOID KERATOSIS
Clinical features

Lichenoid keratoses are rare, usually solitary, well-circumscribed plaques that occur in the dog. The etiology is unknown.

Clinically, individual lesions closely resemble those of psoriasiform-lichenoid dermatosis of the English Springer Spaniel (see preceding discussion). Lichenoid keratoses are scaly or crusted plaques that may appear papillomatous. Erythema is variable and hyperpigmentation may occur. Lesions usually are solitary and are located on the pinnae, groin, and occasionally else-

where. Lichenoid keratoses are asymptomatic. Most lesions have been seen in adult dogs. Breed or sex predilections have not been noted.

Lichenoid keratosis must be differentiated from psoriasiform-lichenoid dermatosis and actinic keratosis. Psoriasiform-lichenoid dermatosis is the more probable diagnosis in the English Springer Spaniel. Actinic keratoses occur only in sun-exposed skin.

Biopsy site selection

Nontraumatized plaques that do not have secondary changes such as erosion, ulceration, or crusting should be selected. Care should be taken during pinnal biopsy procedures not to damage fragile underlying cartilage.

Histopathology (Figure 6-35)

The epidermis shows prominent psoriasiform hyperplasia with generally diffuse hyperkeratosis and multifocal, variably severe parakeratosis. Serocellular crusting may be present. Intraepidermal pustules similar to those of psoriasiform-lichenoid dermatosis are less common but may be identified.

Dermal inflammation is lichenoid (see Chapter 10), and includes lymphocytes, macrophages, and plasma cells. Epidermal and dermal lesions are strikingly similar to psoriasiform-lichenoid dermatosis of English Springer Spaniels (see preceding discussion).

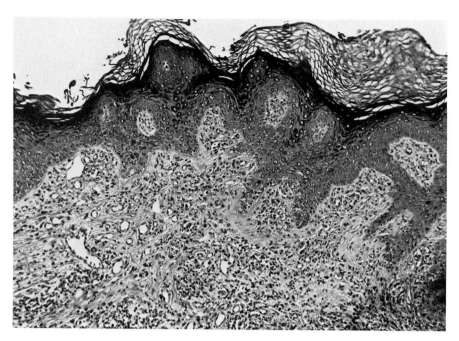

FIGURE 6-35. Lichenoid keratosis in a dog demonstrating marked irregular acanthosis and hyperkeratosis, a diffuse superficial dermal inflammation. (×90.)

Clinical differences allow separation of these entities, since lichenoid keratoses are usually solitary and are found in other breeds.

SUGGESTED READINGS

Fibropruritic nodules

References not available.

Acral lick dermatitis

Walton DW: Psychodermatoses. In Kirk RW, editor: Current veterinary therapy IX, Philadelphia, 1986, WB Saunders, pp 557-559.

White SD: Naltrexone for treatment of acral lick dermatitis in dogs, J Am Vet Med Assoc 196:1073-1076, 1990.

Hypothyroidism

Feldman EC and Nelson RW: Canine and feline endocrinology and reproduction, Philadelphia, 1987, WB Saunders, pp 55-85.

Gross TL and Ihrke PJ: The histologic analysis of endocrine-related alopecia in the dog. In Von Tscharner C and Halliwell REW, editors: Advances in veterinary dermatology, vol 1, London, 1990, Bailliere Tindall, pp 77-88.

Milne KL and Hayes HM: Epidemiologic features of canine hypothyroidism, Cornell Vet 71:3-14, 1981.

Muller GH, Kirk RW, and Scott DW: Small animal dermatology, ed 4, Philadelphia, 1989, WB Saunders, pp 641-653.

Peterson ME and Ferguson DC: Thyroid diseases. In Ettinger SJ, editor: Textbook of veterinary internal medicine, ed 3, Philadelphia, 1989, WB Saunders, pp 1632-1675.

Scott DW: Excessive trichilemmal keratinisation (flame follicles) in endocrine skin disorders of the dog. Vet Dermatol 1:37-40, 1989.

Canine Sertoli cell tumor

Feldman EC and Nelson RW: Canine and feline endocrinology and reproduction, Philadelphia, 1987, WB Saunders, pp 496-497.

Griffin CE: Linear prepucial erythema. Proceedings of the American Academy of Veterinary Dermatology/American College of Veterinary Dermatology, New Orleans, 2:35, 1986.

Gross TL and Ihrke PJ: The histologic analysis of endocrine-related alopecia in the dog. In Von Tscharner C and Halliwell REW, editors: Advances in veterinary dermatology, vol 1, London, 1990, Bailliere Tindall, pp 77-88.

Muller GH, Kirk RW, and Scott DW: Small animal dermatology, ed 4, Philadelphia, 1989, WB Saunders, pp 627-631.

Actinic keratosis

Hargis AM and others: Solar keratosis (solar dermatosis, senile keratosis) and solar keratosis with squamous cell carcinoma, Am J Pathol 94:193-196, 1979.

Lever WF and Schaumburg-Lever G: Histopathology of the skin, ed 7, Philadelphia, 1990, JB Lippincott, pp 542-546.

Madewell BR, Conroy JD, and Hodgkins EM: Sunlight-skin cancer association in the dog: a report of three cases, J Cut Pathol 8:434-443, 1981.

Mason KV: The pathogenesis of solar induced skin lesions in Bull Terriers. Proceedings of the American Academy of Veterinary Dermatology/American College of Veterinary Dermatology, Phoenix, 3:12, 1987.

Schwartz RA and Stoll HL: Epithelial precancerous lesions. In Fitzpatrick TB, Eisen AZ, Wolff K and others, editors: Dermatology in general medicine, ed 3, New York, 1987, McGraw-Hill, pp 733-746.

Acanthosis nigricans of Dachshunds

Anderson RK: Canine acanthosis nigricans, Comp Cont Ed 1:466-471, 1979.

Muller GH, Kirk RW, and Scott DW: Small animal dermatology, ed 4, Philadelphia, 1989, WB Saunders, pp 663-668.

Hyperplastic dermatosis of the West Highland White Terrier

Ihrke PJ: Canine seborrheic disease complex, Vet Clin North Am 9:93-106, 1979.

Power HT: The efficacy of etretinate (Tegison) in the treatment of keratinization disorders in dogs. Proceedings of the American Academy of Veterinary Dermatology/American College of Veterinary Dermatology, St Louis, 5:17, 1989.

Power HT and others: The use of etretinate (Tegison) for the treatment of primary keratinization disorders in Cocker Spaniels, West Highland White Terriers, and Basset Hounds, Manuscript for publication, 1992.

Scott DW and Miller WH: Epidermal dysplasia and *Malassezia pachydermatis* infection in West Highland White Terriers, Vet Dermatol 1:25-36, 1990.

Psoriasiform-lichenoid dermatosis of the Springer Spaniel

Gross TL and others: Psoriasiform lichenoid dermatitis in the Springer Spaniel, Vet Pathol 23:76-78, 1986.

Mason KV and others: Characterization of lichenoid-psoriasiform dermatosis of Springer Spaniels, J Am Vet Med Assoc 8:897-901, 1986.

Lichenoid keratosis

Anderson WI, Scott DW, and Luther PB: Idiopathic benign lichenoid keratosis on the pinna of the ear in four dogs, Cornell Vet 79:179-184, 1989.

Muller GH, Kirk RW, and Scott DW: Small animal dermatology, ed 4, Philadelphia, 1989, WB Saunders, p 941.

CHAPTER 7

Hyperkeratotic diseases
of the epidermis

Hyperkeratotic diseases are characterized by the diffuse accumulation of keratin on the epidermal surface and within superficial hair follicles. Most diseases of this group have a hereditary or metabolic disruption of normal keratinization. Hyperkeratosis or parakeratosis may be present. The epidermis and superficial follicular epithelium may be hyperplastic or of normal thickness; variation may depend in part upon the presence of inflammation.

Other diseases not included in this group may have hyperkeratosis or parakeratosis; for example, similar to sebaceous adenitis, some infectious inflammatory diseases that destroy sebaceous glands (demodicosis or leishmaniasis) can produce secondary hyperkeratosis. Diseases of abnormal follicular growth and differentiation, such as endocrine alopecia and follicular dysplasia, can result in follicular keratosis. Diffuse parakeratosis may be a feature of allergic conditions, such as canine sarcoptic acariasis, or any disease with significant spongiosis. The diseases included in this chapter have the abnormal accumulation of keratin as a predominant and primary pathologic feature.

PRIMARY SEBORRHEA
Clinical features (Figures 7-1 and 7-2)

Seborrhea is a confusing, nonspecific name that has been used to describe the clinical signs of excessive scaling, crusting, and greasiness. The terms *seborrhea sicca* and *seborrhea oleosa* have described the dry, waxy form and the oily form, respectively. Seborrhea has connoted both specific canine keratinization disorders, as well as the scaling and greasiness associated with a number of unrelated skin diseases such as hypothyroidism, demodicosis, sarcoptic acariasis, and flea allergy dermatitis (secondary seborrhea).

The term *primary seborrhea* is used more narrowly to describe inherited keratinization disorders seen in specific breeds of dogs. Keratinization is a series of genetically programmed events by which keratinocytes in the epidermal basal cell layer mature and die, producing the stratum corneum. Defects in this complicated process can lead to different keratinization disorders with variable clinical expression. The terms seborrhea sicca and seborrhea oleosa may still be useful in the clinical characterization of the various forms of primary seborrhea. Seborrheic dermatitis is an additional subgroup characterized by severely inflamed lesions of primary seborrhea (see discussion below).

Clinical signs commonly associated with keratinization disorders include variable scaling, crusting, dryness, waxiness, and oiliness of the skin and haircoat. A ceruminous or waxy otitis externa often is a concomitant feature. A rancid odor is a consistent

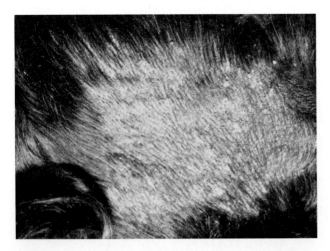

FIGURE 7-1. Primary seborrhea in a black Cocker Spaniel. The area shown has been clipped to allow better visualization of scales.

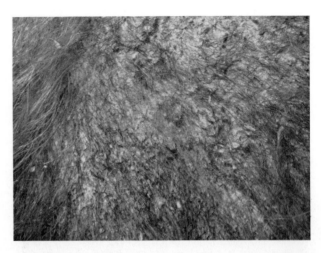

FIGURE 7-2. Severe primary seborrhea in a blond Cocker Spaniel. Adherent keratinous deposits mat the hair remaining within the partially alopecic lesion.

finding in the greasy forms of primary seborrhea. Erythema and alopecia are present in varying degrees in primary seborrhea. Lesions are most commonly located on the trunk. Focally severe lesions also may be present on the pinnae and preen gland. Pruritus is variable. Secondary pyoderma is common. Regional or generalized lymphadenopathy may be present in more severe cases.

Breeds affected include the Cocker Spaniel, English Springer Spaniel, Bassett Hound, Golden Retriever, and Chinese Shar Pei, which usually have seborrhea oleosa; and the Doberman Pinscher, Irish Setter, and German Shepherd Dog, which usually have seborrhea sicca. Seborrhea oleosa is seen most frequently and most severely in the Cocker Spaniel. Clinically similar lesions are seen in the West Highland White Terrier. However, differences in the histopathology of this disease preclude inclusion in the primary seborrhea group (see Chapter 6). Primary seborrhea usually is seen in adult dogs. Sex predilections have not been noted.

Clinical differential diagnoses for primary seborrhea are legion. Visually similar clinical signs are associated with endocrine abnormalities such as hypothyroidism or, less commonly, gonadal hormone aberrations. Clinically identical lesions of scaling and greasiness may be associated with fat deficiency, or, rarely, malabsorption or maldigestion. Scaling and crusting are seen with many other dermatoses, including ectoparasitism, pyoderma, dermatophytosis, autoimmune skin disease, neoplasia, and environmental influences such as dry heat.

Biopsy site selection

Care should be taken to sample lesions with ample and adherent scales and crusts. Since the histopathologic diagnosis depends on the appearance of the stratum corneum, the stratum corneum must be kept intact during biopsy. Severely inflamed lesions should be avoided, if possible, since secondary inflammatory changes may obscure the diagnosis.

Histopathology (Figure 7-3)

Difficulty in the histopathologic evaluation of primary seborrhea arises from the presence of secondary inflammation or seborrheic dermatitis (see following discussion). Seborrheic dermatitis can mimic chronic dermatitis of varying etiology, particularly allergic dermatitis or chronic pyoderma. Since these diseases may be present concurrently in dogs with seborrhea, the histopathologic picture can be very confusing. Thus, convincing evidence of primary seborrhea can often best be obtained from uninflamed skin lesions.

Histopathologic features described here for primary seborrhea are based principally on observation of the disease in the Cocker Spaniel and other spaniels. Hyperkeratosis is the principal feature of uncomplicated (uninflamed) primary seborrhea. Keratin is somewhat amorphous and loosely layered; the typical basket-weave appearance of normal keratin is absent. In Cocker Spaniels, there is often prominent keratin plugging of superficial follicles, which may result in distension of the infundibula, creating a pseudopapillomatous configuration. The epidermis may be normal or slightly acanthotic in uninflamed lesions.

FIGURE 7-3. Primary seborrhea in a Cocker Spaniel. Loosely organized keratin is accumulating on the surface of the skin and is distending the superficial hair follicles. (×100.)

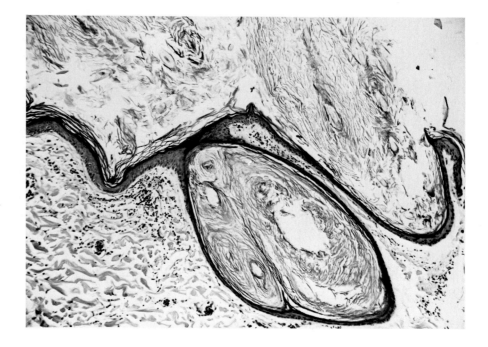

Dermal inflammation is minimal to absent in un-inflamed lesions of primary seborrhea. However, most cases also have lesions of seborrheic dermatitis (see discussion below).

In severe lesions of primary seborrhea with significant follicular keratosis, differentiation from vitamin A–responsive dermatosis must be made. Definitive differentiation between primary seborrhea and vitamin A–responsive dermatosis may be difficult; histologic similarity suggests etiopathogenic overlap of these two syndromes of abnormal keratinization.

Increased epidermal and follicular keratin also are found in many skin diseases, including endocrine dis-orders, follicular dysplasia, and inflammatory diseases that destroy sebaceous glands, such as sebaceous adenitis, demodicosis, and leishmaniasis. The histopathologic diagnosis of primary seborrhea must always be considered in light of the breed affected and concurrent histopathologic evidence of other cutaneous diseases.

SEBORRHEIC DERMATITIS
Clinical features (Figures 7-4 and 7-5)

The term seborrheic dermatitis has been used to describe visually distinctive lesions seen in some dogs with primary seborrhea. Lesions usually occur in dogs

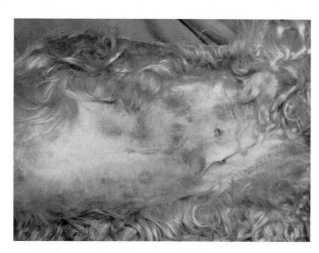

FIGURE 7-4. Seborrheic dermatitis on the ventrum of a blond Cocker Spaniel. Erythematous, well-demarcated, circular plaques with adherent keratinous debris are accompanied by hyperpigmentation.

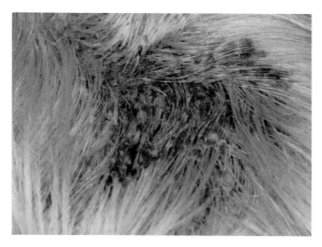

FIGURE 7-5. Seborrheic dermatitis on the lateral thorax of a blond Cocker Spaniel. Waxy keratinous deposits mat the haircoat.

with the greasy, more odoriferous form of seborrhea, termed seborrhea oleosa. Focally severe areas of abnormal keratinization may encourage inflammation, possibly via pruritus-induced self-trauma. Alternatively, some of the clinical and histopathologic differences noted may be due to secondary bacterial involvement. Quantitative and qualitative alteration in the surface lipid film and a subsequent overgrowth of staphylococci may contribute to the clinical signs of seborrheic dermatitis.

Multifocal lesions of seborrheic dermatitis usually are seen in dogs with generalized seborrhea. Erythematous, well-demarcated to coalescing, somewhat circular plaques are characteristic of seborrheic dermatitis. Adherent keratinous debris mats the surrounding hair and varies in color from yellow to brown and in texture from greasy to candle wax–like. Alopecia, lichenification, and hyperpigmentation may be evident in older lesions. Partial central clearing may occur. Lesions are located primarily on the thorax, especially ventrally. Occasionally, generalized seborrheic dermatitis is manifested by widespread erythema, crusting, and lichenification with less obvious plaque formation. Overt pyoderma may be evident. Pruritus is variable but usually is present.

Breed predilections parallel those for seborrhea oleosa (see previous discussion). Seborrheic dermatitis is seen with greatest frequency, and most severely, in the Cocker Spaniel. Adult dogs are affected most commonly and sex predilections have not been noted.

Seborrheic dermatitis should not be expected in dogs without primary seborrhea. Clinical differential diagnoses should include dermatophytosis and focal pyoderma. Vitamin A–responsive dermatosis is clinically similar but is characterized by frond-like follicular keratinous deposits (see later discussion).

Biopsy site selection

Multiple plaques of seborrheic dermatitis should be sampled. Care should be taken that adherent keratinous deposits are not dislodged during procurement.

Histopathology (Figure 7-6)

Seborrheic dermatitis is seen in conjunction with primary seborrhea. The inflammatory features of seborrheic dermatitis are essentially nondiagnostic; it is due to the coexistence of primary seborrhea that a diagnosis of seborrheic dermatitis can be made histopathologically.

There is moderate to severe acanthosis and hyperkeratosis, accompanied by discrete, mound-shaped areas of parakeratosis and crusting. These parakeratotic foci form commonly at the openings ("shoulders") of follicular ostia, particularly in Cocker Spaniels, and have been termed *follicular epaulets*. The formation of follicular epaulets may be the most distinctive histopathologic feature of seborrheic dermatitis, at least in the Cocker Spaniel. Follicular keratosis is the same as that seen in primary seborrhea but may be accompanied by infundibular parakeratosis.

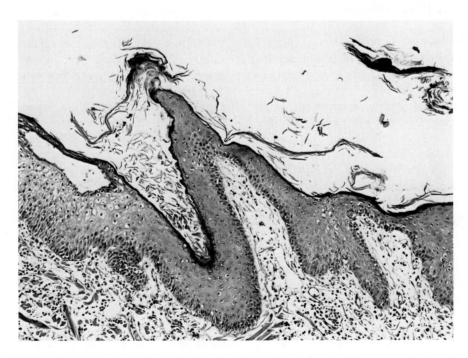

FIGURE 7-6. Seborrheic dermatitis in a dog. Note the parakeratosis in a mound at the edge of a follicular ostium, acanthosis, and superficial dermal inflammation. (×90.)

Dermal inflammation is mixed and variable. Superficial perivascular to interstitial inflammation is composed of a mixed population of cells, including lymphocytes, plasma cells, macrophages, and variable neutrophils. Inflammation often extends around adnexal appendages.

The diagnosis of seborrheic dermatitis should not be difficult if concurrent lesions of primary seborrhea are found; similarly, the diagnosis of seborrheic derma-

titis should not be expected in dogs without primary seborrhea. If typical epidermal and follicular hyperkeratosis is minimal in the specimens available, it may be impossible to separate the lesions of seborrheic dermatitis from those of other chronic dermatitides, particularly chronic superficial spreading pyoderma, and chronic allergic dermatitis. In fact, seborrheic dermatitis may represent secondary pyoderma superimposed upon primary seborrhea, at least in part.

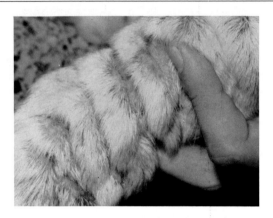

FIGURE 7-7. Seborrheic dermatitis and *Malassezia pachydermatis* infection on the forelimb of a Basset Hound. The affected skin folds are alopecic, erythematous, and exudative.

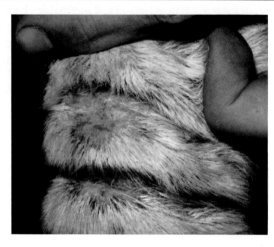

FIGURE 7-8. Closer view of the dog in Fig. 7-7. Exudate is present in the alopecic skin folds.

SEBORRHEIC DERMATITIS AND *MALASSEZIA PACHYDERMATIS* INFECTION

Clinical features (Figures 7-7 and 7-8)

Lesions clinically resembling seborrheic dermatitis have been seen in dogs and are believed to be due to *Malassezia pachydermatis* infection. However, *Malassezia pachydermatis* (formerly *Pityrosporum canis*), a putatively commensal organism, can also be isolated from the ears and skin of dogs and cats without skin disease. Reports indicate that this syndrome is rare. In humans, abnormal selective cell-mediated immune dysfunction has been documented in individuals suffering from recurrent tinea versicolor, a *Pityrosporum orbiculare* infection. A similar selective immunodeficiency in the dog might explain the apparent selective pathogenicity of this ubiquitous, usually commensal organism. Although reports of clinical cure in response to therapy with ketoconazole imply a lack of preexisting disease or other predisposing factors, the authors are suspicious that long-term follow-up may show recrudescence. A possible breed predilection in the Dachshund also suggests that a common, as yet unidentified, predisposing factor, such as genetically determined selective immu-

nodeficiency, may play a role in *Malassezia pachydermatis* infection.

Clinical signs include a generalized, erythematous, mildly exfoliative dermatitis. Focal plaques of slate-colored scale resemble seborrheic dermatitis. Lesions are localized to the chestwall, axillae, groin, and other skin folds. In the Dachshund, lesions restricted to the skin folds on the legs have been seen. Pruritus of variable intensity is a consistent feature.

Dachshunds may be at increased risk. Age or sex predilections have not been noted.

Clinical differential diagnoses include generalized keratinization disorders with seborrheic dermatitis and superficial pyoderma. Identification of the organism via skin scraping, culture, and histopathology, as well as response to appropriate therapy, may allow differentiation.

Biopsy site selection

Selection of an erythematous plaque with marked scaling and crusting is preferred as these lesions are more likely to harbor organisms. Care should be taken to retain scale and crusts during procurement.

FIGURE 7-9. Seborrheic dermatitis and *Malassezia pachydermatis* infection in a dog, showing hyperkeratosis and parakeratotic crust. Numerous yeast organisms are accumulating within the keratin layer *(arrows)*. (×220.)

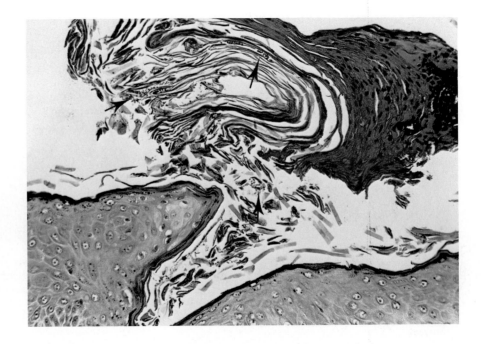

Histopathology (Figures 7-9 and 7-10)

Hyperkeratosis, parakeratosis and acanthosis are similar to primary seborrhea and seborrheic dermatitis (see preceding discussion). Spongiosis is variable and spongiotic pustules may be seen. Hyperkeratosis is interspersed with mounds of parakeratosis or parakeratotic crusts. Numerous budding oval or peanut-shaped *Malassezia* yeasts are embedded in keratin or crusts, but are more easily visualized in keratin. A periodic acid–Schiff stain will accentuate the presence of these organisms and allow easier assessment of their numbers. *Malassezia pachydermatis* may not be present diffusely in the stratum corneum, but the organisms may be seen in randomly distributed, focal accumulations within superficial keratin, including in follicular infundibula.

Dermal inflammation usually is mild and is composed of a variable mixture of neutrophils, lymphocytes, plasma cells, mast cells, macrophages, and occasionally eosinophils. Occasionally, there is mild inflammation around adnexa.

A diagnosis should not be made unless organisms are seen in at least moderate numbers (three to five per 40X field within focal areas of involvement). Even so, a definitive etiologic diagnosis based on histopathology alone should be approached with caution. Response to therapy and absence of other skin disease may be required to confirm a pathogenic role for this organism in the skin. *Malassezia pachydermatis* colonization has been reported by Scott in the West Highland White Terrier. (See hyperplastic dermatosis of the West Highland White Terrier in Chapter 6.)

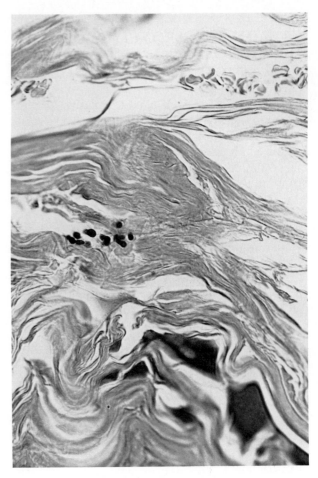

FIGURE 7-10. *Malassezia pachydermatis* within superficial keratin. (Periodic acid–Schiff stain; ×800.)

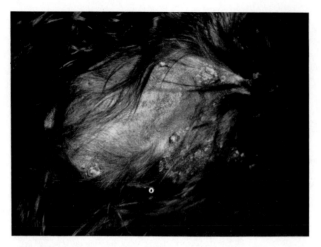

FIGURE 7-11. Vitamin A–responsive dermatosis in a black Cocker Spaniel Dog. Multifocal, well-demarcated, alopecic and scaly plaques are present on the ventral abdomen. *(From Ihrke PJ and Goldschmidt MH: Vitamin A-responsive dermatosis in the dog, J Am Vet Med Assoc 182:688, 1983. Reprinted by permission.)*

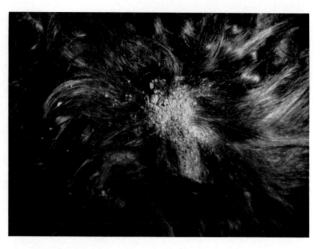

FIGURE 7-12. Closer view of the dog in Fig. 7-11. Follicular fronds are emerging from dilated hair follicles. *(From Ihrke PJ and Goldschmidt MH: Vitamin A-responsive dermatosis in the dog, J Am Vet Med Assoc 182:688, 1983. Reprinted by permission.)*

VITAMIN A–RESPONSIVE DERMATOSIS
Clinical features (Figures 7-11 and 7-12)

Vitamin A–responsive dermatosis is a rare canine keratinization defect seen almost exclusively in the Cocker Spaniel. Marked breed predilection and features in common with other primary keratinization defects suggest a hereditary basis. The relationship between this syndrome and primary seborrhea in the Cocker Spaniel is unclear, since the retinoids (synthetic vitamin A derivatives) have recently been shown to be efficacious in the management of the latter disease.

Vitamin A–responsive dermatosis is characterized by multifocal, alopecic, well-demarcated, erythematous plaques. Severe follicular plugging with tenacious frond-like keratinous debris ("follicular fronds" or "follicular casts") is a characteristic feature. Follicular papules with varying degrees of scaling, crusting, and alopecia are seen in the surrounding skin. Lesions are most prominent on the ventral chest and abdomen. Although most affected dogs have a somewhat dry, dull, disheveled haircoat, generalized primary seborrhea is not seen. A concomitant ceruminous otitis with a rancid "seborrheic" odor may be present.

This syndrome is seen almost exclusively in Cocker Spaniels, but has been identified in other breeds such as the Miniature Schnauzer. Age or sex predilections have not been noted.

The major clinical differential diagnoses are primary seborrhea with seborrheic dermatitis, as seen in Cocker Spaniels. Vitamin A–responsive dermatosis presents as a predominantly ventral, more focal disease that has prominent follicular keratinous deposits.

Biopsy site selection

A plaque with prominent follicular casting should be sampled. Care must be taken so that adherent keratinous debris is not dislodged from the specimen during biopsy.

Histopathology (Figures 7-13 and 7-14)

Severe follicular keratosis is the histopathologic hallmark of vitamin A–responsive dermatosis. Similar follicular lesions occur in vitamin A deficiency in humans and are termed *phrynoderma.* Keratin accumulation in superficial follicles is significantly more severe than in primary seborrhea (see earlier discussion). Distension of follicular ostia and protrusion of massive plugs of keratin (follicular fronds) above the surface of the epidermis are seen. Adjacent dilated follicular infundibula may be mistaken for an uneven or papillated epidermal surface.

Epidermal hyperkeratosis accompanies the follicular changes. The epidermis is mildly to moderately acanthotic. Dermal inflammation varies from minimal to moderate and may resemble the dermal component of seborrheic dermatitis (see earlier discussion).

Differential diagnosis includes primary seborrhea and late-stage sebaceous adenitis. Sebaceous glands are uniformly absent in sebaceous adenitis. Definitive differentiation between primary seborrhea and vitamin A–responsive dermatosis may be difficult; histopathologic similarity suggests etiopathogenic overlap of these two syndromes of abnormal keratinization.

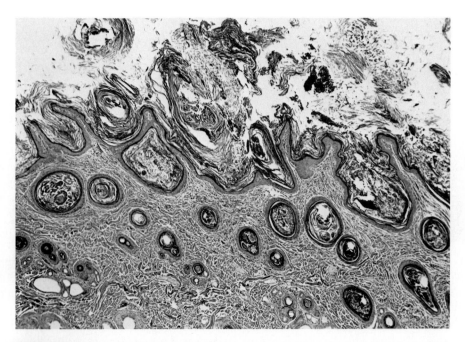

FIGURE 7-13. Vitamin A–responsive dermatosis in a Schnauzer. Note the massive distension of the follicular infundibula with keratin. (×35.)

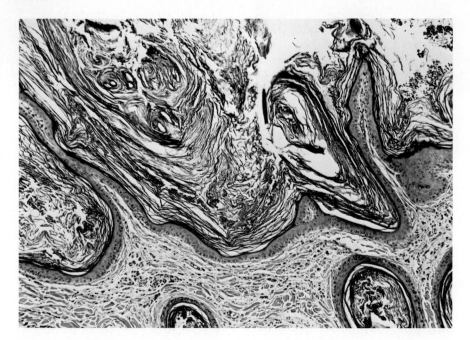

FIGURE 7-14. Higher magnification of keratin-distended follicles shown in Figure 7-13. (×90.)

CANINE EAR MARGIN SEBORRHEA
Clinical features (Figures 7-15 and 7-16)

Canine ear margin seborrhea is a relatively common, aurally confined keratinization defect. Marked breed predilection and features in common with other primary keratinization defects suggest a hereditary basis.

Adherent keratinous deposits are present on both the lateral and medial margins of the pinna. Consider-

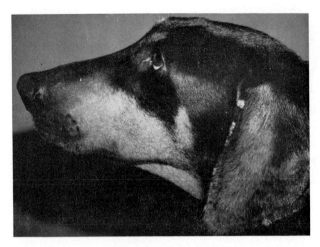

FIGURE 7-15. Ear margin seborrhea in a Doberman Pinscher. Adherent keratinous deposits are present on the partially alopecic margin of the pinna. *(Courtesy HT Power, Santa Cruz, California; case material from the University of California, Davis.)*

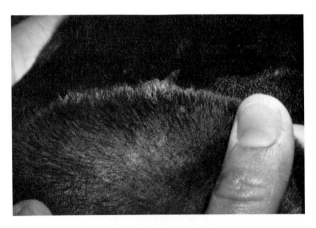

FIGURE 7-16. Closer view of the pinna of the dog in Fig. 7-15. Keratinous deposits entrap hair on the margin of the partially alopecic pinna. *(Courtesy HT Power, Santa Cruz, California; case material from the University of California, Davis.)*

able variation occurs in the character and color of the keratinous accumulations, which vary from greasy to waxy, tenacious to exfoliative, and yellow to brown. Follicular casts or plugs sometimes entrap hair. Partial alopecia of the pinnal margin is common and keratin mats the remaining hair. A waxy, seborrheic odor often is present. The syndrome usually is asymptomatic although pruritus may be seen.

Canine ear margin seborrhea is seen most commonly in Dachshunds, although it may be seen in other breeds of dogs with pendulous ears. Age or sex predilections have not been noted.

Clinical differential diagnoses should include early vasculitis or vasculopathy of the pinnal margin (initially characterized by scaling and hair loss) and early, localized canine sarcoptic acariasis. Vascular diseases cause

some tissue destruction even in the early stages and canine scabies is very pruritic, in contrast to ear margin seborrhea.

Biopsy site selection

A small portion of the margin of the pinna with adherent keratinous deposits should be sampled. Surprisingly good cosmetic acceptability, as well as a representative specimen are obtained when a single-edged razor blade or a scalpel blade is used to amputate a thin or small portion of the rounded edge of the pinna. Care should be taken not to dislodge attached keratinous material.

Histopathology (Figure 7-17)

Ear margin seborrhea is characterized by severe hyperkeratosis and follicular keratosis. Keratin distends follicular ostia and may give the epidermal surface a pronounced pseudopapillomatous appearance. Parakeratosis is variable. Acanthosis is mild to moderate and may not be present diffusely within the specimen.

Superficial perivascular to interstitial, mixed inflammation is variable and may be absent. The inflammatory infiltrate may include lymphocytes, macrophages, and variable neutrophils.

Lesions resemble primary seborrhea or seborrheic dermatitis (see earlier discussion). Differentiation requires knowledge of the location of the clinical lesions.

SCHNAUZER COMEDO SYNDROME
Clinical features

Schnauzer comedo syndrome is a relatively common, usually asymptomatic, skin disease seen exclusively in Miniature Schnauzers. The specific breed predilection is a likely indicator of heritability. Clinical and histopathologic features indicate that this syndrome may be a follicular keratinization defect. Muller, Kirk, and Scott suggest that the syndrome may be due to a developmental dysplasia of hair follicles similar to nevus comedonicus in humans.

Substantial variation in the character and severity of clinical lesions is seen among individual dogs. Lesions may be palpable rather than visual. Occasionally, the principal change is a dorsal band of darkly colored or diffusely erect hair. Crusted papules, small nodules, or frank comedones are associated with hair follicles. Comedones may not appear grossly follicular if the follicular ostia are not dilated. This leads to the visual impression of dense, dark material accumulating in discrete foci beneath the epidermis. Comedones may be very small and require use of a hand lens for identification. More obvious comedones are characterized by peripherally inflamed, dilated hair follicles that contain inspissated, dark, keratinous or caseous debris that may

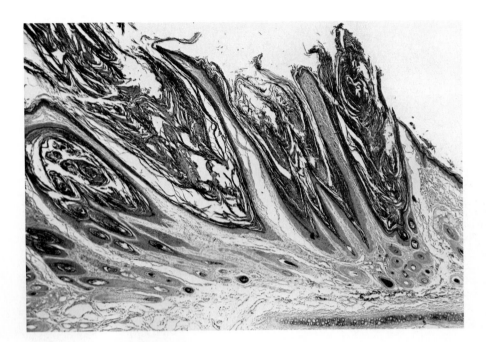

FIGURE 7-17. Ear margin
seborrhea in a dog demonstrating pronounced follicular keratosis. (×22.)

be extruded with digital pressure. Hair is lost from
severely affected follicles. Scaling and erythema are
variable but usually mild. Occasionally, a secondary
bacterial folliculitis accompanied by erythema and scarring is observed. Lesions occur along the midspinal
area from the shoulders to the sacrum, usually within 3
cm of the spine. Pruritus is uncommon.

Schnauzer comedo syndrome is seen only in Miniature Schnauzers and their related crossbreeds. Age or
sex predilections have not been reported. Differential
diagnosis is not problematic because Schnauzer
comedo syndrome is a visually distinctive disease.

Biopsy site selection

Multiple specimens should be taken from severe
skin lesions. Skin biopsy of larger persistent comedones
may be curative for individual more troublesome lesions. If present, pustules should be obtained to confirm the presence of secondary pyoderma.

Histopathology (Figures 7-18 and 7-19)

In Schnauzer comedo syndrome, comedo forma-
tion, or distension of superficial hair follicles with keratin, is the diagnostic histopathologic feature. The size
of the follicular ostium may remain nearly normal,

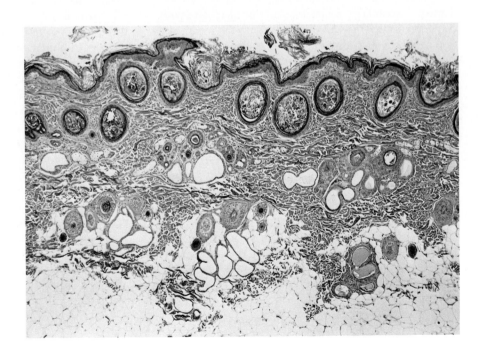

FIGURE 7-18. Schnauzer
comedo syndrome showing diffuse distension of the follicular
infundibula with keratin.
(×22.)

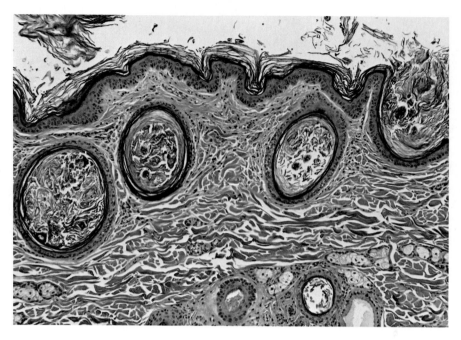

FIGURE 7-19. Higher magnification of the comedones shown in Fig. 7-18. Note the normal keratinization of the epidermis. (×90.)

resulting in a cystic (comedonal) appearance of the keratin-dilated infundibulum. The follicular infundibular wall is generally of normal thickness to moderately acanthotic. Epidermal hyperkeratosis usually is absent to mild. Superficial crusting, originating from secondary pyoderma, may be prominent. Acanthosis is moderate to severe and varies with the degree of secondary inflammation present.

Most specimens submitted for skin biopsy are inflamed. Secondary folliculitis or furunculosis with comedo rupture may be observed. Pustular inflammation may be loosely distributed in the superficial dermis and may involve apocrine sweat glands in severe cases. Chronic lesions have mixtures of neutrophils, macrophages, and plasma cells in superficial and periadnexal distribution.

Comedo formation in Schnauzer comedo syndrome is in contrast to the follicular keratosis of primary seborrhea. In primary seborrhea, follicular ostia are dilated by infundibular engorgement with keratin, whereas in Schnauzer comedo syndrome, follicular ostia remain relatively closed. Other skin diseases with comedo formation include iatrogenic hyperglucocorticoidism, hyperadrenocorticism, and actinic comedones. In diseases of glucocorticoid excess, there is accompanying follicular atrophy and thinning of the infundibular wall. In actinic comedones, a pale concentric layer of collagen usually surrounds the distended

follicle. Clinical features and breed affected also will differentiate Schnauzer comedo syndrome from other skin diseases with histopathologic similarities.

ICHTHYOSIS (Synonym: fish-scale disease)
Clinical features (Figures 7-20 and 7-21)

Ichthyosis is a very rare congenital, hereditary skin disease that has been reported in the dog. Clinical and histopathologic similarities exist between canine ichthyosis and a heterogeneous group of heritable skin diseases in humans termed ichthyosis or ichthyosiform dermatoses. Four principal types of ichthyosis are recognized in humans: ichthyosis vulgaris, X-linked ichthyosis, epidermolytic hyperkeratosis, and lamellar (autosomal recessive) ichthyosis. These genetically and histopathologically diverse skin diseases are united by the common clinical characteristic of the accumulation of large amounts of scale on the surface of the skin. The few cases seen of canine ichthyosis appear to bear closest resemblance to lamellar ichthyosis in humans. Further investigation in the dog also may reveal several heritable forms of ichthyosis.

Tightly adherent, parchment-like, gray or light brown scales cover most areas of the body. Coarse scales give the skin surface a rough, irregular texture that enhances the normal skin markings. These coarse scales are similar visually to dried mud in an empty

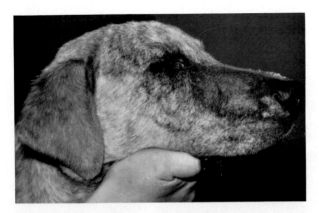

FIGURE 7-20. Canine ichthyosis in a yellow Labrador Retriever. Tightly adherent scales entrap hairs.

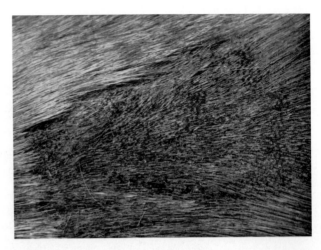

FIGURE 7-21. Closer view of the dog in Fig. 7-20. The affected area was clipped to show the adherent keratinous deposits.

river bed. The haircoat may be sparse and remaining hair is bound in the keratinous deposits. A hand lens may show crateriform enlargements of follicular ostia. Lamellar keratinous projections are prominent, especially on flexural surfaces. Fissures develop in the areas of thickest scale accumulation. Keratinous deposits are shed continuously.

The footpads also are affected as thick deposits build up, fissure, and are shed. Excess keratinous material extends outward from the margins of the pads. The hard keratin of the nails may be affected. Fissuring on the pads and elsewhere leads to secondary bacterial infection. Lymphadenopathy may occur, especially if secondary bacterial infection is present.

Breeds that have been noted to develop ichthyosis include the West Highland White Terrier, Doberman Pinscher, Irish Setter, Collie, Bull Terrier, Boston Terrier, Labrador Retriever, Jack Russell Terrier, and mixed-breed dogs. Most cases of canine ichthyosis have been reported as present from birth. Sex predilections have not been noted.

Clinical differential diagnoses for ichthyosis could include diseases that may exhibit prominent scaling and exfoliation such as primary seborrhea, hyperplastic dermatosis of the West Highland White Terrier, sebaceous adenitis, demodicosis, and dermatophytosis. However, since ichthyosis is a congenital disease, presence of the disease at birth or shortly after birth is a principal differentiating feature. If an adult dog is examined without benefit of historical information regarding age of onset, diagnostic evaluation should include skin scrapings, fungal cultures, and skin biopsy. Histopathology is necessary to confirm a diagnosis of ichthyosis.

Biopsy site selection

Areas of most prominent scaling should be selected, and care should be taken not to dislodge the keratin during procurement of the specimen for biopsy. Multiple specimens should be taken, and ideally skin from an age-matched, breed-matched control also should be sampled.

Histopathology (Figures 7-22 and 7-23)

Most subgroups of ichthyosis in humans exhibit hyperkeratosis. The appearance of the granular layer is variable and may be thickened to absent. The epidermis is of normal thickness to slightly acanthotic. Epidermal vacuolation is seen in epidermolytic hyperkeratosis of humans.

In the few cases of ichthyosis observed by the authors, there is compact hyperkeratosis with mild to moderate acanthosis. Follicular infundibula are affected; hair shafts remain normal and are ensheathed by keratin as they penetrate to the surface. The granular layer is normal to slightly thickened. Scott has described both hypergranulosis and hypogranulosis, in addition to epidermal vacuolation; it is likely that several histopathologic forms exist, as in humans.

Differential diagnoses principally include primary seborrhea. In general, the hyperkeratosis of ichthyosis is more compact than that of primary seborrhea. The onset predominantly in young puppies will allow differentiation of ichthyosis from other hyperkeratotic disorders.

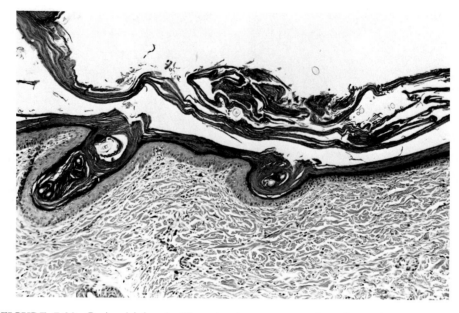

FIGURE 7-22. Canine ichthyosis. Note the dense, compact hyperkeratosis and follicular keratosis. (×90.)

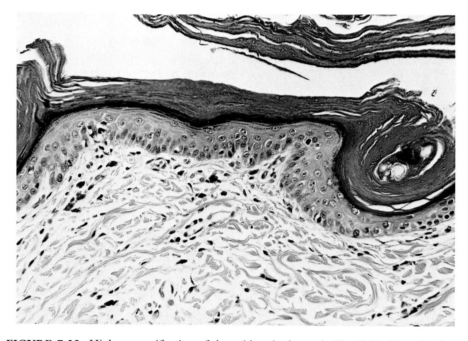

FIGURE 7-23. Higher magnification of the epidermis shown in Fig. 7-22. Note the dense keratin layer, mild acanthosis, and mild hypergranulosis. (×220.)

SEBACEOUS ADENITIS
Clinical features (Figures 7-24 and 7-25)

Sebaceous adenitis is an uncommon canine skin disease of uncertain etiology. A single case of feline sebaceous adenitis has been reported by Scott. Strong breed predilections for clinically and histopathologi-

cally similar but distinct subgroups of sebaceous adenitis suggest a genetic basis. An autoimmune cause also has been suggested. Scaling and follicular plugging, the salient clinical features, probably occur as nonspecific sequelae to the cessation of sebum flow resultant from sebaceous gland inflammation and ablation. Similar secondary hyperkeratosis is seen associated with seba-

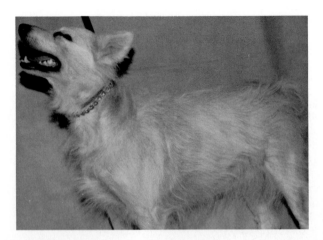

FIGURE 7-24. Sebaceous adenitis in an adult Samoyed. The thinned haircoat is short and disheveled.

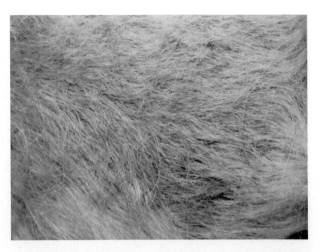

FIGURE 7-25. Closer view of the dog in Fig. 7-24, demonstrating adherent scale. Note the coarse, dry appearance of the remaining haircoat.

ceous gland destruction in generalized demodicosis and cutaneous leishmaniasis. Follicular atrophy or dysplasia may be seen in advanced cases of sebaceous adenitis. It is not clear if there is a causal relationship between loss of sebaceous glands and the development of abnormal follicular maturation, or if these are simply coexistent features of a common inheritable process.

Clinical signs, distribution, and severity of the disease vary substantially among different breeds of dogs. Adherent scale, sometimes forming follicular casts or fronds, is the unifying feature. Coat quality diminishes as the disease progresses, leaving dull, dry, brittle, broken hairs.

In Standard Poodles, keratinous deposits resembling candle-wax drippings that occur on the dorsal muzzle may be the earliest sign. Severe, adherent scale with progressive alopecia is seen in a predominantly dorsal distribution. Frond-like, protruding, keratinous casts may emanate from dilated hair follicles and tenacious keratinous debris ensheathes hairs. Similar lesions to those of the Standard Poodle, but with greater tendency toward plaque formation, are seen in the Samoyed.

In Akitas, lesions are similar to those of Standard Poodles, with the additional feature of more complete alopecia, especially of the secondary hairs. Secondary superficial bacterial folliculitis or deep bacterial folliculitis and furunculosis, manifested as papules, pustules, or nodules, is a prominent feature of sebaceous adenitis in this breed. Fever, malaise, and weight loss may be present as additional, as yet unexplained, systemic features of this disorder.

A markedly different clinical presentation is noted in the Vizsla and occasionally in other short-coated breeds. Focal coalescing nodular lesions and plaques with alopecia and adherent scale are seen predominantly on the trunk.

Strong breed predilections have been noted for Standard Poodles, Samoyeds, Akitas, and Viszlas. However, other purebred dogs (Old English Sheepdog, Toy Poodle, English Springer Spaniel, Lhasa Apso, Boxer, Belgian Sheepdog, Chow Chow, Collie) and mixed-breed dogs have been documented. Young adult dogs most commonly are affected. Sex predilections have not been noted.

Biopsy site selection

Multiple specimens are recommended so that more adnexal units may be observed. Subtle early lesions characterized by adherent scale without alopecia are most useful for documenting active sebaceous gland inflammation. Chronic lesions with extensive alopecia commonly show an absence of sebaceous glands without significant inflammation; multiple specimens are essential to document the widespread absence of sebaceous glands and therefore confirm the diagnosis of sebaceous adenitis.

Histopathology (Figure 7-26)

Most cases exhibit moderate acanthosis and generally severe hyperkeratosis with follicular plugging. Protruding follicular casts of keratin, or follicular fronds, may be prominent, particularly in Standard Poodles. Severe follicular keratosis of this type should always be a signal to the pathologist to search for lesions of the sebaceous glands.

Random sampling of affected dogs (that are most often presented to the practitioner with late-stage dis-

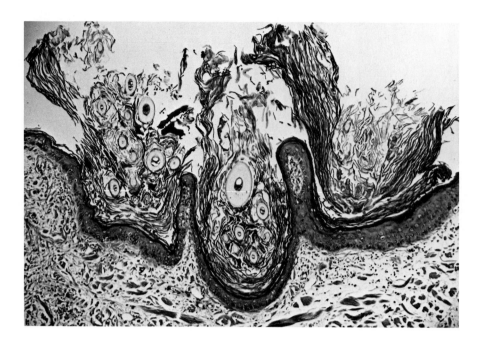

FIGURE 7-26. Sebaceous adenitis in a dog. Hair shafts are engulfed by keratin in the formation of follicular fronds. (×95.)

ease) indicates that diffuse absence of sebaceous glands is the principle histopathologic feature of the chronic disease. A diagnosis of sebaceous adenitis should not be made unless sebaceous glands are completely absent from at least three 4- to 6-mm punch specimens. Associated inflammation is variable (see Chapter 15) and depends on the breed affected and the stage of the disease.

Differential diagnosis of the epidermal lesions includes primary seborrhea or vitamin A–responsive dermatosis. The associated absence of sebaceous glands is the prime differential feature of sebaceous adenitis;

knowledge of the breed affected also allows differentiation from primary keratinization disorders in most cases.

ZINC-RESPONSIVE DERMATOSIS
Clinical features (Figures 7-27 and 7-28)

Zinc-responsive dermatosis is a nutritional skin disease seen uncommonly in the dog. The term *nutrient-responsive dermatosis* is used to encompass syndromes characterized by nutrient deficiency, nutrient imbalances, or the genetic inability to absorb or metabolize a nutrient. Zinc-responsive dermatosis may encompass all three etiologic categories.

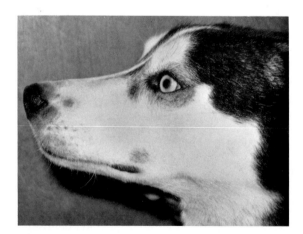

FIGURE 7-27. Zinc-responsive dermatosis in a Siberian Husky. Alopecia, scaling, and crusting are present near the mucocutaneous junctions of the eye, mouth and planum nasale.

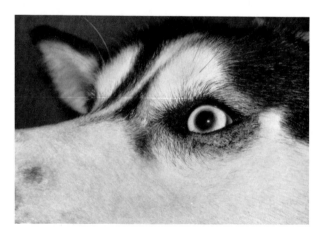

FIGURE 7-28. Closer view of the dog in Fig. 7-27. Crusts adhere to the skin beneath the eye.

Two disease subgroups are reported. Syndrome I, seen primarily in Siberian Huskies and Alaskan Malamutes (also recognized rarely in Great Danes and Doberman Pinschers), may be due to an inheritable impairment in the absorption or metabolism of zinc. This subgroup of zinc-responsive dermatosis is characterized clinically by scaling, crusting, and alopecia. Secondary pyoderma characterized by exudation or suppuration may be present. The most common sites are the perioral and periorbital skin, ears, scrotum, vulva, and perianal area. Pressure points and footpad margins also may be affected. This syndrome may be seen in either puppies or adult dogs.

Syndrome II is seen in rapidly growing large-breed puppies receiving zinc-deficient rations or fed a diet oversupplemented with calcium and other minerals and vitamins. Crusted plaques with erosions or ulcers are seen on the mucocutaneous junctions, planum nasale, footpads, and pressure points. Some dogs have constitutional signs such as anorexia and depression, whereas others have only skin disease; this range of clinical signs may be explained by variability in the severity of zinc deficiency or the presence of a combined trace mineral deficiency. (See following discussion on generic dog food dermatosis.)

Depending on clinical presentation, the differential diagnoses should include superficial necrolytic dermatitis, generic dog food dermatosis, autoimmune skin diseases such as pemphigus foliaceus and systemic lupus erythematosus, demodicosis, dermatophytosis, and pyoderma. Differentiation requires skin scrapings, chemistry screening profiles, fungal culture, an ANA test, and histopathology.

Biopsy site selection

Areas of most severe crusting and scaling should be obtained to maximize epidermal lesions available for histopathologic examination. Care should be taken to avoid areas of erosion or ulceration, since an intact epidermis is necessary to establish a diagnosis.

Histopathology (Figures 7-29 and 7-30)

Moderate to severe acanthosis is present. Parakeratosis may be mild and multifocal to diffuse and moderate. Extension of parakeratosis into hyperplastic follicular infundibula is a characteristic histopathologic feature of zinc-responsive dermatosis. Surprisingly, parakeratosis was not found in two of five dogs with zinc deficiency reported by Van Den Broek.

Serocellular crusting with erosion is variable and may be severe, effacing the parakeratotic layer. Occasionally, dyskeratosis of keratinocytes is seen just beneath the parakeratotic layer. Mild to moderate diffuse spongiosis is present and may also affect superficial follicles. Dermal inflammation is superficial or perivascular to interstitial and comprises lymphocytes, macro-

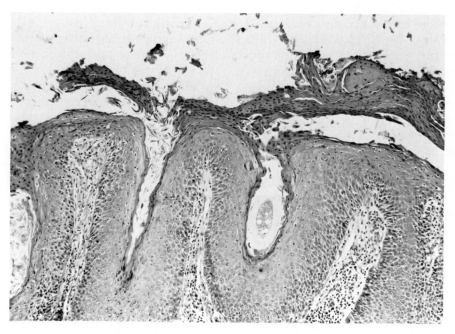

FIGURE 7-29. Zinc-responsive dermatosis in a Siberian Husky. Parakeratosis overlies an acanthotic and spongiotic epidermis, and there is similar involvement of the follicular infundibula. Note the superficial dermal inflammation. (×90.)

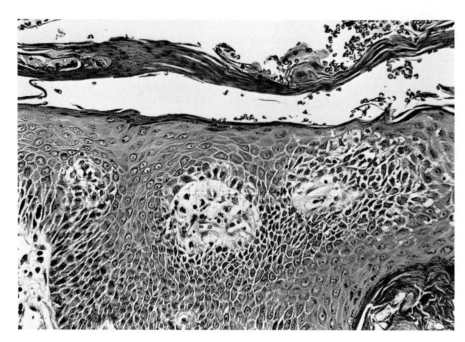

FIGURE 7-30. Higher magnification of zinc-responsive dermatosis in a Siberian Husky, demonstrating spongiosis and parakeratosis. (×220.)

phages, eosinophils, and neutrophils. Inflammation may extend around subjacent adnexal appendages.

Parakeratosis may be a feature of spongiotic inflammation in general, such as that provoked by allergic skin diseases, particularly canine sarcoptic acariasis. Parakeratosis usually is patchy in distribution in allergic skin diseases, but this feature may not always allow differentiation from zinc-responsive dermatosis. Clinical differentiation may be required. Lesions of zinc-responsive dermatosis may resemble chronic lesions of superficial necrolytic dermatitis where parakeratosis is present and necrolysis is absent. Clinical evidence of hepatic disease or diabetes may be required to differentiate chronic superficial necrolytic dermatitis from zinc-responsive dermatosis. Zinc-responsive dermatosis resembles generic dog food dermatosis; however, generic dog food dermatosis generally has superficial epidermal edema or necrolysis in addition to parakeratosis. Zinc-responsive dermatosis also resembles lethal acrodermatitis; however, parakeratosis in lethal acrodermatitis is usually more severe.

GENERIC DOG FOOD DERMATOSIS
Clinical features (Figures 7-31 and 7-32)

Generic dog food dermatosis is a syndrome associated with the exclusive feeding of poor-quality dog food. The frequency of occurrence of this syndrome is controversial. In parts of the world where dogs are fed either good-quality food developed and manufactured

specifically for dogs or balanced diets prepared for human consumption, nutritional skin diseases are uncommon. In other circumstances, where there is feeding of commercial or home-prepared diets that are deficient in nutrients, vitamins, or trace minerals, this dermatosis may be more common. The systemic signs of fever, depression, dependent edema, and lymphadenopathy (coupled with histopathologic findings beyond those seen with zinc-responsive dermatosis) lead one to suspect a deficiency of multiple trace minerals, vitamins, or amino acids. For example, since copper and zinc are required for proper keratinization, conceivably this syndrome could be associated, at least in part, with a combined zinc and copper deficiency.

Clinical signs closely parallel those of dogs that have the more severe manifestations of zinc-responsive dermatosis, syndrome II. Eroded and ulcerated, fissured, well-demarcated annular plaques have an erythematous border and are covered by thick, adherent crusts. Lesions are seen on the muzzle, mucocutaneous junctions, pressure points, and distal extremities. Pain is evident. Lymphadenopathy is common.

Most affected dogs have been less than 1 year of age and in their rapid growth phase. Adult dogs also have been seen occasionally with this syndrome. Dogs in a multiple-dog household being fed the same ration have developed generic dog food dermatosis; however, other dogs in the same environment and fed the same ration have remained normal. Breed or sex predilections have not been noted.

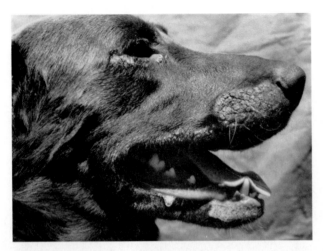

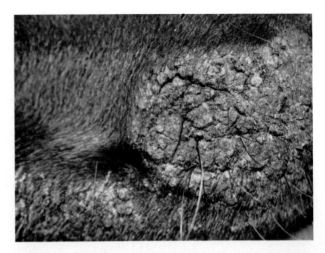

FIGURE 7-31. Generic dog food dermatosis in an adult Chesapeake Bay Retriever. Crusting, scaling, and alopecia are present around the mouth and eye. *(From Sousa CA and others: Dermatosis associated with feeding generic dog food: 13 cases (1981-1982), J Am Vet Med Assoc 192:677, 1983. Reprinted by permission.)*

FIGURE 7-32. Closer view of the dog in Fig. 7-31. Thick, adherent crusts entrap the remaining hair near the mucocutaneous junction of the upper lip.

Clinical differential diagnoses should include zinc-responsive dermatosis, superficial necrolytic dermatitis, autoimmune skin diseases such as pemphigus foliaceus and systemic lupus erythematosus, demodicosis, dermatophytosis, and pyoderma. Generic dog food dermatosis usually is seen in puppies in their rapid growth phase. Differentiation may require skin scrapings, chemistry screening profiles, fungal culture, an ANA test, and histopathology.

Biopsy site selection

Skin biopsy specimens should be obtained from large, annular, and crusted plaques. Areas of erosion and ulceration should be avoided, since an intact epidermis is necessary to establish the diagnosis.

Histopathology (Figures 7-33 and 7-34)

The epidermis is moderately to severely acanthotic. Parakeratosis is moderate and may be interspersed with layers of hyperkeratosis and crusting. In some cases, there is abrupt transition of the superficial epidermis to

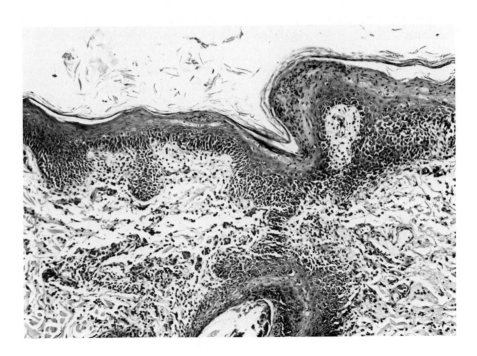

FIGURE 7-33. Generic dog food dermatosis, demonstrating superficial parakeratosis with crusting, subjacent mild epidermal edema and degeneration, and deep spongiosis. (×90.)

FIGURE 7-34. Higher magnification of the epidermis of a dog with generic dog food dermatosis. Superficial crusting and parakeratosis overlie laminar edema and ballooning degeneration of the epidermis. (×220.)

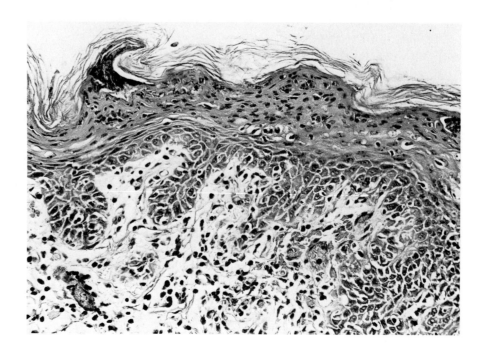

a uniform, eosinophilic layer of compact parakeratosis. Dyskeratosis, characterized by premature keratinization of individual superficial keratinocytes, may be evident. Prominent laminar edema and necrolysis of the superficial epidermis are often observed. The epidermis also may appear slightly dysplastic, characterized by slight loss of normal stratification and uneven size of keratinocytic nuclei. Mild to moderate deep spongiosis may be accompanied by exocytosis of lymphocytes, macrophages, and neutrophils. Epidermal lesions often extend to superficial hair follicles. Intraluminal accumulation of degenerating neutrophils, as well as frank pustular folliculitis are seen. The superficial dermis contains plasma cells, lymphocytes, neutrophils, mast cells, macrophages, and melanophages.

The major histopathologic differential diagnoses are superficial necrolytic dermatitis and zinc-responsive dermatosis. Lesions most closely resemble superficial necrolytic dermatitis, suggesting at least a partially common pathogenesis for the development of the epidermal lesions, possibly via depression in serum amino acids or other nutrients. Zinc-responsive dermatosis does not show epidermal necrolysis, and dyskeratosis is rare.

ACRODERMATITIS OF BULL TERRIERS (Synonym: lethal acrodermatitis of Bull Terriers)

Clinical features (Figures 7-35 through 7-37)

Acrodermatitis of Bull Terriers is an inherited autosomal recessive metabolic disease that may be caused by defects in zinc absorption and metabolism. The syndrome is seen exclusively in white Bull Terriers. The term *lethal acrodermatitis* has been used, since homozygously affected dogs have a median survival age of 7 months and rarely live beyond 18 months of age.

Cutaneous and systemic clinical signs are compatible with severe zinc deficiency. Mundell showed that affected dogs had significantly lowered plasma zinc levels and lowered zinc and copper levels in the kidney and liver. These trace minerals are integral components of over 100 metalloenzymes that participate in many metabolic processes. Decreased serum alkaline phosphatase (ALP) and alanine aminotransferase (ALT; SGPT), increased cholesterol, nonregenerative anemia, a total white blood cell count below 20,000, dysgammaglobulinemia, and decreased lymphocyte blastogenesis reflect the widespread effects of this disease.

Acrodermatitis is characterized clinically by progressive dermatitis of the distal extremities, growth retardation, abnormal behavior, diarrhea, and bronchopneumonia. Affected Bull Terriers develop an erythematous, exfoliative, papular or pustular dermatitis of the distal extremities, skin surrounding the mucocutaneous junctions, and sometimes the mucous membranes at the mucocutaneous junctions by 6 weeks of age. Ulcerated and crusted lesions are prominent on the muzzle and ears. Generalized superficial bacterial folliculitis and ceruminous otitis may be present. Splayed feet show abnormal keratinization of the footpads, which is characterized by villous hypertrophy, fissures, and exfoliation. There is concurrent paronychia and nails may be dystrophic. An abnormally

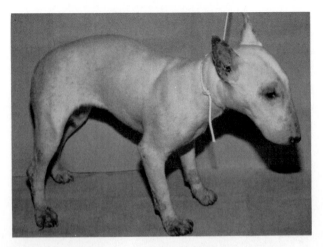

FIGURE 7-35. Acrodermatitis in a Bull Terrier puppy. An erythematous, crusting dermatitis is seen on the distal extremities and surrounding the mucocutaneous junctions of the mouth, eyes, and ears. Note the characteristic splaying of the feet. *(Courtesy AC Mundell, Seattle, Washington; case material from the University of California, Davis.)*

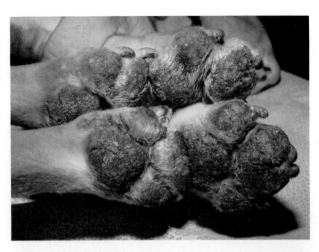

FIGURE 7-37. Closer view of the paws of the dog in Fig. 7-35. The feet show abnormal keratinization of the footpads, characterized by villous hypertrophy, fissures, and exfoliation. *(Courtesy AC Mundell, Seattle, Washington; case material from the University of California, Davis.)*

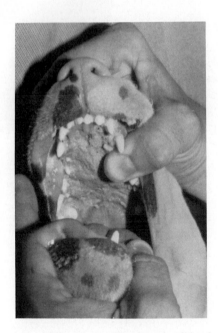

FIGURE 7-36. Closer view of the mouth of the dog in Fig. 7-35. An abnormally arched hard palate is impacted with decayed, malodorous food, which is a characteristic clinical marker for acrodermatitis of Bull Terriers. *(Courtesy AC Mundell, Seattle, Washington; case material from the University of California, Davis.)*

arched hard palate impacted with decayed, malodorous food is a characteristic clinical marker for the disease. Chronic diarrhea and bronchopneumonia are the most serious systemic signs, and bronchopneumonia is the most common cause of death. Sires, dams, and siblings of affected dogs may exhibit an increased frequency of pyoderma, suggesting that heterozygote expression of this genetic disease may increase risk for bacterial skin disease.

The syndrome is seen only in white Bull Terriers and develops shortly after birth. Sex predilections have not been noted. Acrodermatitis of Bull Terriers is clinically distinctive; clinical differential diagnoses are few. Theoretically, generic dog food dermatosis and zinc-responsive dermatosis in Bull Terrier puppies might be similar clinically.

Biopsy site selection

Multiple biopsy specimens should be taken from affected areas. Care must be taken not to dislodge crusts adherent to the specimens.

Histopathology (Figures 7-38 and 7-39)

Acrodermatitis of Bull Terriers is characterized by massive parakeratosis, organized in compact layers. Small-to-moderate–sized serocellular crusts may be embedded in the keratin layer, and entrapped colonies of staphylococci are prominent. The epidermis is moderately to severely acanthotic and occasionally mildly spongiotic. Neutrophils may migrate through the epidermis to form small intraepidermal spongiotic pustules that eventuate in larger superficial pustules and crusts. Erosion and ulceration may be present. Laminar pallor of the superficial epidermis is sometimes observed, but keratinocytes generally appear viable. Rarely, there is loss of nuclear definition or cellular

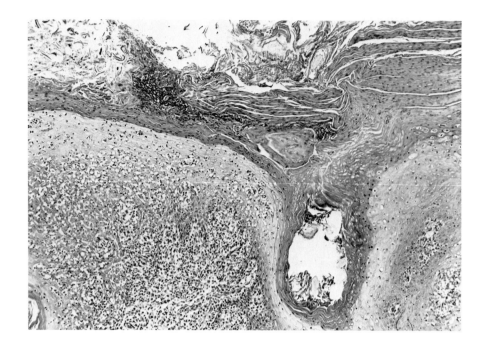

FIGURE 7-38. Acrodermatitis in a Bull Terrier. Massive parakeratosis shows an abrupt transition from the subjacent acanthotic epidermis. Epidermal pallor is in a laminar distribution; neutrophils are migrating to form small spongiotic pustules. Note the involvement of the superficial hair follicle. (×90.)

FIGURE 7-39. High magnification of the epidermis in acrodermatitis. Severe parakeratosis overlies the pale epidermis. (×220.)

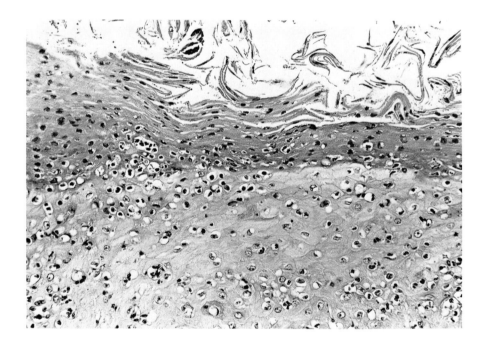

outline; intracytoplasmic vacuolation may be seen. Dyskeratosis occasionally is observed beneath the parakeratotic layer. The deeper keratinocytes may have a slightly gray cast and may appear slightly disordered. Similar histopathologic changes extend to dilated follicular infundibula.

Dermal inflammation is absent or mild to moderate and is composed of lymphocytes, histiocytes, plasma cells, and neutrophils, the latter accumulating beneath overlying foci of pustulation.

Differential diagnosis is generally without difficulty if the characteristic breed occurrence and clinical signs of acrodermatitis are known. Zinc-responsive dermatosis, generic dog food dermatosis, and superficial necrolytic dermatitis are characterized by parakeratosis, but not to the degree observed in acrodermatitis. Generic dog food dermatosis and superficial necrolytic dermatitis are characterized by superficial epidermal necrolysis, which is more striking and prominent than the laminar pallor seen in acrodermatitis.

SUGGESTED READINGS

Primary seborrhea

Carlotti D: Seborrhee canine, Le Point Veterinaire 15:29-38, 1983.

Guaguere E: Le syndrome keratoseborrheique, Pratique Medicale et Chirurgicale de L'Animal de Compagnie 25:117-127, 1990.

Horwitz LN and Ihrke PJ: Canine seborrhea. In Kirk RW, editor: Current veterinary therapy VI, Philadelphia, 1977, WB Saunders Co, pp 519-524.

Ihrke PJ: Canine seborrheic disease complex, Vet Clin North Am 9:93-106, 1979.

Kwochka KW and Rademakers AM: Cell proliferation kinetics of epidermis, hair follicles, and sebaceous glands of Cocker Spaniels with idiopathic seborrhea, Am J Vet Res 50:1918-1922, 1989.

Muller GH, Kirk RW, and Scott DW: Small animal dermatology, ed 4, Philadelphia, 1989, WB Saunders Co, pp 605-612.

Power HT: The efficacy of etretinate (Tegison) in the treatment of keratinization disorders in dogs. Proceedings of the American Academy of Veterinary Dermatology/American College of Veterinary Dermatology, St Louis 5:17, 1989.

Power HT and others: The use of etretinate (Tegison) for the treatment of primary keratinization disorders in Cocker Spaniels, West Highland White Terriers, and Basset Hounds, Manuscript for publication.

Seborrheic dermatitis

Carlotti D: Seborrhee canine, Le Point Veterinaire 15:29-38, 1983.

Guaguere E: Le syndrome keratoseborrheique, Pratique Medicale et Chirurgicale de L'Animal de Compagnie 25:117-127, 1990.

Horwitz LN and Ihrke PJ: Canine seborrhea. In Kirk RW, editor: Current veterinary therapy VI, Philadelphia, 1977, WB Saunders Co, pp 519-524.

Ihrke PJ: Canine seborrheic disease complex, Vet Clin North Am 9:93-106, 1979.

Kwochka KW and Rademakers AM: Cell proliferation kinetics of epidermis, hair follicles, and sebaceous glands of Cocker Spaniels with idiopathic seborrhea, Am J Vet Res 50:1918-1922, 1989.

Muller GH, Kirk RW, and Scott DW: Small animal dermatology, ed 4, Philadelphia, 1989, WB Saunders Co, pp 605-612.

Seborrheic dermatitis and *Malassezia pachydermatis* infection

Mansfield PD and others: Infectivity of *Malassezia pachydermatis* in the external ear canal of dogs, J Am Anim Hosp Assoc 26:97-100, 1990.

Mason KV: Generalized dermatitis associated with *Malassezia pachydermatis* in three dogs. Proceedings of the American Academy of Veterinary Dermatology/American College of Veterinary Dermatology, Phoenix 3:35, 1987.

Mason KV and Evans AG: Dermatitis associated with *Malassezia pachydermatis* in eleven dogs, J Am Anim Hosp Assoc 27:13-20, 1991.

Vitamin A-responsive dermatosis

Guaguere E: Cas clinique: seborrhee primaire respondant a l'administration de vitamine A, Le Point Veterinaire 16:51-53, 1985.

Power HT: The efficacy of etretinate (Tegison) in the treatment of keratinization disorders in dogs. Proceedings of the American Academy of Veterinary Dermatology/American College of Veterinary Dermatology, St Louis 5:17, 1989.

Power HT and others: The use of etretinate (Tegison) for the treatment of primary keratinization disorders in Cocker Spaniels, West Highland White Terriers, and Basset Hounds, Manuscript for publication.

Scott DW: Vitamin A-responsive dermatosis in the Cocker Spaniel, J Am Anim Hosp Assoc 22:125-129, 1986.

Canine ear margin seborrhea

Griffin CE: Pinnal diseases. In: The complete manual of ear care, Lawrenceville, NJ, 1986, Veterinary Learning Systems Co, pp 21-35.

Ihrke PJ: Canine seborrheic disease complex, Vet Clin North Am 9:93-106, 1979.

Muller GH, Kirk RW, and Scott DW: Small animal dermatology, ed 4, Philadelphia, 1989, WB Saunders Co, pp 737-739.

Schnauzer comedo syndrome

Lever WF and Schaumburg-Lever G: Histopathology of the skin, ed 7, Philadelphia, 1990, JB Lippincott Co, p 525.

Muller GH, Kirk RW, and Scott DW: Small animal dermatology, ed 4, Philadelphia, 1989, WB Saunders Co, pp 733-734.

Paradis M and Scott DW: Naevi recemment reconnus chez le chien, Le Point Veterinaire 21:5-9, 1989.

Ichthyosis

August JR, Chickering WR, and Rikihisa Y: Congenital ichthyosis in a dog: comparison with human ichthyosiform dermatoses, Comp Sm Anim 10:40-45, 1988.

Baden HP: Icthyosiform dermatoses. In Fitzpatrick TB, Eisen AZ, Wolff K, and others, editors: Dermatology in general medicine, ed 3, New York, 1987, McGraw-Hill Book Co, pp 506-517.

Guaguere E: Etat ichthyosique congenital chez un Colley, Le Point Veterinaire 20:59-64, 1988.

Lever WF and Schaumburg-Lever G: Histopathology of the skin, ed 7, Philadelphia, 1990, JB Lippincott Co, pp 65-68.

Muller GH: Ichthyosis in two dogs, J Am Vet Med Assoc 169:1313-1316, 1976.

Muller GH, Kirk RW, and Scott DW: Small animal dermatology, ed 4, Philadelphia, 1989, WB Saunders Co, pp 741-747.

O'Neill CS: Hereditary skin diseases in the dog and cat, Comp Cont Ed 3:791-799, 1981.

Scott DW: Congenital ichthyosis in a dog, Comp Anim Pract 19:7-11, 1989.

Sebaceous adenitis

Guaguere E, Alhaidari Z, and Magnol J-P: Adenite sebacee granulomateuse a propos de trois cas, Pratique Medicale et Chirurgicale de L'Animal de Compagnie 25:169-175, 1990.

Power HT and Ihrke PJ: Synthetic retinoids in veterinary dermatology, Vet Clin North Am, 6:1525-1539, 1990.

Rosser EJ and others: Sebaceous adenitis with hyperkeratosis in the Standard Poodle: a discussion of ten cases, J Am Anim Hosp Assoc 23:341-345, 1987.

Scott DW: Adenite sebacee pyogranulomateuse sterile chez un chat, Le Point Veterinaire 21:7-11, 1989.

Scott DW: Granulomatous sebaceous adenitis in dogs, J Am Anim Hosp Assoc 22:631-634, 1986.

Zinc-responsive dermatosis

Fadok VA: Nutritional therapy in veterinary dermatology. In Kirk RW, editor: Current veterinary therapy IX, Philadelphia, 1986, WB Saunders Co, pp 591-596.

Huber TL and others: Variations on digestibility of dry dog foods with identical label guaranteed analysis, J Am Anim Hosp Assoc 22:571-575, 1986.

Kunkle GA: Zinc-responsive dermatoses in dogs. In Kirk RW, editor: Current veterinary therapy VII, Philadelphia, 1980, WB Saunders Co, pp 472-476.

Sanecki RK, Corbin JE, and Forbes RM: Tissue changes in dogs fed a zinc-deficient ration, Am J Vet Res 43:1642-1646, 1982.

Van Den Broek AHM and Thoday KL: Skin disease in dogs associated with zinc deficiency: a report of five cases, J Small Anim Pract 27:313-323, 1986.

Generic dog food dermatosis

Huber TL and others: Variations on digestibility of dry dog foods with identical label guaranteed analysis, J Am Anim Hosp Assoc 22:571-575, 1986.

Sousa CA and others: Dermatosis associated with feeding generic dog food: 13 cases (1981-1982), J Am Vet Med Assoc 192:676-680, 1983.

Acrodermatitis of Bull Terriers

Jezyk PF and others: Lethal acrodermatitis in Bull Terriers, J Am Vet Med Assoc 188:833-839, 1986.

Muller GH, Kirk RW, and Scott DW: Small animal dermatology, ed 4, Philadelphia, 1989, WB Saunders Co, pp 674-675.

Mundell AC: Mineral analysis in Bull Terriers with lethal acrodermatitis. Proceedings of the American Academy of Veterinary Dermatology/American College of Veterinary Dermatology, Washington DC, 4:22, 1988.

Diseases of the dermis

Perivascular diseases of the dermis

Perivascular dermatitis is a relatively nonspecific inflammatory pattern in the skin characterized by infiltrates of inflammatory cells around vessels of the dermis. Inflammation does not remain strictly around vessels in advanced cases of perivascular dermatitis but also spreads to the adjacent dermal interstitium. The majority of the diseases in this group have an allergic cause; histopathologic differentiation among them may be difficult. Identification of the primary inflammatory cell present may allow partial differentiation; however, the definitive diagnosis will depend heavily upon clinical assessment, including response to therapy. Most of these diseases also are characterized by acanthosis (see chronic hyperplastic dermatitis in Chapter 6).

Most inflammatory diseases of the skin are characterized by perivascular infiltrates at some stage in the histogenesis of the lesions because blood vessels are the source of all inflammation in tissue. The diseases included in this chapter are those which have perivascular inflammation as the primary and predominant pattern.

SUPERFICIAL SPREADING PYODERMA
Clinical features (Figures 8-1 and 8-2)

See Chapter 1.

Biopsy site selection

Specimens for skin biopsy should be obtained from the advancing edge of circular, scaling, and erythematous lesions. The central alopecic area that is sometimes hyperpigmented is older and less likely to yield diagnostic results. Care should be taken to ensure that scales or crusts remain intact on the specimen. If present, pustules also should be sampled.

Histopathology (Figures 8-3 and 8-4)

Epidermal lesions were described in Chapter 1. Dermal inflammation consists of superficial perivascular neutrophils that predominate in early lesions and usually are intermingled with macrophages and lymphocytes. Plasma cells are seen in chronic lesions. Mild to moderate edema may be present. Vessels may be mildly dilated.

Chronic superficial spreading pyoderma may be indistinguishable from chronic hyperplastic dermatitis, if typical epidermal lesions are lacking in the specimen for biopsy. A predominance of plasma cells may suggest chronic superficial spreading pyoderma but dermal inflammation alone is not sufficient to indicate the diagnosis.

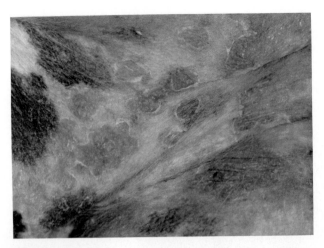

FIGURE 8-1. Superficial spreading pyoderma in a Border Collie. Multiple coalescing erythematous macules with peripheral collarettes cover the glabrous skin of the ventral abdomen. Macular hyperpigmentation is the sequela to prior infection.

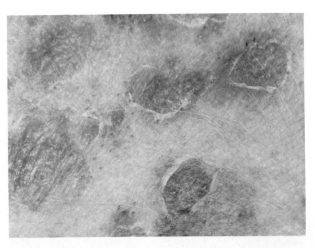

FIGURE 8-2. Closer view of Fig. 8-1. Collarettes peel peripherally from the margins of the macules. Pustules are not present.

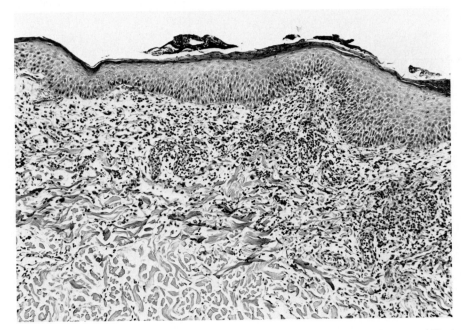

FIGURE 8-3. Superficial spreading pyoderma in a dog. Superficial dermal neutrophilic inflammation is accompanied by epidermal acanthosis, spongiosis, and crusting. (×90.)

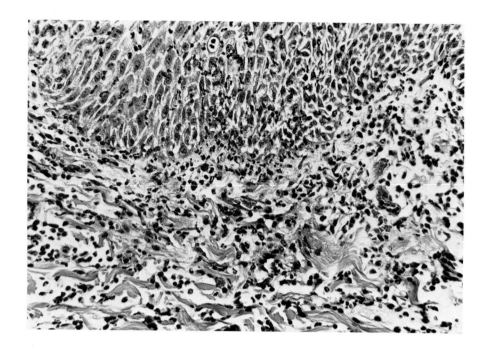

FIGURE 8-4. Superficial dermal inflammation in superficial spreading pyoderma. Neutrophils are intermingled with fewer mixed mononuclear cells. Note the migration of neutrophils into the spongiotic epidermis. (×220.)

ATOPY (Synonyms: allergic inhalant dermatitis, atopic disease)

Clinical features (Figures 8-5 through 8-7)

Atopy is a common, heritable type I hypersensitivity to pollens and other environmental allergens. Genetically predisposed individuals inhale or possibly percutaneously absorb various allergens, which provoke allergen-specific immunologic events in the dermis, leading to the release of pharmacologically active compounds from mast cells. Atopy is well documented in the dog and incompletely characterized in the cat. Reaginic antibodies, IgE and IgGd, have been demonstrated in the dog. The reaginic antibody responsible for feline atopy as yet has not been identified.

Pruritus is the principal clinical feature. Primary skin lesions are rare in canine atopy; most skin lesions are due to secondary self-trauma. Self-trauma leads to variable degrees of erythema, alopecia, and excoriation. Lichenification and hyperpigmentation are observed in

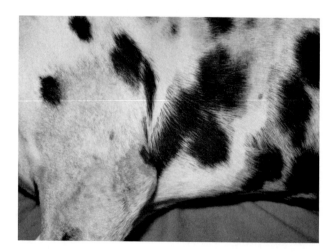

FIGURE 8-5. Atopy in a Dalmatian. Areas of erythema and self-traumatic alopecia are seen periorally and on the forelimbs, distal extremities, lateral thorax, and ventral abdomen.

FIGURE 8-6. Closer view of the dog in Fig. 8-5. Excoriations are present on the elbow and lateral thorax. Note the absence of primary lesions.

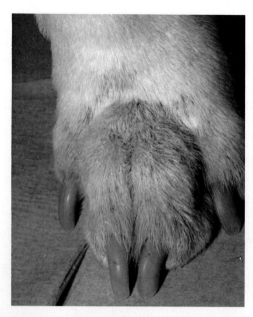

FIGURE 8-7. Atopy in a Bull Terrier. Pruritus has prompted self-traumatic alopecia on the dorsum of a forepaw.

chronically affected dogs. Greasiness or hyperhidrosis also may be present. Salivary staining of the haircoat occurs in dogs with light coat color. The face, dorsum of the feet, and ears are the most common sites, but involvement of the ventrum, particularly the axillae and groin, also is observed. Lesions may be generalized. Uncommonly, pinnal inflammation characterized by erythema and swelling may be the only feature of canine atopy and may be seen in conjunction with otitis externa. Secondary pyoderma is common.

Feline atopy is less well understood. Erythema and excoriation may be localized to the face or ears or may be generalized. Additionally, a wide variety of specific skin manifestations have been reported by many authors, including miliary dermatitis, indolent ulcer, and eosinophilic plaque.

Canine breed predilections include small terriers (West Highland White Terrier, Wirehaired Fox Terrier, Cairn Terrier, and Scottish Terrier), Golden Retriever, Dalmatian, Boxer, Pug, Irish Setter, English Setter, Miniature Schnauzer, Lhasa Apso, and Chinese Shar Pei. Female dogs may be at slightly higher risk. The peak incidence occurs between 1 and 3 years of age; clinical signs of atopy rarely begin before 6 months of age or after 7 years of age. An exception is the Chinese Shar Pei, in which atopy has been documented as early as 3 months of age. Initially, most dogs manifest atopy as a summer-fall pruritus, with the time of involvement tending to lengthen each year. Age, breed, or sex predilections have not been reported with feline atopy.

Canine clinical differential diagnoses include flea allergy dermatitis, food allergy, pruritic superficial pyoderma, and irritant or allergic contact dermatitis. Differential diagnosis may be hampered by the frequent coexistence of flea allergy dermatitis and atopy. Flea allergy dermatitis has a primary papular eruption with prominent dorsal lumbosacral distribution. Pruritus frequently is limited to the rear one-half of the body. Food allergy is nonseasonal and less corticosteroid responsive than is canine atopy. Primary lesions, such as papules and pustules, are seen with pruritic pyoderma, and response to proper antibiotic therapy should be complete. Contact dermatitis is rare and usually is limited to ventral, sparsely haired skin.

Feline clinical differential diagnoses include flea allergy dermatitis, food allergy, and feline psychogenic alopecia. Miliary dermatitis with rump and neck involvement is seen with flea allergy dermatitis. Food allergy is nonseasonal, less corticosteroid responsive, and often involves primarily the head and neck. Inflammation is not a feature of feline psychogenic alopecia.

Biopsy site selection

Biopsy is employed primarily to rule out other more histopathologically specific skin diseases. Areas of erythema with minimal self-trauma should be selected. Chronic areas of lichenification and hyperpigmentation are frequently complicated by secondary pyoderma.

Histopathology (Figures 8-8 and 8-9)

Epidermal lesions are those of chronic hyperplastic dermatitis due to allergy (see Chapter 6). Mild to severe acanthosis, which also involves follicular infundibula, is present. The epidermis may have patchy, mild spongiosis with exocytosis of lymphocytes. Focal parakeratosis and crusting is variable but usually mild. Dense, brightly eosinophilic, compact keratin is observed; this type of keratinization may reflect persistent self-trauma. There may be mild follicular keratosis.

The dermis is characterized by a superficial perivascular infiltrate that generally is mild in lesions of atopy that are not complicated by superficial pyoderma. The inflammatory infiltrate principally consists of mixtures of lymphocytes and macrophages. Mast cells may be prominent, but eosinophils are rare. Neutrophils and plasma cells are seen in small numbers, and their presence may depend on the extent of secondary pustulation and crusting induced by self-trauma (impetiginization). Superficial dermal blood vessels often are dilated and may be congested. Edema is variable but usually is mild.

Sebaceous gland hyperplasia may be seen in any long-standing pruritic skin disease of dogs, including atopy. Sebaceous glands enlarge and proliferate loosely in the dermis, and this alteration may correlate directly

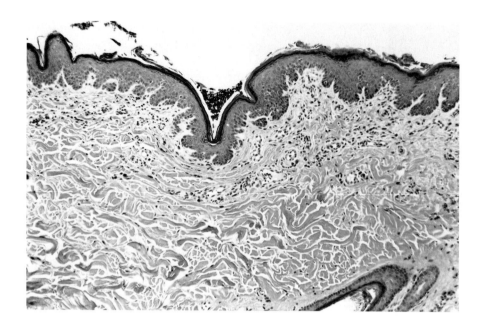

FIGURE 8-8. Atopy in a dog. Irregular acanthosis overlies mild superficial dermal inflammation. Note the mild vascular ectasia. (×90.)

FIGURE 8-9. Atopy in a dog. Mild accumulations of mononuclear cells are oriented around superficial blood vessels. (×220.)

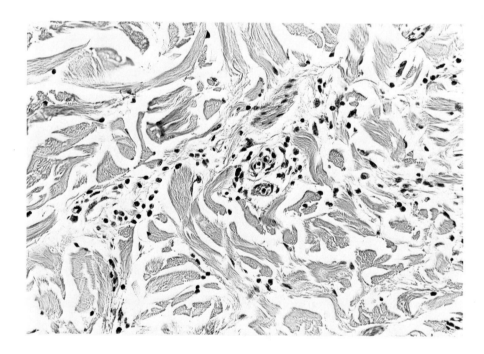

with the degree of oily seborrhea observed. There also may be squamous metaplasia of sebaceous glands, in which individual sebaceous glands are replaced by squamous epithelium, usually expanding outward from the ductular region. Apocrine sweat glands may be dilated and lined by hyperplastic epithelium; this change is another nonspecific feature of chronic pruritus and may correlate clinically with hyperhidrosis.

Differential diagnoses include other allergic skin diseases or skin diseases that evoke persistent self-trauma. Identification of primary lesions, such as pus-

tules in pruritic superficial spreading pyoderma, is helpful; however, superficial spreading pyoderma may accompany atopy. Atopy may be the tentative histopathologic diagnosis for the pruritic dog when superficial perivascular inflammation is minimal and does not include eosinophils. However, inflammation of canine flea allergy dermatitis may obscure the subtle inflammation of atopy in dogs with concurrent conditions. Clinical correlation and appropriate confirmatory testing always are required, since histopathologic findings are not etiologically diagnostic for atopy.

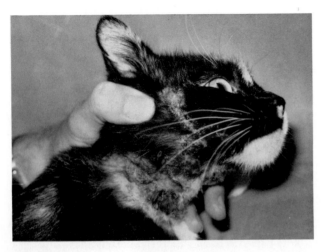

FIGURE 8-10. Food allergy in a cat. Severe self-trauma to the head and neck has created extensive alopecia, ulceration, and crusting.

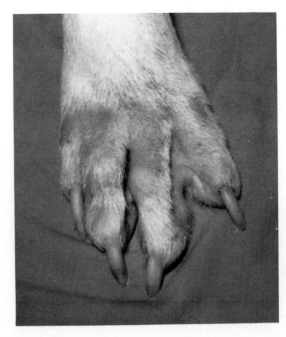

FIGURE 8-11. Food allergy in a Dalmatian. Self-traumatic alopecia and erythema are noted on the dorsum of a forepaw.

FOOD ALLERGY
Clinical features (Figures 8-10 and 8-11)

Food allergy is an uncommon allergic skin disease seen in the dog and cat that is presumed to be a hypersensitivity reaction to ingested allergens. The immunologic basis of food allergy in domestic animals is not known. In humans, type I hypersensitivity most frequently is documented, but types III and IV hypersensitivities also have been implicated. Dermatologic and gastrointestinal signs of food allergy may coexist both in animals and in humans. It has been estimated by most authors that less than 20% of animals with dermatologic signs of food allergy have coexistent gastrointestinal signs and vice versa. Food allergy is seen more frequently in animals with other allergic diseases. Food allergy has been characterized as being both very rare and very common! This disparate information on the reported incidence of food allergy may be associated with the prioritization of diagnostic tests for allergic disease and the threshold phenomenon.

Clinically, food allergy is one of the most pleomorphic skin diseases encountered in clinical veterinary practice. In both dogs and cats, primary skin lesions frequently are not present, as in atopy. When present, primary lesions may include erythematous papules, wheals, and pustules with crusts. Secondary erosion, ulceration, and excoriation with alopecia may be seen, particularly if pruritus is severe. Affected cats may present with allergic miliary dermatitis; Scott (1987) has documented associated eosinophilic plaque and indolent ulcer in cats with miliary dermatitis due to food allergy.

Lesions may be generalized or localized to the face,

feet, or ears. In feline food allergy, head and neck lesions predominate; erosions and ulcers may be prominent. Pruritus is a consistent clinical feature; however, cases of canine food allergy with minimal pruritus have been documented.* Feline food allergy is one of the most pruritic feline skin diseases. In the dog, food allergy may be an underlying cause of recurrent pyoderma.

The Miniature Schnauzer, Golden Retriever, West Highland White Terrier, and Chinese Shar Pei may be at increased risk for food allergy. Canine food allergy can commence as early as 6 months of age but may occur at any age. Sex predilection has not been reported in the dog. Breed, age, or sex predilections have not been reported in cats.

Major clinical differential diagnoses include other highly pruritic skin diseases such as atopy, flea allergy dermatitis, sarcoptic or notoedric acariasis, and feline mosquito-bite hypersensitivity. Feline mosquito-bite hypersensitivity is localized to the dorsal muzzle and ears and is markedly seasonal. Food allergy is nonseasonal and is one of the least glucocorticoid responsive of the allergic skin diseases.

Biopsy site selection

Primary lesions, if present, and lesions with minimal self-trauma are preferred sites. In the cat, it is

_____
* Kunkle GA: Personal communication, 1986.

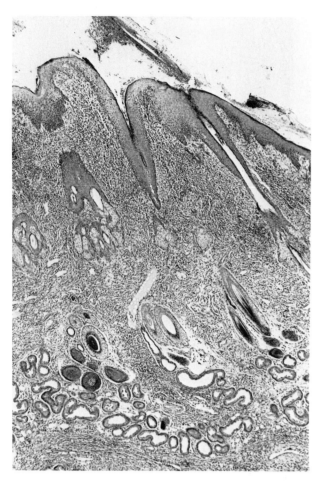

FIGURE 8-12. Food allergy in a cat. Severe inflammation is diffusely present in the dermis. (×35.)

especially important to avoid ulcers. If feline food allergy is suspected in cases with severe head and neck pruritus and self-trauma, the area at the back of the neck between the shoulder blades is an ideal site for biopsy, since cats cannot easily reach this location to traumatize the skin.

Histopathology (Figures 8-12 through 8-14)

Epidermal lesions include those of chronic hyperplastic dermatitis caused by allergy (see Chapter 6). Acanthosis may be severe and there may be patchy spongiosis. Secondary superficial crusting and erosion may be extensive in this intensely pruritic disease, particularly in the cat, and ulcers are not uncommon.

The dermis has a superficial perivascular pattern of inflammation that may become diffuse in more severely inflamed lesions. Inflammation is mixed in dogs and may include lymphocytes, macrophages, eosinophils, and mast cells. Neutrophils and plasma cells may be prominent, depending on the degree of self-trauma–induced epidermal damage and inflammation. Vessels are dilated and congested, and there may be mild to moderate superficial dermal edema. Inflammation may extend mildly down around subjacent adnexal appendages. Chronic lesions may be characterized by sebaceous gland and apocrine gland hyperplasia (see earlier discussion on atopy).

In cats, lesions may be similar to miliary dermatitis (see later discussion). Mast cells may be present in large numbers throughout the superficial and middle dermis. In some instances, lesions of feline food allergy have been confused with cutaneous mast cell neoplasia.

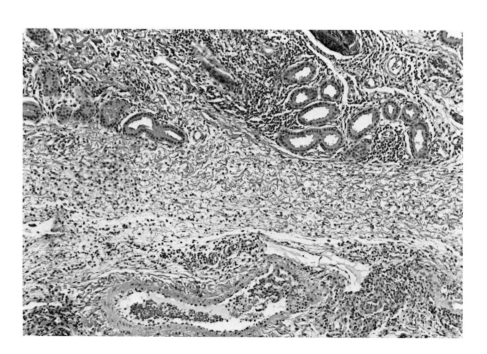

FIGURE 8-13. Food allergy in a cat. The deep dermis contains inflammation oriented around blood vessels. (×90.)

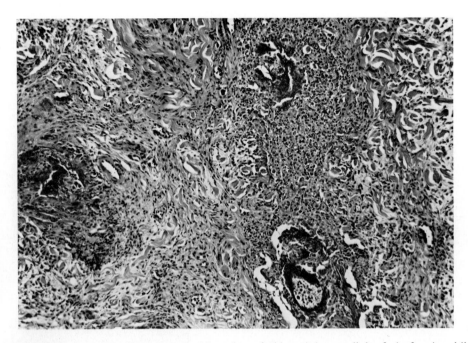

FIGURE 8-14. Food allergy in a cat. Note three darkly staining, acellular foci of eosinophil degranulation and collagen degeneration. ($\times$90.)

Eosinophils are usually present. Eosinophilic infiltrates may extend to surround vessels of the deep dermis and upper layers of the panniculus; this deep extension of eosinophilic inflammation is highly suggestive of food allergy, particularly when found in lesions known to be confined to the head and neck. However, Scott (1980) and more recently White (1989, 1990) have described a superficial inflammatory infiltrate without eosinophils, consisting of mononuclear cells alone or admixed with neutrophils, in cats with food allergy.

The authors have recently recognized small foci of collagen degeneration and eosinophil degranulation in a case of feline food allergy characterized by severe eosinophilic dermatitis. Eosinophilic folliculitis and furunculosis, characterized by the degranulation of eosinophils in and around follicles, also has been observed.

Differential diagnoses in the dog and cat include other allergic skin diseases, particularly those characterized by eosinophils, such as canine flea allergy dermatitis and feline allergic miliary dermatitis, feline mosquito-bite hypersensitivity, or sarcoptic and notoedric acariasis. Canine atopy is generally less inflamed and does not include significant numbers of eosinophils, as do most cases of canine food allergy. In the cat a predominance of mast cells or severe and deep extension of eosinophilic inflammation is suggestive of food allergy, particularly when lesions are known to be confined to the head and neck. However, the deep eosino-

philic inflammation of feline mosquito-bite hypersensitivity can be virtually identical. Feline mosquito-bite hypersensitivity may have prominent eosinophil degranulation and collagen degeneration, in contrast to feline food allergy, in which these lesions are rare and mild. Specific histopathologic delineation of food allergy in dogs and cats usually is not possible, and clinical differentiation is required.

CANINE FLEA ALLERGY
DERMATITIS (Synonyms: FAD, canine flea-bite hypersensitivity)
Clinical features (Figures 8-15 through 8-17)

Canine flea allergy dermatitis is an extremely common pruritic skin disease caused by hypersensitivity to salivary antigens of the flea. Type I immediate hypersensitivity, type IV delayed hypersensitivity, and cutaneous basophil hypersensitivity all have been documented by Halliwell (1987, 1989) as immunologic participants. A late-phase IgE-mediated reaction also may contribute to the pathogenesis. Flea allergy dermatitis is the most common cause of canine skin disease on a worldwide basis.

The single most important clinical sign is pruritus that is predominantly localized to the caudal half of the dog. Crusted papules occur in a somewhat bilaterally symmetric pattern and involve the dorsal lumbosacral region, tailbase, perineum, and medial and caudal

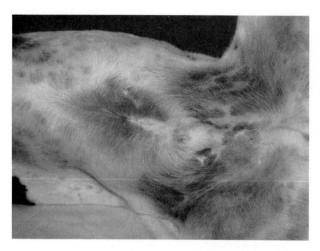

FIGURE 8-15. Acute canine flea allergy dermatitis. Salivary staining, erythema, and small papules are present somewhat symmetrically on the ventral abdomen. Note the characteristic involvement of the umbilicus. *(Courtesy MD Song; case material from the University of California, Davis.)*

thighs. The umbilical fold commonly is affected in male dogs. Lesions vary from subtle to severe. Alopecia, lichenification, and hyperpigmentation may be present in chronic cases and are contingent on the degree of self-trauma. Fibropruritic nodules may form in susceptible individuals (see Chapter 6). Occasionally, pruritus may be generalized. Flea allergy can predispose to recurrent pyoderma.

Breeds at increased risk for the development of flea allergy dermatitis include the Cairn Terrier, Irish Setter, West Highland White Terrier, Border Collie, Scottish Terrier, and Lhasa Apso.* Flea allergy develops most often in dogs between 1 and 3 years of age but may commence later in life in dogs that have had previous minimal flea exposure. Rarely, signs may be seen in dogs younger than 6 months of age. A definite seasonality (summer and fall) is seen with flea allergy dermatitis in areas of the world with cold winters. There is no sex predilection.

Major clinical differential diagnoses include pruritic superficial spreading pyoderma, atopy, and food allergy. In superficial spreading pyoderma, pustules are the primary lesion, the axilla and groin commonly are involved, and lesions spread peripherally and form collarettes. Atopy and food allergy both have more facial and pedal involvement and pruritus is not localized to the caudal one-half of body.

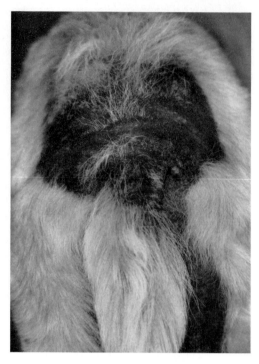

FIGURE 8-16. Chronic flea allergy dermatitis in a Samoyed crossbreed. Classic lesions, consisting of somewhat symmetric alopecia, hyperpigmentation, and lichenification, are seen in the dorsal lumbosacral region.

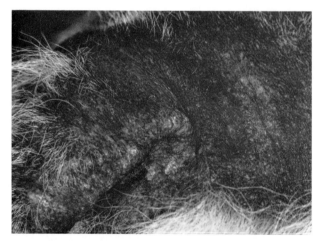

FIGURE 8-17. Closer view of the lateral tail fold of the dog in Figure 8-16. The papules of acute flea allergy dermatitis are superimposed on chronic skin lesions.

Biopsy site selection

Areas of papular eruption and erythema with minimal self-trauma are preferred sites for skin biopsy. Sites of secondary pyoderma should be avoided.

* Sischo WM and Ihrke PJ: Unpublished data, 1990.

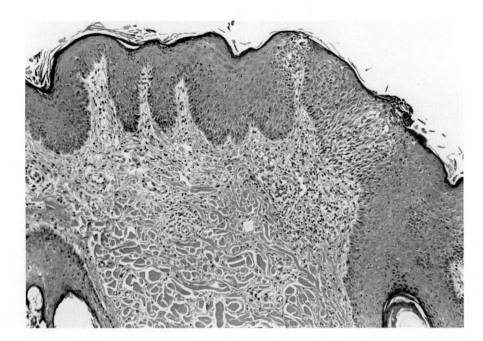

FIGURE 8-18. Canine flea allergy dermatitis. Irregular acanthosis accompanies superficial perivascular inflammation. Note the discrete spongiotic foci with crusting. (×95.)

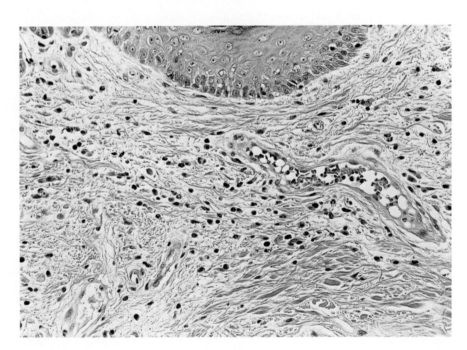

FIGURE 8-19. Canine flea allergy dermatitis. Eosinophils are accumulating around superficial dermal blood vessels. (×220.)

Histopathology (Figures 8-18 and 8-19)

Epidermal lesions are those of chronic hyperplastic dermatitis caused by allergy (see Chapter 6) and include irregular acanthosis with patchy spongiosis, serocellular crusting, and parakeratosis.

In experimentally induced flea-bite hypersensitivity in dogs, eosinophils and edema predominated early in the immediate response (15 minutes to 4 hours); eosinophils persisted and were accompanied by mononuclear cells in late reactions (24 to 48 hours). This

biphasic pattern of inflammation supports both type I and type IV hypersensitivity in canine flea allergy dermatitis. Additionally, Halliwell (1987) has shown that cutaneous basophils are a significant component of the delayed response to flea bites in dogs, implicating cutaneous basophil hypersensitivity. Basophils are not identifiable by routine processing and staining of skin biopsy specimens.

In specimens from natural cases of flea allergy dermatitis, dermal inflammation is superficial, perivascular to diffuse, and generally mild to moderate. Eosinophils and mast cells are mixed with lymphocytes and macrophages. Neutrophils and plasma cells also may be prominent, and the presence of these cells may depend on the degree of secondary self-trauma. Melanophages may be observed. There are variable superficial edema and vascular ectasia. Inflammation frequently extends around adnexal appendages. Sebaceous gland and apocrine gland hyperplasia may be present in chronic lesions (see earlier discussion on atopy). Rarely, fibropruritic nodules are present (see Chapter 6); however, these lesions are not routinely obtained for histopathologic confirmation of flea allergy.

Lesions of flea allergy dermatitis closely resemble those of other allergic dermatitides. Eosinophils may be a key differential feature in separating flea allergy from atopy, since specimens from cases of uncomplicated atopy usually do not exhibit eosinophils. Food allergy may be indistinguishable. Other parasitic allergic diseases, such as sarcoptic acariasis or hookworm dermatitis, will closely resemble flea allergy dermatitis (if parasites are not found in tissue), and clinical differentiation is required.

FELINE ALLERGIC MILIARY DERMATITIS

Clinical features (Figure 8-20)

See Chapter 5.

Biopsy site selection

Nontraumatized, recently erupted, crusted papules are ideal for biopsy. If pruritus is extreme, special care should be taken to avoid traumatized lesions. If lesions

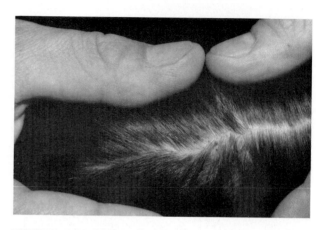

FIGURE 8-20. Feline allergic miliary dermatitis. Minute, discrete, crusted papules are seen where the haircoat is parted.

are present between the shoulder blades, this site is recommended for biopsy, since self-trauma is not readily accomplished in this location.

Histopathology (Figure 8-21)

Epidermal lesions, described in Chapter 5, include discrete serocellular crusts or spongiotic eosinophilic pustules associated with variable erosion and acanthosis. The dermal inflammatory infiltrate is mild to moderate and consists of eosinophils, mast cells, and fewer lymphocytes and macrophages. Dermal inflammation is perivascular to interstitial and extends from the superficial to the middle (follicular) dermis. Perivascular inflammation of the deep dermis also may be present and, when severe, may be suggestive of food allergy (see earlier discussion). Neutrophils may be prominent

FIGURE 8-21. Feline allergic miliary dermatitis. Eosinophils are accumulating in the superficial dermis. (×220.)

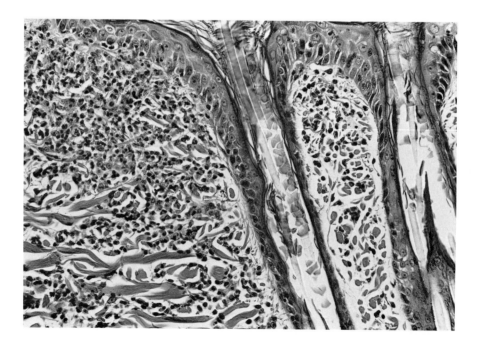

beneath epidermal erosion or ulceration. Edema of the superficial dermis may occur and vessels may be dilated. Superficial dermal fibrosis is a feature of chronically or severely self-traumatized lesions.

Eosinophilic folliculitis and furunculosis are additional histopathologic findings in some cats with severe allergic miliary dermatitis. The etiopathogenesis of eosinophilic folliculitis in the cat is not yet known; recently, food allergy and mosquito-bite hypersensitivity have been documented by the authors in cats with eosinophilic folliculitis of the face.

Histopathologic differential diagnoses are few, but many types of allergic skin disease of cats can be manifested histopathologically as allergic miliary dermatitis. Eosinophilic plaque resembles allergic miliary dermatitis and is characterized by more intense but qualitatively similar lesions. Eosinophilic plaque may represent a more severe and localized manifestation of allergic skin disease in cats.

CANINE SARCOPTIC ACARIASIS
(Synonyms: canine scabies, sarcoptic mange)
Clinical features (Figures 8-22 through 8-24)

Canine sarcoptic acariasis is a highly contagious, intensely pruritic, transmissible skin disease caused by the burrowing epidermal mite *Sarcoptes scabiei* var. *canis*. The mite is relatively host specific but can cause at least transient pruritic disease in other host species, including cats and humans. Scabies of canine origin in humans is the most common pruritic zoonosis. The scabies mite of humans, *Sarcoptes scabiei* var. *hominis*, induces a complex hypersensitivity reaction involving both humoral and cell-mediated hypersensitivity and the formation of circulating immune complexes. Immunoglobulins IgM, IgE, and complement factor 3 have been demonstrated in vessel walls and at the dermal-epidermal junction. The presence of positive skin test reactivity to house dust mite extract in some dogs with sarcoptic acariasis and proteinuria presumptively associated with immune complex glomerulonephritis indicate the likelihood of a complex immunologic etiopathogenesis. Individual variation in the intensity of the immunologic reaction to mites is characterized by variability in severity of clinical signs, the existence of asymptomatic carriers, and a decrease in mite numbers as the disease progresses. Dogs with compromised immune systems (from coexistent immunosuppressive disease or injudicious therapy with corticosteroids or cytotoxic drugs) may harbor much larger populations of mites in the condition of so-called Norwegian scabies, named after the disease seen in human patients with immunosuppressive diseases such as acquired immunodeficiency syndrome.

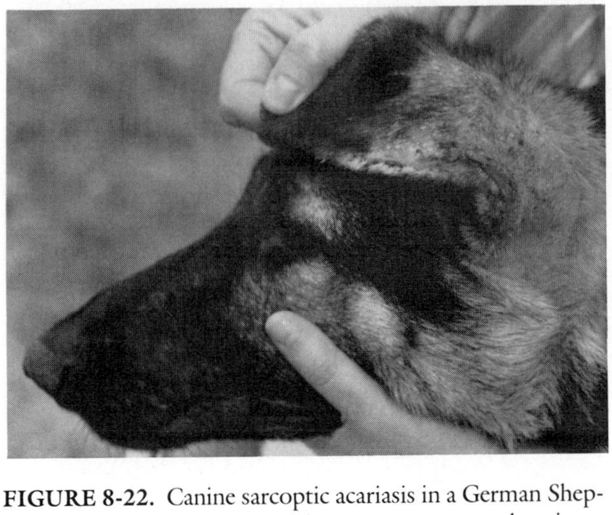

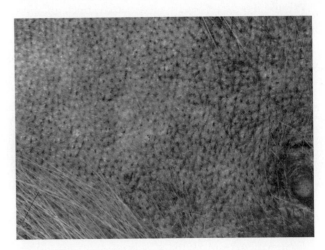

FIGURE 8-23. Close-up of the lesions of sarcoptic acariasis on the ventral abdomen of a dog. A maculopapular rash is present.

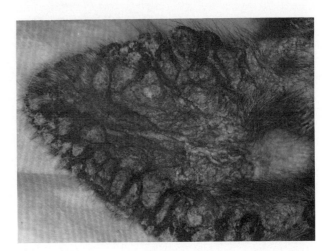

FIGURE 8-24. Ear of an Akita with severe, chronic sarcoptic acariasis. Thick, adherent crusts cover the almost totally alopecic pinna.

FIGURE 8-22. Canine sarcoptic acariasis in a German Shepherd Dog. Alopecia and crusting are present on the pinna.

An erythematous maculopapular eruption with crusting and alopecia is accompanied by secondary self-traumatic excoriations of variable severity. The crusts are often thick and yellowish white. Extensive alopecia, lichenification, and hyperpigmentation may be seen in chronic cases. The preference of mites for sparsely haired skin results in a predominantly ventral distribution. The margins of the pinnae are most often affected and may be the initial site of involvement, especially in young dogs. The ventral abdomen and chest and lateral elbows also are involved commonly. Generalized dermatopathic lymphadenopathy often is present. Somewhat surprisingly, secondary pyoderma is not common. Corticosteroid administration in antiinflammatory dosages may impede clinical diagnosis by decreasing the severity of lesions.

Norwegian scabies exhibits much more florid clinical signs in conjunction with large mite populations. Affected dogs have severe, generalized, thick adherent crusts with marked alopecia.

The Labrador Retriever, Cocker Spaniel, and Doberman Pinscher are at statistically significant increased risk for being diagnosed as having canine sarcoptic acariasis.* This marked breed predilection for a contagious disease probably is explained by a greater likelihood of dogs of these breeds developing the hypersensitivity reaction that yields the characteristic clinical features. The Cocker Spaniel may be at increased risk for the development of Norwegian scabies. This apparent predilection might be explained by a breed-based specific immunologic defect. An age predilection for young dogs is seen and may correlate with increased

* Sischo WM and Ihrke PJ: Unpublished data, 1989.

opportunity for exposure in large breeding farms and pet stores. Immunologic factors also could favor young dogs developing obvious clinical disease. There is no sex predilection.

Clinical differential diagnoses should include pruritic skin diseases such as canine flea allergy dermatitis and pruritic superficial pyoderma, both of which may present with similar crusted papules as seen in sarcoptic acariasis. Other pruritic canine skin diseases such as atopy and food allergy usually do not exhibit primary lesions. The typical site predilections for canine sarcoptic acariasis (margins of the pinnae, ventral abdomen and chest, and lateral elbows) will aid in the differentiation from other pruritic skin diseases. Skin scrapings and fecal flotation are recommended diagnostic procedures. Since scabies mites may be difficult to demonstrate in skin scrapings, empirical treatment for canine sarcoptic acariasis based on clinical impression is a useful diagnostic tool.

Biopsy site selection

Erythematous papules from sparsely haired areas, such as the ventrum, are ideal biopsy sites. Biopsy site selection also should include crusted lesions, since these may be more likely to reveal the offending parasite. Multiple specimens should be obtained to increase the potential for finding mites in tissue. Excoriated lesions or frank pustules indicative of secondary pyoderma should be avoided. Ear margins should not be selected for biopsy, unless exclusively affected, since sampling may result in scarring and distortion of the pinna.

Histopathology (Figure 8-25)

The epidermis has moderate to severe acanthosis and variable spongiosis, accompanied by hyperkerato-

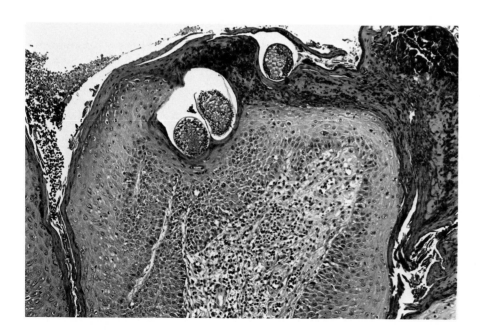

FIGURE 8-25. Canine sarcoptic acariasis. Mites are embedded in the superficial epidermis and overlying crust. Note the superficial inflammatory infiltrate. (×120.)

sis and patchy parakeratosis. In some cases mild to moderate parakeratosis is diffusely present. Serocellular crusting may be multifocally evident. Rarely, in a fortuitously procured specimen, cross-sections of *Sarcoptes scabiei*; var. *canis* (200 to 400 μm) or their oval eggs (100 to 150 μm) are discovered embedded in the keratin layer or superficial cell layers of the epidermis. Large numbers of mites embedded in extensive, thick crusts may be present in patients with severe infestation caused by immunologic compromise (Norwegian scabies).

Dermal lesions bear strong resemblance to those of canine flea allergy dermatitis (see earlier discussion). Eosinophils and mast cells are intermingled in a mild to moderate superficial perivascular inflammatory infiltrate of lymphocytes and macrophages. Neutrophils and plasma cells may be prominent in specimens obtained from sites of epidermal erosion and crusting due to self-trauma.

Differential diagnoses principally include other parasitic allergic diseases, particularly canine flea allergy dermatitis. Clinical differentiation by discovery of the offending mites or by response to appropriate therapy usually is required unless parasites are discovered in tissue section. Lesions of sarcoptic acariasis that are characterized by diffuse parakeratosis and that have no organisms present may closely resemble zinc-responsive dermatosis.

FELINE NOTOEDRIC ACARIASIS

(Synonyms: feline scabies, notoedric mange, head mange)

Clinical features (Figure 8-26)

Feline notoedric acariasis is a highly contagious, intensely pruritic transmissible skin disease caused by the burrowing epidermal mite *Notoedres cati*. The disease is rare in most parts of North America but may be found in localized enzootic areas. As with canine sarcoptic acariasis, the mite is relatively host specific but can cause pruritic disease in other host species, including dogs and humans. A complex hypersensitivity reaction similar to that proposed in canine sarcoptic acariasis is suspected (see preceding discussion).

An erythematous papular rash rapidly eventuates in thick, adherent, yellowish gray crusts. Severe self-trauma produces excoriation. Alopecia is progressive and may be severe. Lichenification varies with chronicity. Similar to canine sarcoptic acariasis, the margins of the pinnae are most often affected initially. Lesions spread rapidly over the face and neck as areas of involvement increase by peripheral extension. Cats who remain untreated may develop generalized disease. Pruritus is intense. Generalized dermatopathic lymphadenopathy is a consistent feature. Breed, age, or sex predilections have not been noted.

Clinical differential diagnoses should include other pruritic skin diseases with a predilection for the face and ears. Otodectic acariasis, food allergy, pemphigus foliaceus, and atopy should be considered. Skin scrapings and fecal flotations should be performed. Skin scrapings may be a more useful diagnostic tool than in canine sarcoptic acariasis, since notoedric mites may be more prevalent on affected cats and hence may be easier to demonstrate by scraping. Empirical treatment for feline notoedric acariasis based on clinical impression also is considered a useful diagnostic tool.

Biopsy site selection

Biopsy site selection should include severely crusted lesions, since they may reveal the offending parasite. Multiple sites should be sampled to increase the potential for finding mites in tissue. Areas of severe excoriation should be avoided.

Histopathology (Figure 8-27)

Hyperkeratosis and parakeratosis overlie moderate acanthosis. Parakeratosis with inflammatory debris (scale-crust) is often distributed in mounds. Mild spongiosis is present. Histopathologically, parasites are discovered more readily in feline notoedric acariasis than in canine sarcoptic acariasis. *Notoedres cati* may be seen in variable numbers embedded in the superficial layers of the epidermis. *Notoedres cati* are slightly smaller than *Sarcoptes scabiei*.

The dermis has superficial, perivascular to diffuse, mild to moderate inflammation composed of eosinophils, macrophages, mast cells, neutrophils, and lymphocytes. Mild edema and vascular ectasia may be present.

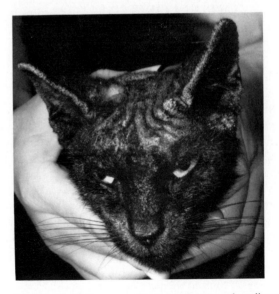

FIGURE 8-26. Feline notoedric acariasis. Note the adherent crusts, alopecia, and excoriations. *(Courtesy IJ Ameti, Orange, California.)*

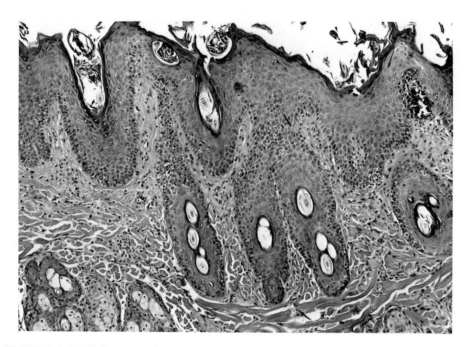

FIGURE 8-27. Feline notoedric acariasis. Mites are embedded in the superficial acanthotic epidermis and in keratin. Mild superficial dermal inflammation is evident. (×100.)

The dermal inflammation is not specifically diagnostic and resembles that of other allergic skin diseases in cats. Dermal inflammation of food allergy is often more severe and deeply extensive than the inflammation of notoedric acariasis. Feline allergic miliary dermatitis caused by fleas or atopy may be indistinguishable from notoedric acariasis. Discovery of mites in tissue is the key differential feature.

CHEYLETIELLOSIS (Synonym: *Cheyletiella* dermatitis)

Clinical features (Figures 8-28 and 8-29)

Cheyletiellosis is a mild, variably pruritic, transmissible skin disease caused by surface-living mites of the genus *Cheyletiella*. The mite appears to be only partially host specific. Dogs are believed to be parasitized primarily by *Cheyletiella yasguri*, cats by *Cheyletiella blakei*, and rabbits by *Cheyletiella parasitovorax*. However, multiple mammalian species (including humans) in the same environment may be parasitized by the same species of *Cheyletiella* mites. Cheyletiellosis is an underreported zoonosis. Although the entire life cycle is completed on the host, adult female mites may be able to survive in the environment transiently, thus increasing the likelihood of transmission to other animals. Infestations may be enzootic in catteries. Cheyletiellosis is seen most commonly in areas of the world where vigorous flea control is either not necessary or not prac-

ticed, because the mites usually are sensitive to parasiticides.

The immunology of cheyletiellosis is largely unexplored. Although host access to antigen probably is less, since the mite does not burrow into living epidermis, the potential may exist for a complex hypersensitivity reaction similar to that seen with the sarcoptiform mites. It is likely that host immune response is an important factor in the clinical expression of the disease because mite counts are much higher and cheyletiellosis is clinically most severe in kittens or puppies less than 3 months of age.

Feline cheyletiellosis is characterized clinically by mild scaling and crusting with minimal to absent underlying skin changes. Allergic miliary dermatitis may be seen in more severe cases (see Chapter 5). Inapparent carriers are common. The dorsal trunk is most commonly affected but lesions may be generalized. Mites and their eggs may be visible to the naked eye or with the use of a hand lens. Entrance and egress of the mites from the nostrils of cats has been seen by Stein.* The activity of the mites may increase in the evening, and they are best observed traversing the dorsal muzzle. Pruritus is variable but often is absent.

In dogs, scaling and mild crusting are predomi-

* Stein BS: As presented, Annual Meeting of The American Academy of Veterinary Dermatology/American College of Veterinary Dermatology, 1982.

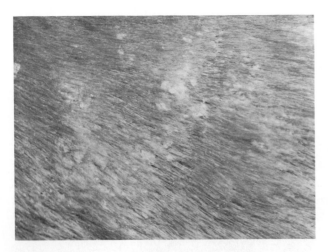

FIGURE 8-28. Cheyletiellosis in a Cocker Spaniel. Moderate scaling and crusting on the trunk are the only clinical signs of the disease.

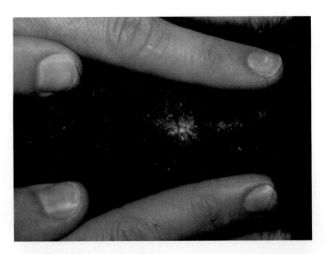

FIGURE 8-29. Cheyletiellosis in a dog. Mild scaling without erythema is noted on the dorsal trunk.

nantly on the dorsal trunk but may generalize. Mild lymphadenopathy may be noted. Pruritus usually is mild.

Breed or sex predilections have not been noted. Clinical disease is noted most commonly in dogs and cats less than 6 months of age. Infested adults are more likely to be inapparent carriers.

The scaling and crusting caused by cheyletiellosis must be differentiated from seborrhea, from the scaling and crusting caused by nutritional deficiency or endoparasitism in young animals, from feline allergic miliary dermatitis due to other causes, and from other ectoparasitic diseases such as mild flea allergy dermatitis, pediculosis, and chigger infestation. Primary seborrhea is rare in dogs less than 6 months of age. Superficial skin scrapings, acetate tape preparations, and fecal flotations are useful in establishing a definitive diagnosis; generally *Cheyletiella* mites are found more readily than those in most other ectoparasitic contagious skin diseases. However, the mites may be more difficult to demonstrate if some ectoparasite control is being practiced. Response to therapy may be employed as a diagnostic tool if cheyletiellosis is suspected.

Biopsy site selection

Areas of maximal scaling and crusting should be selected. Care should be taken not to dislodge surface crusting because that is the habitat of the mite.

Histopathology (Figures 8-30 and 8-31)

The epidermis is irregularly acanthotic and moderately to severely hyperkeratotic. Variable numbers of *Cheyletiella* mites, measuring 350 to 500 μm in length, are entrapped in the keratin. Eggs are observed rarely and measure 200 μm.

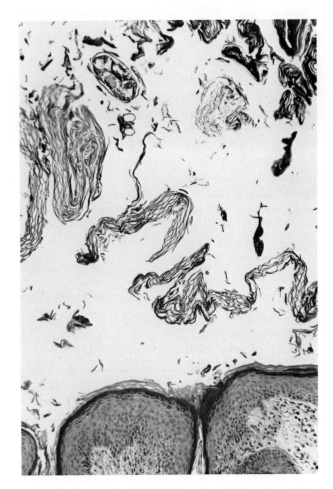

FIGURE 8-30. Cheyletiellosis in a dog. Note mite within abundant hyperkeratotic scale. (×100.) (*Case material from NK Gulbas, Phoenix, Arizona.*)

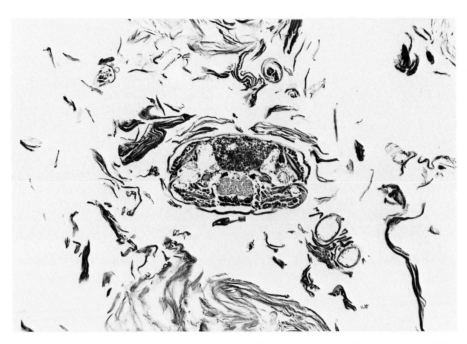

FIGURE 8-31. Higher power magnification of the mite shown in Figure 8-30. (×220.)

The superficial dermis has a mixed inflammatory infiltrate that is perivascular to interstitial and includes eosinophils, lymphocytes, macrophages, and plasma cells. Variable superficial dermal edema is present.

Differential diagnoses principally include sarcoptic acariasis in dogs and notoedric acariasis in cats. Hyperkeratosis may be more prominent in cheyletiellosis than in sarcoptic or notoedric acariasis. On average, adult sarcoptic and notoedric mites are smaller and of a more round configuration than the elongated mites of *Cheyletiella* species. Additionally, large numbers of mites are suggestive of cheyletiellosis in dogs, because mites are rare in random specimens from dogs with sarcoptic acariasis.

CUTANEOUS DIROFILARIASIS

(Synonym: heartworm dermatitis)

Clinical features (Figures 8-32 and 8-33)

Cutaneous dirofilariasis is a very rare skin disease seen in dogs in conjunction with *Dirofilaria immitis*. The presumed mechanism is a hypersensitivity reaction to microfilaria. Two dissimilar syndromes have been reported. In the syndrome reported by Scott, a multifocal nodular dermatitis with prominent facial involvement was seen. A second syndrome reported by Halliwell described a highly pruritic papular dermatitis clinically resembling canine sarcoptic acariasis. In addition to these two syndromes, solitary cavitating nodules harboring aberrant migrating adult heartworms have been reported in dogs and humans. The authors have seen two cases of microfilaria-related skin disease in dogs that were negative for *Dirofilaria immitis* infection using direct and enzyme-linked immunosorbent assays. One animal had a pruritic plaque on the head; the second had generalized pruritic, erythematous, and papular skin disease. The second case was positive for *Dipetalonema reconditum*.

Multifocal nodular dermatitis with erosion and ulceration was reported by Scott. Erythematous papules coalesced and eventuated in firm alopecic nodules. The lesions were chronic, slowly progressive, and mildly pruritic. The dorsum of the muzzle, lips, and pinnae were affected most frequently but lesions also were seen on the trunk and limbs. The cases described by Halliwell exhibited a generalized, maculopapular, erythematous eruption with severe pruritus. In both syndromes, complete resolution of the skin disease in response to therapy for heartworms was used as a method of validating the diagnosis.

Case sampling has been too small to infer breed, age, or sex data. However, the cases seen by Scott were mature, large-breed dogs.

Clinical differential diagnoses for the syndrome reported by Scott should include diseases such as subcutaneous and deep mycoses, nocardiosis, actinomycosis, and sterile granulomatous diseases, which may cause progressive, multifocal, alopecic nodules. Sarcoptic acariasis and other pruritic skin diseases of similar distribution should be considered for the syndrome reported by Halliwell. The diagnosis of cutaneous dirofilariasis is supported by compatible clinical and histopathologic findings coupled with response to therapy.

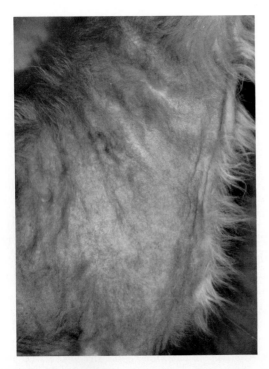

FIGURE 8-32. Shoulder and neck of a Collie with cutaneous dirofilariasis. A finely papular eruption with alopecia is present.

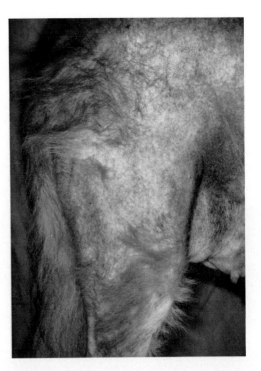

FIGURE 8-33. Caudal thighs of the dog in Figure 8-32. Note the hyperpigmentation as a chronic manifestation of this pruritic skin disease.

Biopsy site selection

Multiple specimens should be obtained from well-developed nodular lesions or generalized papular eruptions.

Histopathology (Figures 8-34 and 8-35)

Histopathology was not available for the syndrome described by Halliwell. Lesions described by Scott and the histopathology of the pruritic plaque observed by

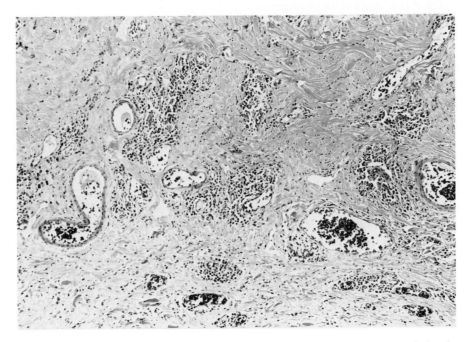

FIGURE 8-34. Cutaneous dirofilariasis in a dog. Inflammatory cells are accumulating in a tightly perivascular pattern. Fragments of microfilaria were sparsely present (not shown). (×90.) *(Case material from JR Hill, Mountainview, California.)*

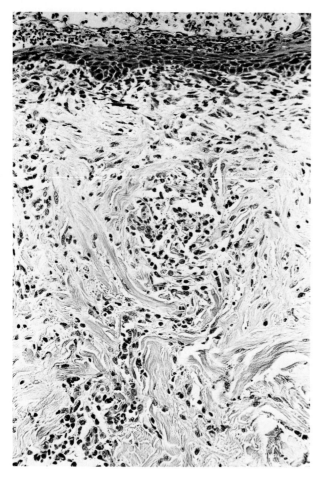

FIGURE 8-35. Cutaneous dirofilariasis in a dog. Mononuclear cells (macrophages and lymphocytes) form a nodular pattern around superficial dermal vessels. The overlying epidermis contains a vesicopustule. (×220.) *(Case material from JR Hill, Mountainview, California.)*

The formation of extravascular or perivascular granulomas suggests cutaneous dirofilariasis. In this respect, lesions resemble those of cutaneous onchocerciasis of horses, a microfilaria-induced skin disease. Discovery of microfilaria in tissue may be difficult. Identification of organisms in intravascular spaces only is not diagnostic; intravascular microfilaria may be incidental findings in dogs living in enzootic areas of *Dirofilaria immitis* and *Dipetalonema reconditum* infection. Microfilaria must be found at the centers of inflammatory foci. Response to therapy, involving eradication of all stages of heartworms or other filarial parasites, is the best method of definitive diagnosis in these cases.

HOOKWORM DERMATITIS (Synonyms: cutaneous ancylostomiasis, cutaneous uncinariasis)
Clinical features (Figures 8-36 and 8-37)

Hookworm dermatitis is an uncommon skin disease incidental to larval migration associated with the normal life cycle of the hookworms, *Ancylostoma braziliense*, *Ancylostoma caninum*, and *Uncinaria stenocephala*. It is presumed to be due to a hypersensitivity reaction to migrating larvae; coexistent arthritis, as reported by Baker (1981), suggests a more complex immunologic etiopathogenesis. Third-stage larvae enter the skin in soil contact areas, principally the distal extremities. Hookworm dermatitis is reported to occur more frequently in association with *Uncinaria stenocephala* and is more common in Ireland, southwestern England, the southeastern United States, and other humid areas of the world where hookworms are common.

The clinical features have been described in detail by Baker (1970, 1981). Erythematous papules are the initial lesions and are followed by lichenification and alopecia. Characteristic changes in the texture of the footpads occur. The pad margins become soft and friable and sometimes separate from the underlying dermis. Nail deformation and paronychia with loss of the nail are seen in chronic cases. The distal extremities often are most severely affected, but other areas of soil contact such as the xiphoid, posterior sternal region, ventral abdomen, and the skin over bony prominences may be affected. Pruritus is mild to moderate. Concomitant arthritis of the distal interphalangeal joint also has been reported by Baker (1981).

Breed, age, and sex data are not available. However, hookworm dermatitis is predominantly a disease of sporting dogs kenneled on earth or grass runs with poor sanitation.

Clinical differential diagnoses should include other ectoparasitic diseases such as demodicosis, *Pelodera* (rhabditic) dermatitis, and canine sarcoptic acariasis. Irritant or allergic contact dermatitis could present

one author* (which was heartworm negative; see above) are similar.

The epidermis is moderately acanthotic or ulcerated. Epidermal pustulation and crusting may be present. The dermis is characterized by superficial and deep perivascular infiltrations of macrophages, eosinophils, neutrophils, lymphocytes, and plasma cells. Macrophages predominate and often form nodular or granulomatous configurations around or near vessels. Segments of microfilaria are seen, usually in small numbers, within vessels, as well as within extravascular inflammatory foci.

Differential diagnoses include other skin diseases characterized by eosinophilic perivascular dermatitis.

---

* Thelma Lee Gross.

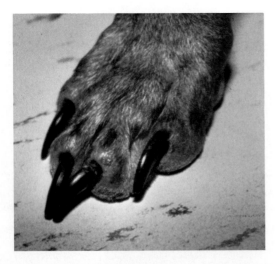

FIGURE 8-36. Hookworm dermatitis on the dorsum of the paw of a Doberman Pinscher. Erosions and ulcerations are present around the margins of the nail beds. *(Courtesy GA Kunkle, Gainesville, Florida.)*

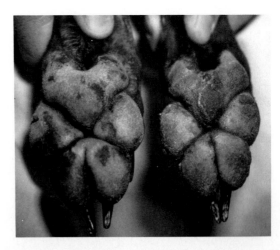

FIGURE 8-37. Ventral paw of the Doberman Pinscher with hookworm dermatitis in Fig. 8-36. Note the ulcers on the footpads. *(Courtesy GA Kunkle, Gainesville, Florida.)*

with similar clinical features. A history of poor housing and sanitation in an enzootic area should increase suspicion of hookworm dermatitis.

Biopsy site selection

Affected sites with maximal ground contact that exhibit erythema, papules, alopecia, and lichenification should be selected for skin biopsy. Multiple samples will increase the likelihood of diagnosis. Submission of fresh tissue to a parasitologist for maceration and examination is ideal for identifying the parasites.*

Histopathology

The epidermis is acanthotic and may be eroded. Multifocal spongiosis, parakeratosis, and serocellular crusts are common features. Tracts caused by migration of larvae have been described by Muller, Kirk, and Scott and are characterized by linear accumulations of neutrophils and eosinophils that extend through the epidermis to the dermis.

The dermis is characterized by a superficial, mild to moderate, perivascular to interstitial, eosinophilic dermatitis. Neutrophils, lymphocytes, and macrophages are present in variable numbers. Larvae rarely are discovered in tissue section but may be recovered via maceration and dissection of skin specimens, best undertaken by a parasitologist.

Differential diagnoses include allergic dermatitides that feature eosinophils, such as other parasitic skin

diseases (canine flea allergy dermatitis, canine sarcoptic acariasis), and food allergy. Geographic location and opportunity for exposure must be considered in the diagnosis of hookworm dermatitis if etiologic agents cannot be demonstrated in tissue.

ALLERGIC CONTACT DERMATITIS
Clinical features (Figures 8-38 through 8-40)

See Chapter 4.

Biopsy site selection

Erythematous macules or papules represent early stages of the disease and, if present, should be sampled for biopsy. Newer lesions should be chosen over chronic lesions characterized by hyperpigmentation and lichenification, which are not diagnostic histopathologically. Lesions with severe self-trauma also should be avoided. The best lesions for histopathology can be obtained from positive patch tests at 24 to 48 hours.

Histopathology (Figure 8-41)

Acute and chronic lesions of the epidermis, described in Chapter 4, consist of spongiotic vesicles that progress to mild crusting and acanthosis. Dermal inflammation is superficial and perivascular and is generally mild. Lymphocytes, macrophages, and rarely a few eosinophils are seen. Mast cells may be prominent. Neutrophils are rare unless there is severe erosion or ulceration due to secondary self-trauma. Edema may be present.

Chronic allergic contact dermatitis mimics chronic dermatitis of any cause. Atopy, which also is character-

---

* Kunkle GA: Personal communication, 1990.

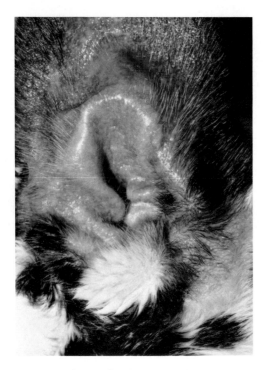

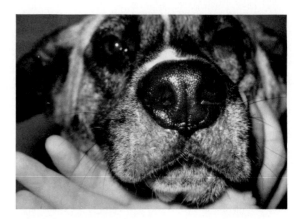

FIGURE 8-39. Allergic contact dermatitis in a dog. Note the alopecia and hyperpigmentation of the muzzle.

FIGURE 8-38. Acute allergic contact dermatitis of the ear of a Dalmatian caused by the neomycin in a topical otic preparation. An exudative and vesicular papular eruption extends beyond the confines of the ear canal.

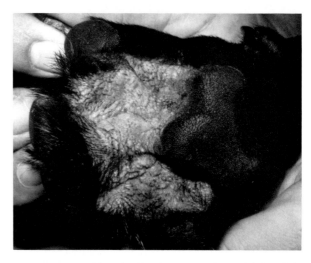

ized by mild inflammation in which eosinophils are rare, may be most similar. Clinical differentiation is required; histopathologic changes, unless from known positive patch tests, do not allow definitive diagnosis.

FIGURE 8-40. Chronic allergic contact dermatitis involving the ventral interdigital web of a Labrador Retriever. Lichenification, alopecia, and erythema are present. *(Courtesy CE Griffin, Garden Grove, California; case material from the University of California, Davis.)*

SUGGESTED READINGS

Superficial spreading pyoderma
See Chapter 1.

Atopy
Carlotti D: La dermatite atopique du chien, Le Point Veterinaire 17:5-17, 1985.

McDougal BJ: Allergy testing and hyposensitization for three common feline dermatoses, Mod Vet Pract 81:629-633, 1986.

Reedy LM: Results of allergy testing and hyposensitization in selected feline skin diseases, J Am Anim Hosp Assoc 18:618-623, 1982.

Reedy LM and Miller WH: Allergic skin diseases of dogs and cats, Philadelphia, 1989, WB Saunders, pp 23-109.

Schwartzman RM: Atopy in the dog, Arch Dermatol 96:418-422, 1967.

Scott DW: Feline dermatology 1983-1985, J Am Anim Hosp Assoc 23:255-274, 1987.

Scott DW: Observations on canine atopy, J Am Anim Hosp Assoc 17:91-100, 1981.

Sousa CA: Atopic dermatitis, Vet Clin North Am 18:1049-1059, 1988.

Willemse A: Investigations on canine atopic dermatitis, doctoral thesis, Utrecht, Netherlands, 1984, Drukkerij Elinkwijk, pp 1-163.

Food allergy
August JR: Dietary hypersensitivity in dogs: cutaneous manifestations, diagnosis, and management, Comp Cont Ed 7:469-477, 1985.

Baker E: Food allergy, Vet Clin North Am 4:79-89, 1974.

Carlotti DN, Remy I, and Prost C: Food allergy in dogs and cats: a review and report of 43 cases, Vet Dermatol 1:55-62, 1990.

Kettelhut BV and Metcalfe DD: Adverse reactions to food. In Middleton EM, Reed CE, Ellis EF, and others, editors: Allergy: principles and practice, St Louis, 1988, CV Mosby, pp 1481-1502.

Medleau L, Latimer KS, and Duncan JR: Food hypersensitivity in a cat, J Am Vet Med Assoc 189:692-693, 1986.

Reedy LM and Miller WH: Allergic skin diseases of dogs and cats, Philadelphia, 1989, WB Saunders, pp 147-158.

Scott DW: Feline dermatology 1900-1978: a monograph, J Am Anim Hosp Assoc 16:380-381, 1980.

Scott DW: Feline dermatology 1983-1985: "the secret sits," J Am Anim Hosp Assoc 23:261, 1987.

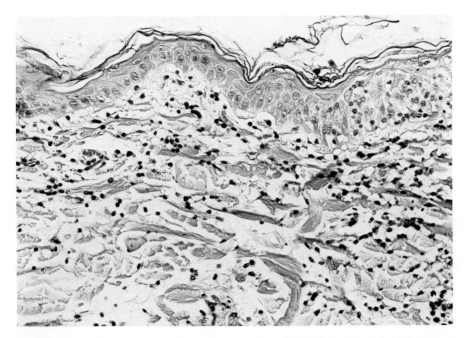

FIGURE 8-41. Allergic contact dermatitis in a dog. Superficial perivascular inflammation consists principally of mixed mononuclear cells. Note the epidermal spongiotic vesiculation at right. (×220.)

Strombeck DR and Guilford WG: Small animal gastroenterology, ed 2, Davis, Calif, 1990, Stonegate Publishing, pp 344-356.

Walton GS: Skin responses in the dog and cat to ingested allergens: observations on 100 confirmed cases, Vet Rec 81:709-713, 1967.

White SD: Difficult dermatologic diagnosis, J Am Vet Med Assoc 196:225, 1990.

White SD: Food hypersensitivity in 30 dogs, J Am Vet Med Assoc 188:695-698, 1986.

White SD and Mason IS: Dietary allergy. In Von Tscharner C and Halliwell REW, editors: Advances in veterinary dermatology, vol 1, London, 1990, Bailliere Tindall, pp 404-406.

White SD and Sequoia D: Food hypersensitivity in cats: 14 cases (1982-1987), J Am Vet Med Assoc 194:692-695, 1989.

Canine flea allergy dermatitis

Bevier DE: Fleas and flea control. In Kirk RW, editor: Current veterinary therapy X, Philadelphia, 1989, WB Saunders, pp 586-592.

Carlotti D and Heripret D: La dermatite par allergie aux piqures de puce chez le chien, Pratique Medicale et Chirurgicale de l'Animal de Compagnie, 6:(Suppl)1-64, 1986.

Halliwell REW and Gorman NT: Veterinary clinical immunology, Philadelphia, 1989, WB Saunders, pp 264-267.

Halliwell REW and Schemmer KR: The role of basophils in the immunopathogenesis of hypersensitivity to fleas (Ctenocephalides felis) in dogs, Vet Immunol Immunopathol 15:203-215, 1987.

Reedy LM and Miller WH: Allergic skin diseases of dogs and cats, Philadelphia, 1989, WB Saunders, pp 171-187.

Scheidt VJ: Flea allergy dermatitis, Vet Clin North Am 18:1023-1042, 1988.

Feline allergic miliary dermatitis

See Chapter 5.

Canine sarcoptic acariasis

Ackerman AB: Histologic diagnosis of inflammatory skin diseases, Philadelphia, 1978, Lea & Febiger, pp 295-301.

Anderson RK: Canine scabies, Comp Cont Ed 1:687-693, 1979.

Anderson RK: Norwegian scabies in a dog: a case report, J Am Anim Hosp Assoc 17:101-104, 1981.

Baker BB and Stannard AA: A look at canine scabies, J Am Anim Hosp Assoc 10:513-515, 1974.

Halliwell REW and Gorman NT: Veterinary clinical immunology, Philadelphia, 1989, WB Saunders, pp 269-270.

Lever WF and Schaumburg-Lever G: Histopathology of the skin, ed 7, Philadelphia, 1990, JB Lippincott, pp 237-238.

Feline notoedric acariasis

Lever WF and Schaumburg-Lever G: Histopathology of the skin, ed 7, Philadelphia, 1990, JB Lippincott, pp 237-238.

Muller GH, Kirk RW, and Scott DW: Small animal dermatology, ed 4, Philadelphia, 1989, WB Saunders, pp 396-407.

Cheyletiellosis

Alexander MM and Ihrke PJ: Cheyletiella dermatitis in small animal practice: a review, Cal Vet 3:9-12, 1982.

Foxx TS and Ewing SA: Morphologic features, behavior, and life history of Cheyletiella yasguri, Am J Vet Res 30:269-285, 1969.

McKeever PJ and Allen SK: Dermatitis associated with Cheyletiella infestation in cats, J Am Vet Med Assoc 174:718-720, 1979.

Muller GH, Kirk RW, and Scott DW: Small animal dermatology, ed 4, Philadelphia, 1989, WB Saunders, pp 369-376.

Paradis M, Scott DW, and Villeneuve A: Efficacy of ivermectin against Cheyletiella blakei infestation in cats, J Am Anim Hosp Assoc 26:125-128, 1990.

Rivers JK, Martin J, and Pukay B: Walking dandruff and Cheyletiella dermatitis, J Am Acad Dermatol 15:1130-1133, 1986.

Cutaneous dirofilariasis

Elkins AD amd Berkenblit M: Interdigital cyst in the dog caused by an adult *Dirofilaria immitis,* J Am Anim Hosp Assoc 26:71-72, 1990.

Halliwell REW and Gorman NT: Veterinary clinical immunology, Philadelphia, 1989, WB Saunders, pp 278.

Lever WF and Schaumburg-Lever G: Histopathology of the skin, ed 7, Philadelphia, 1990, JB Lippincott, pp 239.

Scott DW and Vaughn TC: Papulonodular dermatitis in a dog with occult filariasis, Comp Anim Pract 1:31-35, 1987.

Hookworm dermatitis

Baker KP: Clinical aspects of hookworm dermatitis, Br Vet Dermatol Study Group Newsletter 6:69-74, 1981.

Baker KP and Grimes TD: Cutaneous lesions in dogs associated with hookworm infestations, Vet Rec 87:376-379, 1970.

Muller GH, Kirk RW, and Scott DW: Small animal dermatology, ed 4, Philadelphia, 1989, WB Saunders, pp 347-350.

Allergic contact dermatitis

See Chapter 4.

Vascular diseases of the dermis

Vascular diseases of the dermis, as classified here, include those in which cutaneous vessels are the primary target. Urticaria is generally manifested predominantly by edema as a result of the direct or immune-mediated vascular effects of allergens or physical agents; however, some clinical cases of urticaria may be characterized histopathologically by vasculitis. For simplicity, vascular diseases are grouped here by histomorphologic characteristics and not by clinical appearance.

Vasculitis is characterized by vascular inflammation, as well as vascular alterations, including frank necrosis, fibrinoid change, endothelial swelling, and thrombosis. Most cutaneous vasculitides of animals may be attributed to immune-mediated mechanisms that are triggered by drugs, systemic collagen vascular diseases, or, commonly, undiscovered stimuli. A smaller group of vasculitides results from systemic infectious diseases.

URTICARIA AND ANGIOEDEMA (Synonym: hives)
Clinical features (Figures 9-1 through 9-3)

Urticaria and angioedema are edematous cutaneous reaction patterns characterized by the formation of wheals. Urticaria is distinguished by edema that is limited to the dermis. Extension of edema to the subjacent subcutaneous tissue is seen with angioedema. Both reaction patterns are uncommon in the dog and rare in the cat. Urticaria may be initiated by immunologic or nonimmunologic factors. Angioedema is almost always associated with hypersensitivity reactions. In addition, angioedema may proceed to anaphylaxis and consequently is of graver concern. The most frequently reported immunologic causes of urticaria and angioedema include drug reactions, food allergy, stinging or biting arthropods, vaccines, bacterins, blood transfusions, infections, plants, and atopy. Nonimmunologic or physical causes include heat, cold, sunlight, and water. Dermatographism is a rare subgroup of urticaria in which pressure to the skin produced by a blunt instrument initiates wheals. Muller, Kirk, and Scott indicate that dermatographism has been seen in the dog. Details were not given.

A wheal is a discrete, well-demarcated, erythematous, edematous swelling with a flat top and steep walled margins. Overlying hair may stand erect if wheals are present in haired areas. Wheals vary from small (< 1 cm in diameter) circular lesions to lesions many centimeters in diameter and may enlarge by peripheral extension to become confluent. Bizarre geographic (map-like) configurations may be seen. Angioedema is physically similar but considerably less well demarcated, since the edema is not confined to the dermis. Pruritus is highly variable. If pruritus is present, primary lesions may be obscured by self-trauma. Sites of involvement are contingent on the cause. Urticaria from venomous arthropods is seen more commonly on the face and on the comparatively glabrous areas such as the groin. Angioedema from an injection usually occurs at

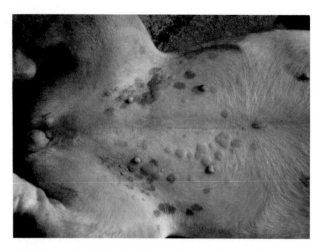

FIGURE 9-1. Urticaria due to insect bites on the ventral abdomen of an English Bulldog. Multiple, erythematous, well-demarcated wheals are present.

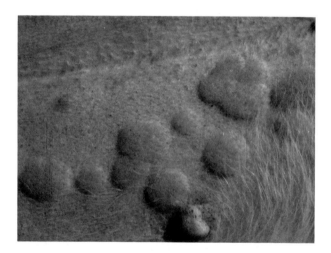

FIGURE 9-2. Closer view of dog in Figure 9-1. Several steep-walled wheals have coalesced.

the site of injection, but may extend widely to surrounding areas. Cold- or water-induced urticaria occurs at the sites of contact.

Breed, age, or sex predilections have not been substantiated. Short-coated breeds such as the English Bulldog, Bull Terrier, Doberman Pinscher, and Dalmatian may be at increased risk. However, this clinical impression may be due to the fact that truncal urticaria is more easily noticed in short-coated dogs, since short hairs standing erect over wheals are striking; additionally, all of these breeds have comparatively glabrous abdomens.

Superficial bacterial folliculitis is the major clinical differential diagnosis, since hairs standing erect as a result of perifollicular inflammation may mimic wheals.

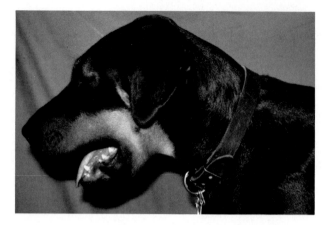

FIGURE 9-3. Angioedema of the face of a Doberman Pinscher puppy caused by a stinging insect. The eyes are swollen shut, and the muzzle is severely distorted by edema.

In addition, early erythema multiforme, vasculitis, and mast cell tumors all may be characterized by wheals or wheal-like lesions.

Biopsy site selection

Expeditious skin biopsy is recommended, since wheals are transient lesions. If pruritus is present, wheals may be obscured by secondary self-trauma. The inclusion of a biopsy specimen from adjacent normal skin may be helpful, since the dermal edema of urticaria may be subtle.

Histopathology (Figures 9-4 and 9-5)

Epidermal changes usually are not present in nontraumatized wheals. Dermal histopathologic changes may be subtle. Edema may widen the spaces between collagen fibers in the upper one half to one third of the dermis but easily can be missed if it is not severe. Urticaria should be suspected in any case for which no obvious histopathologic changes are present in tissue. In more severe urticaria, prominent edema may expand the superficial dermis and result in secondary dermal-epidermal separation. Angioedema may be characterized by severe edema that extends to the subcutis.

Inflammation may be present, and lesions may mimic Ackerman's urticarial allergic eruption. This type of urticaria may be more common in Bull Terriers and Bulldogs and is characterized by superficial and perivascular mast cells, eosinophils, neutrophils, and fewer lymphocytes and macrophages. The epidermis may be moderately acanthotic, and there may be occasional superficial pustulation and spongiosis. The type and degree of inflammatory infiltrate may depend on the underlying cause of the urticarial eruption. Muller, Kirk, and Scott, and Lever have described leukocyto-

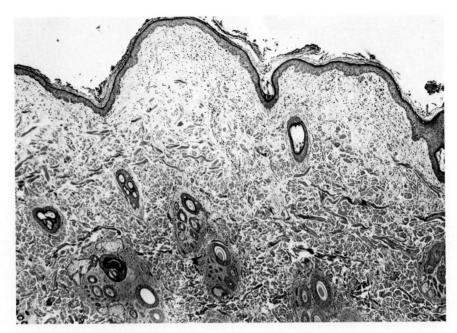

FIGURE 9-4. Urticaria in a dog. Edema imparts a pallor to the superficial dermis. Note the mild superficial inflammation. (×35.)

clastic vasculitis in urticaria of dogs and humans, respectively. (See following discussion.)

Urticaria is distinctive. On the other hand, urticarial allergic eruption may resemble other superficial perivascular skin diseases histopathologically but has more prominent dermal edema. In particular, severe lesions of superficial spreading pyoderma or acute lesions of parasitic allergy may be similar.

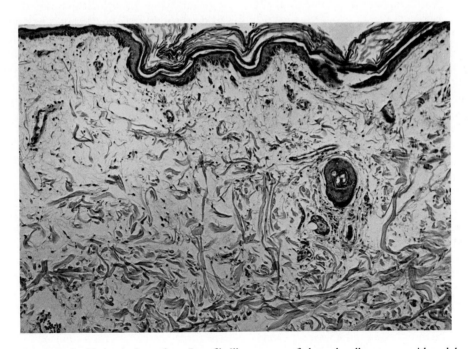

FIGURE 9-5. Urticaria in a dog. Interfibrillar spaces of dermal collagen are widened by edema. (×100.)

IMMUNE-MEDIATED VASCULITIS
Clinical features (Figure 9-6)

Immune-mediated vasculitis is a rare syndrome of multifactorial etiology seen in dogs and cats. Inflammatory changes in the walls of blood vessels lead to swelling, purpura, and necrosis. Most immune-mediated vasculitides are probably caused by immune-complex disease (type III hypersensitivity). The offending antigen is rarely identified. Connective tissue diseases and drugs may be precipitating factors, although many cases are idiopathic. Visceral lesions may be seen contingent on the underlying cause.

Swelling, erythema, purpura, hemorrhagic bullae, necrosis, and ulceration are seen. Devitalized tissue is firm and discolored and may slough. Areas of less extensive collateral circulation such as the pinnae, paws, tail tip, lips, oral mucosa, and antecubital region most commonly are affected. Pain is variable but usually is present if tissue necrosis is marked. Systemic signs such as fever, malaise, and anorexia may be noted.

According to Scott, Dachshunds and Rottweilers may be at increased risk. Although age and sex predilections have not been established, vasculitis is probably more common in older animals.

Clinical differential diagnoses should include septic vasculitis, disseminated intravascular coagulation, cold agglutinin disease, cryoglobulinemia, frostbite, and ischemic necrosis associated with toxins. History, environment, laboratory findings, and evidence of systemic disease may aid in the differentiation of these clinically similar diseases.

Biopsy site selection

Early lesions of hemorrhage and swelling are preferred over chronic lesions of ulceration for histopathologic examination. Frequently, deep specimens are required to detect vasculitis centered in the deep dermis or panniculus. Consequently, wedge biopsy is preferred over punch biopsy. Multiple specimens should be submitted, if possible, because diagnostic lesions of vasculitis may be difficult to find in tissue.

Histopathology (Figures 9-7 and 9-8)

Primary epidermal lesions are not a feature of vasculitis. Exudation, crusting, erosion, and ulceration may develop secondary to hypoxic tissue damage induced by loss of subjacent vascular integrity.

Most cases of immune-mediated vasculitis involve small vessels of the dermis. Rarely, vasculitis also may affect vessels of the panniculus, as in erythema nodosum–like panniculitis (vasculitic septal panniculitis; see Chapter 20). In so-called leukocytoclastic vasculitis, which is perhaps the most common morphologic type of immune-mediated vasculitis, neutrophilic inflammation centers in and around dermal

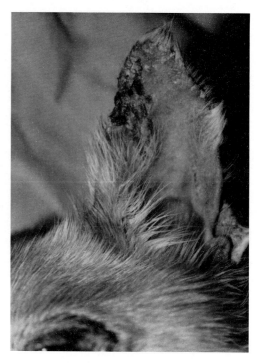

FIGURE 9-6. Immune-mediated vasculitis affecting the ear of a Chihuahua. Necrosis and ulceration have led to loss of tissue along the pinnal margin; note accompanying crusting.

venules. Leukocytoclasia is manifested by fragmented neutrophilic debris around vessels ("nuclear dust"). Fibrinoid change of vessels is common, and intravascular fibrin thrombi may be present rarely. Perivascular hemorrhage and edema may occur.

Vasculitis may be nonleukocytoclastic and may include lymphocytic and histiocytic infiltrates, possibly as a result of cell-mediated immunologic activity. Variation in the inflammatory infiltrate may depend on the type of immunologic reaction that the inciting antigen induces.

Histopathologic evidence of vascular inflammation and necrosis may be difficult to document in cases of clinically suspected vasculitis. Suspicion for vasculitis may be based on histopathologic evidence of ischemic necrosis, prominent and closely oriented perivascular inflammation, or severe dermal hemorrhage and edema.

Histopathologic differential diagnoses are few if vascular inflammation and necrosis are found. Septic vasculitis is rare and should include a predominantly neutrophilic infiltrate. (See discussion below.) Cutaneous vascular necrosis and inflammation can be seen in the rare canine lymphomatoid granulomatosis, a poorly understood lymphohistiocytic proliferative disease that may precede frank lymphoma (see Chapter 31), or rarely in leukemia cutis where neoplastic myeloid or erythroid cells invade dermal vessels.

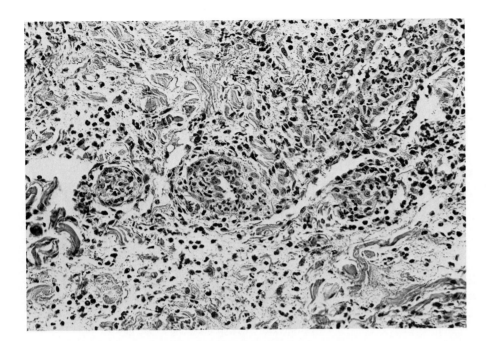

FIGURE 9-7. Immunemediated vasculitis in a dog. Vessel walls contain neutrophils, and endothelial cells are swollen. (×220.)

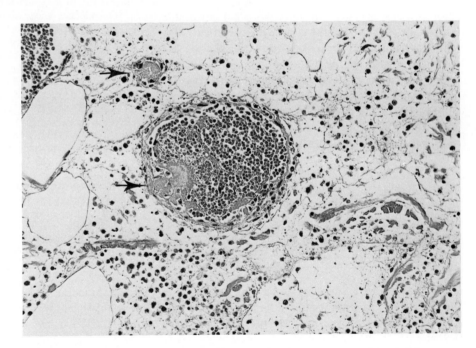

FIGURE 9-8. Vasculitis in a dog, demonstrating acute fibrinoid necrosis of the vessel wall. Note the early fibrin thrombus in a large necrotic vessel and small adjacent venule *(arrows)*. (×220.)

SEPTIC VASCULITIS
Clinical features (Figure 9-9)

Septic vasculitis is characterized by inflammatory changes in the walls of blood vessels secondary to catastrophic bacterial infection. It is rare in both the dog and the cat. Septic vasculitis may occur as a sequela to severe, canine deep pyoderma, especially when the bacterial infection is secondary to generalized demodicosis or a defect in host immune response. Rocky Mountain spotted fever is an additional uncommon cause of vasculitis in dogs. Vasculitis associated with ehrlichiosis

and vasculitis caused by systemic infection with *Erysipelothrix rhusiopathiae* were each described in separate canine cases by Crawford.

Clinical signs partially parallel cutaneous immunemediated vasculitis. Swelling, erythema, purpura, hemorrhagic bullae, necrosis, and ulceration may be generalized or localized to areas of less extensive collateral circulation, such as the distal extremities and pinnae. Cellulitis and deep folliculitis and furunculosis may be present, especially if septic vasculitis is secondary to demodicosis. Fistulous tracts may be seen. Devitalized tissue may be firm and discolored if the vasculitis is not

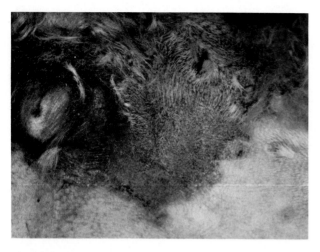

FIGURE 9-9. Septic vasculitis of the ventral abdomen of a dog secondary to septicemia. Firm and discolored devitalized tissue is surrounded by a margin of erythema, swelling, and ulceration.

accompanying primary skin infection. Pain is variable but usually is present if tissue necrosis is marked. Systemic signs such as fever, malaise, and anorexia are common features and may indicate coexistent visceral septic vasculitis affecting multiple internal organs. Coma and death are possible sequelae.

Specific breed, age, and sex predilections have not been noted for septic vasculitis. Septic vasculitis secondary to demodicosis would have breed and age predilections similar to demodicosis alone.

Clinical differential diagnoses should include immune-mediated vasculitis, severe deep bacterial folliculitis and furunculosis, disseminated intravascular coagulation, and ischemic necrosis associated with toxins. Generalized skin lesions and documentation of sepsis by blood culture are suggestive of septic vasculitis.

Biopsy site selection

Early lesions, characterized by erythema or petechial hemorrhage, are preferred over advanced lesions with extensive necrosis and ulceration. Wedge biopsy specimens are more likely to yield a diagnosis, because the punch technique may result in disruption of friable, devitalized lesions. If distal extremities are sampled, the collateral circulation must be adequate to nourish distal tissue and provide for healing of the biopsy site.

Histopathology

Primary epidermal lesions are not a feature of septic vasculitis. Secondary necrosis and ulceration are common in advanced lesions as a result of hypoxic tissue damage.

Dermal vascular lesions may resemble those of immune-mediated vasculitis but often are more severe. (See preceding discussion.) A primarily neutrophilic inflammation occurs in and around vessels. Vascular necrosis and fibrin thrombi may be prominent. Severe hemorrhage and edema and dermal and epidermal necrosis (infarction) are common and may be extensive. Rarely, bacterial emboli may be present in florid cases. In cases of septic vasculitis secondary to generalized demodicosis with deep pyoderma, features of that disease also are present. (See Chapter 16.)

SUGGESTED READINGS

Urticaria and angioedema

Ackerman AB: Histologic diagnosis of inflammatory skin diseases, Philadelphia, 1978, Lea & Febiger, pp 180-183, 305.

Kaplan AP: Urticaria and angioedema. In Middleton EM, Reed CE, Enis EF, and others, editors: Allergy: principles and practice, St Louis, 1988, CV Mosby, pp 1377-1401.

Lever WF and Schaumburg-Lever G: Histopathology of the skin, ed 7, Philadelphia, 1990, JB Lippincott, pp 152-153.

Mueller DL and Noxon JO: Anaphylaxis: pathophysiology and treatment, Comp Cont Ed 12:157-170, 1990.

Muller GH, Kirk RW, and Scott DW: Small animal dermatology, ed 4, Philadelphia, 1989, WB Saunders, pp 447-449.

Reedy LM and Miller WH: Allergic skin diseases of dogs and cats, Philadelphia, 1989, WB Saunders, pp 23-31.

Stafford CT: Urticaria as a sign of systemic disease, Ann Allergy 64:264-272, 1990.

Immune-mediated vasculitis

Crawford MA and Foil CS: Vasculitis: clinical syndromes in small animals, Comp Cont Ed 11:400-415, 1989.

Halliwell REW and Gorman NT: Veterinary clinical immunology, Philadelphia, 1989, WB Saunders, pp 280-281.

Jones RE and others: Questions to the editorial board and other authorities (vasculitis), Am J Dermatopathol 7:181-187, 1985.

Lever WF and Schaumburg-Lever G: Histopathology of the skin, ed 7, Philadelphia, 1990, JB Lippincott, pp 188-193.

Muller GH, Kirk RW, and Scott DW: Small animal dermatology, ed 4, Philadelphia, 1989, WB Saunders, pp 533-535.

Randall MG and Hurvitz AI: Immune-mediated vasculitis in five dogs, J Am Vet Med Assoc 183:207-211, 1983.

Scott DW and others: Immune-mediated dermatoses in domestic animals: ten years after. II, Comp Cont Ed 9:539-553, 1987.

Septic vasculitis

Crawford MA and Foil CS: Vasculitis: clinical syndromes in small animals, Comp Cont Ed 11:400-415, 1989.

Jones RE and others: Questions to the editorial board and other authorities (vasculitis), Am J Dermatopathol 7:181-187, 1985.

Lever WF and Schaumburg-Lever G: Histopathology of the skin, ed 7, Philadelphia, 1990, JB Lippincott, 323-325.

Lichenoid (interface) diseases of the dermis

Lichenoid and interface diseases of the dermis are characterized by superficial dermal inflammation that is oriented along the dermal-epidermal junction. The terms *lichenoid* and *interface* are often used interchangeably. For descriptive clarity, the authors prefer to define *interface dermatitis* as mild, superficial dermal inflammation that is oriented tightly to and often obscures the dermal-epidermal junction; whereas *lichenoid dermatitis* is characterized by dense, laminar or band-like inflammation within the superficial dermis, which may or may not obscure the dermal-epidermal junction.

Lichenoid or interface dermatitides often have as their proven or proposed pathogenic mechanism an immune-mediated damage to components of the overlying epidermis, in particular, basal cells, the basement membrane, or melanocytes. Histopathologic differentiation of the diseases of this group will depend upon differences in the epidermal lesions, as well as variation in the composition of the dermal infiltrate.

MUCOCUTANEOUS PYODERMA
Clinical features (Figures 10-1 and 10-2)

Mucocutaneous pyoderma is an uncommon syndrome seen in the dog, characterized by erythema, crusting, and swelling around mucocutaneous junctions. The syndrome is seen most commonly on the lips and perioral skin. Similar lesions may be seen less commonly at other mucocutaneous sites, such as the vulva, prepuce, and anus. Mucocutaneous pyoderma may affect the mucocutaneous margin of one naris or occasionally both nares. Lip lesions usually are bilaterally symmetric and gradual in onset. Depigmentation of the lips and adjacent skin may be seen in chronic cases. Perioral mucocutaneous pyoderma may coexist with lip-fold pyoderma in some cases. Regional lymphadenopathy is variable. Pruritus or pain may be noted and self-trauma is common. Signalment predilections have not been documented; however, German Shepherd Dogs may be affected more frequently.

Discoid lupus erythematosus is the major clinical differential diagnosis. In discoid lupus erythematosus, partially symmetric lesions usually are present also on the dorsum of the muzzle and the planum nasale. Perioral demodicosis may be considered, but generally is seen in younger dogs and has a more rapid onset. Lip-fold pyoderma also may mimic (and can accompany) mucocutaneous pyoderma. Lesions of lip-fold pyoderma are confined to a triangular fold on either side of the lower lip; lip-fold pyoderma is seen primarily in spaniels.

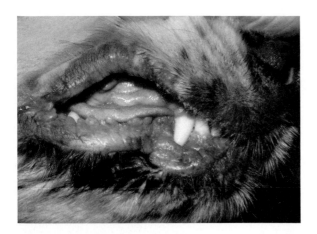

FIGURE 10-1. Mucocutaneous pyoderma in a Brittany Spaniel. Note erythema, swelling, and crusting involving the lips and adjacent skin of the muzzle. Salivary staining is present on the haircoat ventral to the lower lip.

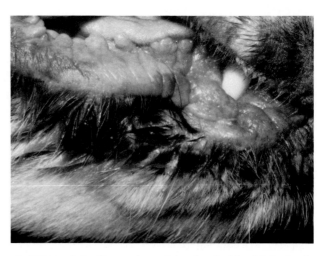

FIGURE 10-2. Closer view of the dog in Fig. 10-1. Swelling is extensive where the upper canine tooth contacts the lower lip. Exudate mats the hair surrounding the lesions.

Biopsy site selection

Areas of inflammation and crusting without ulceration are recommended sites for biopsy. Punch biopsies are preferred because scarring of delicate mucosal tissue is minimized by this technique.

Histopathology (Figures 10-3 and 10-4)

The epidermis is hyperplastic and often has superficial pustulation and crusting. Exocytosis of neutrophils may be accompanied by spongiosis. In areas complicated by self-trauma, erosion or ulceration are observed.

The dermis contains a dense, lichenoid band of superficial inflammation composed of plasma cells, which often predominate, as well as mixtures of lymphocytes, neutrophils, and macrophages. There is close approximation to the overlying epidermis by the inflammatory infiltrate, but the dermal-epidermal interface is not obscured. Pigmentary incontinence may be present. If specimens are obtained from haired skin, milder similar inflammation often surrounds subjacent adnexal appendages.

Plasmacellular subepidermal or submucosal inflammation may be the principal histopathologic feature of

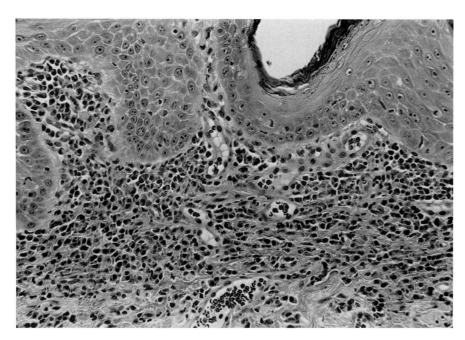

FIGURE 10-3. Mucocutaneous pyoderma. A lichenoid band of inflammation in the superficial dermis contains prominent plasma cells. (×90.)

FIGURE 10-4. Mucocutaneous pyoderma demonstrating many plasma cells in the superficial dermal infiltrate. (×350.)

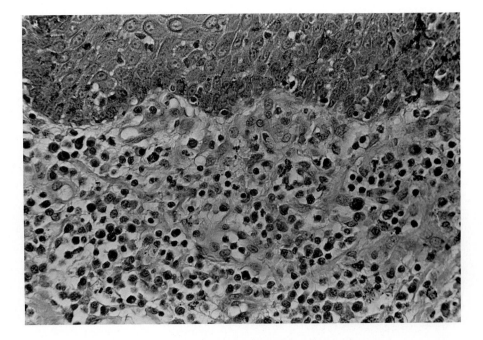

mucocutaneous inflammation regardless of the underlying cause. Intertrigo (skin-fold pyoderma) located near mucocutaneous junctions (lip fold and vulvar fold) is histopathologically similar, but may exhibit fewer plasma cells. Clinical separation of these entities is required.

Discoid lupus erythematosus is the major differential diagnosis for the perioral or nasal forms of mucocutaneous pyoderma. In contrast to discoid lupus erythematosus, basal cell degeneration is not observed in perioral mucocutaneous pyoderma. Plasma cells are clearly prominent in mucocutaneous pyoderma, whereas lymphocytes and macrophages usually predominate in discoid lupus erythematosus.

DISCOID LUPUS ERYTHEMATOSUS
Clinical features (Figures 10-5 and 10-6)

See Chapter 2.

Biopsy site selection

Areas of early depigmentation, characterized by graying or partial loss of pigment, are optimal sites for skin biopsy. Traumatized lesions or lesions with severe crusting, ulceration, or scarring should be avoided.

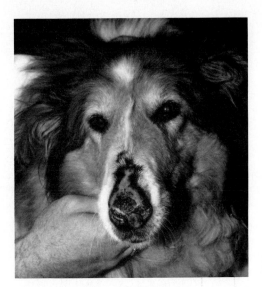

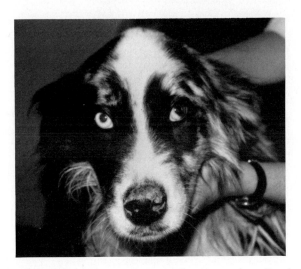

FIGURE 10-5. Discoid lupus erythematosus in a Border Collie. Lesions consist of depigmentation, ulceration, and crusting involve only the planum nasale.

FIGURE 10-6. Chronic, severe discoid lupus erythematosus in a Collie. Depigmentation, ulceration, and crusting affect the dorsal muzzle and the planum nasale. Necrosis of the epithelium and the underlying connective tissue has altered the conformation of the planum nasale.

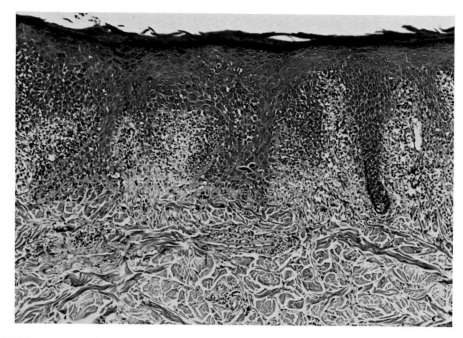

FIGURE 10-7. Discoid lupus erythematosus of the planum nasale. Lichenoid inflammation partially obscures the dermal-epidermal junction. (×110.)

Early lesions of the lip and dorsal muzzle are more likely to yield diagnostic results. Difficulties with hemostasis and scarring may be additional reasons to avoid the planum nasale or pinnae unless other more suitable sites for biopsy are not affected.

Histopathology (Figures 10-7 and 10-8)

Epidermal lesions and immunofluorescent findings have been discussed in Chapter 2 and principally include basal cell degeneration and deposition of immunoglobulin and complement at the basement mem-

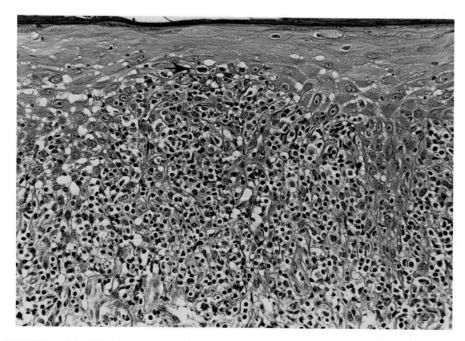

FIGURE 10-8. High-power magnification of discoid lupus erythematosus demonstrating mixed mononuclear inflammation at the dermal-epidermal junction. Note the basilar vacuolar degeneration and focal necrotic basal keratinocyte *(arrow)*. (×220.)

brane zone. The superficial dermis contains a dense, band-like lichenoid infiltrate or occasionally a milder interface infiltrate. Inflammation consists of lymphocytes, macrophages, and fewer plasma cells that abut and partially obscure the overlying dermal-epidermal interface. Plasma cells may be more prominent if lesions from the lip are examined. There may be exocytosis of lymphocytes into the lower layers of the epidermis. Pigmentary incontinence, characterized by coarsely clumped melanin in superficial dermal macrophages, is often marked and reflects previous damage to the basal cell layer of the epidermis. Neutrophils are variable in the dermis, and their numbers reflect the degree of overlying epidermal erosion and superficial crusting. Often a characteristic nodular pattern of inflammation (mixed mononuclear cells) surrounds follicles and adnexal glands in specimens obtained from haired skin.

Rosenkrantz demonstrated that groups of dogs with discoid lupus erythematosus had increased mucin deposition (acid mucopolysaccharide) intraepithelially and intradermally when compared to groups of dogs with other skin diseases. Caution in the use of mucin deposition as a diagnostic aid is advised; strict adherence to the pH requirements of routine mucin stains (Alcian blue at pH 2.5) is critical. In addition, individual cases of other inflammatory skin diseases may show significant mucin deposition. Eosinophilic plaque may have striking epidermal and superficial follicular mucinosis, and furunculosis and other severe dermal inflammatory diseases may show deposition of dermal mucin.

Discoid lupus erythematosus may be indistinguishable from systemic lupus erythematosus, particularly

when dermal inflammation is mild. (See discussion below.) Other differential diagnoses include perioral and nasal mucocutaneous pyoderma, and Vogt-Koyanagi-Harada–like syndrome. Basal cell degeneration is a feature of discoid lupus erythematosus that is absent in mucocutaneous pyoderma, and plasma cells are usually not as prominent in discoid lupus erythematosus as they are in mucocutaneous pyoderma. Vogt-Koyanagi-Harada–like syndrome generally will have a greater preponderance of large macrophages in the dermal infiltrate. Finer melanin granulation is seen within macrophages in Vogt-Koyanagi-Harada–like syndrome in comparison to the heavy clumping of melanin observed in discoid lupus erythematosus.

SYSTEMIC LUPUS ERYTHEMATOSUS
Clinical features (Figures 10-9 and 10-10)
See Chapter 2.

Biopsy site selection
Care should be taken to avoid ulcers or erosions, since an intact epidermis is necessary to substantiate the diagnosis. Erythematous areas adjacent to ulcers may yield diagnostic results. If panniculitis is suspected, a full-thickness wedge technique is recommended to ensure that subcutaneous fat is included in the specimen. Oral specimens rarely are beneficial, since ulcers, which are inherently nondiagnostic, are common in this location. In addition, the mucosa may be disrupted easily from the submucosa in apparently intact lesions.

Histopathology (Figures 10-11 and 10-12)
The histopathologic findings of systemic lupus erythematosus may be nondiagnostic, a dilemma that also

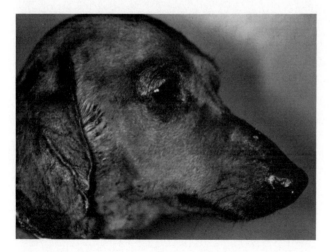

FIGURE 10-9. Systemic lupus erythematosus in an aged Dachshund. Necrosis leading to scarring affects the muzzle, periorbital skin, and pinnae somewhat symmetrically. *(Courtesy AM Hargis, Seattle, Washington; case material from the University of California, Davis.)*

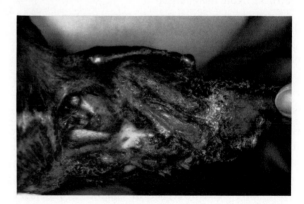

FIGURE 10-10. Systemic lupus erythematosus affecting the inner surface of the pinnae of the Dachshund seen in Figure 10-9. Extensive tissue necrosis is caused by vasculitis. *(Courtesy AM Hargis, Seattle, Washington; case material from the University of California, Davis.)*

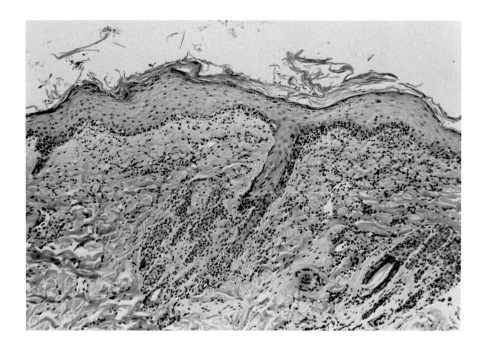

FIGURE 10-11. Systemic lupus erythematosus in a cat. Interface dermatitis is accompanied by mild periadnexal inflammation. (*Case material from WS Rosenkrantz, Garden Grove, California.*) (×90.)

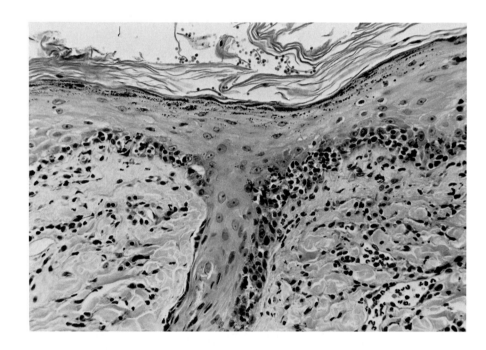

FIGURE 10-12. Higher magnification of the dermal-epidermal junction shown in Figure 10-11. Note the interface inflammation, which obscures the basement membrane zone. Vacuolar degeneration of the basal cell layer is prominent. (×220.)

is encountered in human medicine. Classically, histopathologic and immunofluorescent or immunohistochemical findings are similar to those of discoid lupus erythematosus. (See preceding discussion.) Epidermal lesions have been discussed in Chapter 2 and principally include basal cell degeneration.

Inflammation in sytemic lupus erythematosus is usually not as intense as in discoid lupus erythematosus; the orientation of inflammatory cells is generally interface rather than lichenoid in pattern. Plasma cells are not as prominent as in many cases of discoid lupus

erythematosus; lymphocytes and macrophages may predominate. The outer root sheaths of superficial hair follicles may be similarly affected. Mucin may be prominent. (See preceding discussion on discoid lupus erythematosus.)

Panniculitis attributed to systemic lupus erythematosus has been observed in the dog and cat and has been compared to lupus profundus or lupus panniculitis in humans. In lupus panniculitis, lymphocytes and plasma cells predominate in a lobular to diffuse pattern, and lymphoid follicles may be present.

PEMPHIGUS ERYTHEMATOSUS
Clinical features (Figure 10-13)

See Chapter 1.

Biopsy site selection

Because of the fragile and transient nature of primary lesions in pemphigus erythematosus, early lesions (pustules and vesicopustules) should be obtained promptly. Diagnostic histopathology may not be forthcoming from older crusted lesions. If only crusted lesions are available, these should be procured carefully, and the pathology service should be instructed to include any dissociated crusts in the slide preparation.

Histopathology (Figure 10-14)

Epidermal lesions have been described in Chapter 1 and are principally those of pemphigus foliaceus (superficial pustulation with acantholysis). Basal cell degeneration, as seen in discoid lupus erythematosus, also may be present. (See Chapter 2.)

Dermal lesions resemble those of discoid lupus erythematosus (see preceding discussion) and include a lichenoid infiltrate of lymphocytes, macrophages, and plasma cells. Inflammation often obscures the dermal-epidermal interface. Pigmentary incontinence is mild to moderate.

The lichenoid inflammation observed in lesions of chronic facial pemphigus foliaceus is histopathologically indistinguishable from that of pemphigus erythematosus. A question as to whether some cases of

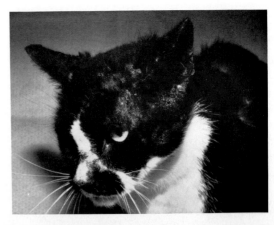

FIGURE 10-13. Pemphigus erythematosus in a cat. Partially bilaterally symmetric vesicopustules, accompanied by later stage erosions and ulcerations with adherent crusts, affect the planum nasale, dorsal muzzle, ears, and forehead. *(Courtesy AC Mundell, Seattle, Washington; case material from the University of California, Davis.)*

chronic facial pemphigus foliaceus are in fact pemphigus erythematosus exists in the mind of the authors. However, according to the currently accepted definition in veterinary dermatology, the ANA test should be positive, and immunofluorescent or immunohistochemical testing should show deposition of immunoglobulin at *both* the basement membrane zone and the intercellular spaces of the epidermis in order to confirm a diagnosis of pemphigus erythematosus.

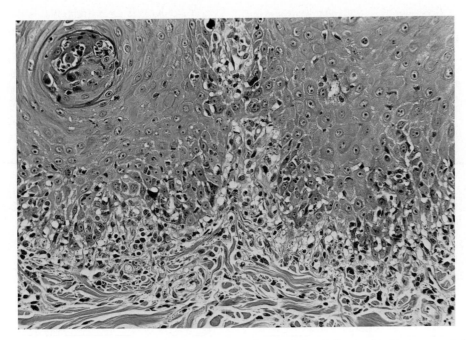

FIGURE 10-14. Pemphigus erythematosus in a dog. Interface inflammation is accompanied by vacuolation of the basilar epidermis. Note the small intraepidermal pustule containing free keratinocytes at left. (×220.)

VOGT-KOYANAGI-HARADA-LIKE SYNDROME (Synonyms: VKH, cutaneous depigmentation and uveitis in dogs)

Clinical features (Figures 10-15 through 10-17)

Vogt-Koyanagi-Harada–like syndrome in the dog is a rare syndrome of probable autoimmune etiology characterized by a concurrent granulomatous uveitis and symmetric facial depigmentation. A type IV hypersensitivity to melanin has been demonstrated in humans with Vogt-Koyanagi-Harada syndrome. Similar mechanisms have been postulated for the dog. In contrast to the syndrome seen in humans, deafness and neurologic signs suggestive of meningeal involvement have not been reported in the dog.

Clinically, uveitis usually either precedes or occurs concurrently with skin disease. Rarely, skin disease may precede uveitis. The ophthalmologic component of the disease usually holds greater portent than the cutaneous component, since blindness may be the sequela. Skin disease may be largely asymptomatic and is primarily cosmetically disfiguring. Consequently, diagnosis of the skin disease may bear greatest importance as a marker for the ophthalmologic disease.

Symmetric facial leukoderma is accompanied by variable erythema and crusting. Leukotrichia and alopecia are less common. The dorsal muzzle, periorbital region, planum nasale, and lips are the predominant sites of involvement. Male dogs commonly have scrotal lesions and female dogs may have vulvar lesions. Lesions also may be seen on the footpads and perianally. On rare occasion, as reported by Campbell, depigmentation of the skin and haircoat may become generalized. Pruritus is variable but may be marked. Regional lymphadenopathy is common. Photoaggravation of skin lesions has been noted.

Akitas, Samoyeds, Siberian Huskies, Alaskan Malamutes, Chow Chows, and their related cross breeds are at increased risk. Vogt-Koyanagi-Harada–like syndrome also has been seen in the Shetland Sheepdog, white German Shepherd Dog, Irish Setter, Ainu, and Shiba. Age or sex predilections have not been established.

Vogt-Koyanagi-Harada–like syndrome must be differentiated from facially oriented autoimmune skin diseases (discoid lupus erythematosus, systemic lupus

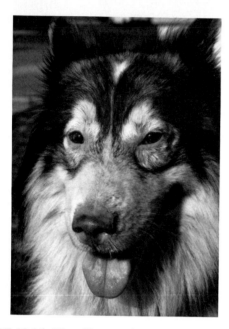

FIGURE 10-15. Vogt-Koyanagai–Harada-like syndrome in an Alaskan Malamute. Partially bilaterally symmetric leukotrichia and vitiligo are accompanied by erythema and alopecia.

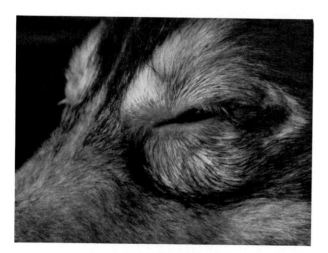

FIGURE 10-16. Closer view of periorbital area of dog in Figure 10-15. Note the swelling, and squinting indicative of photophobia associated with uveitis.

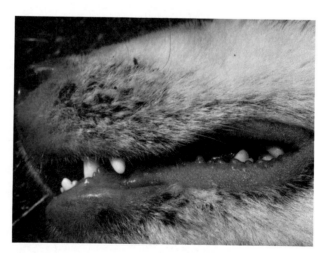

FIGURE 10-17. Closer view of the muzzle of dog in Figure 10-15. Diffuse erythema and crusting are present. The depigmented lips were uniformly black before the onset of disease.

erythematosus, pemphigus foliaceus, and pemphigus erythematosus) and vitiligo. An ANA test should be performed to aid in differentiating systemic lupus erythematosus. An ophthalmologic examination should be performed, since concurrent uveitis is highly suggestive of Vogt-Koyanagi-Harada–like syndrome. Histopathology frequently will aid in differentiation.

Biopsy site selection

Areas of depigmentation, erythema, and scaling, preferably of recent development, are beneficial sites for skin biopsy. As in other facial skin diseases, the lips and dorsal muzzle are preferred sites, since sampling is not difficult and scarring is not likely. Secondarily infected or self-traumatized lesions should be avoided.

Histopathology (Figures 10-18 through 10-20)

The epidermis is acanthotic and there may be secondary superficial crusting with variable erosion or ulceration. Melanin in the basal layer may be decreased or absent in chronic lesions; decreased numbers of epidermal melanocytes, as reported by Kern, may be de-

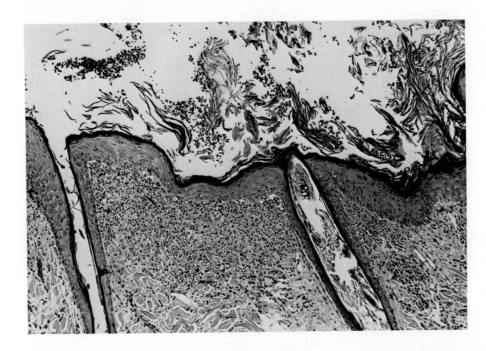

FIGURE 10-18. Vogt-Koyanagi-Harada–like syndrome. A lichenoid band of predominantly histiocytic inflammation is within the superficial dermis. (×90.)

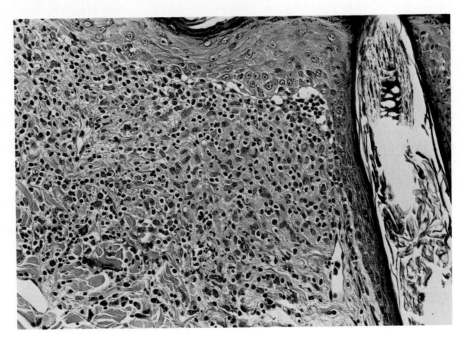

FIGURE 10-19. Higher magnification of the lichenoid inflammation shown in Figure 10-18. Note the predominance of large epithelioid macrophages, some of which contain a fine, dustlike scattering of intracytoplasmic melanin. (×220.)

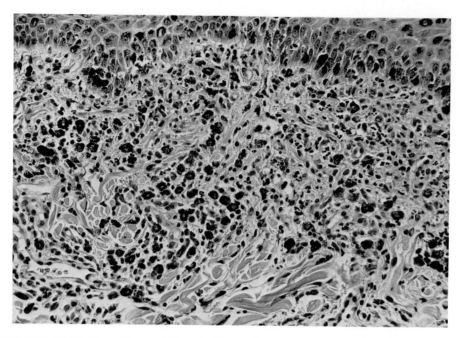

FIGURE 10-20. Vogt-Koyanagi-Harada–like syndrome. Melanin granules are distributed abundantly in macrophages. (×220.)

tected. Exocytosis of mononuclear cells may be evident. Basal cell degeneration is rare.

Chronic lesions of Vogt-Koyanagi-Harada–like syndrome may show only minimal dermal inflammation in the face of decreased or absent epidermal melanin. In early lesions, melanin alteration is often subtle and dermal inflammation pronounced. Early dermal lesions are characterized by a dense band of inflammation that lies immediately subjacent to the epidermis, touching but rarely obscuring the overlying basal cell layer. Inflammatory cells consist of large, often pale macrophages and fewer lymphocytes and plasma cells. Macrophages often contain finely granular melanin pig-

ment. Occasionally, similar inflammation in a nodular pattern may be found surrounding adnexa. The presence of neutrophils in the dermal infiltrate depends on the degree of overlying epidermal erosion or ulceration.

Vogt-Koyanagi-Harada–like syndrome must be differentiated principally from discoid lupus erythematosus. The predominance of large macrophages and the finely granular appearance of the melanin pigment contained within them are key differentiating features from discoid lupus erythematosus. In addition, basal cell degeneration is typical of discoid lupus erythematosus but rare in Vogt-Koyanagi-Harada–like syndrome.

VITILIGO (Synonym: idiopathic leukoderma)
Clinical features (Figures 10-21 through 10-24)

Vitiligo is an acquired melanocytopenic disorder characterized by progressive, usually well-circumscribed, loss of pigmentation. With the exception of idiopathic depigmentation of the planum nasale ("Dudley nose"), a condition that may or may not be due to similar mechanisms, vitiligo is relatively uncommon in the dog and very rare in the cat. Marked breed predilections indicate that vitiligo in the dog may be heritable. Vitiligo in humans is a heritable disease of autosomal dominance and variable expression. Similar genetics have been hypothesized by Mahaffey for vitiligo of the Belgian Tervuren Dog.

The etiopathogenesis of vitiligo in domestic animals and humans is unclear. Serum antimelanocyte antibodies documented in affected Belgian Tervurens by Naughton suggest an autoimmune basis for vitiligo. However, composite research data from human medicine indicates that vitiligo may have a complex pathogenesis, involving the lack of normal protective mechanisms that eliminate toxic melanin precursors, neurochemical mediators that inhibit melanogenesis or destroy melanocytes, and the induction of autoantibodies against various antigens in the melanogenic system.

Depigmented macules gradually develop on the planum nasale, lips, muzzle, buccal mucosa, and elsewhere on the face. Footpads may be affected. Erythema

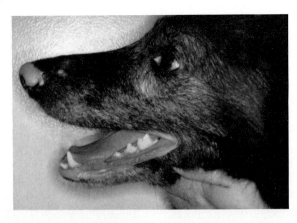

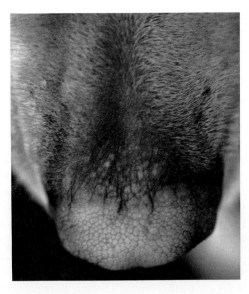

FIGURE 10-21. Vitiligo in a Belgian Tervuren. Note the depigmentation of the planum nasale, muzzle, lips, and periorbital skin, and the pigment loss from the facial haircoat. *(Courtesy BA Atlee, Davis, California; case material from the University of California, Davis.)*

FIGURE 10-23. Vitiligo affecting only the planum nasale and the adjacent muzzle in a Labrador Retriever. This specific type of vitiligo has been termed "Dudley nose" by dog breeders.

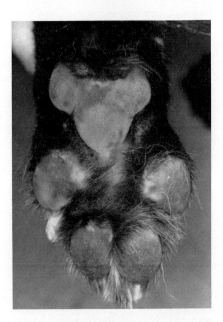

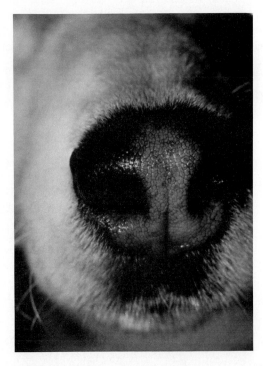

FIGURE 10-22. Vitiligo of the paw pads in the Belgian Tervuren seen in Figure 10-21. A mottled loss of pigmentation has occurred on all footpads. *(Courtesy BA Atlee, Davis, California; case material from the University of California, Davis.)*

is uncommon and scaling or crusting are not seen. Leukotrichia and depigmentation of the nails may accompany leukoderma. Partial facial symmetry is typical. The lesions are asymptomatic; pruritus or pain are not noted. The evolution of the syndrome is unpredictable. Affected areas may repigment, remain unchanged, or wax and wane. According to Mahaffey, the full extent of hypopigmentation occurred within 3 to 6 months of onset.

FIGURE 10-24. Vitiligo affecting only the planum nasale in a Siberian Husky Dog. Focal loss of pigmentation was the only abnormality noted.

Vitiligo may be a marker for visceral metabolic abnormalities: a high incidence of coexistent metabolic diseases, including diabetes mellitus, and various thyroid diseases (such as hypothyroidism, hyperthyroidism, and thyroiditis) have been seen in humans. Recently, Scott reported concurrent vitiligo and juvenile-onset diabetes mellitus in a Dachshund.

Pigment loss limited to the planum nasale ("Dudley nose") also has been termed vitiligo. In some dogs, depigmentation and subsequent repigmentation have occurred in a cyclic manner.

A marked breed predilection exists for the Belgian Tervuren. Other breeds at increased risk include the German Shepherd Dog, Rottweiler, and Doberman Pinscher. Vitiligo also has been seen in the Collie, Old English Sheepdog, and Dachshund. A syndrome apparently similar to vitiligo has been seen in Siamese cats by Guaguere and Holzworth.* Vitiligo develops most frequently in animals less than 3 years of age. Sex predilections have not been noted. Idiopathic depigmentation of the planum nasale ("Dudley nose") occurs most frequently in the Golden Retriever, yellow Labrador Retriever, and Arctic breeds such as the Siberian Husky and the Alaskan Malamute.

Vitiligo must be differentiated from Vogt-Koyanagi-Harada–like syndrome, discoid lupus erythematosus, and systemic lupus erythematosus. Vitiligo is a syndrome seen during young adulthood and is asymptomatic. Differentiating diagnostic aids include detection of uveitis by ophthalmologic examination

* Holzworth J: Personal communication, 1990.

(Vogt-Koyanagi-Harada–like syndrome) or a positive ANA test (systemic lupus erythematosus). Histopathology may aid in differentiation. A general physical examination, complete blood count, chemical screening profile, and possibly thyroid function tests are recommended to rule out coexistent disease.

Biopsy site selection

Skin biopsy is recommended as early as possible in the development of the disease. Ideal sites include those from junctions of lesions and adjacent normally pigmented skin. The wedge technique will best allow the evaluation of the lesion, transition zone, and adjacent normal skin.

Histopathology (Figures 10-25 and 10-26)

The affected epidermis is characterized by marked reduction to complete absence of epidermal melanocytes and melanin. Comparison with adjacent pigmented skin is often striking. Other epidermal lesions are not observed.

The dermis is often normal. However, recently the authors have observed mild interface accumulations of lymphocytes and fewer macrophages in specimens from affected Belgian Tervurens and Rottweilers. These lesions are presumed to be early, but temporal correlation with the clinical lesions was not made. Lymphocytes are closely applied to the dermal-epidermal junction and migrate into the overlying epi-

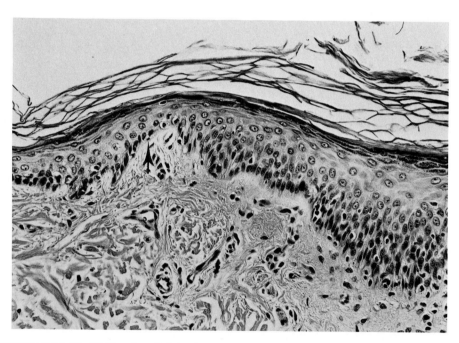

FIGURE 10-25. Vitiligo in a Belgian Tervuren. Note the relative absence of melanin in the basilar epidermis to right of the arrow. Normal pigmentation is seen to the left of the arrow. (×230.)

FIGURE 10-26. Depigmented footpad from same dog as in Figure 10-25. Lymphocytes are present in the basilar epidermis and around vessels of the superficial dermis. (× 230.)

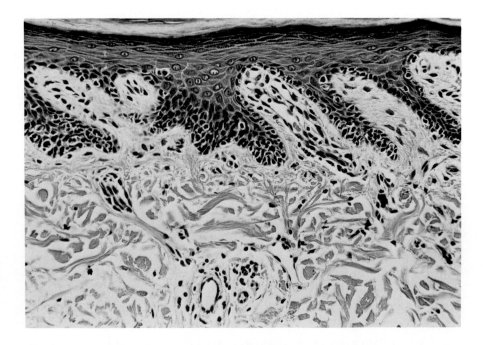

dermis. These inflammatory changes support the possibility of an autoimmune-mediated trigger for vitiligo in some dogs. Similar inflammation has been observed by Moellmann and Bhawan in normal-appearing skin at the border of vitiliginous lesions in humans.

Differential diagnoses are not known for specimens characterized by loss of epidermal melanocytes and melanin. Since these lesions can mimic normal nonpigmented skin (in which melanocytes are inapparent), knowledge of the clinical or gross lesions is critical to the histopathologic diagnosis. In inflamed lesions of vitiligo, discoid or systemic lupus erythematosus should be considered. Basal cell degeneration is absent in vitiligo but present in lupus erythematosus; the inflammation observed in vitiligo has not been as severe as in most cases of lupus erythematosus.

ERYTHEMA MULTIFORME
Clinical features (Figure 10-27)

See Chapter 3.

Biopsy site selection

Areas of erythema without crusting or ulceration are ideal sites for skin biopsy. An intact epidermis is crucial for the diagnosis of this syndrome.

Histopathology (Figures 10-28 and 10-29)

The epidermal lesions have been discussed in Chapter 3; individual keratinocyte necrosis is the key diagnostic feature. The superficial dermis contains an interface infiltration of lymphocytes and histiocytes,

which may obscure the overlying dermal-epidermal junction. Often lymphocytes migrate into the overlying epidermis where they surround necrotic keratinocytes (satellitosis). Neutrophils are variable and reflect the degree of secondary ulceration or erosion. Vessels may be dilated and congested.

The superficial pattern of lymphocytic and histiocytic inflammation seen in erythema multiforme may resemble systemic or possibly discoid lupus erythematosus. In erythema multiforme, the individual keratinocyte necrosis seen at all levels of the epidermis is distinctive and allows differentiation.

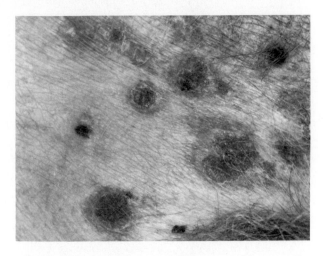

FIGURE 10-27. Erythema multiforme caused by a reaction to trimethoprim-sulfa in a dog. Note the well-demarcated, erythematous, coalescing target lesions with erythematous borders.

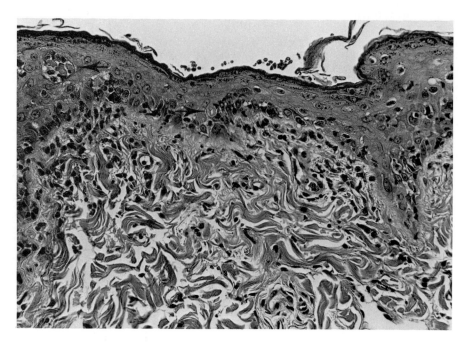

FIGURE 10-28. Erythema multiforme in a dog. Mild superficial inflammation is accompanied by mild basal cell vacuolation and degeneration. Note the individual necrosis of keratinocytes within the more superficial layers of the epidermis *(arrows)*. (×220.)

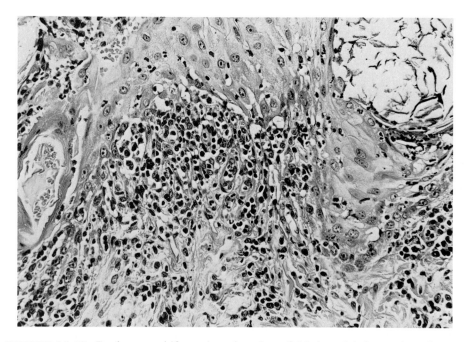

FIGURE 10-29. Erythema multiforme in a dog. Superficial dermal inflammation obscures the dermal-epidermal interface. Note the prominent basal cell vacuolation. (×220.)

ACTINIC KERATOSIS (Synonyms: solar keratosis, squamous cell carcinoma in situ)
Clinical features (Figure 10-30)

See Chapters 6 and 21.

Biopsy site selection

Specimens for biopsy should be obtained from different stages of the disease. If present, samples should include discolored macules, areas of erythema, crusted plaques, nodules, and margins of erosions or ulcerations in order to reveal the spectrum of disease present and to uncover possible neoplasia. If possible, solitary lesions should be resected in their entirety to prevent possible progression to overt neoplasia.

Histopathology (Figures 10-31 through 10-33)

Epidermal lesions have been described in Chapter 6 and principally include hyperplasia and dysplasia (also see Chapter 21). In dogs, the dermis often contains a dense lichenoid band of inflammation that partially obscures the dermal-epidermal interface. Plasma cells and lymphocytes predominate and are accompanied by variable numbers of neutrophils. Laminar dermal fibrosis begins superficially and may extend deeply to replace hair follicles. Superficial dermal vessels may be proliferative and ectatic. Lichenoid dermatitis generally is not observed in actinic lesions of cats; inflammation is mild and perivascular. However, some feline

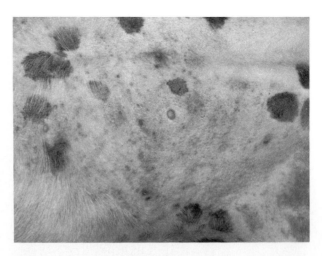

FIGURE 10-30. Actinic keratosis in a Staffordshire Terrier. Subtle crusting and scaling are accompanied by a diffuse papular eruption (secondary pyoderma) on the ventral abdomen of a dog with a history of sunbathing. *(Courtesy AM Hargis, Seattle, Washington; case material from the University of California, Davis.)*

cases of actinic keratosis have more intense dermal inflammation with fibrosis.

Solar elastosis may be seen in dogs or, rarely, in cats. Degeneration of collagen and elastic fibers of the superficial dermis leads to replacement by thickened, wavy, basophilic fibers of elastotic material. van Gie-

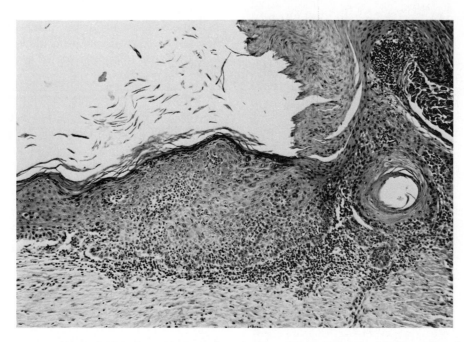

FIGURE 10-31. Actinic keratosis in a dog. A dense lichenoid band of inflammation is accompanied by subjacent fibrosis. Note the epidermal dysplasia and characteristic stacked parakeratosis. (×90.)

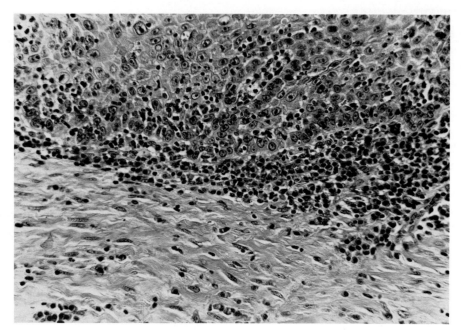

FIGURE 10-32. Higher magnification of the dermal inflammation shown in Figure 10-31. Laminar fibrosis is seen beneath accumulations of lymphocytes and plasma cells. (×90.)

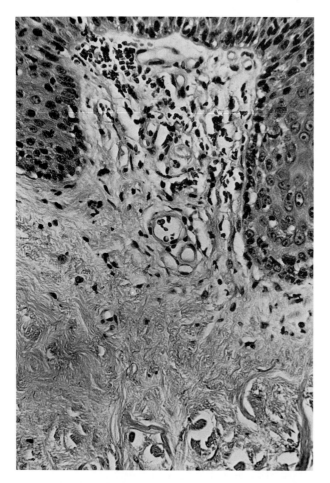

FIGURE 10-33. Solar elastosis in a dog with actinic keratosis. Thick, wavy, dark fibers of elastotic material are seen within altered, homogenized dermal collagen. (×250.)

son's stain will accentuate subtle elastotic changes as foci of tangled, silver-dense fibers in a background of degenerated, homogenized dermal connective tissue. Follicular lesions also may be found in dogs with solar keratosis and consist of comedone formation with pyoderma (see Chapter 16).

The lichenoid inflammation of actinic keratosis may mimic other dermatoses, including psoriasiform-lichenoid dermatosis and lichenoid keratosis. The characteristic epidermal dysplasia of actinic keratosis will allow differentiation.

PSORIASIFORM-LICHENOID DERMATOSIS OF THE SPRINGER SPANIEL (Synonym: lichenoid-psoriasiform dermatosis of Springer Spaniels)

Clinical features (Figure 10-34)

See Chapter 6.

Biopsy site selection

Solitary plaques with minimal crusting and erosion are preferred sites for biopsy. Multiple specimens from lesions in varying stages of development are ideal. Care must be taken with pinnal biopsy procedures not to damage fragile underlying cartilage.

Histopathology (Figure 10-35)

Epidermal lesions have been described in Chapter 6 and consist of psoriasiform hyperplasia with intraepidermal pustulation. The dermis contains a dense superficial band consisting primarily of plasma cells. Fewer lymphocytes, histiocytes, neutrophils, and eosinophils are present. Inflammation tends to obscure the dermal-epidermal interface. Mild pigmentary incontinence may be present.

Principal differential diagnoses include discoid lupus erythematosus and mucocutaneous pyoderma. Although dermal lesions are somewhat similar to discoid lupus erythematosus, plasma cells are more prominent in psoriasiform-lichenoid dermatosis, and epidermal lesions of the two diseases are distinctly different (see Chapters 2 and 6). Dermal lesions of psoriasiform-lichenoid dermatosis also resemble those of canine mucocutaneous pyoderma. However, in addition to the striking clinical differences between these two diseases, the epidermal lesions of psoriasiform-lichenoid dermatosis will allow differentiation.

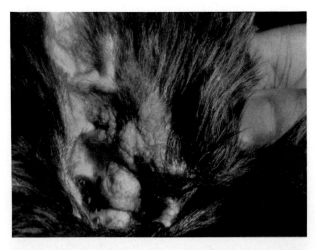

FIGURE 10-34. Psoriasiform-lichenoid dermatosis of the Springer Spaniel. Waxy, crusted, lichenoid plaques are present on the medial surface of the pinnae. *(Courtesy REW Halliwell, Edinburgh.)*

FIGURE 10-35. Psoriasiform-lichenoid dermatosis of the Springer Spaniel. Lichenoid dermatitis is accompanied by irregular acanthosis and discrete intraepidermal pustules. (×90.)

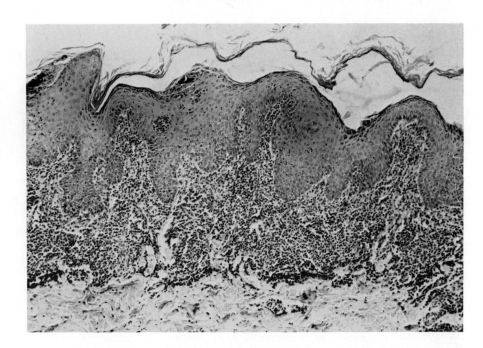

LICHENOID KERATOSIS
Clinical features

See Chapter 6.

Biopsy site selection

Nontraumatized plaques without secondary changes such as erosion, ulceration, or crusting should be selected. Care should be taken with pinnal biopsy procedures not to damage fragile underlying cartilage.

Histopathology (Figure 10-36)

Epidermal lesions principally include psoriasiform hyperplasia (see Chapter 6). Lichenoid dermal inflam-

mation is band-like and predominantly lymphocytic and plasmacytic. Variable numbers of macrophages and neutrophils are present. Inflammation may obscure the dermal-epidermal interface and may extend around subjacent adnexal appendages or deep dermal vessels.

Dermal inflammation may be similar to that of psoriasiform-lichenoid dermatosis and shares its histopathologic differential diagnoses, discoid lupus erythematosus and mucocutaneous pyoderma. Differences in epidermal lesions and clinical distinctions will allow separation.

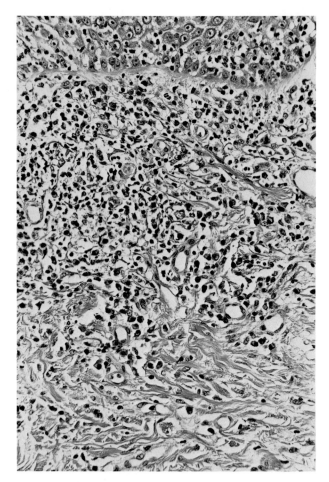

FIGURE 10-36. Lichenoid keratosis in a dog. Note the dense band of mixed inflammation with prominent plasma cells in the superficial dermis. (×220.)

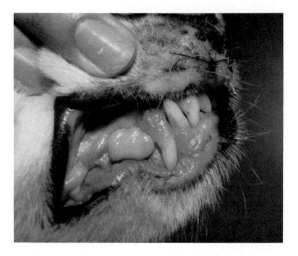

FIGURE 10-37. Mycosis fungoides in an aged Spitz. Coalescing, depigmented, erythematous plaques accompanied by cicatricial alopecia involve the lips, muzzle, and planum nasale. (*Courtesy AH Werner, Los Angeles, California; case material from the University of California, Davis.*)

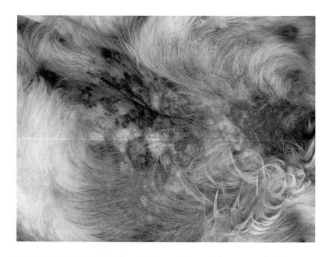

FIGURE 10-38. Mycosis fungoides of the ventral abdomen of a dog. Coalescing pleomorphic lesions consist of erythematous plaques and nodules with erosion, ulceration, and crusting. Note the alteration in pigmentation and alopecia. (*Courtesy AH Werner, Los Angeles, California; case material from the University of California, Davis.*)

MYCOSIS FUNGOIDES (Synonyms: cutaneous epitheliotropic malignant lymphoma, cutaneous T-cell lymphoma)

Clinical features (Figures 10-37 through 10-40)

Mycosis fungoides is a malignancy of T-lymphocyte origin seen uncommonly in the dog and rarely in the cat. In humans, mycosis fungoides has been shown to be a neoplasm of helper T cells. The term *mycosis fungoides,* an archaic and confusing misnomer, refers to the initial clinical characterization of skin tumors as resembling mushrooms. Mycosis fungoides is included in this chapter, since early lesions can mimic inflammatory skin disease, both clinically and histopathologically. (See Chapter 31 for additional discussion of epitheliotrophic malignant lymphoma.)

Clinically, mycosis fungoides is a remarkably pleomorphic disease. In the dog, generalizing erythematous exfoliative dermatitis (exfoliative erythroderma) with variable alopecia may be the most frequent initial presentation. Formation of solitary or multiple ulcerated plaques in the oral mucosa, lips, and perioral muzzle is another common early manifestation of mycosis fungoides. Multiple (rarely solitary), coalescing, erythematous plaques or nodules, may develop in haired skin, sometimes as an initial sign but more often following exfoliative erythroderma. Crusting and ulceration of skin lesions are common. Ulceration with depigmentation may be seen on or around the lips or other muco-cutaneous junctions in later stages of mycosis fungoides, regardless of the initial presentation. Facial lesions may be strikingly bilaterally symmetric and center around the philtrum between the planum nasale and the upper lip. Solitary lesions, especially of the philtrum or oral mucosa, may remain indolent. Pruritus is variable but is most often associated with generalized exfoliative dermatitis. Lymphadenopathy commonly is present in later stages.

Feline mycosis fungoides presents most often as exfoliative erythroderma with alopecia and crusting, especially of the neck and head. Erythematous plaques

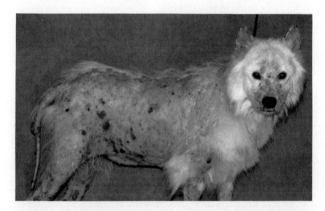

FIGURE 10-39. Advanced, generalized mycosis fungoides in an aged Samoyed. Ulcerated erythematous plaques and nodules are disseminated within a background of erythema, exfoliation, and extensive alopecia. *(Courtesy MA McMurdy.)*

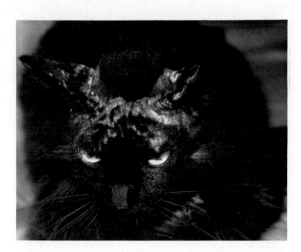

FIGURE 10-40. Mycosis fungoides in a cat. Coalescing, erythematous, small plaques and nodules are present somewhat symmetrically on the forehead and ears. Affected areas were partially alopecic but additional hair was clipped to enhance visualization.

and nodules also may be observed. Hyperpigmentation and lichenification may be noted. Oral or mucocutaneous involvement is less common than in dogs.

Similar to most neoplasms, mycosis fungoides usually affects older animals. An average age of 11 years has been reported in dogs, but dogs as young as 2 years of age have been affected. Breed or sex predilections have not been reported.

Clinical differential diagnoses are legion and are contingent on the clinical presentation. Oral lesions may resemble inflammatory stomatitis or autoimmune diseases such as pemphigus vulgaris or bullous pemphigoid. Facial disease, especially if symmetric and depigmenting, may mimic autoimmune skin diseases such as discoid lupus erythematosus and Vogt-Koyanagi-Harada–like syndrome. Severely exfoliative mycosis fungoides is often misdiagnosed as a keratinization defect or allergic skin disease, particularly if pruritus is present. Feline mycosis fungoides most often is confused clinically with dermatophytosis. Histopathology will establish the diagnosis in well-developed lesions.

Biopsy site selection

Skin specimens should be taken from plaques, nodules, or areas of exfoliative erythroderma. In the oral cavity, plaques are more likely than ulcers to yield a definitive diagnosis. Multiple specimens are especially important in early cases, since histopathologic diagnosis may be difficult. If initial specimens are suggestive but not diagnostic for mycosis fungoides, periodic rebiopsy is recommended. One author* has seen a cat with generalized exfoliative skin disease for which a definitive diagnosis of mycosis fungoides could not be made until after periodic biopsy had been performed for over a year.

Histopathology (Figures 10-41 and 10-42)

Histopathology is variable, depending on the stage of the disease. In dogs, early exfoliative lesions may contain small numbers of intraepithelial lymphocytes that are not overtly neoplastic cytologically. As the disease progresses to plaque and nodule stages in the dog, lymphocytes increase in number and become cytologically more malignant, characterized by large, pale nuclei with a convoluted contour. The skin of cats with mycosis fungoides tends to retain morphologically well-differentiated lymphocytes in the advanced stages of illness, which can make histopathologic diagnosis more difficult.

In typical diagnostic lesions, the epidermis is acanthotic and contains infiltrating lymphocytes, usually in

* Peter J. Ihrke.

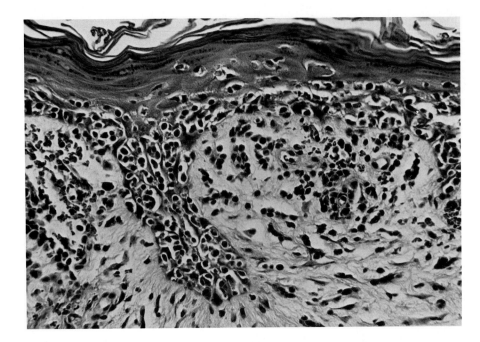

FIGURE 10-41. Mycosis fungoides in a dog. Uniform lymphocytes of mature appearance are invading the epidermis and superficial follicle and are intermingled with fewer inflammatory cells in the superficial dermis. (×220.)

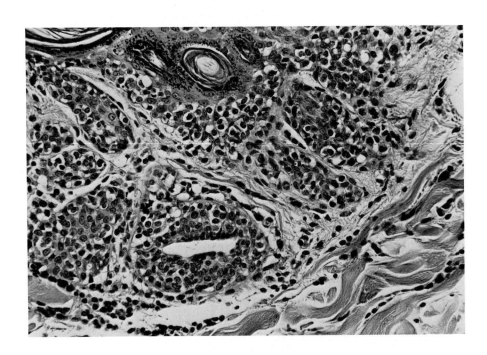

FIGURE 10-42. Mycosis fungoides in a dog. Large neoplastic lymphocytes are infiltrating the adnexal appendages. (×220.)

moderate to large numbers. There may be small clear zones around individual lymphocytes or groups of lymphocytes within the epidermis. These clusters of neoplastic lymphocytes are termed *Pautrier's microabscesses* after the original observer in human dermatopathology. Similar intraepithelial infiltrations of neoplastic lymphocytes also are observed within the epithelium of hair follicles and apocrine sweat glands. In the dog, adnexal involvement may precede epidermal involvement. Epidermal necrosis may be seen.

The dermis contains similar neoplastic lymphocytes, and these frequently obscure the dermal-epidermal interface as cells migrate into the overlying epidermis. In the dog, mixed inflammatory infiltrates, including mature lymphocytes, also may be found around superficial dermal blood vessels. As the disease progresses, neoplastic lymphocytes form dense infiltrates in the superficial dermis (plaque stage) or infiltrates that extend into the deep dermis and panniculus (nodular or tumor stage; see Chapter 31). Hair follicles and apocrine sweat glands are often destroyed by neoplastic lymphocytes. Careful examination may reveal the outer glassy membrane surrounding neoplastic lymphocytes within the framework of a previous follicle. There may be regression of individual lesions, characterized by a decrease in numbers of neoplastic lymphocytes and severe dermal fibrosis with ablation of hair follicles.

In cats, lymphocytes may retain a mature, nonneoplastic appearance, both in epithelial and nonepithelial locations, throughout the course of the disease. Epithelial and adnexal involvement may be sparse. The presence of a monotonous population of lymphocytes and the migration of lymphocytes into epithelial tissues without spongiosis are supportive of mycosis fungoides in the cat.

The prime differential feature of mycosis fungoides is the presence of a monotonous population of lymphocytes in epithelial locations. In early lesions, differentiation from predominantly lymphocytic inflammatory dermatoses, such as alopecia areata, some allergic reactions (including contact dermatitis), or feline dermatophytosis, may be difficult. Lymphocytic infiltration of epithelial tissues in mycosis fungoides is not usually associated with spongiosis, in contrast to most inflammatory diseases.

SUGGESTED READINGS

Mucocutaneous pyoderma
References not available.

Discoid lupus erythematosus
Rosenkrantz WS and others: Histopathological evaluation of acid mucopolysaccaride (mucin) in canine discoid lupus erythematosus, J Am Anim Hosp Assoc 22:577-584, 1986.
See also Chapter 2.

Systemic lupus erythematosus
See Chapter 2.

Pemphigus erythematosus
See Chapter 1.

Vogt-Koyanagi-Harada–like syndrome
Asakura I: Harada syndrome (uveitis diffusa acuta) in the dog, Jpn J Vet Med 673:445-455, 1977.
Bussanich MN, Rootman J, and Dolman CL: Granulomatous pan-uveitis and dermal depigmentation in dogs, J Am Anim Hosp Assoc 18:131-138, 1982.
Campbell KL, McLaughlin SA, and Reynolds HA: Generalized leukoderma and poliosis following uveitis in a dog, J Am Anim Hosp Assoc 22:121-124, 1986.
Fabries L: Syndrome "VKH" chez le chien au sujet de deux cas clinique. Pratique Medicale et Chirurgicale de l'Animal de Compagnie 19:393-397, 1984.
Kern TJ and others: Uveitis associated with poliosis and vitiligo in six dogs, J Am Vet Med Assoc 187:408-414, 1985.
Lorincz AL: Disturbances of melanin pigmentation. In Moschella SL and Hurley HJ, editors: Dermatology. Philadelphia, 1985, WB Saunders, pp 1296-1297.

Mosher DB and others: Disorders of pigmentation. In Fitzpatrick TB, Eisen AZ, Wolff K, and others, editors, Dermatology in general medicine, New York, 1987, McGraw-Hill, pp 834-836.
Muller GH, Kirk RW, and Scott DW: Small animal dermatology, ed 4, Philadelphia, 1989, WB Saunders, pp 542-544.
Romatowski J: A uveodermatological syndrome in an Akita dog, J Am Anim Hosp Assoc 21:777-780, 1985.
Sugiura S: Vogt-Koyanagi-Harada disease, Jpn J Ophthalmol 22:9-35, 1978.

Vitiligo
Bhawan J and Bhutani LK: Keratinocyte damage in vitiligo, J Cutan Pathol 10:207-212, 1983.
Guaguere E and Alhaidari Z: Pigmentary disturbances. In Von Tscharner C and Halliwell REW, editors: Advances in veterinary dermatology, vol 1, London, 1990, Bailliere Tindall, pp 395-398.
Guaguere E and Alhaidari Z: Disorders of melanin pigmentation in the skin of dogs and cats. In Kirk RW, editor: Current veterinary therapy X, Philadelphia, 1989, WB Saunders, pp 628-632.
Guaguere E, Alhaidari Z, and Ortonne J-P: Troubles de la pigmentation melanique en dermatologie des carnivores. II. Hypomelanoses et amelanoses, Le Point Veterinaire 18:5-14, 1986.
Lever WF and Schaumburg-Lever G: Histopathology of the skin, ed 7, Philadelphia, 1990, JB Lippincott, pp 490-491.
Mahaffey MB, Yarbrough KM, and Munnell JF: Focal loss of pigment in the Belgian Tervuren Dog, J Am Vet Med Assoc 173:390-396, 1978.
Moellmann G and others: Extracellular granular material and degeneration of keratinocytes in the normally pigmented epidermis of patients with vitiligo, J Invest Dermatol 79:321-330, 1982.
Mosher DB and others: Disorders of pigmentation. In Fitzpatrick TB, Eisen AZ, Wolff K, and others, editors: Dermatology in general medicine, New York, 1987, McGraw-Hill, pp 810-821.
Muller GH, Kirk RW, and Scott DW: Small animal dermatology, ed 4, Philadelphia, 1989, WB Saunders, pp 705-714.
Naughton GK and others: Antibodies to surface antigens of pigmented cells in animals with vitiligo, Proc Soc Exp Biol Med 181:423-426, 1986.
Scott DW and Randolph JF: Vitiligo in two Old English Sheepdog littermates and in a Dachshund with juvenile-onset diabetes mellitus, Comp Anim Pract 19:18-22, 1989.

Erythema multiforme
See Chapter 3.

Actinic keratosis
See Chapter 6.

Psoriasiform-lichenoid dermatosis of the Springer Spaniel
See Chapter 6.

Lichenoid keratosis
See Chapter 6.

Mycosis fungoides
Baker JL and Scott DW: Mycosis fungoides in two cats, J Am Anim Hosp Assoc 25:97-101, 1989.
Caciolo PL and others: A case of mycosis fungoides in a cat and literature review, J Am Anim Hosp Assoc 19:505-512, 1983.
DeBoer DJ, Turrel JM, and Moore PF: Mycosis fungoides in a dog: demonstration of T-cell specificity and response to radiotherapy, J Am Anim Hosp Assoc 26:566-572, 1990.
Doe R, Zackheim HS, and Hill JR: Canine epidermotropic cutaneous lymphoma, Am J Dermatopathol 10:80-86, 1988.
Kelly DF, Halliwell REW, and Schwartzman RM: Generalized cutaneous eruption in a dog with histologic similarity to human mycosis fungoides, Br J Dermatol 86:164-171, 1972.

Lever WF and Schaumburg-Lever G: Histopathology of the skin, ed 7, Philadelphia, 1990, JB Lippincott, pp 819-827.

Muller GH, Kirk RW, and Scott DW: Small animal dermatology, ed 4, Philadelphia, 1989, WB Saunders, pp 921-922.

Shadduck JA and others: A canine cutaneous lymphoproliferative disease resembling mycosis fungoides in man, Vet Pathol 15:716-724, 1978.

Walton DK: Canine epidermotropic lymphoma. In Kirk RW, editor: Current veterinary Therapy IX, Philadelphia, 1986, WB Saunders Co, pp 609-614.

Infectious nodular and diffuse granulomatous and pyogranulomatous diseases of the dermis

Nodular and diffuse granulomatous and pyogranulomatous diseases of the dermis are characterized by multifocal nodular inflammation, which tends toward confluence or a diffuse pattern. Diffuse inflammatory infiltrates often obscure the normal dermal architecture and may extend to the underlying panniculus as well. Granulomatous inflammation is composed principally of macrophages, with or without giant cells, which tend toward formation of granulomas. The presence of discrete granulomas is not a requisite for the interpretation of inflammation as "granulomatous." Pyogranulomatous inflammation has a more prominent component of neutrophils; pyogranulomas are formed from central accumulations of neutrophils that are rimmed by macrophages. Diseases included in this chapter are those in which infectious agents incite the inflammatory reaction; differential diagnosis is facilitated through identification of the offending agent in tissue.

ACTINOMYCOSIS AND NOCARDIOSIS
Clinical features (Figures 11-1 through 11-4)

Nocardiosis and actinomycosis are rare cutaneous (and visceral) diseases seen in the dog and cat that are caused by actinomycetes ("higher" bacteria). These two diseases share substantial clinical and histopathologic similarities. *Actinomyces* species are gram-positive, non-acid fast, filamentous anaerobic or microaerophilic rods, and *Nocardia* species are gram-positive, partially acid fast, filamentous, aerobic rods. *A. viscosus* and *A. hordeovulnaris* are commensal inhabitants of the oral cavity and gastrointestinal tract in many mammals. *N. asteroides*, *N. brasiliensis*, and *N. caviae* are common saprophytes found in soil and fresh water. Actinomycosis and nocardiosis are opportunistic infections created most commonly through wound contamination. Differentiation between the two diseases may be difficult both clinically and histopathologically. In the past, nocardiosis may have been overdiagnosed; newer methods of microbiologic differentiation most often identify *Actinomyces* species in cases where both clinical and histopathologic characteristics did not allow differentiation.

Actinomycosis results from contamination of penetrating wounds, such as those caused by grass awns, quills, cactus spines, and other foreign bodies. Infection may

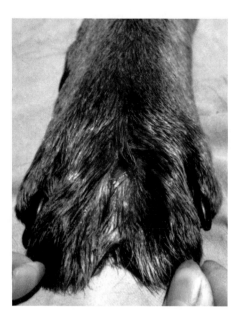

FIGURE 11-1. Actinomycosis secondary to interdigital grass awn implantation in a dog. A fistulous tract drains sparse purulent debris.

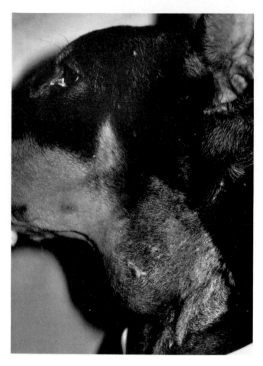

FIGURE 11-3. Nocardiosis in a Doberman Pinscher. A large nodule is accompanied by severe soft tissue swelling. Note surface defects indicating sites of drainage.

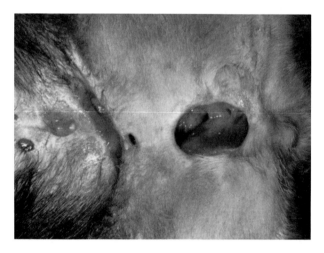

FIGURE 11-2. Nocardiosis in a cat. Fistulous tracts within inflamed tissue are seen on the ventral abdomen. *(Courtesy LP Schmeitzel, Knoxville, Tennessee.)*

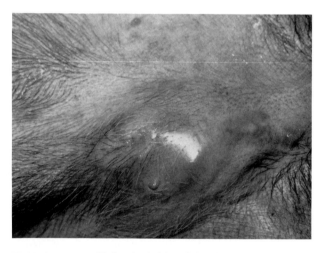

FIGURE 11-4. Abdominal skin of the dog in Figure 11-3. The firm, multiloculated nodule has surface ulceration. The overlying skin is erythematous to bluish.

occur through the creation of an anaerobic inflammatory environment that is conducive to the replication of previously existent commensal organisms. Nocardiosis may be associated with wound contamination, inhalation, or ingestion. Both actinomycosis and nocardiosis are facilitated in animals with impaired host defense mechanisms.

Draining fistulous tracts, abscesses, and ulcerated dermal and subcutaneous nodules are seen in actinomycosis and nocardiosis. The character of the exudate is highly variable and may range from serosanguineous to sanguinopurulent. Yellow "sulfur granules" or

"grains" in the exudate are suspicious for actinomycosis since the most common agent of nocardiosis, *N. asteroides*, generally does not form granules. Conversely, *N. caviae* and *N. braziliensis* may produce grains. Lesions tend to be grouped; progression is by gradual local extension. The distal extremities, face, and neck are the most commonly affected sites, since these areas most frequently interface with the environment and thus are most susceptible to trauma.

Regional lymphadenopathy is common with both actinomycosis and nocardiosis. Actinomycotic osteomyelitis and pulmonary nocardiosis are the most frequent concurrent infections. Systemic signs may be seen with either disease contingent on the portal of entry and the coexistence of visceral infection. Young male outdoor dogs of active large breeds are reported to be at greater risk because of the increased likelihood of exposure to penetrating wounds and foreign body implantation.

Clinical differential diagnoses should include systemic mycoses, cryptococcosis, cutaneous infections of other opportunistic fungi and algae, opportunistic mycobacterial infection, and infection by other aerobic or anaerobic bacteria. Differentiation is accomplished by routine and special culture techniques, cytologic examination of exudates, and histopathology. Fungal culture should not be performed until systemic mycoses are ruled out by impression smear and histopathology since attempted culture of systemic fungi may be dangerous (see later discussion).

Biopsy site selection

Identification of organisms histopathologically is contingent upon obtaining adequate tissue samples from affected areas. An aggressive wedge technique is recommended to obtain deep nodules and tissue surrounding and beneath fistulous tracts. Radical surgical ablation of solitary lesions may be curative. Impression smears should be made from the cut surface of a nodule and submitted for special staining in an attempt to identify organisms.

Histopathology (Figures 11-5 and 11-6)

The epidermis is variably acanthotic, and ulceration may be present. The dermis and often the subcutis are heavily infiltrated with neutrophils and macrophages in confluent pyogranulomatous configuration. Pyogranulomas are generally large and are formed by focally extensive accumulations of neutrophils surrounded by cuffs of large epithelioid macrophages. Lymphocytes and plasma cells are present at the periphery of chronic lesions, and there is variable fibrosis surrounding the inflammatory foci.

Organisms may be difficult to identify because they are often not in abundance. Small to large, often radiating clusters of tangled, filamentous and branched bacteria may be found at the centers of pyogranulomas. Grains, seen commonly in actinomycosis, are formed by the deposition of brightly eosinophilic, radiating, and clubbed deposits (Splendore-Hoeppli reaction, which is an antigen-antibody reaction to infectious agents or parasites) at the periphery of organized aggregates of bacteria. The most commonly implicated organism in nocardiosis, *N. asteroides*, rarely is associated with tissue grains. *Actinomyces* species are gram-positive and are not acid fast; *Nocardia* species are gram-positive, are partially or weakly acid fast, and may be beaded. A Fite-Faraco modification of the acid-fast stain is used for identification of *Nocardia* species. This stain employs peanut oil to prevent excessive decolorization of organisms during the staining process. Caution is advised when additional sectioning for special staining is performed; sectioning that is too deep may pass through available colonies. If bacteria are not

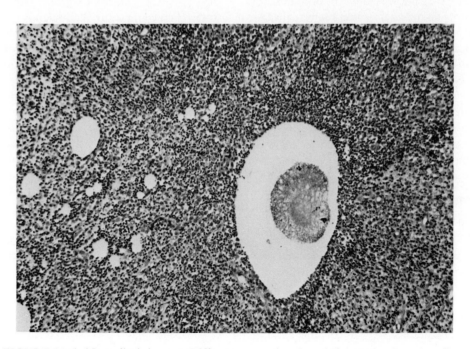

FIGURE 11-5. Nocardiosis in a cat. Diffuse pyogranulomatous inflammation is surrounding a large colony of organisms within a large clear zone. (×90.)

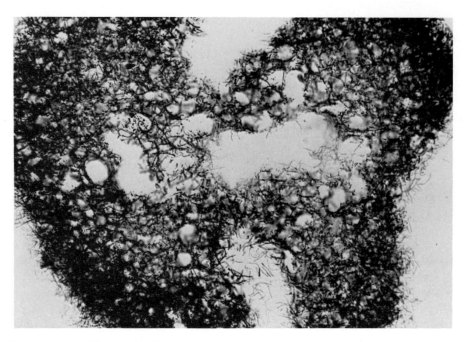

FIGURE 11-6. Higher magnification of the colony shown in Figure 11-5 revealing tangled, filamentous, and beaded bacteria that were culturally identified as *Nocardia asteroides*. (Brown-Hopps stain; ×560.)

present in deeper tissue, the original hematoxylin and eosin-stained section may be decolorized and stained.

Differential diagnoses include foreign body reactions, deep mycotic infections, infection caused by opportunistic mycobacteria, botryomycosis, or other chronic bacterial infections. Botryomycosis, which is nodular clinically, is characterized by the accumulation of Splendore-Hoeppli material around bacteria (usually staphylococci) to form grains in tissue, thus superficially resembling actinomycosis. The characteristic morphology and staining characteristics of *Nocardia* species and *Actinomyces* species in tissue usually allow differentiation from most other infectious agents. *Nocardia* species may slightly resemble opportunistic mycobacteria in tissue section, but accumulate in larger tangled colonies, are only partially or weakly acid fast, and elicit a more prominent neutrophilic response than do the opportunistic mycobacteria.

FELINE LEPROSY
Clinical features (Figures 11-7 and 11-8)

Feline leprosy is a rare granulomatous mycobacterial skin disease caused by an acid-fast bacteria that cannot be cultured using routine laboratory methods. Although transmission was not achieved in one study by Schiefer using two cats, *Mycobacterium lepraemurium*, the rat leprosy bacteria, may be the etiologic

agent. The mode of transmission is not known. The frequent localization to the head and neck have led to speculation that the organism may be transmitted by bite wounds from either rats or other cats. Credence is given to the theory of transmission of *M. lepraemurium* from rats by the predominant occurrence of feline leprosy in seaport cities of western North America, Australia, France, and the Netherlands. The leprosy bacillus of humans has been identified in fleas, mosquitoes, and ticks. Consequently, these vectors also could be involved in the transmission of feline leprosy. Leprosy in humans commonly is associated with immunodeficiency. Data reflecting the status of the immune system of affected cats are not available.

Single or multiple, grouped, well-circumscribed, alopecic nodules (5 to 20 mm in diameter) develop slowly in the skin or the subjacent subcutis. Although nodules may gradually increase in size, new lesions generally do not appear. Larger nodules ulcerate and scant exudation is seen. The margins of the ulcers usually are firm and slightly elevated. Less commonly, fistulas may be present. The face, forelimbs, and trunk are the most common sites. Rarely, lesions may involve the facial mucocutaneous junctions. Typically, lesions are asymptomatic. However, cats may groom ulcerated nodules, especially of the forelimbs. Regional lymphadenopathy is common.

Young adult cats are affected most frequently.

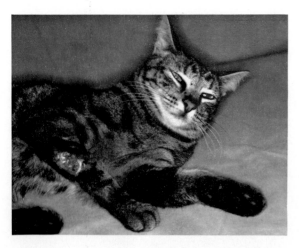

FIGURE 11-7. Feline leprosy in a young, male, outdoor cat from the San Francisco seaport. A large and a small ulcerated nodule are present on the right forelimb.

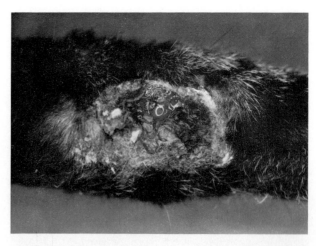

FIGURE 11-8. Closer view of the cat in Figure 11-7. A well-demarcated, ulcerated nodule with slightly elevated margins drains a sparse exudate.

Breed or sex predilections have not been reported, but feline leprosy may be more common in roaming intact male cats.

Clinical differential diagnoses include cryptococcosis, other opportunistic fungal infections, systemic mycoses, sporotrichosis, sterile granuloma and pyogranuloma syndrome, and neoplasms such as mast cell tumor or fibrosarcoma. Differentiation is accomplished by routine and special culture techniques, cytologic examination of exudates, and histopathology. Fungal culture should not be performed until systemic mycoses are ruled out by impression smears and histopathology, since attempted culture of systemic fungi may be dangerous (see later discussion). Signs referable to disseminated disease usually are seen with systemic mycoses but are absent in feline leprosy. The nodules of feline sporotrichosis have draining fistulous tracts (containing abundant organisms easily identified by direct smears) in contrast to the scantily exudative lesions of feline leprosy.

Biopsy site selection

If feline leprosy is suspected, an intact nodule should be excised surgically using the wedge technique. If a solitary lesion is present, complete excision may provide the added benefit of a surgical cure.

Histopathology (Figures 11-9 through 11-11)

The epidermis is mildly to moderately acanthotic. The dermis and often the subcutis contain diffuse infiltrates of predominantly large, pale, foamy, or epithelioid macrophages. Inflammation obscures the normal dermal architecture. Large vacuoles may be present

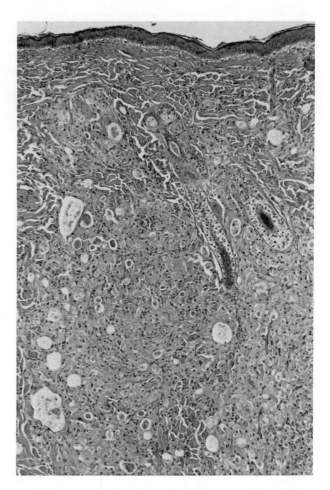

FIGURE 11-9. Feline leprosy. Diffuse granulomatous inflammation is characterized by foamy, vacuolated macrophages. (×90.)

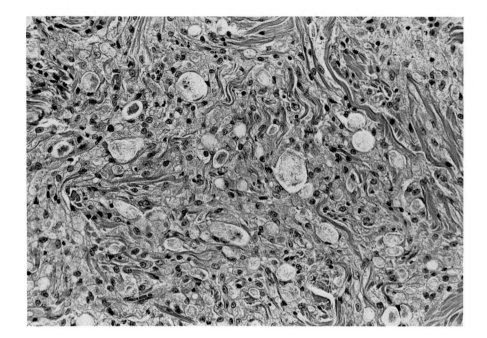

FIGURE 11-10. Feline leprosy. Note pale vacuolated macrophages; the large, clear spaces contain numerous organisms that are poorly visualized with hematoxylin and eosin. (×220.)

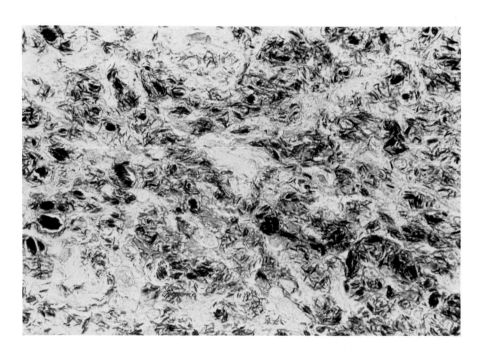

FIGURE 11-11. Feline leprosy. Large numbers of acid-fast rods fill the cytoplasm of macrophages and are seen densely in extracellular spaces. (Ziehl-Neelsen stain; ×560.)

among macrophages. Smaller numbers of neutrophils or lymphocytes may be interspersed. Giant cells usually are not seen. Using a routine acid fast stain, such as Ziehl-Neelsen, numerous acid-fast bacilli are identified within macrophages or dermal vacuoles; organisms are also silver positive. The presence of these organisms in the face of a negative mycobacterial culture confirms the diagnosis of feline leprosy, since cultural isolation of this organism is not possible under routine laboratory conditions.

Differential diagnoses include cutaneous xanthoma, preauricular xanthogranuloma of cats (a type of sterile granuloma and pyogranuloma), and cutaneous infections caused by opportunistic mycobacteria. Xanthomas are characterized by similar infiltrations of foamy macrophages but usually have deposition of more obvious lipid, seen as pale lakes within tissue. Preauricular xanthogranuloma may contain more prominent giant cells; organisms are not identified in this sterile lesion. In opportunistic mycobacterial infection caused by the fortuitum-chelonei complex (see following discussion), only scant organisms are seen in tissue section and inflammation is distinctly pyogranulomatous. In the single reported feline case of systemic *M. avium* infection with cutaneous involvement (see following discussion), the inflammatory infiltrate was similar to that of feline leprosy, and large numbers of organisms were seen in the tissue section. However, unlike the mycobacterium of feline leprosy, *M. avium* can be identified by culture.

OPPORTUNISTIC MYCOBACTERIAL INFECTION (Synonyms: opportunistic mycobacterial granulomas, atypical mycobacteriosis, nontuberculous mycobacterial infection)

Clinical features (Figures 11-12 and 11-13)

Opportunistic mycobacterial infections are seen uncommonly in cats and very rarely in dogs and are caused by the traumatic implantation of facultatively pathogenic mycobacteria. Causative organisms include the rapidly growing Runyon group IV mycobacteria: *Mycobacterium fortuitum, M. chelonei, M. smegmatis, M. phlei, M. xenopi,* and *M. thermoresistable.* A single cat with disseminated *M. avium-intracellulare* (Runyon group III) infection and subcutaneous nodules was reported by Buergelt. In cats and dogs, *M. fortuitum* and *M. chelonei* are isolated most frequently as facultative pathogens. These organisms exist worldwide in wet environments. Runyon group IV mycobacterial infection is assumed to be associated with infected wounds (cat fights), other trauma, or injections. In humans, disseminated opportunistic mycobacterial infection occurs in immunocompromised individuals, whereas localized skin and subcutaneous infection is seen in normal individuals.

In the cat, largely asymptomatic cutaneous and subcutaneous abscesses progress to nonhealing ulcers that have well-demarcated margins and undermine adjacent normal-appearing skin. The lesions are moist, but little drainage occurs. Lesions are not as proliferative as those of many other infectious feline skin diseases. Skin flaps at the edges of the ulcer remain surprisingly minimally thickened. If prior surgery has been performed, irregular scarring may obscure the more characteristic lesions. The groin is the most common site. Lesions may be seen elsewhere on the trunk or less commonly on the head or neck. Lesions develop slowly over weeks or months. Excessive grooming of the affected area may be noted. Regional lymphadenopathy is variable, but constitutional signs are absent or rare.

In dogs, focal or grouped, cutaneous and subcutaneous nodules or large, firm swellings ulcerate and drain. The subcutaneous undermining that is characteristic of opportunistic mycobacterial infection in the cat is not observed in the dog. One author* has examined lesions from a dog with multiple facial papules and nodules and from another dog with a solitary nodule of the ear; these contained large numbers of organisms histopathologically (not typical of the fortuitum-chelonei complex). Culture was not performed because of removal of the entire nodule without prior knowledge of its cause in one case, and spontaneous regres-

* Thelma Lee Gross.

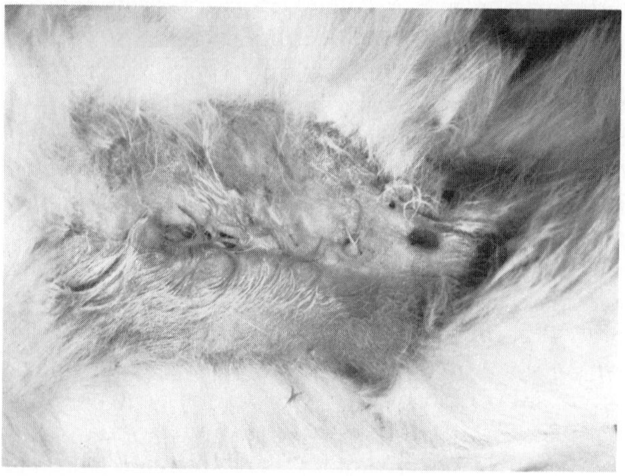

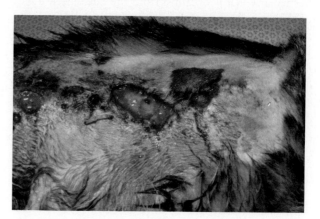

FIGURE 11-12. Opportunistic mycobacterial infection in a cat caused by *Mycobacterium fortuitum.* Abscesses have progressed to the nonhealing ulcers and fistulas seen here. (*Courtesy AH Werner, Los Angeles, California; case material from the Univeristy of California, Davis.*)

FIGURE 11-13. Severe opportunistic mycobacterial infection in a cat caused by *Mycobacterium fortuitum.* Nonhealing ulcers have well-demarcated margins and undermine adjacent normal-appearing skin. (*Courtesy AC Mundell, Seattle, Washington; case material from the University of California, Davis.*)

sion of the remaining facial lesions following biopsy in the second case. Breed, age, and sex predilections have not been reported.

Differential diagnosis in the cat should include bite wound abscesses, deep mycotic infections, and sterile nodular panniculitis. Greater local tissue reaction, pain, or signs of systemic illness are more common with bite wound abscesses and systemic mycoses. Sterile nodular panniculitis is extremely rare in the cat and must be differentiated by histopathology and culture.

Differential diagnosis in the dog may be more problematic, since the proliferative tissue response seen in canine opportunistic mycobacterial infections may mimic many other bacterial or fungal infectious diseases of the skin, including actinomycosis or nocardiosis, deep bacterial folliculitis and furunculosis, systemic mycoses, cryptococcosis, or cutaneous infections of other opportunistic fungi and algae.

Differentiation is accomplished by routine and special culture techniques, cytologic examination of exudates, and histopathology. Fungal culture should not be performed until systemic mycoses are ruled out by impression smear and histopathology, since attempted culture of systemic fungi may be dangerous (see later discussion). Direct smears of exudate and bacterial culture may more be more rewarding than histopathology in identifying the etiologic agent in opportunistic mycobacterial infections.

Biopsy site selection

Specimens should be taken by wedge technique from dermal and subcutaneous tissue at the deep advancing border of the lesion. Punch biopsy is not sufficient to obtain deep tissue. Overlying skin alone may not contain characteristic inflammation and organisms, particularly if it is obtained from the devitalized edges of the wound. If opportunistic mycobacterial infection is suspected in resectable lesions, lesions should be removed with wide margins, since surgical extirpation offers the best chance of cure. After the lesion is resected, a final outer excision well into unaffected tissue should be performed using freshly sterile instruments.

Touch preparations from freshly incised biopsy specimens or smears of exudate may be useful in identifying organisms. Acid-fast stains should be requested for all microbiologic or cytologic specimens submitted to the laboratory.

Histopathology (Figures 11-14 and 11-15)

The epidermis is usually acanthotic or ulcerated. Typically, multinodular to diffuse pyogranulomatous dermatitis and panniculitis are present. Small pyogranulomas with central clear zones, corresponding to residual lipid from degenerating adipose tissue of the

panniculus, are surrounded by a thin rim of neutrophils and a wider outer zone of epithelioid macrophages. Pyogranulomas often are confluent and are interspersed with diffuse inflammation composed of macrophages and neutrophils. Giant cells usually are not present.

Organisms are characteristically difficult to find in tissue section. A Fite-Faraco modification of the acid-fast stain is most beneficial for identification of the mycobacteria. The staining process employs peanut oil to prevent excessive decolorization of organisms. Frozen sections of formalin-fixed specimens may enhance discovery of the organisms because xylene and alcohol (lipid solvents used during routine processing of tissue) are circumvented except for brief immersion after staining and before application of the coverslip. Small numbers of filamentous, sometimes tangled, and slightly beaded, acid-fast rods are found in the clear centers of deep pyogranulomas, where staining may be preserved because of the presence of protective fat of the panniculus. Organisms also may be found in small numbers within macrophages.

Demonstration of typical acid-fast organisms in the central clear spaces of pyogranulomas suggests an opportunistic mycobacterial infection, but the diagnosis should be confirmed by culture.

In the single report of *M. avium* infection in a cat, systemic as well as cutaneous and subcutaneous lesions were present. This type of infection differs from opportunistic mycobacterial infections of the fortuitum-chelonei complex in that diffuse infiltrations of foamy macrophages containing large numbers of organisms were present, similar to feline leprosy. A histopathologically similar feline case with cutaneous and visceral dissemination and large numbers of organisms in tissue was described by Donnelly; culture was not performed.

The facial and aural lesions in dogs, observed by one author,* were characterized by diffuse pyogranulomatous inflammation (without discrete pyogranulomas containing clear vacuoles). Large numbers of delicate acid-fast bacteria were demonstrated; culture was not performed.

Differential diagnoses of the opportunistic mycobacterial infections include foreign body reactions and other deep infections caused by bacteria or fungi. The typical small pyogranulomas surrounding clear central spaces are very suggestive of opportunistic mycobacterial infection. The opportunistic mycobacteria of the fortuitum-chelonei complex may resemble *Nocardia* species in tissue. Larger clusters of bacteria characterize nocardiosis, and neutrophils are more prominent in the inflammatory infiltrate.

---

* Thelma Lee Gross.

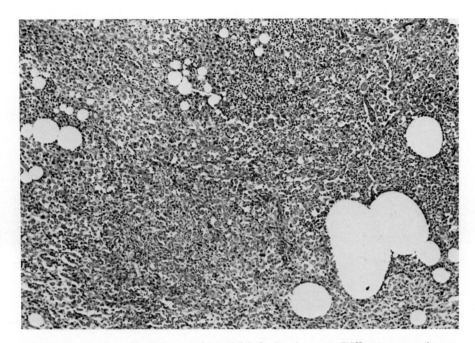

FIGURE 11-14. Opportunistic mycobacterial infection in a cat. Diffuse pyogranulomatous inflammation is punctuated by clear spaces that previously contained lipid. (×90.)

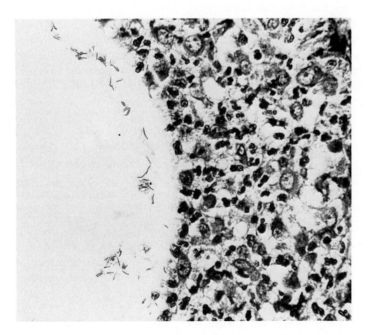

FIGURE 11-15. Higher magnification of Figure 11-14. Neutrophils and macrophages surround a central clear space in which filamentous mycobacteria are present. (Ziehl-Neelsen stain; ×560.)

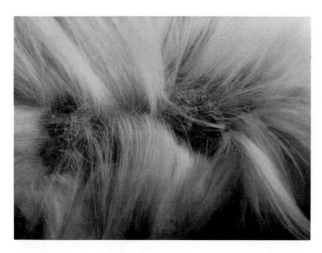

FIGURE 11-16. Feline dermatophytic mycetoma caused by *Microsporum canis* in the scapular region of a Persian cat. Crusted and hyperpigmented nodules have an irregular contour.

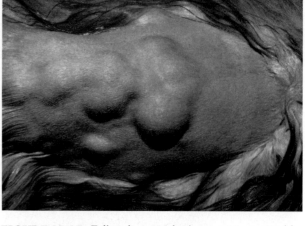

FIGURE 11-17. Feline dermatophytic mycetoma caused by *Microsporum canis* on the dorsal trunk of a Persian cat. Note the irregularly shaped, coalescing, subcutaneous and dermal nodules. *(Courtesy AC Mundell, Seattle, Washington; case material from the University of California, Davis.)*

FELINE DERMATOPHYTIC MYCETOMA (Synonym: dermatophytic pseudomycetoma)

Clinical features (Figures 11-16 and 11-17)

Feline dermatophytic mycetomas are uncommon deep dermal and subcutaneous fungal infections caused by dermatophytes. Genetically preprogrammed, selective immunodeficiency may play a role in the development of these lesions since the syndrome has been seen almost exclusively in Persian cats. *Microsporum canis* has been isolated in most cases where fungal culture was performed. Presumably, the infection begins with more typical follicular dermatophyte colonization. Frequent localization of lesions to the dorsal thorax in outdoor cats may indicate the possibility of traumatic implantation of organisms into the dermis and subcutis from colonized hairs. This traumatic implantation could result from cat fights. Positive dermatophyte cultures from normal-appearing areas distant from the dermatophytic mycetoma indicate that affected cats may previously have been inapparent carriers.

Firm, irregularly shaped nodules (5 to 20 mm in diameter) develop and gradually enlarge and coalesce in the dermis or the underlying subcutaneous tissue. Larger lesions may ulcerate and discharge a seropurulent to granular material. Chronic lesions may hyperpigment. Alopecia may be a feature if the syndrome coexists with more typical feline dermatophytosis. Lesions usually are grouped but may be solitary. Lymphadenopathy may be present but systemic signs are uncommon.

The syndrome is seen almost exclusively in Persian cats. Age and sex predilections have not been noted.

Clinical differential diagnoses should include systemic mycoses, cryptococcosis, cutaneous infections of other opportunistic fungi, sporotrichosis, and neoplasia. The marked breed predilection for Persian cats is helpful in increasing the index of suspicion for dermatophytic mycetoma. Histopathology and fungal culture of a biopsy specimen are required for differentiation. Fungal culture should not be performed until systemic mycoses are ruled out by impression smear and histopathology because attempted culture of systemic fungi may be dangerous (see following discussion). A positive fungal culture from distant sites, fluorescence with a Wood's lamp, or a positive microscopic hair analysis for dermatophytosis increases the likelihood of a focal nodular lesion being a dermatophytic mycetoma.

Biopsy site selection

An entire nodule should be removed using the wedge resection technique. If the lesion is solitary, as in early cases, this technique has the added benefit of providing a surgical cure. If a dermatophytic mycetoma is suspected clinically, a deep portion of the lesion should be submitted for dermatophyte culture, after the overlying epidermis has been removed using sterile technique.

Histopathology (Figures 11-18 and 11-19)

The overlying epidermis and superficial dermis may be unremarkable, except for mild to moderate acanthosis, or minimal perivascular or periadnexal mixed inflammation. Ulceration may be present. Often

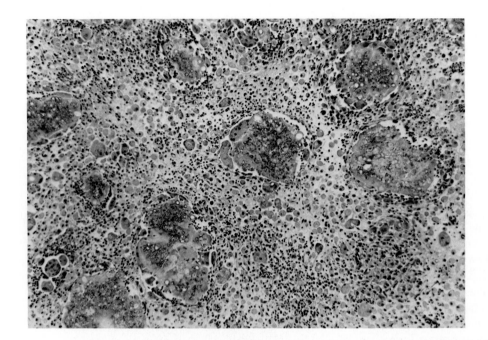

FIGURE 11-18. Feline dermatophytic mycetoma caused by *Microsporum canis*. Granules composed of discrete colonies of dermatophytes are surrounded and interspersed by granulomatous inflammation. (×90.)

FIGURE 11-19. Higher magnification of a granule of dermatophytic mycetoma. Irregular hyphae with bulbous, spore-like dilations are embedded in amorphous material. Note the thin rim of neutrophils surrounding the granule and large epithelioid macrophages in the outer zone of inflammation. (×220.)

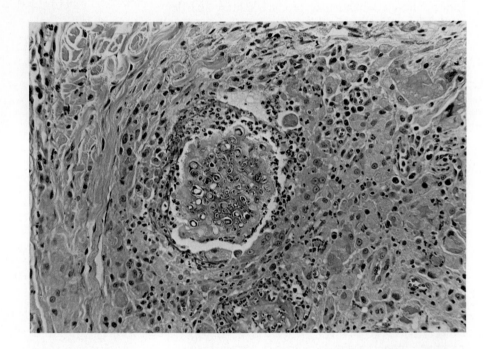

there is some colonization of hair shafts by dermatophytic spores and hyphae.

Diagnostic lesions are found in the subfollicular dermis and panniculus. Large amorphous aggregates are composed of tight clusters of somewhat refractile, pleomorphic fungal hyphae with bulbous, thick-walled dilatations, resembling spores. These fungal aggregates are embedded in amorphous eosinophilic material resembling a Splendore-Hoeppli reaction (an antigen-antibody complex in reaction to infectious agents or parasites) to form large granules; such granule forma-

tion around fungi is histopathologically characteristic of a mycetoma. The granules are cuffed by large macrophages and fewer giant cells; neutrophils and lymphocytes are present in small numbers. Proliferating fibroblastic tissue may surround the outer aspect of the lesions. Organisms are strongly positive using periodic acid–Schiff and Gomori's methenamine-silver stains. The organisms of dermatophytic mycetoma bear no morphologic resemblance to dermatophytes in hair follicles; however, culture confirms the presence of dermatophytes, generally *Microsporum canis*.

Histopathologic appearance is distinctive, but dermatophytic mycetoma must be differentiated from other fungal infections. Most of the systemic and opportunistic fungi affecting cats and dogs are smaller and more uniform in appearance in tissue section and do not form granules in tissue.

CUTANEOUS INFECTIONS OF SYSTEMIC FUNGI (Diseases: histoplasmosis, blastomycosis, coccidioidomycosis)
Clinical Features (Figures 11-20 through 11-22)

Histoplasmosis, blastomycosis, and coccidioidomycosis are systemic mycoses that occasionally disseminate secondarily to the skin. The organisms that cause these systemic mycoses, *Histoplasma capsulatum, Blastomyces dermatitidis,* and *Coccidioides immitis,* are able to invade the normal immunocompetent host, usually via inhalation of conidia, and are thus differentiated from the opportunistic fungal infections, including cryptococcosis. Very rarely, direct inoculation of fungal organisms into a wound may produce solitary skin lesions. The dog is a natural host for systemic mycoses. All three diseases are rare in the cat. Canine blastomycosis is the most common systemic mycosis seen in small animal practice; skin lesions are seen in up to 40% of affected dogs. Cutaneous involvement is much less common in histoplasmosis and coccidioidomycosis. The systemic mycoses are considered regional dermatoses with geographic restrictions to certain endemic areas (Table 11-1).

The lungs are often the primary site of infection in systemic mycoses. Skin lesions seen with systemic my-

coses are generally of much less consequence than the underlying, often life-threatening visceral disease. The reader is referred to standard texts in veterinary dermatology and mycology for further information about visceral manifestations of the systemic mycoses.

There is a commonality of skin lesions among the

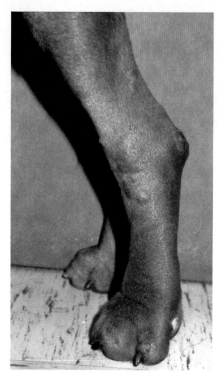

FIGURE 11-21. Multiple nodules and soft-tissue swelling on the hindlimb of the dog in Figure 11-20. *(Courtesy VA Fadok, Denver, Colorado.)*

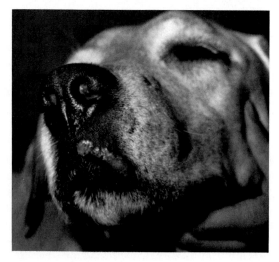

FIGURE 11-20. Cutaneous blastomycosis in a dog. Well-demarcated nodules of the muzzle have coalesced and ulcerated. *(Courtesy VA Fadok, Denver, Colorado.)*

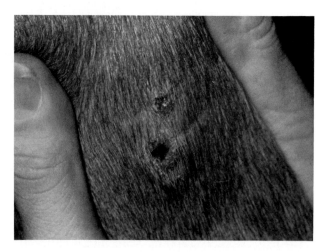

FIGURE 11-22. Closer view of an ulcerated nodule on the hindlimb of the dog in Figure 11-21. Drainage is minimal. *(Courtesy VA Fadok, Denver, Colorado.)*

TABLE 11-1. Ecology of the systemic mycoses

Disease	Ecologic niche	Endemic areas (U.S.)
Blastomycosis	Moist soil enriched with organic debris, waterways, water	East, Mississippi-Ohio River Valley
Coccidioidomycosis	Desert soil	Southwest
Histoplasmosis	Bird or bat droppings	Mississippi-Ohio River Valley

systemic mycoses. Variability is contingent on the host species, organism, and anatomic site of infection. Papular to nodular lesions become abscessed or ulcerated, and draining fistulous tracts may develop. Draining fluid may be either serosanguineous or purulent. Other lesions may be proliferative without drainage. According to Legendre (1981, 1990), the planum nasale, face, and nail beds may be preferred sites for blastomycosis. Barsanti indicates that in coccidioidomycosis, skin lesions are almost always found over sites of infected bone.

Breed, age, or sex predilections have not been reported for blastomycosis. According to Wolf (1990), histoplasmosis is seen most commonly in young (under 4 years) dogs and cats; Pointers, Weimaraners, and Brittanys may be overrepresented. Maddy has reported a greater prevalence of disseminated coccidioidomycosis following respiratory tract infection in Boxers and Doberman Pinschers; the authors also have noted an apparent predilection in Boxers. Selby has reported a possible predilection for coccidioidomycosis in male dogs.

Clinical differential diagnoses include cutaneous cryptococcosis, cutaneous infections of other opportunistic fungi and algae, sporotrichosis, feline leprosy, opportunistic mycobacterial infection, sterile granuloma and pyogranuloma, cutaneous histiocytosis, and neoplasia. Cytology or histopathology are required for definitive diagnosis. Fungal culture is not recommended for veterinary practices or most diagnostic laboratories because of the substantial danger of infection from the mycelial forms of these fungal organisms. Baum has reported primary pulmonary blastomycosis

in a laboratory worker exposed to a culture of the mycelial form of *B. dermatitidis*.

Biopsy site selection

If present, intact nodules should be surgically excised for histopathology. Impression smears for cytology should be made from freshly cut biopsy specimens and exudates. Clinicians and laboratory personnel should wear protective gloves when handling fresh specimens if systemic mycoses are suspected. Although systemic mycoses are not considered to be contagious diseases, localized skin lesions have been reported in humans in conjunction with the direct inoculation of infective material via contaminated needles or scalpels. Blastomycosis has been seen secondary to bites from an infected dog. Fortunately, systemic dissemination of these accidental skin infections has not been reported.

Histopathology (Figures 11-23 through 11-25)

The epidermis may be acanthotic or ulcerated and exudative. The dermis contains a diffuse infiltration of large macrophages, admixed with variable neutrophils, lymphocytes, and plasma cells. Discrete granulomas or pyogranulomas may be present. Necrosis may be observed. Organisms are identified in tissue as yeasts. In the yeast phase, these organisms have single- or double-contoured walls; fungal stains such as periodic acid–Schiff or Gomori's methenamine silver will selectively stain the wall. Tissue identification depends on recognition of typical morphologic features of the individual organisms (Table 11-2). Numbers of organisms vary from moderate in blastomycosis

TABLE 11-2. Histopathologic features of the systemic mycoses

Organism	Morphology	Location
Blastomyces dermatitidis	Spherical; 8 to 20 μ; double wall; broad-based budding	Free and in macrophages
Histoplasma capsulatum	Egg-shaped; 2 to 4 μ; clear halo within single wall	In macrophages
Coccidioides immitis	Spherules with endospores; 10 to 80 μ; double wall	Free

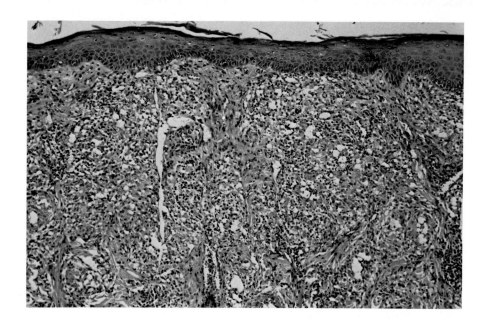

FIGURE 11-23. Cutaneous coccidioidomycosis demonstrating diffuse pyogranulomatous inflammation of the dermis. (×90.)

FIGURE 11-24. *Blastomyces dermatitidis* in a skin lesion from a dog. (×560.)

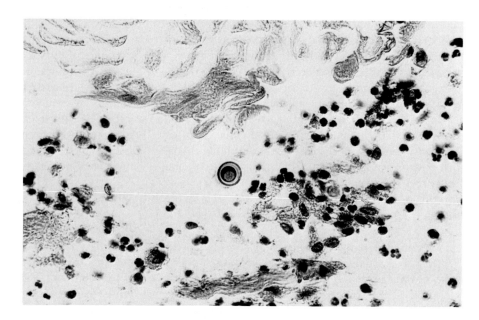

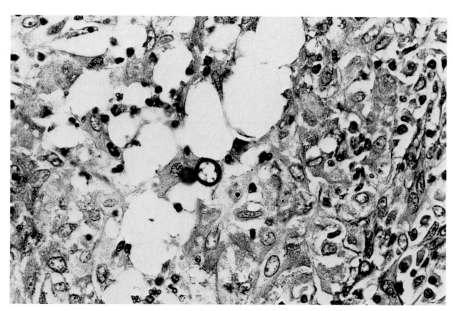

FIGURE 11-25. *Coccidioides immitis* in a skin lesion from a dog. (×560.)

or histoplasmosis to scarce in coccidioidomycosis.

Differential diagnosis is not difficult because the morphologic characteristics of these organisms generally are diagnostic. Blastomycosis may resemble cryptococcosis; *B. dermatitidis* lacks the outer capsule of *C. neoformans* and shows broad-based rather than narrow-based budding. *Sporothrix schenckii* displays budding in tissue, but is smaller and generally more pleomorphic than *B. dermatitidis*; additionally, organisms are difficult to find in specimens from cases of canine sporotrichosis, but *B. dermatitidis* is easily identified in tissue.

CUTANEOUS CRYPTOCOCCOSIS
Clinical features (Figure 11-26)

Cryptococcosis is a systemic mycosis caused by the encapsulated yeast-like fungus, *C. neoformans*. *C. neoformans* is a ubiquitous saprophyte found in nitrogen-rich debris but is isolated most commonly from soil contaminated with pigeon droppings. Cutaneous cryptococcosis is very rare in the dog. Although uncommon, cryptococcosis is the most frequently diagnosed systemic mycosis in the cat. The respiratory tract, skin, central nervous system, and eyes are affected most commonly in the cat. According to Medleau and Barsanti, skin lesions are seen in approximately 40% of cats with cryptococcosis. Inhalation of airborne organisms is considered to be the most likely route of infection. The upper respiratory tract is believed to be the usual portal of entry. Intranasal granulomatous disease is the most common initial infection, and skin disease is believed to be a sequela of either hematogenous or lymphogenous spread or self-inoculation. Cryptococcosis is seen most frequently in humid, subtropical regions of the world.

Individual serotypes exhibit marked differences in virulence. The organism generally is considered to be an opportunist and is seen primarily in association with coexistent debilitating or immunosuppressive diseases such as neoplasia, diabetes mellitus, and feline leukemia virus (FeLV) or feline immunodeficiency virus (FIV) infection in cats. In addition, cryptococcosis is seen as a sequela to iatrogenic immunosuppression caused by glucocorticoids or cytotoxic chemotherapy.

Well-circumscribed, usually grouped, dermal or subcutaneous, firm or fluctuant nodules typically characterize cutaneous cryptococcosis. Lesions ulcerate and drain a scant to copious, serous to mucoid exudate. Less commonly, lesions may be solitary or widely disseminated. The head, neck, and ears are affected most frequently. Regional lymphadenopathy is common. If present, visceral disease can cause a variety of systemic signs, including fever, inappetence, weight loss, general malaise, and neurologic signs.

Breed, age, or sex predilections have not been reported. Clinical differential diagnoses should include

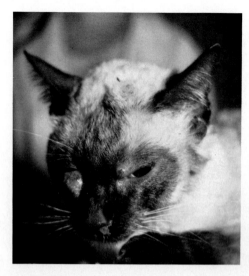

FIGURE 11-26. Cutaneous cryptococcosis in a cat with FeLV infection. Well-circumscribed, dermal nodules involve the periorbital skin and base of the ears. Concurrent intranasal granulomatous disease is present (note nasal exudate).

other systemic mycoses, infections caused by other opportunistic fungi and algae, sporotrichosis, feline leprosy, sterile granuloma and pyogranuloma syndrome, cutaneous histiocytosis, and neoplasia. Diagnosis is confirmed by impression smears of exudate, histopathology, culture on Sabouraud's dextrose agar, or the cryptococcal antigen latex agglutination test. Fungal culture should not be performed until other systemic mycoses are ruled out by impression smear and histopathology, since attempted culture of other systemic fungi may be dangerous (see preceding discussion). The culture of *C. neoformans* is not a public health hazard because only the yeast form is routinely isolated.

Biopsy site selection

Wedge biopsy specimens should be taken from intact or recently ulcerated nodules. Impression smears for cytology should be made from freshly cut biopsy specimens and exudates. Extensive necrosis may complicate the histopathologic diagnosis in older lesions. In contrast to the other systemic fungi, contact with infected tissue is not a risk to clinicians or laboratory personnel because the yeast form is not infective and does not aerosolize from tissue.

Histopathology (Figures 11-27 and 11-28)

The epidermis is normal, slightly acanthotic, or ulcerated. Generally, large numbers of oval or spherical yeasts are present diffusely in the dermis and subcutis. *Cryptococcus neoformans* organisms measure 5 to 20 μ and are surrounded by a wide clear capsule that increases the overall diameter to a maximum of 30 μ. Narrow-based budding often is visible. Large numbers

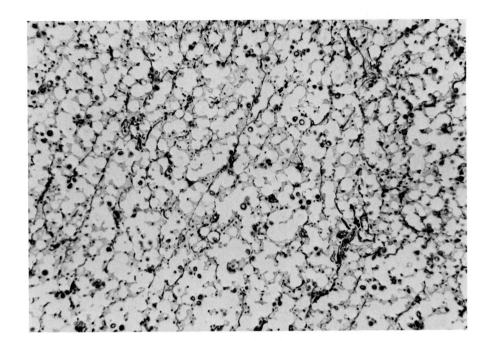

FIGURE 11-27. Feline crypto-coccosis. Note the diffuse accumulation of yeast-like organisms. Scant inflammation and prominent capsulation of the organisms create a foamy or bubbly appearance. (×90.)

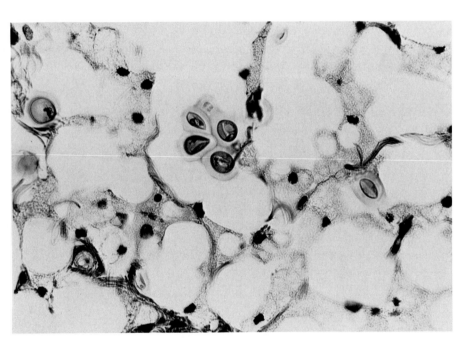

FIGURE 11-28. *Cryptococcus neoformans* in a skin lesion from a dog. (×560.)

of organisms with confluent capsules create a pale, foamy, or "soap bubble" appearance to the tissue, which is highly characteristic of cryptococcosis. Mucicarmine stain will define the capsule. There may be artifactual loss or collapse of capsular material, leaving a dense, mucicarmine-positive zone immediately surrounding the central body and an outer unstained zone where the capsule existed before tissue processing. In rare cases, poor capsule formation may be present.

Inflammation often is scant to absent, but may be mild to moderate. In inflamed lesions, large macrophages, many of which have engulfed organisms, are accompanied by variable numbers of neutrophils. Lymphocytes may occasionally be evident.

Cryptococcosis generally is typical histopathologically. Occasionally, differentiation from blastomycosis may be required, particularly in infections caused by strains exhibiting poor capsulation. *B. dermatitidis* lacks a capsule, has broad-based rather than narrow-based budding, and usually evokes more inflammation in tissue than does *C. neoformans*.

CUTANEOUS INFECTIONS OF OTHER OPPORTUNISTIC FUNGI AND ALGAE (Diseases: aspergillosis, paecilomycosis, protothecosis, phaeohyphomycosis, zygomycosis, mycetoma)

Clinical features (Figures 11-29 through 11-32)

Skin infection caused by other opportunistic fungi and algae is uncommon in the cat and very rare in the dog. The causative organisms of this group of diseases include *Aspergillus* species (aspergillosis); *Paecilomyces* species (paecilomycosis or hyalohyphomycosis); *Prototheca wickerhamii* (the alga of protothecosis); *Alternaria alternata, Cladosporium* species, *Dreschlera specifera, Exophiala jeanselmei, Moniliella suaveolens, Phialophora verrucosa, Pseudomicrodochium suttonii, Scolecobasidium humicola, Stemphylium* species, and *Xylohypha emmonsii*

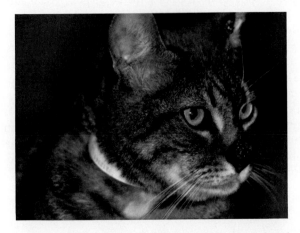

FIGURE 11-29. Opportunistic fungal infection (phaeohyphomycosis) in a cat caused by *Alternaria* species. Ulcerated, firm nodules are present on the planum nasale and pinna.

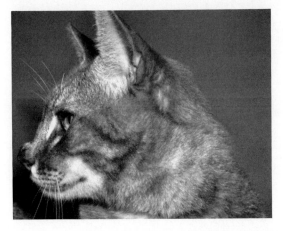

FIGURE 11-30. Side view of the cat in Figure 11-29. A large nodule is deforming the planum nasale.

(phaeohyphomycosis); *Basidiobolus haptosporus* and *Conidiobolus coronatus* (zygomycosis); *Curvularia geniculata* and *Madurella grisea* (black-grain mycetomas); and *Pseudallescheria boydii* and *Acremonium hyalinum* (white-grain mycetomas).

Primary cutaneous infection occurs most commonly as a result of trauma. Immunologic incompetence is documented most frequently in animals with systemic opportunistic infection. Primary cutaneous or subcutaneous infection most commonly characterizes phaeohyphomycosis and zygomycosis. Skin disease secondary to systemic infection occurs with aspergillosis, protothecosis, and white-grain mycetomas. Skin infection in paecilomycosis (hyalohyphomycosis) can be primary or secondary to systemic infection.

Similar to the systemic mycoses, there is a commonality of the clinical lesions seen with the opportunistic fungal and algal diseases. Grouped papules, nodules, or erythematous macules coalesce and enlarge slowly by local extension. Ulceration may result in chronic nonhealing abscesses, draining fistulous tracts,

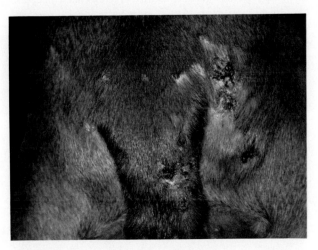

FIGURE 11-31. Widespread opportunistic fungal infection (phaeohyphomycosis) in a Viszla. Multiple ulcerated plaques and nodules are present on the rump.

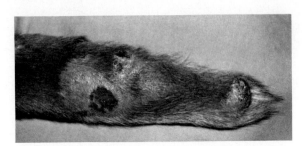

FIGURE 11-32. Closer view of the tail of the dog in Figure 11-31. Alopecic nodules have coalesced and ulcerated.

or coalescing shallow ulcers. Additionally, tissue grains or granules are seen in mycetomas. Variation in other associated clinical signs is extreme and is contingent on the host species, organism, and the site of entry. The reader is referred to standard texts in veterinary dermatology and mycology for further information.

Little data are available on breed, age, or sex predilections for opportunistic fungal and algal infections; this may reflect the infrequency of these diseases. Since acquired immunologic incompetence is more common in older animals, these animals may be at greater risk for opportunistic fungal and algal infection. Limited evidence indicates that German Shepherd Dogs may be at increased risk for aspergillosis.

Clinically, infections of these opportunistic fungi and algae may resemble other systemic mycoses, feline leprosy, opportunistic mycobacterial infection, sterile granuloma and pyogranuloma syndrome, cutaneous histiocytosis, foreign body reactions, and neoplasia. Impression smears from exudates may demonstrate the offending agent. Fungal culture and histopathology are required to establish a diagnosis. Fungal culture should not be performed until systemic mycoses are ruled out by impression smear and histopathology since attempted culture of these fungi may be dangerous (see earlier discussion).

Biopsy site selection

Nonulcerated lesions should be removed using the wedge resection technique. Impression smears for cytology should be made from freshly cut biopsy specimens and exudates. If only fistulated nodules or chronic abscesses are present, care should be taken to obtain a deep, representative sample. Clinicians and laboratory personnel should wear protective gloves when handling infected tissue. These organisms can cause opportunistic infections in humans by direct inoculation, similar to the systemic fungi (see earlier discussion).

Histopathology (Figures 11-33 and 11-34)

The epidermis is acanthotic and occasionally may be ulcerated. In opportunistic fungal infection the dermis and usually the underlying panniculus are diffusely infiltrated with large epithelioid or foamy macrophages. Variable numbers of neutrophils and lymphocytes are present, and multinucleated giant cells may be found. Close examination may reveal ghosts of fungal organisms within or among macrophages, which subsequent periodic acid–Schiff or Gomori's methenamine silver staining will delineate; these ghosts create the vacuolated or foamy appearance of the macrophages. Organisms may be pigmented in phaeohyphomycosis. Many of the opportunistic fungi have branching, septate hyphae. Morphology of the specific organism responsible will vary, depending on the species of fungus present. The reader is referred to standard textbooks on medical mycology. Histopathology alone cannot specifically identify these organisms; fungal culture is required.

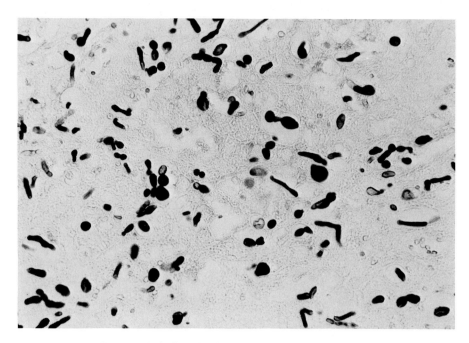

FIGURE 11-33. Opportunistic fungal infection in a cat caused by *Curvularia* species. Note the irregular hyphae containing arthrospore-like swellings. (Gomori's methenamine silver stain; × 350.)

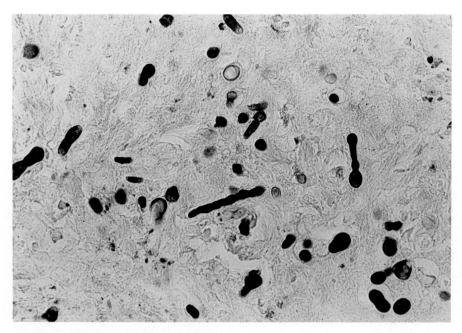

FIGURE 11-34. Opportunistic fungal infection in a cat. Irregular, septate hyphae have bulbous swellings. (Gomori's methenamine silver stain; ×560.)

Infection with the colorless alga *Prototheca* produces a characteristic histopathologic picture. The organisms are unique and easily identified in tissue. *Prototheca* species are round to oval and measure 3 to 20 μ in diameter. Characteristic daughter cells, or endospores, create a subdivided or "cut pie" appearance to the organism. Tissue reaction may be minimal, or there may be diffuse inflammation composed of macrophages, lymphocytes, and occasional neutrophils.

Differential diagnosis principally involves definitive identification of the etiologic agent, which is not possible using histopathology alone. Fungal or algal culture is required. The opportunistic infections that are characterized by infiltrations of vacuolated macrophages may mimic cutaneous xanthoma, or feline leprosy. Generally, ghosts of opportunistic fungi are apparent on close examination of hematoxylin-and-eosin stained sections. Special stains will also allow differentiation from mycobacterial infection or cutaneous xanthoma.

SPOROTRICHOSIS
Clinical features (Figure 11-35)

Sporotrichosis is an uncommon, subacute or chronic, granulomatous disease seen in the cat and dog, which is caused by the dimorphic fungus, *Sporothrix schenckii*. The organism is worldwide in distribution and grows as a saprophytic mycelial fungus in moist organic debris. Access to the host is accomplished by puncture wound contamination. The organism establishes infection as a yeast at body temperature in the dermis and subcutis and may ascend to regional lymph nodes. Rarely, visceral dissemination may occur. Dissemination may be limited to immunocompromised individuals in the dog and has been associated with glucocorticoid therapy. In cats, visceral dissemination may occur in healthy individuals.

Sporotrichosis in cats, unlike in other host species, is characterized by large numbers of organisms in draining fluids and in tissue. For this reason, cats with

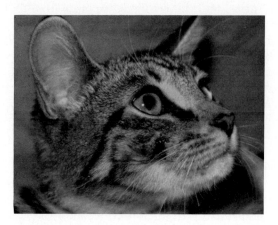

FIGURE 11-35. Sporotrichosis in a cat. A firm, alopecic nodule on the face has ulcerated and fistulated, discharging serosanguineous fluid that contained large numbers of organisms on direct smear.

sporotrichosis may more readily infect humans, and extreme caution must be exercised by all handlers of infected animals or fresh tissue. Dunstan reported that the motile organisms may penetrate intact human skin.

Skin lesions of dogs and cats develop at the site of inoculation. Lesions tend to be grouped and localized. Firm, alopecic, nonpainful nodules ulcerate and fistulate to discharge a light-brown, serosanguineous fluid. Satellite lesions may form near the primary puncture wound. Individual nodules may appear verruciform. The head and limbs are the most common sites of infection. Disseminated cutaneous lesions have been seen in the Doberman Pinscher. Regional lymphadenopathy is common and affected lymph nodes may fistulate.

Breed, age, or sex predilections have not been reported for the cat or dog. However, Doberman Pinschers may be at increased risk for the development of multicentric cutaneous sporotrichosis.

Clinically, solitary or grouped lesions of sporotrichosis must be differentiated from systemic mycoses, cryptococcosis and other opportunistic fungal infections, feline leprosy, bacterial abscesses, foreign body reactions, and neoplasms. Multicentric lesions, as seen in the Doberman Pinscher, may resemble deep bacterial folliculitis and furunculosis or systemic mycoses. Impression smears of exudate and histopathology should be performed. Fungal culture from tissue specimens may be required to establish a diagnosis in dogs. Fungal culture should not be performed until the systemic mycoses are ruled out by impression smear and histopathology, since attempted culture of systemic fungi may be dangerous (see earlier discussion).

Biopsy site selection

Deep punch or wedge biopsy specimens should be obtained, preferably from nondraining lesions. Impression smears for cytology should be made from freshly cut biopsy specimens and exudates. Since feline sporotrichosis has marked zoonotic potential, veterinarians or laboratory personnel handling the cat or fresh specimens from the cat should wear gloves and wash thoroughly with fungicidal antiseptics such as povidone-iodine or chlorhexidine. Fungal culture of biopsy specimens may be beneficial in suspected cases of canine sporotrichosis, since organisms may be sparse.

Histopathology (Figures 11-36 through 11-39)

The epidermis in both feline and canine sporotrichosis is acanthotic to ulcerated. There may be variable exudation and crusting. Inflammation is diffuse throughout the superficial and deep dermis and may extend to the panniculus.

Feline sporotrichosis differs markedly from canine

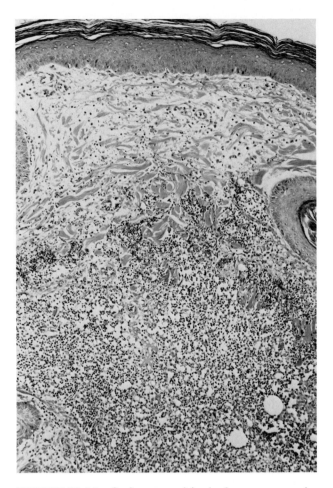

FIGURE 11-36.   Canine sporotrichosis. Severe pyogranulomatous inflammation is oriented in the middle and deep dermis. *(Case material from MB Calderwood Mays, Gainesville, Florida.) (×90.)*

sporotrichosis in that organisms are abundant and easily visible, even on routine staining with hematoxylin and eosin. Macrophages are diffusely present and are intermingled with fewer neutrophils in a nodular to diffuse pyogranulomatous pattern; occasional lymphocytes are seen. Elongated, "cigar-shaped" organisms ("dot"-shaped in cross section), 4 to 9 μ in length and 1 to 2 μ in diameter, are present in profusion, both free and within macrophages.

In canine sporotrichosis the dermis and usually the panniculus are diffusely infiltrated with large numbers of neutrophils and macrophages. Fewer lymphocytes and plasma cells are intermingled. Discrete pyogranulomas may be present. Necrosis with cavitation and hemorrhage are variable, but may be severe. Usually, very small numbers of organisms are scattered throughout the inflammatory infiltrate, but may be more abundant in dogs that have received recent corticosteroid

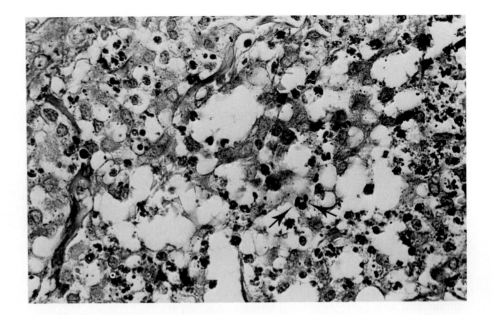

FIGURE 11-37. Higher magnification of Figure 11-36. Focal oval and budding organisms *(arrows)* are present within pyogranulomatous infiltrate. (Periodic acid–Schiff stain; ×560.)

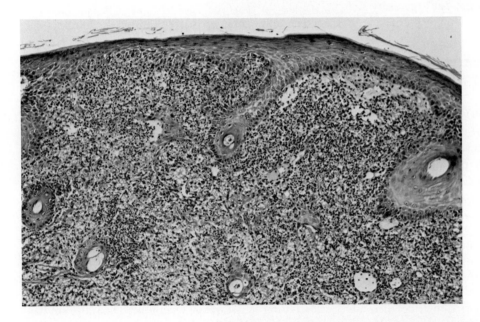

FIGURE 11-38. Feline sporotrichosis. Severe diffuse pyogranulomatous inflammation is interspersed by hypocellular gray zones that contain numerous organisms (not visible at this power). (×90.)

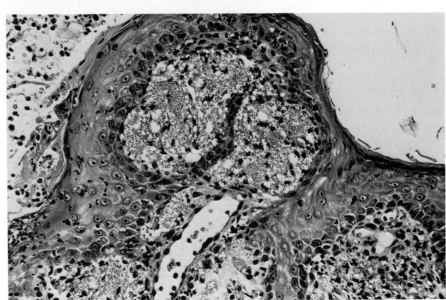

FIGURE 11-39. Feline sporotrichosis. Note myriads of small, elongated or dot-like *Sporothrix schenckii.* (×220.)

therapy. *S. schenckii* is best visualized in dogs using a periodic acid–Schiff or Gomori's methenamine silver stain. Organisms in tissue are pleomorphic, round or oval, occasionally budding yeasts that measure 3 to 8 μ in diameter. When demonstration of organisms in tissue is not successful, the diagnosis may be problematic unless cytologic evaluation of smears of exudate reveals the fungus. Fluorescent antibody testing to detect organisms in biopsy specimens also has been used.

Differential diagnosis is exceedingly more difficult in the dog than in the cat because of the relative paucity of organisms in canine cases. Histopathologic differential diagnoses in the dog include infections by opportunistic or systemic fungi, foreign body reactions, and severe bacterial pyoderma. Demonstration of fungi or foreign material will allow differentiation. Additionally, the inflammation of canine sporotrichosis is less suppurative and more pyogranulomatous than most cases of bacterial pyoderma. In the cat, organisms are highly characteristic in tissue and allow definitive diagnosis.

CUTANEOUS PYTHIOSIS (Synonyms:

phycomycosis, oomycosis)
Clinical features (Figure 11-40)

Cutaneous pythiosis is a rare, ulcerative, pyogranulomatous skin disease seen in the dog. *Pythium* species are protozoan plant pathogens that are fungus-like, aquatic, dimorphic, and flagellate. The natural habitat of *Pythium* species is stagnant water containing a high content of organic debris. Affected animals probably have previously existing trauma and acquire the organism when swimming or wading in infested water. The disease is seen primarily in warm humid climates such as the Gulf Coast of the United States. An increased incidence is noted in the summer and early fall.

The initial lesion is a poorly circumscribed dermal nodule. Progression is rapid as the lesion expands peripherally and subcutaneously, leading to the formation of satellite nodules. Nodules become necrotic, ulcerate, and develop fistulous tracts that drain purulent or serosanguineous exudate. The legs, face, and lumbosacral area are the most common sites. Dorsal lumbosacral infection may be secondary to trauma from flea allergy dermatitis. Pruritus is marked and commonly initiates severe self-trauma. Viscerally disseminated disease in a dog has been reported by Foil (1984).

Although statistical evaluation of signalment data is not available, pythiosis reportedly is more common in young adult, large-breed dogs. German Shepherd Dogs may be at increased risk.

Clinically, pythiosis may resemble deep bacterial infection (deep pyoderma, opportunistic mycobacterial

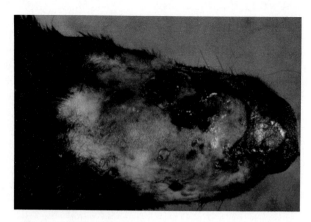

FIGURE 11-40. Cutaneous pythiosis on the muzzle of a dog. Multiple, coalescing, necrotic and ulcerated nodules have adherent, dried serosanguineous exudate. (*Courtesy CS Foil, Baton Rouge, Louisiana.*)

infection, actinomycosis, nocardiosis), fungal infections (systemic mycoses, cryptococcosis, cutaneous infections of opportunistic fungi), demodicosis, neoplasms, or acral lick dermatitis (if on a distal extremity). Histopathology will aid in the diagnosis. Culture on vegetable extract agar is required to grow *Pythium* species, but should not be attempted until systemic mycoses are ruled out by cytology or histopathology because of the attendant danger of cultural isolation of the systemic fungi (see earlier discussion). Definitive diagnosis requires the identification of motile zoospores; special techniques are required to induce zoospore formation. Since peripheral eosinophilia is seen in approximately 50% of dogs with pythiosis, this is an additional aid in the differential diagnosis.

Biopsy site selection

Both intact and ulcerated nodules should be excised using sterile wedge technique. The subjacent panniculus should be included in the specimen. If pythiosis is suspected in a solitary lesion, wide surgical extirpation is recommended and offers the additional advantage of a potential cure. The zoonotic potential of pythiosis is as yet unknown but probably is minimal. However, reasonable caution such as the wearing of gloves is recommended.*

Histopathology (Figures 11-41 and 11-42)

Acanthosis or severe ulceration of the epidermis is seen. The dermis and often the panniculus are diffusely and severely inflamed. Necrosis is present and may be extensive. Pyogranulomatous inflammation is punctuated by discrete, often large foci of degenerating

* Foil CS: Personal communication, 1990.

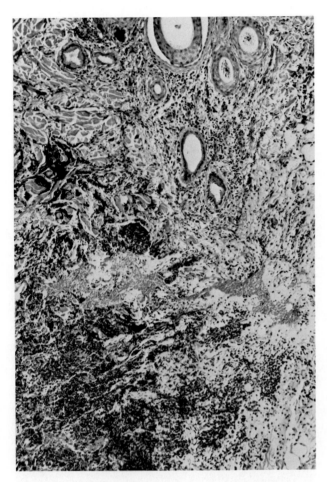

FIGURE 11-41. Canine cutaneous pythiosis. Darkly staining lakes of degranulated, eosinophilic debris are accompanied by hemorrhage and inflammation. (×90.)

eosinophils (similar to "kunkers" of equine pythiosis). These eosinophilic foci are surrounded by intact eosinophils, neutrophils, macrophages, and rare multinucleated giant cells. Organisms are seen with special staining in eosinophilic foci or in other areas of necrosis and inflammation. *Pythium* species have broad, usually nonseptate, branching hyphae, which measure 4 to 8 μ in diameter. Occasional vascular necrosis and thrombosis are present and may be attended by hyphae within devitalized vessel walls. Edema and hemorrhage are variable.

Organisms usually are not visible in hematoxylin and eosin-stained sections. The periodic acid–Schiff stain also usually will not detect *Pythium* species in tissue; this stain is superior in detecting living organisms, and *Pythium* organisms are often devitalized in specimens obtained for histopathology. Gomori's methenamine silver will stain the wall of living or dead fungi and must be utilized in any suspected case of pythiosis or the diagnosis may be overlooked. Brown has recently described a technique utilizing indirect immunoperoxidase to specifically identify *Pythium* species in tissue.

Differential diagnosis includes deep bacterial or fungal infections or foreign body reactions, particularly those characterized by severe necrosis. Necrotizing inflammation caused by deep arthropod trauma (spider bites) also may be considered. Demonstration of the organism in tissue will differentiate pythiosis from noninfectious or bacterial diseases. Opportunistic fungal infections may closely resemble pythiosis. Differentiation from the morphologically very similar zygo-

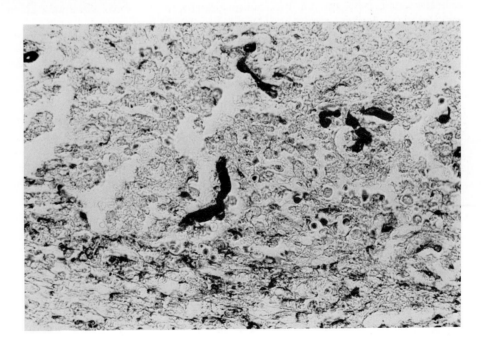

FIGURE 11-42. Canine cutaneous pythiosis. Note the silver-positive, irregular fungal hyphae. (Gomori's methenamine silver stain; ×560.)

mycetes is particularly difficult; however, in contrast to *Pythium* species, zygomycetes often may be visible with hematoxylin and eosin alone. Foci of degenerating eosinophils and vascular necrosis may be other helpful histopathologic morphologic clues in the differential diagnosis of pythiosis. Identification of the organism by immunohistochemistry or culture of clinical specimens is required for definitive diagnosis.

CUTANEOUS LEISHMANIASIS
Clinical features (Figures 11-43 and 11-44)

Leishmaniasis is a cutaneous and systemic disease seen uncommonly in dogs and very rarely in cats. The disease is caused by obligatory intracellular protozoa of the genus *Leishmania,* which are transmitted by sandflies. In the dog, *L. donovani* is reported most commonly, although *L. chagasi* also has been documented. The insect vectors in North America are the bloodsucking sandflies of the genus *Lutzomyia,* whereas the European vectors are *Phlebotomus* species. Dogs, wild canids, and rodents are the natural reservoirs.

The distribution of leishmaniasis is characterized by marked geographic restriction. Canine leishmaniasis is rare in the United States; enzootic foci are located only in Oklahoma and Texas. European distribution is along the Mediterranean coast, particularly in southern France, Portugal, Spain, Greece, and Italy. With increased pet mobility, more cases are being seen in nonendemic areas after pets return from distant locales.

Little is known about the pathogenesis of leishmaniasis in dogs. Local infection of the skin is followed by dissemination of the parasites. In humans, defects in T cell–associated host defense mechanisms determine susceptibility. Recent work by Slappendel (1988, 1990) suggests that circulating immune complexes may play an important role in the pathogenesis of leishmaniasis by inducing polyarthritis, bleeding tendencies, and renal failure.

Typical clinical features include a nonpruritic, generalized exfoliative dermatitis with alopecia. Silvery-white, asbestos-like, adherent scales are a distinctive feature. Nodules and focal ulcerations may occur as the disease progresses. The muzzle, periorbital region, and ears are common initial sites and often are more severely affected. Facial bilateral symmetry may be marked. Periorbital rings of alopecia and scaling are common. Depigmentation of the planum nasale and muzzle may be seen. Generalized peripheral lymphadenopathy is a common feature. Systemic signs such as fever, malaise, weight loss, muscle atrophy, coagulopathy, polyarthritis, and renal failure may be present in advanced cases.

Perhaps because of the likelihood of exposure to

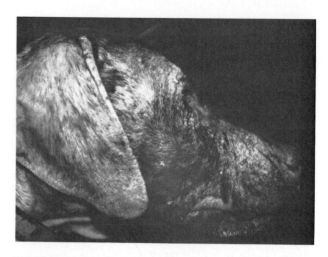

FIGURE 11-43. Cutaneous leishmaniasis in a dog. Generalized scaling is present on the face and ears. *(Courtesy Z Alhaidari, Roquefort-les-Pins, France.)*

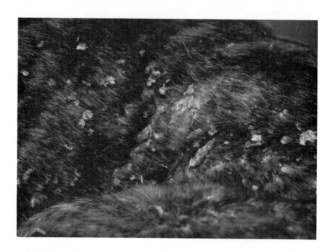

FIGURE 11-44. Cutaneous leishmaniasis in a dog. Distinctive silvery-white, asbestos-like adherent scales are distributed in the haircoat. *(Courtesy Z Alhaidari, Roquefort-les-Pins, France.)*

the vector, cutaneous leishmaniasis is more common in active young adult dogs. Slappendel (1988, 1990) reported the median age as 4 years; male dogs were at increased risk. Breed predilection has not been noted.

Clinical differential diagnoses should include autoimmune skin diseases with frequent facial involvement (discoid lupus erythematosus, pemphigus foliaceus, pemphigus erythematosus), mycosis fungoides, dermatophytosis, and zinc-responsive dermatosis. Vesicles or pustules characterize pemphigus; involvement of the footpads is common in pemphigus foliaceus, but rare in leishmaniasis. Systemic or discoid lupus erythematosus may closely mimic leishmaniasis, particularly when depigmentation is present, but scaling usually is a less striking feature. Zinc-responsive dermatosis exhibits more frequent mucocutaneous involvement. Skin biopsy is mandatory for the differentiation of these diseases.

Biopsy site selection

Biopsy specimens should be taken from multiple areas of adherent scale. Nodules, if present, should be sampled. Chronic lesions are more likely to yield diagnostic results. Cytology of bone marrow or lymph node aspirates, or biopsy of lymph nodes may aid in establishing the diagnosis.

Histopathology (Figures 11-45 and 11-46)

The epidermis is characterized by moderate acanthosis and moderate to severe hyperkeratosis or parakeratosis with crusting. The dermis has multinodular to diffuse infiltrations of foamy macrophages, and fewer lymphocytes, plasma cells, and neutrophils. Nodular inflammation may be oriented around adnexal append-

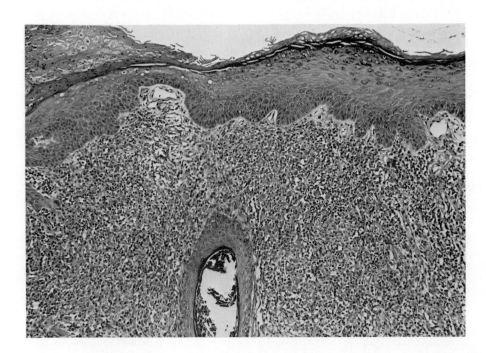

FIGURE 11-45. Cutaneous leishmaniasis in a dog. The dermis is diffusely and severely inflamed. (×90.)

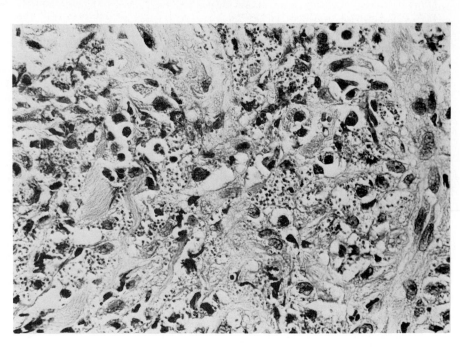

FIGURE 11-46. High magnification of cutaneous leishmaniasis in a dog demonstrates numerous, small intracytoplasmic *Leishmania donovani* within macrophages. (×560.)

ages in earlier lesions. Sebaceous glands may be swept up and obliterated by the inflammation, which may explain the development of hyperkeratosis (see sebaceous adenitis, Chapter 7). Variable numbers of *Leishmania* species, which are round to oval, 1 to 2 μ in width, and 2 to 4 μ in length, may be present either within macrophages or extracellularly. Organisms are visible with hematoxylin and eosin but are accentuated with Giemsa staining. A round basophilic nucleus and a typical rod-shaped kinetoplast are clustered near one end of the organism. Identification of organisms in tissue by histopathology or cytology is required for definitive diagnosis.

Periadnexal inflammation in cutaneous leishmaniasis might be confused with the periadnexal subtype of sterile granuloma and pyogranuloma syndrome or with the granulomatous forms of sebaceous adenitis as seen in Viszlas. Differential diagnosis is not difficult when typical organisms are identified in tissue. Organisms occasionally may be difficult to find in skin specimens. When clinical and historic suspicion is high, lymph node biopsy and bone marrow aspirates may be required to establish proof of leishmaniasis.

SUGGESTED READINGS

Actinomycosis and nocardiosis

Ackerman N, Grain E, and Castleman W: Canine nocardiosis, J Am Anim Hosp Assoc 18:147-153, 1982.

Brennan KE and Ihrke PJ: Grass awn migration in dogs and cats: a retrospective study of 182 cases, J Am Vet Med Assoc 182:1201-1204, 1983.

Davenport DJ and Johnson GC: Cutaneous nocardiosis in a cat, J Am Vet Med Assoc 188:728-729, 1986.

Foil CS: Cutaneous fungal diseases. In Nesbitt GH, editor: Dermatology: contemporary issues in small animal practice, New York, 1987, Churchill Livingstone, pp 135-138.

Hardie EM: Actinomycosis and nocardiosis. In Greene CE, editor: Infectious diseases of the dog and cat, Philadelphia, 1990, WB Saunders, pp 585-591.

Lever WF and Schaumburg-Lever G: Histopathology of the skin, Philadelphia, 1990, JB Lippincott, pp 385-387.

Muller GH, Kirk RW and Scott DW: Small animal dermatology, ed 4, Philadelphia, 1989, WB Saunders, pp 278-282.

Feline leprosy

Kunkle GA: Feline leprosy. In Greene CE, editor: Infectious diseases of the dog and cat, Philadelphia, 1990, WB Saunders, pp 567-569.

McIntosh DW: Feline leprosy: a review of forty-four cases from western Canada, Can Vet J 23:291-295, 1982.

Schiefer HB and Middleton DM: Experimental transmission of a feline mycobacterial skin disease (feline leprosy), Vet Pathol 20:460-471, 1983.

White SD and Ihrke PJ: Pyoderma. In Nesbitt GH, editor: Dermatology: contemporary issues in small animal practice, New York, 1987, Churchill Livingstone, p 110.

Opportunistic mycobacterial infection

Alhaidari Z, Leclerc JM, and Terreau Y: Mycobacteriose chez un chat, Pratique Medicale Chirurgicale de l'Animal de Compagnie 20:325-327, 1985.

Buergelt CD, Fowler JL, and Wright PJ: Disseminated avian tuberculosis in a cat, Cal Vet 10:13-15, 1982.

Donnelly TM, Jones MR, and Wickam N: Diffuse cutaneous granulomatous lesions associated with acid-fast bacilli in a cat, J Small Anim Pract 23:99-105, 1982.

Gross TL and Connelly MR: Nontuberculous mycobacterial skin infections in two dogs, Vet Pathol 20:117-119, 1983.

Kunkle GA: Atypical mycobacterial infections. In Greene CE, editor: Infectious diseases of the dog and cat, Philadelphia, 1990, WB Saunders, pp 569-572.

Kunkle GA and others: Rapidly growing mycobacteria as a cause of cutaneous granulomas: report of five cases, J Am Anim Hosp Assoc 19:513-521, 1983.

Lever WF and Schaumburg-Lever G: Histopathology of the skin, Philadelphia, 1990, JB Lippincott, pp 332-333.

White SD and others: Cutaneous atypical mycobacteriosis in cats, J Am Vet Med Assoc 182:1218-1222, 1983.

Willemse T and others: *Mycobacterium thermoresistibile*: extrapulmonary infection in a cat, J Clin Microbiol 21:854-856, 1985.

Feline dermatophytic mycetoma

Miller WH and Goldschmidt MH: Mycetomas in the cat caused by a dermatophyte: a case report, J Am Anim Hosp Assoc 22:255-260, 1986.

Tuttle PA and Chandler FW: Deep dermatophytosis in a cat, J Am Vet Med Assoc 183:1106-1108, 1983.

Yager JA and others: Mycetoma-like granuloma in a cat caused by *Microsporum canis*, J Comp Pathol 96:171-175, 1986.

Cutaneous infections of systemic fungi

Barsanti JA and Jeffery KL: Coccidioidomycosis. In Greene CE, editor: Infectious diseases of the dog and cat, Philadelphia, 1990, WB Saunders, pp 696-706.

Baum GL and Lerner PI: Primary pulmonary blastomycosis: a laboratory-acquired infection, Ann Intern Med 73:263-265, 1970.

Breider MA and others: Blastomycosis in cats: five cases (1979-1986), J Am Vet Med Assoc 193:570-572, 1988.

Clinkenbeard KD, Cowell RL, and Tyler RD: Disseminated histoplasmosis in cats: 12 cases (1981-1986), J Am Vet Med Assoc 190:1445-1448, 1987.

Fadok VA: Dermatologic manifestations of subcutaneous and deep mycoses, Comp Cont Ed 6:506-514, 1980.

Foil CS: Cutaneous fungal diseases. In Nesbitt GH, editor: Dermatology: contemporary issues in small animal practice, New York, 1987, Churchill Livingstone, 146-155.

Jones TC and Hunt RD: Veterinary pathology, Philadelphia, 1983, Lea & Febiger, pp 669-688.

Legendre AM: Blastomycosis. In Greene CE, editor: Infectious diseases of the dog and cat, Philadelphia, 1990, WB Saunders, pp 669-678.

Legendre AM and others: Canine blastomycosis: a review of 47 clinical cases, J Am Vet Med Assoc 178:1163-1168, 1981.

Lever WF and Schaumburg-Lever G: Histopathology of the skin, Philadelphia, 1990, JB Lippincott, pp 373-383.

Maddy KT: Disseminated coccidioidomycosis of the dog, J Am Vet Med Assoc 132:483-489, 1958.

Miller PE, Miller LM, and Schoster JV: Feline blastomycosis: a report of three cases and literature review (1961-1988), J Am Anim Hosp Assoc 26:417-424, 1990.

Selby LA, Becker SV, and Hayes HW: Epidemiologic risk factors associated with canine systemic mycoses, Am J Epidemiol 113:133-139, 1981.

Wolf AM: Histoplasmosis. In Greene CE, editor: Infectious diseases of the dog and cat, Philadelphia, 1990, WB Saunders, pp 679-686.

Wolf AM: Primary cutaneous coccidioidomycosis in a dog and a cat, J Am Vet Med Assoc 174:504-506, 1979.

Wolf AM and Belden MN: Feline histoplasmosis: a literature review and retrospective study of 20 new cases, J Am Anim Hosp Assoc 20:995-998, 1984.

Cutaneous cryptococcosis

Foil CS: Cutaneous fungal diseases. In Nesbitt GH, editor: Dermatology: contemporary issues in small animal practice, New York, 1987, Churchill Livingstone, pp 150-153.

Hubert B and Magnol J-P: Cryptococcose cutanee chez un chat infecte par le virus leucemogene, Pratique Medicale et Chirurgicale de l'Animal de Compagnie 20:253-256, 1985.

Lever WF and Schaumburg-Lever G: Histopathology of the skin, Philadelphia, 1990, JB Lippincott, pp 379-381.

MacDonald DW and Stretch HC: Canine cryptococcosis associated with prolonged corticosteroid therapy, Can Vet J 23:200-202, 1982.

Medleau L and others: Clinical evaluation of a cryptococcal antigen latex agglutination test for diagnosis of cryptococcosis in cats, J Am Vet Med Assoc 196:1470-1473, 1990.

Medleau L and others: Cutaneous cryptococcosis in three cats, J Am Vet Med Assoc 187:169-170, 1985.

Medleau L and Barsanti JA: Cryptococcosis. In Greene CE, editor: Infectious diseases of the dog and cat, Philadelphia, 1990, WB Saunders, pp 687-695.

Cutaneous infections of other opportunistic fungi and algae

Beale KM and Pinson D: Phaeohyphomycosis caused by two different species of *Curvularia* in two animals from the same household, J Am Anim Hosp Assoc 26:67-70, 1990.

Dhein CR and others: Phaeohyphomycosis caused by *Alternaria alternata* in a cat, J Am Vet Med Assoc 193:1101-1103, 1988.

Foil CS: Miscellaneous fungal infections. In Greene CE, editor: Infectious diseases of the dog and cat, Philadelphia, 1990, WB Saunders, pp 731-741.

Foil CS: Cutaneous fungal diseases. In Nesbitt GH, editor: Dermatology: contemporary issues in small animal practice, New York, 1987, Churchill Livingstone, pp 138-155.

Kwochka KW and others: Canine phaeohyphomycosis caused by *Drechslera spicifera*: a case report and literature review, J Am Anim Hosp Assoc 20:625-633, 1984.

Lever WF and Schaumburg-Lever G: Histopathology of the skin, Philadelphia, 1990, JB Lippincott, pp 371-387.

McKenzie RA and others: Subcutaneous phaeohyphomycosis caused by *Moniliella suaveolens* in two cats, Vet Pathol 21:582-586, 1984.

Muller GH, Kirk RW, and Scott DW: Small animal dermatology, ed 4, Philadelphia, 1989, WB Saunders, pp 319-341.

Neer TM: Disseminated aspergillosis, Comp Anim Pract 10:465-471, 1988.

Sousa CA and Ihrke PJ: Subcutaneous phaeohyphomycosis (*Stemphylium* sp. and *Cladosporium* sp.) in a cat, J Am Vet Med Assoc 185:673-675, 1984.

Tyler DE: Protothecosis. In Greene CE, editor: Infectious diseases of the dog and cat, Philadelphia, 1990, WB Saunders, pp 742-748.

Sporotrichosis

Dunstan RW, Reimann KA, and Langham RF: Feline sporotrichosis, J Am Vet Med Assoc 189:880-883, 1986.

Dunstan RW and others: Feline sporotrichosis: a report of five cases with transmission to humans, J Am Acad Dermatol 15:37-45, 1986.

Foil CS: Cutaneous fungal diseases. In Nesbitt GH, editor: Dermatology: contemporary issues in small animal practice, New York, 1987, Churchill Livingstone, pp 141-144.

Lever WF and Schaumburg-Lever G: Histopathology of the skin, Philadelphia, 1990, JB Lippincott, pp 383-385.

Rosser EJ and Dunstan RW: Sporotrichosis. In Greene CE, editor: Infectious diseases of the dog and cat, Philadelphia, 1990, WB Saunders, 707-710.

Cutaneous pythiosis

Brown CC and others: Use of immunohistochemical methods for diagnosis of equine pythiosis, Am J Vet Res 49:1866-1868, 1988.

Campbell CK: Pythiosis, Equine Vet J 22:227-228, 1990.

English PB and Frost AJ: Phycomycosis in a dog, Aust Vet J 61:291-292, 1984.

Foil CS: Miscellaneous fungal infections. In Greene CE, editor: Infectious diseases of the dog and cat, Philadelphia, 1990, WB Saunders, pp 731-741.

Foil CS: Cutaneous fungal diseases. In Nesbitt GH, editor: Dermatology: contemporary issues in small animal practice, New York, 1987, Churchill Livingstone, pp 144-146.

Foil CS and others: A report of subcutaneous pythiosis in five dogs and a review of the etiologic agent *Pythium* sp., J Am Anim Hosp Assoc 20:959-966, 1984.

Lever WF and Schaumburg-Lever G: Histopathology of the skin, Philadelphia, 1990, JB Lippincott, pp 371-372.

Miller RI and Campbell RSF: The comparative pathology of equine cutaneous phycomycosis, Vet Pathol 21:325-332, 1984.

Troy GC: Canine phycomycosis: a review of twenty-four cases, Calif Vet March/April:12-17, 1985.

Cutaneous leishmaniasis

Bourdeau P: Elements pratiques du diagnostic de la leishmaniose canine, Le Point Veterinaire 15:43-50, 1983.

Groulade P and others: Special leishmaniose, Pratique Medicale et Chirurgicale de l'Animal de Compagnie: 5(suppl):5-156, 1988.

Permez C and others: Canine American cutaneous leishmaniasis: a clinical and immunological study in dogs naturally infected with *Leishmania braziliensis* in an endemic area in Rio de Janeiro, Brazil, Am J Trop Med Hyg 38:52-58, 1988.

Schawalder P: Leishmaniose bei Hund und Katze, Kleintier Praxis 22:237-246, 1977.

Slappendel RJ: Canine leishmaniasis: a review based on 95 cases in the Netherlands, Vet Quarter 10:1-16, 1988.

Slappendel RJ and Greene CE: Leishmaniasis. In Greene CE, editor: Infectious diseases of the dog and cat, Philadelphia, 1990, WB Saunders, pp 769-777.

CHAPTER 12

Noninfectious nodular and diffuse granulomatous and pyogranulomatous diseases of the dermis

Nodular and diffuse granulomatous and pyogranulomatous diseases of the dermis are characterized by multifocal nodular inflammation that tends toward confluence or a diffuse pattern. Granulomatous inflammation is composed principally of macrophages, with or without giant cells, that are often but not exclusively organized as discrete granulomas. Pyogranulomatous inflammation has a more prominent component of neutrophils; pyogranulomas are formed by central accumulations of neutrophils that are surrounded by macrophages. A third category, typified by cutaneous histiocytosis, is characterized by diffuse infiltrations of histiocytes in sheet-like or tumor-like configurations. Morphologic overlap of these three types of inflammatory patterns is often encountered within the individual diseases described in this chapter.

Diseases included in this chapter are not the result of infectious agents but occur because of foreign body penetration, metabolic aberrations, or idiopathic factors. Differentiation from infectious processes of similar appearance may be required through the use of special stains.

FOREIGN BODY REACTIONS (Synonym: foreign body granuloma)
Clinical features (Figures 12-1 and 12-2)

Foreign body reactions are seen commonly in dogs but uncommonly in cats, which is probably due to the propensity of cats to meticulously groom the haircoat. Lesions are associated with penetration by a variety of foreign matter, usually plant in origin. Types of penetrating foreign material include grass awns, cactus spines, porcupine quills, and fiberglass fibers. The foxtail, *Hordeum jubatum,* is the most common foreign body seen in North America. Other barbed awns from the genuses *Hordeum, Stipa,* and *Setaria* are distributed worldwide.

Distinctive sharp anterior florets on the awn penetrate the skin or body orifice after being retained in the haircoat of the animal. Barbs on the awn prevent retrograde migration, and anterograde motion is encouraged by muscular movement. Secondary bacterial infection is common; actinomycosis and nocardiosis may be induced as the direct result of foreign body penetration.

Erythema and mild exudation are the initial clinical signs at the time of penetration

190

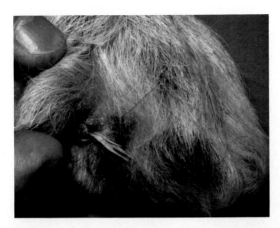

FIGURE 12-1. Interdigital foreign body reaction in a dog caused by grass awns. A firm nodule in the dorsal interdigital web has fistulated, and another grass awn has begun penetration.

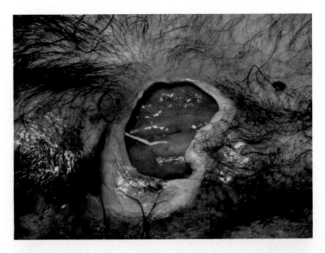

FIGURE 12-2. Severe foreign body reaction caused by a grass awn on the prepuce of a dog. The lesion has fistulated, discharging the grass awn and associated necrotic debris.

by the foreign body. As the foreign body migrates inward, firm nodules or abscesses form, fistulate, and drain seropurulent or serosanguineous exudate. Nonbarbed foreign bodies and some grass awns are shed by this process. Nodular areas of scar tissue may surround the fistulas as the lesions progress. The dorsal interdigital webs are the most common sites for lesions caused by grass awns, although penetration can occur at any site, including the oral cavity. Multiple lesions are common. Lesions associated with other foreign bodies do not exhibit site predilections. Deep pyoderma aggravates the process, which is due in part to follicular rupture with release of keratin and hair. Hair and keratin also may be carried into deep tissue by the inciting puncture.

Young dogs of hunting and working breeds are at greater risk, since exposure is more likely in these breeds. Sex predilections have not been noted.

Clinical differential diagnoses should include deep bacterial folliculitis and furunculosis without foreign bodies (particularly interdigital pyoderma), mycotic infection, ruptured follicular cysts, or neoplasms. Deep pyoderma without associated foreign body penetration is usually more disseminated in distribution. Fistulous tracts associated with grass awns commonly are deeper (as determined by probing) than cavitating or necrotizing lesions caused by deep pyoderma or ruptured follicular cysts that fistulate. Clinical or histologic identification of foreign material is required for a definitive diagnosis.

Biopsy site selection

Solitary lesions should be removed in their entirety if surgically feasible. If multiple lesions are present,

representative specimens should be taken from multiple sites. Ideally, both closed and open lesions should be sampled. Deep wedge resection is recommended, since the foreign body may be located beneath the dermis.

Histopathology (Figures 12-3 and 12-4)

The epidermis is often severely acanthotic and exudative. Ulceration may be present.

The dermis, panniculus, and occasionally the underlying skeletal muscle are diffusely and severely inflamed and often fibrotic. Large central or multicentric foci of frank suppuration or pyogranulomatous inflammation, sometimes including eosinophils, are observed. Necrosis may be severe and can be accompanied by cavitation caused by loss of devitalized tissue. At the periphery of the lesion there are mixed mononuclear cells that usually include prominent plasma cells. Granulation tissue proliferation and mature areas of fibrosis often subtend and surround the inflammatory core or cores. Fistula formation is frequent and is characterized by linear or curvilinear spaces, lined with neutrophils and surrounded by fibrosis. Fibrosis may predominate in chronic lesions. Foreign material, usually of plant origin, occasionally may be found within fistulas or neutrophilic foci, but its presence is not required to suggest the diagnosis, since the pattern of inflammation is quite characteristic. Plant foreign bodies usually appear in tissue sections as polygonal or linear structures that have very pale eosinophilic or amphophilic staining properties. The plant fragment may contain yellow or brown pigment. The plant cell walls have a honeycomb-like configuration when

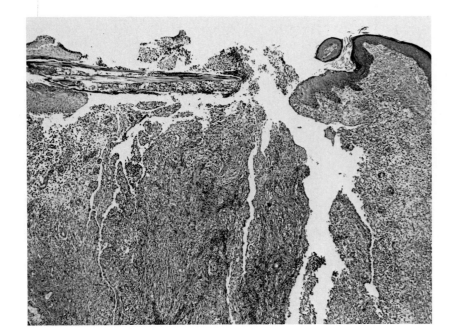

FIGURE 12-3. Foreign body reaction in a dog. Note the cutaneous fistula with a fragment of plant spicule in the surface opening. (×35.)

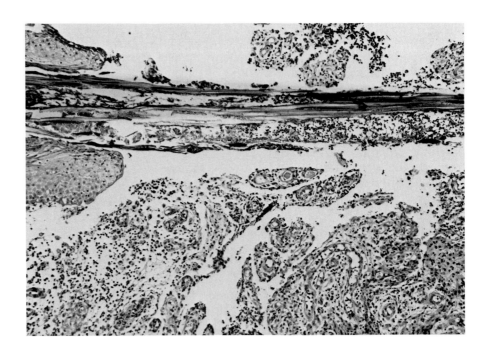

FIGURE 12-4. Higher magnification of the foreign body reaction in Figure 12-3. Neutrophils surround the spicule. Subjacent inflamed granulation tissue proliferates in opening of fistula. (×90.)

viewed in cross section, and the cells have little internal structure. Colonies of bacteria are often present within the plant cells. Free hair and keratin may be present and may aggravate the inflammatory process.

Differential diagnoses include penetrating wounds without foreign body retention, deep bacterial folliculitis and furunculosis with ruptured hair follicles, or ruptured follicular cysts. Puncture wounds without penetration of foreign material may produce a similar lesion, particularly if bacteria or follicular tissue is introduced. Ruptured furuncles or follicular cysts may lead to a similar but more shallow pattern of inflammation, since keratin and hair essentially act as endogenous foreign bodies when released from hair follicles.

CUTANEOUS XANTHOMA
Clinical features (Figure 12-5)

Cutaneous xanthomas are benign, typically multifocal, granulomatous lesions containing lipoprotein-derived deposits. Xanthomas are rare in the cat and very rare in the dog. Usually, formation of xanthomas reflects abnormal plasma concentrations of cholesterol or triglycerides, termed *dyslipoproteinemia*. Dyslipoproteinemias may occur either in conjunction with heritable defects in lipid metabolism or secondary to diseases such as diabetes mellitus. Xanthomas in cats as a result of hereditary hyperchylomicronemia have been reported by Jones (1983, 1986). Xanthomas also have been seen secondary to naturally occurring and megestrol acetate–induced diabetes mellitus in cats and secondary to diabetes mellitus in a dog. Reedy reported cutaneous xanthomas in one dog secondary to an experimental high-cholesterol diet. Multiple cutaneous xanthomas in adult Siamese cats without hypercholesterolemia, evidence of lipemic serum, or diabetes mellitus were reported by Fawcett, and recently two additional cases have been observed.* Solitary, idiopathic, nodular xanthomas without concomitant dyslipoproteinemia also have been observed rarely in the dog and cat. These solitary xanthomas may actually represent benign histiocytic or fibrohistiocytic proliferations that have a xanthomatous component of unknown derivation (see benign fibrous histiocytoma, Chapter 28).

Multiple pale yellow-to-white plaques, nodules, or papules with erythematous borders develop in the dermis and may extend to the subjacent subcutaneous tissue. Larger masses may ulcerate and discharge inspissated, amorphous, necrotic material. Skin lesions in the dog reported by Chastain were seen on the face, ears, and ventrum. In the cat, lesions have been noted on the face, legs, and trunk; over bony prominences; and in the footpads. Cutaneous xanthomas are asymptomatic. Xanthomas seen in conjunction with inherited hyperchylomicronemia may exhibit peripheral neuropathy believed to be due to nerve compression from lipid deposits.

Breed, age, or sex predilections have not been established. Clinically, xanthomas must be differentiated from infectious and noninfectious granulomas and pyogranulomas, as well as neoplasms. Histopathology is required to differentiate these diseases. A chemical screening panel should be performed to evaluate for diabetes mellitus, hypercholesterolemia, or elevated plasma triglycerides.

---

* Case material and laboratory data from Carr SH: Clearwater, Florida, 1990.

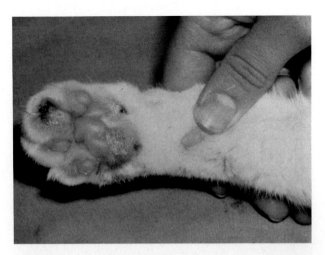

FIGURE 12-5. Cutaneous xanthoma on the footpads of a cat following long-term therapy with megestrol acetate. *(From Kwochka KW and Short BG: Cutaneous xanthomatosis and diabetes mellitus following long-term therapy with megestrol acetate in a cat, Comp Cont Ed 6:185-192, 1984. Reprinted with permission.)*

Biopsy site selection

Punch or wedge biopsy specimens should be taken from plaques or nodules prior to ulceration, since secondary inflammation or necrosis may impede evaluation. If possible, footpad lesions should be avoided because healing may be prolonged if the underlying reason for dyslipoproteinemia is not medically manageable.

Histopathology (Figures 12-6 through 12-8)

The epidermis may be moderately acanthotic. In the typical xanthoma resulting from hyperlipoproteinemia, the dermis is diffusely filled with large macrophages containing abundant, foamy cytoplasm. Giant cells are observed. There are often small lakes of extracellular, amorphous, and pale-staining material, and there are usually acicular cholesterol clefts. Oil-red-O staining of frozen tissue reveals lipid within macrophages and giant cells and in extracellular lakes. Neutrophils are interspersed in small numbers; a few lymphocytes may be observed.

In xanthomas of Siamese cats without evidence of hyperlipoproteinemia, numerous large, foamy macrophages are intermingled with lymphoid nodules and prominent accumulations of eosinophils. Giant cells may be massive; up to 10 nuclei may be present. Extracellular lakes and acicular deposits are observed.

Solitary idiopathic nodular xanthomas are more circumscribed histopathologically, have a relative absence of free lipid in tissue, and have a higher propor-

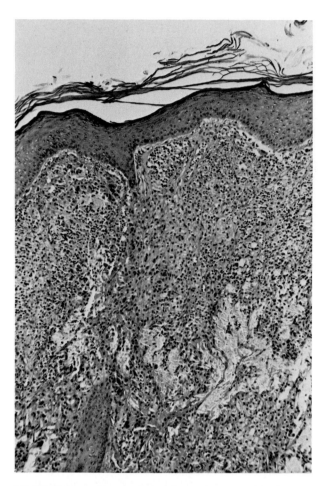

FIGURE 12-6. Cutaneous xanthoma in a cat with diabetes mellitus. Diffuse pyogranulomatous inflammation is interspersed with large, pale, acellular lakes of lipid. (×90.)

tion of nonfoamy histiocytes than do typical cutaneous xanthomas. These lesions may be histopathologic variants of benign fibrous histiocytoma (see Chapter 28).

The principal differential diagnosis in the cat is cutaneous infection of opportunistic fungi or feline leprosy, both of which may have diffuse infiltrations of pale or foamy macrophages. Demonstration of organisms will allow differentiation. In addition, preauricular xanthogranuloma, a form of sterile granuloma and pyogranuloma syndrome in cats, may have similar foamy macrophages. Most cutaneous xanthomas have extracellular deposits of lipid or cholesterol clefts, whereas sterile (nonmetabolic) and infectious granulomas that contain foamy macrophages do not.

STERILE GRANULOMA AND PYOGRANULOMA SYNDROME

(Synonym: idiopathic periadnexal multinodular granulomatous dermatitis)

Clinical features (Figures 12-9 and 12-10)

Sterile granuloma and pyogranuloma syndrome is a heterogeneous group of diseases united by similar histopathologic features. The syndrome is relatively common in dogs and rare in cats. The histiocytic nature of the inflammation, coupled with the often dramatic response to glucocorticoids, suggest the likelihood of an immune dysfunction, perhaps associated with persistent antigenic drive. As more clinical and histopathologic information is gained, subtypes may emerge that are based on the breed affected, distribution of lesions, response to therapy, and specific histopathologic or immunohistologic features.

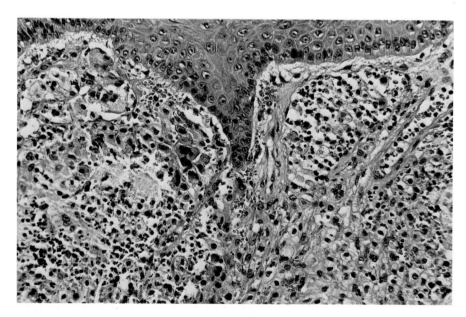

FIGURE 12-7. Higher magnification of the superficial dermis shown in Figure 12-6. Note the diffuse distribution of neutrophils, foamy macrophages and giant cells. (×220.)

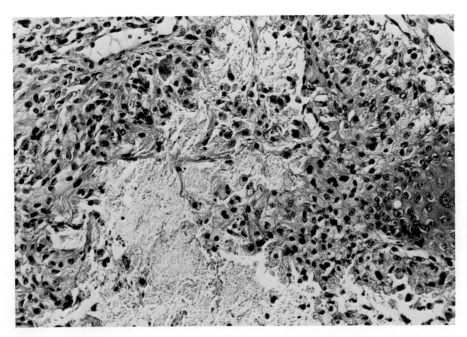

FIGURE 12-8. Cutaneous xanthoma in the same cat as in Figure 12-6. Note the pale lakes of extracellular lipid. (×220.)

The clinical appearance in dogs may vary with the breed affected. Lesions consist of multiple, firm, well demarcated, partially alopecic nodules (measuring 0.5 to 2 cm in diameter) or plaques that initially occur most commonly on the muzzle. Lesions may form on the pinnae, face, neck, trunk, and occasionally on the distal extremities. A single case reviewed by one author,* which was histopathologically very similar to cutaneous sarcoidosis (a noninfectious granulomatous

disease of humans), was described clinically as multifocal nodules on the face.* Sterile granuloma and pyogranuloma syndrome is asymptomatic. Lesions may regress spontaneously or they may wax and wane.

Several authors have reported canine syndromes with clinical and histopathologic features compatible with sterile granuloma and pyogranuloma syndrome. Dogs reported by Carpenter as having idiopathic peri-

* Case material from JO Noxon, Ames, Iowa, 1984.

* Thelma Lee Gross.

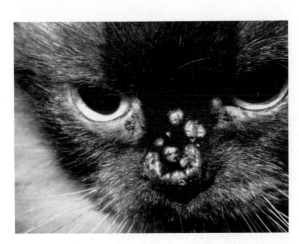

FIGURE 12-9. Sterile granuloma and pyogranuloma syndrome on the muzzle of a cat. Well-demarcated, coalescing, hairless nodules are present.

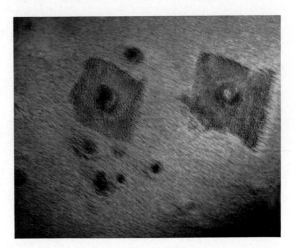

FIGURE 12-10. Sterile granuloma and pyogranuloma syndrome in a Great Dane. Multiple alopecic nodules are present on the lateral thorax. Several nodules have had surrounding hair clipped to enhance visibility.

adnexal multinodular granulomatous dermatitis exhibited similar clinical signs; however, nodules were described as haired. A subgroup of dogs with cutaneous histiocytosis, reported by Calderwood Mays, had lesions clinically and histopathologically similar to sterile granuloma and pyogranuloma syndrome.

Firm, well-demarcated to coalescing, hairless nodules (2 to 10 mm in diameter) have been observed in cats. Lesions are often restricted to the muzzle, but also may affect the footpads or surrounding skin. Scott (1990, 1991) has recently reported an apparently similar syndrome in cats, characterized by "multiple erythematous-to-violaceous papules, nodules, and plaques" confined to the head and pinnae.

A second localized feline syndrome identified by the authors and also recently reported by Scott (1990, 1991) features slightly orange, bilaterally symmetric plaques confined to the preauricular regions, which may be termed *preauricular xanthogranuloma*. The lesions bruise easily, and hemorrhage may be extensive.

Sterile granuloma and pyogranuloma syndrome may be seen more frequently in the Great Dane, Boxer, English Bulldog, Dachshund, and Golden Retriever but may affect any breed. Age or sex predilections have not been noted. Age, sex, or breed predilections have not been evident in the few feline cases seen.

Clinical differential diagnoses include other granulomatous and pyogranulomatous disorders caused by bacteria, fungi, or foreign bodies. Cutaneous xanthomas and neoplasms also must be considered.

Clinical similarities are shared with cutaneous histiocytosis; however, distinct granulomas or pyo-granulomas are not seen histopathologically in cutaneous histiocytosis. Vigorous efforts must be made to attempt to culture bacteria and fungi from aseptically obtained biopsy specimens, since some organisms may be difficult to identify histopathologically in granulomatous skin lesions. Additional proof of the diagnosis of sterile granulomatous or pyogranulomatous skin disease is obtained retrospectively if the syndrome responds to glucocorticoid therapy.

Biopsy site selection

Multiple biopsy specimens should be obtained from intact lesions. Specimens obtained utilizing sterile surgical technique should be submitted for aerobic, anaerobic, mycobacterial, and fungal culture.

Histopathology (Figures 12-11 through 12-13)

Common features of the sterile granuloma and pyogranuloma syndrome include a normal to moderately acanthotic epidermis with occasional ulceration and granulomatous or pyogranulomatous dermal to subcutaneous inflammation. Lesions may be discrete and nodular, but may progress to a diffuse pattern. Granulomas or pyogranulomas are devoid of foreign material or infectious agents that can be detected by currently utilized techniques.

The histopathologically variable diseases within this group are currently united principally by the common feature of "sterile" granulomatous or pyogranulomatous inflammation of the skin and subcutis. A few histopathologic types of sterile granuloma and pyogranuloma syndrome in the dog and cat are recognized

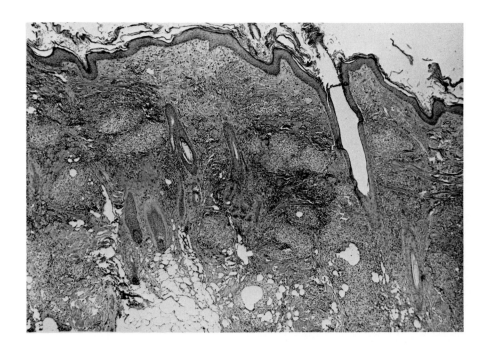

FIGURE 12-11. Sterile granuloma and pyogranuloma syndrome in a dog. Pale, discrete-to-confluent granulomas and pyogranulomas are disseminated throughout the dermis and panniculus. (×35.)

by the authors and others and include the pyogranulo-matous type, the periadnexal type, and the preauricular xanthogranuloma of cats. Cutaneous sarcoidosis-like disease is an additional rare subtype. Variation in the microscopic pattern may depend on the species and breed in which the disorder is expressed. Further clinical separation of this complex is required so that the pathologist may determine which morphologic variations may be used to obtain more specific histopathologic diagnoses.

The pyogranulomatous type is characterized by distinct pyogranuloma formation. Lesions are diffusely oriented in the dermis and panniculus. Pyogranulomas are discrete to confluent and contain central neutrophils and peripheral cuffs of macrophages. Lymphocytes and plasma cells are seen in small numbers.

The periadnexal type is characterized by prominent granulomatous inflammation around adnexal appendages; the superficial dermis is generally spared. Both Calderwood Mays and Carpenter reported that periadnexal accumulations of histiocytes, lymphocytes, and neutrophils coalesced to form more diffuse infiltrations in the later stages of the disease; thus separation of this subgroup from cutaneous histiocytosis may be artificial (see following discussion). Sausage-shaped configurations, as described by Muller, Kirk, and Scott (and observed by the authors most characteristically in Great Danes) may follow or track hair follicles.

Preauricular xanthogranuloma of cats is characterized by diffuse infiltrations of pale, slightly spindled-to-epithelioid, often foamy histiocytes, usually intermingled with prominent giant cells. Hemorrhage often is

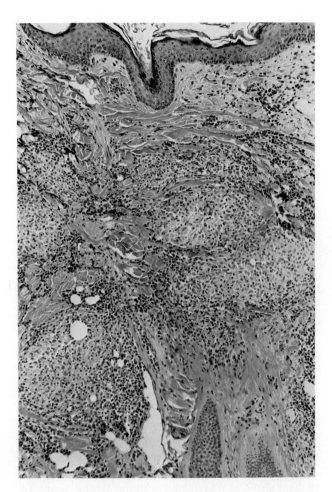

FIGURE 12-12. Higher magnification of granulomas shown in Figure 12-11. (×90.)

FIGURE 12-13. Feline preauricular xanthogranuloma. Large histiocytic cells and numerous giant cells diffusely fill the dermis. Note hemorrhage at the left. (×220.)

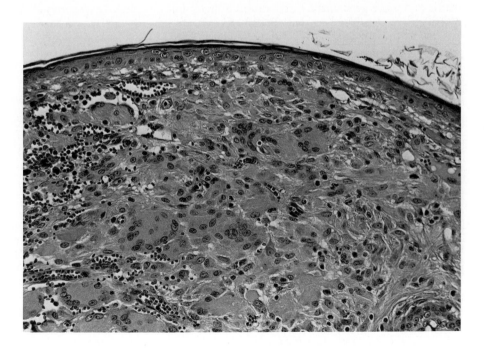

present multifocally throughout the lesion. A thin grenz zone (zone of uninvolved superficial dermis) may be seen. Superficial dermal fibrosis is present in chronic lesions, probably as a sequela to ulceration. Occasionally, macrophages may palisade around collagen fibers but collagen degeneration has not been observed. Patchy clusters of lymphocytes and plasma cells are present; neutrophils may be prominent if the overlying epidermis is ulcerated.

Sarcoidal granulomas, resembling the granulomas in human cutaneous sarcoidosis, are characterized by multifocal to confluent "naked tubercles" or granulomas comprising predominantly epithelioid macrophages. A few lymphocytes or neutrophils may be intermingled. Giant cells are rare.

Differential diagnoses vary with histopathologic type. The periadnexal type is distinctive, but milder cases may be confused with the nodular granulomatous form of sebaceous adenitis, as seen in Viszlas. Advanced lesions of this subgroup, which are characterized by more diffuse infiltration of the skin, resemble cutaneous histiocytosis; in fact, the separation of these two syndromes may be artificial. The pyogranulomatous subtype may be similar to infectious diseases such as opportunistic myobacterial infection or fungal infections; culture and special staining allow differentiation. The xanthogranulomatous form, best typified by the preauricular lesions in cats, may closely mimic cutaneous xanthomas (see above) or feline leprosy. Xanthomas generally have extracellular accumulations of pale lipid within the dermis; feline leprosy is characterized by large numbers of acid-fast bacteria in tissue.

CUTANEOUS HISTIOCYTOSIS
Clinical features (Figures 12-14 through 12-16)

Cutaneous histiocytosis is a term used to group a number of uncommon to rare, benign proliferative disorders of dogs that are characterized by histiocytic inflammation. Clinical and histopathologic similarities are shared with sterile granuloma and pyogranuloma syndrome; however, the principal differentiating feature is that distinct granulomas or pyogranulomas are not seen histopathologically in cutaneous histiocytosis. Both syndromes may represent proliferative disorders of histiocytes as a result of immune dysfunction and persistent antigenic drive.

Clinical variability is marked. Multiple, haired or alopecic plaques or nodules develop in localized clusters or in a more generalized distribution. Solitary ini-

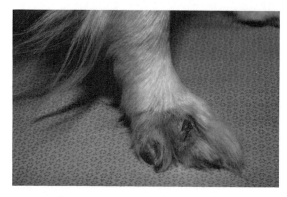

FIGURE 12-15. Cutaneous histiocytosis in a Shetland Sheep Dog. An alopecic nodule on the dorsal digit has ulcerated. *(Courtesy AC Mundell, Seattle, Washington; case material from the University of California, Davis).*

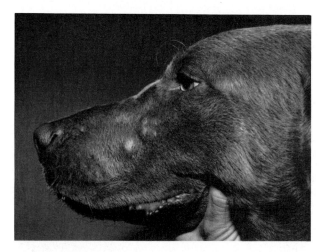

FIGURE 12-14. Cutaneous histiocytosis in a Chesapeake Bay Retriever. Multiple, partially alopecic nodules are present on the face. *(Courtesy AC Mundell, Seattle, Washington; case material from the University of California, Davis).*

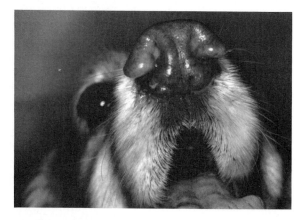

FIGURE 12-16. Cutaneous histiocytosis in a dog. Diffuse infiltration of the planum nasale has resulted in a "clown nose" appearance.

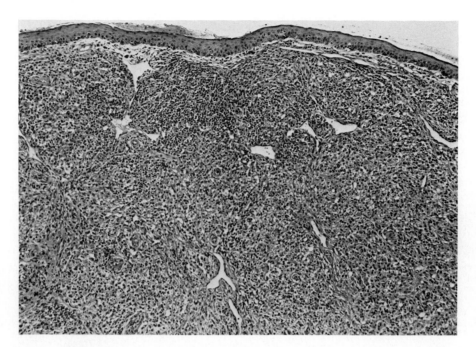

FIGURE 12-17. Cutaneous histiocytosis in a dog. Note the diffuse infiltration of the dermis. (×90.)

tial lesions or multiple, grouped nodules may resemble cutaneous histiocytomas. Rapidly growing, infiltrating nodules and plaques may clinically mimic malignant neoplasms. Larger nodules may umbilicate or ulcerate. Older lesions may regress spontaneously, even as new lesions are developing. Periods of total remission may be observed. Nasal mucosal involvement has been seen and is characterized by swollen mucosa of the nares, difficulty in breathing, and "bubble blowing." Several dogs seen by one author* have had visually striking lesions limited to a diffuse enlargement of the planum nasale, resulting in a "clown nose" appearance.

The Shetland Sheepdog and Collie may be at increased risk for cutaneous histiocytosis. However, the syndrome has been identified in a wide variety of purebred and mixed-breed dogs. Age or sex predilections have not been noted.

Clinical differential diagnoses should include neoplasms, particularly canine cutaneous histiocytomas and cutaneous lymphoma (including mycosis fungoides), as well as other granulomatous or pyogranulomatous dermatoses. Clinical overlap with sterile granuloma and pyogranuloma syndrome may be seen. Sterility of these lesions should be proven with culture if necessary. Empirical treatment with corticosteroids may be helpful diagnostically, since most neoplasms are poorly responsive, and cutaneous histiocytosis may respond readily.

* Peter J. Ihrke.

Biopsy site selection

Multiple biopsy specimens should be obtained from intact lesions. Specimens should be submitted for aerobic and anaerobic bacterial culture and fungal culture to rule out an infectious process.

Histopathology (Figures 12-17 through 12-19)

Cutaneous histiocytosis shares features in common with sterile pyogranuloma and granuloma syndrome, since both syndromes are sterile proliferations of histiocytes. These two entities may both represent different types of proliferative disorders that are triggered by unknown antigenic stimuli acting on the histiocytic and lymphocytic arms of the immune system.

In one less common form of cutaneous histiocytosis, multiple lesions that are virtually identical to solitary canine cutaneous histiocytoma are found (see Chapter 30). The overlying epidermis is ulcerated or acanthotic. Sheets of uniform histiocytes with oval granular nuclei and pale eosinophilic or amphophilic cytoplasm are accompanied by smaller numbers of mature lymphocytes, particularly at deep margins. The mitotic rate may be brisk (up to 3 mitotic figures per 40 × field).

Cutaneous histiocytosis is more often characterized by a heterogeneous mixture of histiocytes, lymphocytes, and neutrophils. Large epithelioid or vacuolated (xanthomatous) histiocytes are organized in sheets and obscure the normal dermal architecture and adnexa. Infiltrates may extend into the underlying panniculus.

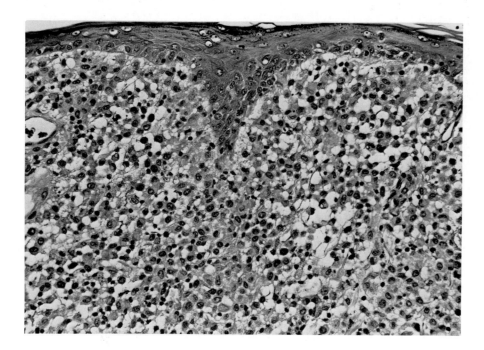

FIGURE 12-18. Cutaneous histiocytosis in a dog. Note the diffuse infiltration of large histiocytic cells. (×220.)

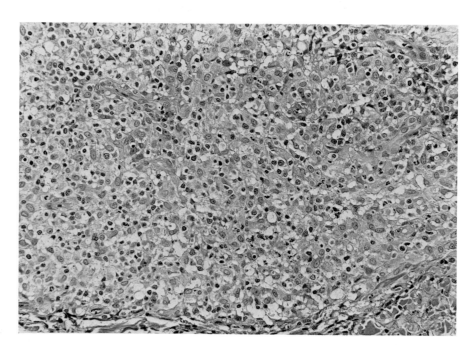

FIGURE 12-19. Cutaneous histiocytosis in a dog. Large, pale histiocytic cells are intermingled with fewer lymphocytes and neutrophils. (×220.)

Mitotic figures vary from few to many. Lymphocytes and neutrophils are intermingled in varying numbers in all cases and may be prominent. Discrete granulomas or pyogranulomas are not present.

Recently, histopathologic documentation of nasal involvement was made by one author* in two dogs with cutaneous histiocytosis (both dogs were clinically

"bubble blowers").* Infiltrations of histiocytes, lymphocytes, and neutrophils—as seen in the skin—were present in the distal squamous mucosa of the nasal cavity and resulted in occlusion of the nares.

The principal differential diagnosis for the histiocytoma-like form of cutaneous histiocytosis is malignant lymphoma. Some cases have required the

---

* Thelma Lee Gross.

* Case material from one dog from Stallings B: Hemet, California, 1990.

use of T-cell and histiocytic markers for differentiation.* Cutaneous lymphoma tends to involve the panniculus more heavily ("bottom-heavy" infiltrate). The heterogeneous form of cutaneous histiocytosis is distinctive, but in some cases may be confused with fungal infection. Special staining and culture allow differentiation. Additionally, this form of cutaneous histiocytosis resembles late-stage lesions of the periadnexal form of sterile pyogranuloma and granuloma syndrome, and separation of these two entities may be artificial.

SYSTEMIC HISTIOCYTOSIS OF THE BERNESE MOUNTAIN DOG
Clinical features (Figures 12-20 and 12-21)

Systemic histiocytosis is a rare familial histiocytic proliferative disorder seen in Bernese Mountain Dogs. The cause of the syndrome is unknown. Systemic histiocytosis involves cells of monocyte-macrophage lineage and shares clinical and histopathologic features with the histiocytosis X complex in humans. X-linked recessive inheritance is unlikely even though the syndrome is seen predominantly in males, since transmission via paternal lines has been noted. An autosomal recessive mode of inheritance has been postulated by Moore (1984). The syndrome exhibits a marked predilection for the skin and lymph nodes but widespread visceral involvement also is seen. A second histiocytic proliferative disorder, termed *malignant histiocytosis,* also reported by Moore (1986), occurred in the same family line as the dogs seen with systemic histiocytosis. Malignant histiocystosis is predominantly a visceral disease, although multiple subcutaneous masses have been seen.

Multiple, erythematous papules, plaques, and nodules develop over large areas of the body. Most nodules are dermal, but extension into the subcutis may be noted. Hair is lost progressively from enlarging lesions and the normal surface topography is ablated. Larger lesions erode and ulcerate. Mottled hyperpigmentation is seen with chronicity. Older ulcerated lesions may develop characteristic peripheral thickening, creating a crateriform appearance. The lesions are seen most commonly and with greatest density on the muzzle, planum nasale, eyelids, and scrotum. Conjunctival lesions may be present. Regional or generalized lymphadenopathy is noted.

The clinical course of systemic histiocytosis is variable. Some cases are characterized by periods of exacerbation and partial remission. Other cases proceed

* Courtesy Moore PF: Department of Pathology, University of California, Davis.

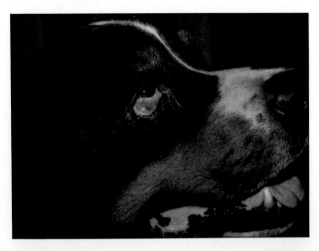

FIGURE 12-20. Systemic histiocytosis of the Bernese Mountain Dog. Multiple dermal nodules are present on the muzzle and in the conjunctiva.

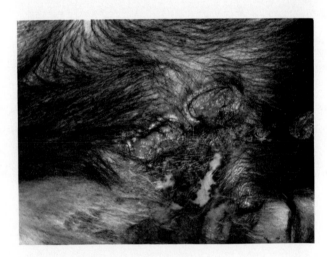

FIGURE 12-21. Systemic histiocytosis of the Bernese Mountain Dog. Chronic ulcers on the ventral abdomen have characteristic peripheral thickening, creating a crateriform appearance.

rapidly and aggressively without remissions. Most dogs with this syndrome eventually are euthanized. Necropsy shows widespread histiocytic infiltration affecting the skin, lymph nodes, lung, liver, bone marrow, spleen, kidneys, testes, and orbital soft tissue.

This characteristic form of systemic histiocytosis has been seen in the Bernese Mountain Dog only. Adult males less than 8 years of age are affected most frequently.

Systemic histiocytosis of the Bernese Mountain Dog must be differentiated clinically from aggressive cutaneous neoplasms, such as malignant lymphoma, and from other histiocytic proliferative diseases, such as

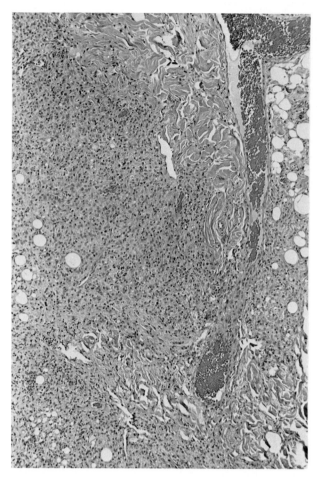

FIGURE 12-22. Systemic histiocytosis of the Bernese Mountain Dog. Diffuse infiltration of pale histiocytes is present in the deep dermis. (×95.)

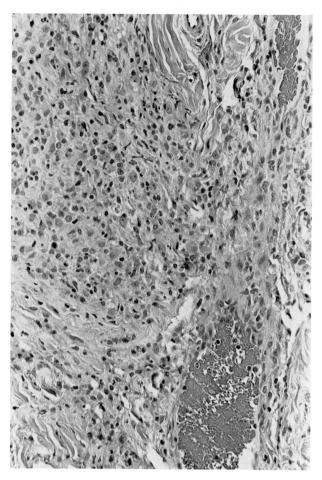

FIGURE 12-23. Higher magnification of the dermis in Figure 12-22. Large, pale histiocytes are accompanied by fewer lymphocytes and occasional neutrophils. (×220.)

cutaneous histiocytosis. Breed is a key feature in differentiation. Histopathology is required to differentiate this syndrome from cutaneous neoplasia.

Biopsy site selection

Multiple biopsy specimens should be taken from well-developed lesions. Lesions of the eyelid should be avoided unless other sites are not available because healing may be prolonged in this location.

Histopathology (Figures 12-22 and 12-23)

The epidermis is normal to acanthotic. The deep dermis and panniculus have multinodular to diffuse accumulations of large histiocytic cells. The infiltrates were reported by Moore to be more severe and diffuse in scrotal and nasal lesions. Histiocytes are intermingled with smaller numbers of neutrophils, lymphocytes, and occasional plasma cells or eosinophils. Giant

cells are rare. Mild invasion of arrector pili muscles is present. Adnexal appendages and adipose tissue of the panniculus are compressed. The infiltrate may extend mildly between collagen fibers or around vessels of the middle and superficial dermis, but often completely spares these areas. In the cases described by Moore, histiocytic cells infiltrated blood vessel walls, resulting in some thrombosis and ischemic necrosis; fibrosis characterized chronic lesions.

Differential diagnoses principally include cutaneous histiocytosis and advanced lesions of periadnexal sterile granuloma and pyogranuloma syndrome. In contrast to these other sterile histiocytic disorders, the infiltrates of systemic histiocytosis are more abundant in the deep dermis and panniculus, creating a "bottom-heavy" silhouette. Vascular infiltration has not been observed in cutaneous histiocytosis or the sterile granuloma and pyogranuloma syndrome.

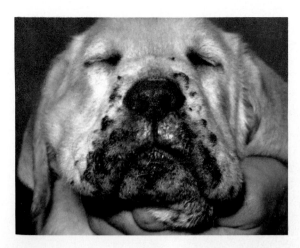

FIGURE 12-24. Juvenile sterile granulomatous dermatitis and lymphadenitis in a Labrador Retriever. Pustules and nodules accompanied by edema and crusting have developed rapidly on the muzzle in a partially bilaterally symmetric pattern.

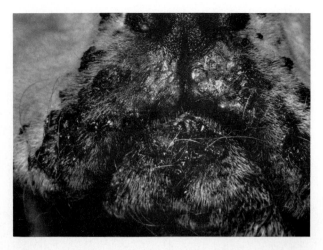

FIGURE 12-25. Closer view of dog in Figure 12-24. Perioral fistulas are draining copious purulent material.

JUVENILE STERILE GRANULOMATOUS DERMATITIS AND LYMPHADENITIS (Synonyms: juvenile cellulitis, juvenile pyoderma, puppy strangles, "big head")

Clinical features (Figures 12-24 and 12-25)

Juvenile sterile granulomatous dermatitis and lymphadenitis is an uncommon canine skin disease of unknown etiology, characterized by severe granulomatous dermatitis and lymphadenitis. Bacterial involvement, when present, is secondary. Suppression of in vitro lymphocyte blastogenesis secondary to a serum factor has been documented by Scott* and one author.† The dramatic response to immunosuppressive dosages of glucocorticoids indicates the likelihood of an underlying immune dysfunction. Heritability is supported by an increased occurrence in certain breeds and a genetic study of an affected family of Dachshunds by Prieur.

Mandibular lymphadenopathy often is the initial presenting clinical sign of juvenile sterile granulomatous dermatitis and lymphadenitis. Pustules and nodules develop rapidly, accompanied by edema and crusting. Lesions may fistulate and drain copious purulent material. Epidermal fragility may be marked. Cicatricial alopecia is a sequela in severe cases. The muzzle, periorbital region of the face, and ears are affected most commonly. A concomitant, highly purulent, otitis ex-

* Scott DW: Personal communication, 1982.
† Peter J. Ihrke.

terna is seen frequently. Occasionally, the prepuce and perianal area may be affected. White (1989) reported fever, anorexia, and joint pain as less consistent findings, and sterile suppurative arthritis was found. Lethargy and general malaise are common.

Breed predilections may exist for Golden Retrievers, Dachshunds, yellow Labrador Retrievers, and Lhasa Apsos. However, juvenile sterile granulomatous dermatitis also has been seen in Brittanys, English Pointers, Chesapeake Bay Retrievers, Weimaraners, Miniature Poodles, Rottweilers, and mixed-breed dogs. Juvenile sterile granulomatous dermatitis usually is seen in dogs older than 3 weeks but less than 4 months of age. Single or multiple puppies in a litter may be affected. On rare occasion, a clinically and histopathologically identical disease has been seen in adult dogs. Sex predilection has not been noted.

Juvenile sterile granulomatous dermatitis must be differentiated from fulminating generalized demodicosis, severe pyoderma secondary to immunodeficiency, drug eruption, and facial angioedema. Multiple skin scrapings should be obtained to rule out demodicosis, as should smears from intact pustules to rule out primary bacterial infection. Histopathology of early lesions is necessary for definitive diagnosis.

Biopsy site selection

Multiple punch biopsy specimens (4 or 6 mm in diameter) should be taken from early, nontraumatized intact pustules or nodules. Wedge biopsy technique or 8-mm biopsy punches are not recommended, since the devitalized tissue is quite friable, and sutures may not maintain tissue integrity if defects larger than 6 mm in diameter are created.

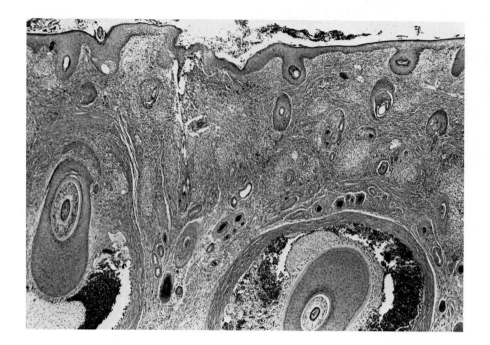

FIGURE 12-26. Juvenile sterile
granulomatous dermatitis and
lymphadenitis revealing diffuse
pale-staining granulomas and
pyogranulomas in the periadnexal dermis of the muzzle.
(×35.)

Histopathology (Figures 12-26 through 12-28)

The epidermis may be normal, acanthotic, or ulcerated in severe lesions. Superficial exudation may be severe.

The dermis is characterized by multiple discrete or confluent granulomas and pyogranulomas, comprised of nodular clusters of large epithelioid macrophages with variably-sized cores of neutrophils. Pyogranulomas are oriented around follicles and do not invade follicular walls but often obliterate sebaceous glands and sweat glands. Pyogranulomas may extend to the panniculus. In severe lesions, inflammation is predominantly suppurative, and large lakes of neutrophils may be present in the superficial dermis, in and around ruptured follicles, and in the subjacent panniculus. It is not known whether these lesions represent secondary bacterial abscesses or simply reflect the inflammatory spectrum of this disease.

Differential diagnoses include other infectious and noninfectious granulomatous and pyogranulomatous diseases, including granulomatous periadnexitis caused by demodicosis, the pyogranulomatous type of sterile granuloma and pyogranuloma syndrome, and sterile nodular panniculitis. Demodicosis occasionally may present with a similar histopathologic appearance, but fragments of mites at the centers of granulomas allows separation of these entities, and demodectic granulomas are generally less severe and do not extend to the panniculus. Discrete perifollicular and subcutaneous pyogranulomas without evidence of foreign material or infectious agents are suggestive of juvenile sterile granulomatous dermatitis and lymphadenitis, particularly in puppies. Without knowledge of the age affected, differ-

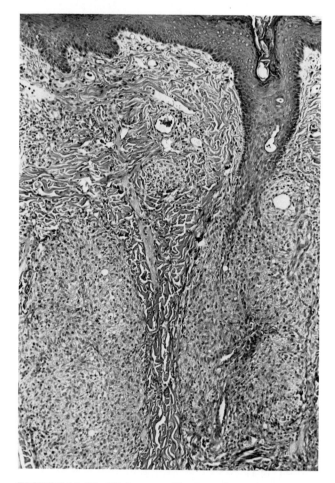

FIGURE 12-27. Higher magnification of granulomatous inflammation in juvenile sterile granulomatous dermatitis and lymphadenitis. A large granuloma surrounds the deep aspect of a follicle at the right. (×90.)

FIGURE 12-28. Juvenile sterile granulomatous dermatitis and lymphadenitis, demonstrating involvement of the panniculus. Inflammation is diffuse and contains a prominent component of neutrophils. ($\times$90.)

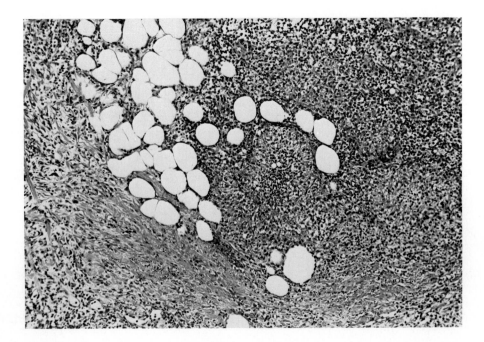

entiation from the pyogranulomatous subtype of sterile pyogranuloma and pyogranuloma syndrome may be impossible. The subcutaneous pyogranulomas of juvenile sterile granulomatous dermatitis closely resemble those of sterile nodular panniculitis; it is of interest to note that the Dachshund is at increased risk for both diseases.

SUGGESTED READINGS

Foreign body reactions

Brennan KE and Ihrke PJ: Grass awn migration in dogs and cats: a retrospective study of 182 cases, J Am Vet Med Assoc 182:1201-1204, 1983.

Fadok VA: Granulomatous dermatitis in dogs and cats, Semin Vet Med Surg 2:186-194, 1987.

Greene RT, Harling DE, and Dillman RC: Fiberglass-induced pyogranulomatous stomatitis in a dog, J Am Anim Hosp Assoc 23:401-404, 1987.

Lever WF and Schaumburg-Lever G: Histopathology of the skin, Philadelphia, 1990, JB Lippincott, pp 243-248.

Cutaneous xanthoma

Brewer HB and Fredrickson DS: Dyslipoproteinemias and xanthomatoses. In Fitzpatrick TB, Eisen AZ, Wolff K, and others, editors: Dermatology in general medicine, New York, 1987, McGraw-Hill, pp 1722-1738.

Chastain CB and Graham CL: Xanthomatosis secondary to diabetes mellitus in a dog, J Am Vet Med Assoc 172:1209-1211, 1978.

Fawcett JF, Demaray SY, and Altman N: Multiple xanthomatosis in a cat, Feline Pract 5:31-33, 1977.

Jones BR and others: Inherited hyperchylomicronemia in the cat, Feline Pract 16:7-12, 1986.

Jones BR and others: Cutaneous xanthomata associated with diabetes mellitus in a cat, J Small Anim Pract 26:33-41, 1985.

Jones BR and others: Occurrence of idiopathic, familial hyperchylomicronaemia in a cat, Vet Rec 112:543-547, 1983.

Kwochka KW and Short BG: Cutaneous xanthomatosis and diabetes mellitus following long-term therapy with megestrol acetate in a cat, Comp Cont Ed 6:185-192, 1984.

Reedy LM: Xanthomatosis in a dog on a high cholesterol diet, Proceedings of the American Academy of Veterinary Dermatology/American College of Veterinary Dermatology, New Orleans 2:7, 1986.

Rhodes KH, Baer K, and Everds N: Cutaneous xanthomatosis associated with persistent hyperlipidemia in a cat, Proceedings of the American Academy of Veterinary Dermatology/American College of Veterinary Dermatology, San Francisco 6:16-17, 1990.

Sterile granuloma and pyogranuloma syndrome

Carpenter JL and others: Idiopathic periadnexal multinodular granulomatous dermatitis in dogs, Vet Pathol 24:5-10, 1987.

Conroy JD: An overview of immune-mediated mucocutaneous diseases in the dog and cat, Am J Dermatopathol 5:595-599, 1983.

Fadok V: Granulomatous dermatitis in dogs and cats, Semin Vet Med Surg 2(3):186-194, 1987.

Muller GH, Kirk RW, and Scott DW: Small animal dermatology, ed 4, Philadelphia, 1989, WB Saunders, pp 552-555.

Panich R: Canine cutaneous sterile pyogranuloma/granuloma syndrome: a retrospective analysis of 29 cases (1976-1988), Proceedings of the American Academy of Veterinary Dermatology/American College of Veterinary Dermatology, San Francisco 6:33, 1990.

Scott DW: Idiopathic sterile granulomatous and pyogranulomatous dermatitis in cats, Proceedings of the American Academy of Veterinary Dermatology/American College of Veterinary Dermatology, San Francisco 6:59, 1990.

Scott DW, Buerger RG, and Miller WH: Idiopathic sterile granulomatous and pyogranulomatous dermatitis in cats, Vet Dermatol 1:129-137, 1991.

Cutaneous histiocytosis

Calderwood Mays MB and Bergeron JA: Cutaneous histiocytosis in dogs, J Am Vet Med Assoc 188:377-381, 1986.

Fadok V: Granulomatous dermatitis in dogs and cats, Semin Vet Med Surg 2(3):186-194, 1987.

Muller GH, Kirk RW, and Scott DW: Small animal dermatology, ed 4, Philadelphia, 1989, WB Saunders, pp 552-555.

Systemic histiocytosis of the Bernese Mountain Dog

Moore PF: Systemic histiocytosis of Bernese Mountain Dogs, Vet Pathol 21:554-563, 1984.

Moore PF and Rosin A: Malignant histiocytosis of Bernese Mountain Dogs, Vet Pathol 23:1-10, 1986.

Muller GH, Kirk RW, and Scott DW: Small animal dermatology, ed 4, Philadelphia, 1989, WB Saunders, pp 907-911.

Juvenile sterile granulomatous dermatitis and lymphadenitis

Carlotti D, Fourrier P, and Magnol J-P: Les pseudopyodermites, Pratique Medicale et Chirurgicale de l'Animal de Compagnie 23:499-503, 1988.

Prieur DJ and Hargis AM: A severe form of juvenile pyoderma with an inherited component, Fed Proc Am Soc Exp Biol 41:696, 1982.

Reimann KA and others: Clinicopathologic characterization of canine juvenile cellulitis, Vet Pathol 26:499-504, 1989.

White SD and Ihrke PJ: Pyoderma. In Nesbitt GH, editor: Dermatology: contemporary issues in small animal practice, New York, 1987, Churchill Livingstone, pp 112-113.

White SD and others: Juvenile cellulitis in dogs: 15 cases (1979-1988), J Am Vet Med Assoc 195:1609-1611, 1989.

Nodular and diffuse diseases of the dermis with prominent eosinophils or plasma cells

This group of diseases is characterized by prominent eosinophils (or plasma cells in plasma cell pododermatitis) within a diffuse dermal infiltrate. This type of inflammation tends to obscure the normal dermal architecture and may compress or replace adnexal appendages. Collagen degeneration may accompany eosinophilic inflammation. These diseases are suspected of having an allergic basis in many cases; however, eosinophilic granuloma is believed to be the result of eosinophil dysfunction, which may have a hereditary cause.

ARTHROPOD-BITE GRANULOMA (Synonym: insect-bite granuloma)
Clinical features (Figure 13-1)

Arthropod-bite granuloma occurs in the dog and cat as a sequela to the bite or sting of various arthropods. Ticks are the most commonly documented cause; this may be the result of the propensity of the tick to remain attached to the host after the initial insult, thus aiding in discovery by the owner. Arthropod-bite granuloma rarely is reported. Because of the difficulty in establishing cause and effect, the true frequency is unknown. Types III and IV hypersensitivity are the proposed causes of similar lesions in humans. Other aggressively biting and stinging arthropods may produce similar lesions. Focal eosinophilic granuloma of dogs may be a manifestation of arthropod bites in some cases and is discussed separately in the section on canine eosinophilic granuloma.

Focal erythema and swelling are the initial clinical signs of arthropod bites. These may be the sole clinical signs in many cases. Lesions vary from 5 to 20 mm in diameter and usually are circular. A firm nodule, the clinically typical arthropod-bite "granuloma," may form as a chronic sequela to often surprisingly minimal acute lesions. Alternatively, the acute erythematous lesions may worsen rapidly, leading to necrosis with ulceration, alopecia, and crusting. Scarring with striae, permanent alopecia, and hyperpigmentation may efface the normal surface architecture of the affected cutaneous site. Affected areas usually are pruritic or painful. Site predilections follow the biting habits of the various arthropods. Tick-bite hypersensitivity is seen most frequently on the muzzle, periorbital region, ears, and interdigital webs. Breed, age, or sex predilections have not been noted.

Clinical differential diagnoses for early arthropod-bite reactions (swelling and erythema) are legion but should include drug eruption, kerion, and trauma. The

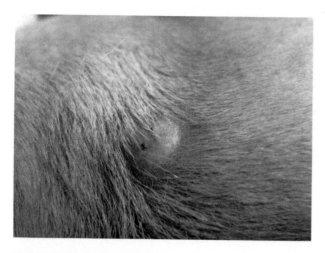

FIGURE 13-1. Chronic arthropod-bite granuloma caused by a tick. The well-demarcated nodule has a central punctate ulcer.

late-stage, or true arthropod-bite granuloma, must be differentiated from foreign body reactions, other granulomas, and neoplasms. A clinical history and histopathology may be required for differentiation.

Biopsy site selection

If multiple lesions are present, punch or wedge specimens should be taken from representative lesions. Solitary nodules should be removed in their entirety.

Histopathology (Figures 13-2 through 13-4)

The epidermis is necrotic, ulcerated, and exudative in acute lesions. Acanthosis or ulceration occurs in chronic lesions.

Early arthropod-bite reactions, as typified by ticks, have extensive necrosis and inflammation, which may occasionally occur in the classic triangular or "wedge-shaped" configuration with the apex near the panniculus. Inflammation is perivascular to diffuse and includes numerous eosinophils, lymphocytes, and macrophages. Edema and hemorrhage may be prominent.

In chronic nodular lesions, or true arthropod-bite granulomas, macrophages, lymphocytes, mast cells, eosinophils, and plasma cells densely infiltrate the dermis and subcutis, obscuring the normal architecture. Nodular accumulations of lymphocytes, resembling lymphoid follicles, may be prominent. Fibrovascular tissue is intermingled with inflammatory cells among the lymphoid follicles.

Differential diagnoses are few for the acute arthropod-bite reactions, particularly if the typical wedge-shaped configuration is seen. Foreign body reactions or reactions to injection of medicaments or vaccines must be considered as possible differential diagnoses for late-stage arthropod-bite granulomas. In granulomas, arthropod insult may be suggested by a localized inflammatory nodule, which includes lymphocytes, often in follicular arrangement, and eosinophils.

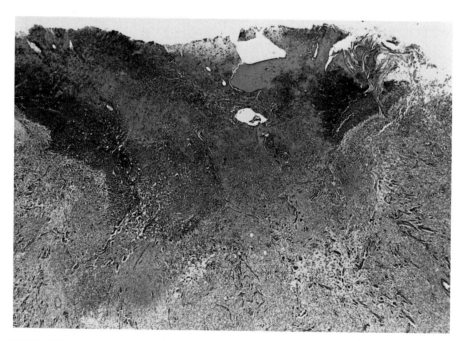

FIGURE 13-2. Acute arthropod-bite granuloma in a cat. Note the prominent wedge-shaped necrosis and superficial crusting. ($\times 35$.)

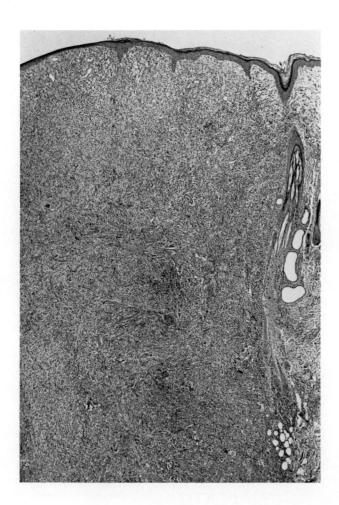

FIGURE 13-3. Chronic arthropod-bite granuloma (insect-bite granuloma) in a dog. Mixed inflammation fills the dermis and subcutis. (×35.)

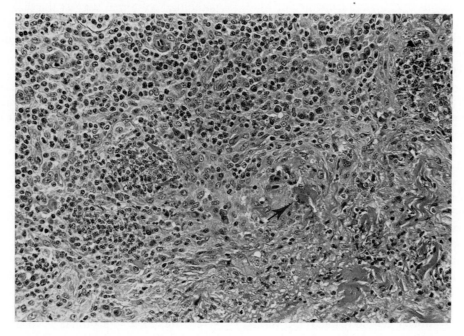

FIGURE 13-4. Higher magnification of the arthropod-bite granuloma shown in Figure 13-3 reveals a dense population of mixed mononuclear cells and fewer eosinophils. Note the small focus of collagen degeneration *(arrow)*. (×220.)

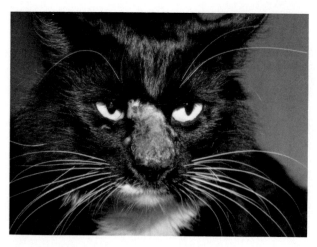

FIGURE 13-5. Feline mosquito-bite hypersensitivity. A visually striking, well-demarcated, erythematous lesion with swelling, alopecia, erosion, ulceration, and exudation developed rapidly on the dorsal muzzle. Note that the planum nasale is affected.

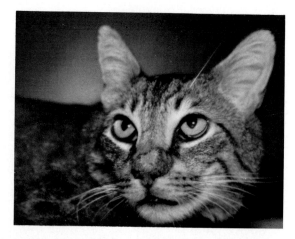

FIGURE 13-6. Feline mosquito-bite hypersensitivity demonstrating focal swelling, erosion, and ulceration of the dorsal muzzle and planum nasale accompanied by alopecia.

FELINE MOSQUITO-BITE HYPERSENSITIVITY (Synonym: feline insect-bite hypersensitivity)
Clinical features (Figures 13-5 and 13-6)

Feline mosquito-bite hypersensitivity is a visually distinctive, uncommon, predominantly facial, and presumably allergic skin disease that is associated with mosquito bites. Lesions have been documented by Mason (1988, 1991) to occur at the exact site of previous mosquito bites. It is not known currently if the same reaction pattern can be seen with the bite of other flying insects. The syndrome follows the classic seasonal pattern of mosquito-bite hypersensitivity in humans, characterized by development of lesions in the summer and regression the following winter. Furthermore, the syndrome has been seen only in cats allowed outdoors, and lesions resolve when strict indoor confinement is instituted.

A partially symmetric, erythematous facial eruption with papules and crusting is noted initially. In severe, acute cases, a visually striking well-demarcated lesion characterized by swelling, alopecia, erosion, ulceration, and exudation develops rapidly on the dorsal muzzle. Hyperpigmentation or hypopigmentation may be seen as a sequela to active disease, and firm, hyperpigmented nodules may be present in chronic cases. The planum nasale, periorbital region, and pinnae also may be affected. Symmetry can be marked. Occasionally, facial disease may be more widespread, and footpads may be affected. The affected areas are relatively less haired and presumably are attractive targets for flying insects. Regional lymphadenopathy is common.

Pruritus is variable but usually is moderate. Occurrence of the disease coincides with the mosquito season, and lesions may increase in severity over subsequent years of exposure.

Breed, age, or sex predilections have not been noted. Clinical differential diagnoses could include other cutaneous hypersensitivities such as food allergy, autoimmune diseases such as pemphigus foliaceus, and possibly notoedric acariasis. However, feline mosquito-bite hypersensitivity is a very distinctive disease. Histopathology will often suggest the diagnosis, but definitive diagnosis is based on the resolution of clinical signs following elimination of exposure to mosquitos.

Biopsy site selection

Multiple specimens should be taken from affected areas. Because lesions are mostly confined to sparsely haired, highly vascular facial areas that bleed easily and readily show scars, small specimens should be procured carefully. Four-millimeter biopsy punches are cosmetically advantageous for obtaining specimens from the muzzle or pinna of cats. Care should be taken not to damage underlying cartilage if the pinna is sampled. Periorbital lesions should not be sampled to avoid scarring at the lid margins.

Histopathology (Figures 13-7 through 13-9)

Moderate acanthosis with variable but frequently severe erosion, ulceration, and exudation is seen. The superficial dermis and the deep dermis are usually severely inflamed. Inflammation begins perivascularly but soon spreads diffusely into the interstitium. Eosinophils predominate and are accompanied by lymphocytes, mast cells, macrophages, and neutrophils in variable numbers. Edema and sometimes hemorrhage

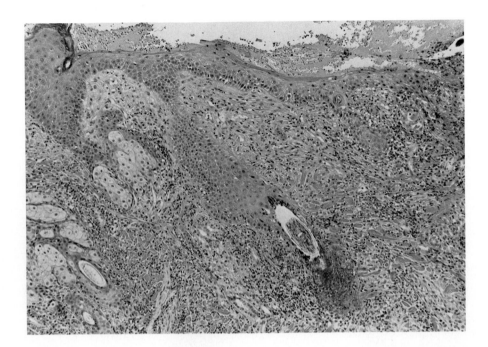

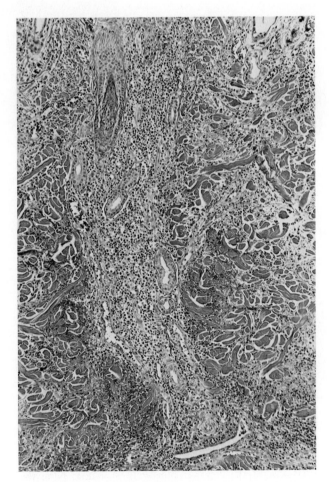

FIGURE 13-7. Feline mosquito-bite hypersensitivity. Diffuse inflammation is punctuated by eosinophilic folliculitis. (×90.)

are present. Small to moderately sized foci of eosinophil degranulation may be seen around collagen fibers and resemble flame figures or eosinophilic granulomas. There may be similar degranulating eosinophils in and around hair follicles (eosinophilic folliculitis) or within and surrounding vessels.

Histopathologically, lesions of mosquito-bite hypersensitivity are more severe than those of most other allergic skin diseases of cats. Mosquito-bite hypersensitivity resembles some cases of feline food allergy and eosinophilic plaque, both of which may feature severe and deep eosinophilic inflammation. Both food allergy and mosquito-bite hypersensitivity may show eosinophilic folliculitis with degranulation, as well as foci of collagen degeneration; however, these lesions probably are more common and more prominent in cases of mosquito-bite hypersensitivity. Foci of eosinophil degranulation and collagen degeneration are similar to those seen in idiopathic eosinophilic granuloma. Large areas of amorphous degenerating collagen and degranulated eosinophils, as seen in most cases of idiopathic feline eosinophilic granulomas, are not generally a feature of mosquito-bite hypersensitivity. Additionally, degranulating eosinophils involving follicles (eosinophilic folliculitis), as seen in mosquito-bite hypersensitivity, are not a feature of idiopathic feline eosinophilic granuloma. It is important to stress that severe eosinophilic inflammation of *any* kind (for example, that seen in some mast cell tumors) can evoke secondary degranulation and damage to collagen. Clinical features, which are distinctive, are required to differentiate mosquito-bite hypersensitivity from other histopathologically similar eosinophilic diseases of the cat.

FIGURE 13-8. Feline mosquito-bite hypersensitivity. Several foci of eosinophil degranulation and mild collagen degeneration are intermingled with diffuse eosinophilic inflammation. (×90.)

FIGURE 13-9. Feline mosquito bite hypersensitivity. Large numbers of eosinophils are accumulating around vessels of the deep dermis. (×220.)

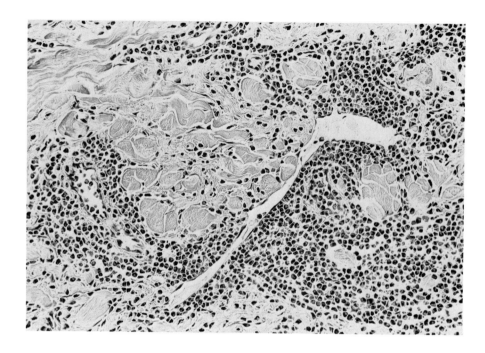

SPIDER BITES
Clinical features (Figure 13-10)

Spider bites cause a spectrum of skin disease in the dog and cat, which ranges from local swelling to life-threatening tissue necrosis. Woodpiles and undisturbed areas of old buildings are favorite habitats of spiders. Spider bites rarely are reported in veterinary medicine. The secretive behavior of spiders makes it difficult to confirm their bites. The species of spiders most often implicated in spider bites in North America include the

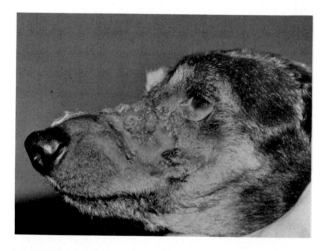

FIGURE 13-10. Putative spider bite in a dog. Note the drip-like configuration of the necrotic lesion, which characterizes a heavy molecular weight necrotoxin. *(Courtesy CS Foil, Baton Rouge, Louisiana.)*

brown recluse *(Loxosceles reclusus)*, the black widow *(Latrodectus mactans)*, the red widow *(Latrodectus bishopi)*, and the common brown spider *(Loxosceles unicolor)*.

The genera *Latrodectus* produces primarily systemic effects via neurotoxins, whereas the genera *Loxosceles* mainly produces local tissue damage through the release of necrotoxins. The necrotoxin produced by the brown recluse spider causes the most severe tissue damage. Other North American spiders capable of producing necrotic skin lesions include the running spiders *(Chiracanthium* species), black jumping spiders *(Phidippus* species), golden orb weavers *(Argiope* species*)*, wolf spiders *(Lycosa* species), green lynx spider *(Peucetia viridans)*, and funnel-web spider *(Atarx* species*)*.

The brown recluse spider produces inapparent small puncture marks followed by a central papule with surrounding erythema. Blister formation and skin necrosis occur within 6 to 12 hours. Tissue damage is extensive and results in a dark, necrotic, indolent, non-healing ulcer. The face and forelegs most commonly are affected. Pain or pruritus rarely is present. Systemic effects, including disseminated intravascular coagulopathy, renal failure, and death, are reported in the human literature.

The black widow spider produces minimal skin damage, usually limited to erythema. Systemic signs occur within 1 to 8 hours after envenomation.

Breed, age, or sex predilections are not available. However, active and inquisitive animals with access to spider habitats are at increased risk. Brown recluse spider bites occur primarily between March and October

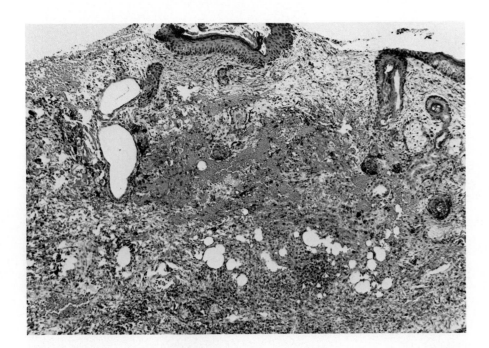

FIGURE 13-11. Putative spider bite in a dog. Diffuse and severe mixed inflammation is accompanied by severe hemorrhage, noted centrally. (×90.)

in North America, since this spider hibernates in the winter.

Clinical differential diagnoses for necrotizing spider bites include lesions caused by venomous insects, poisonous snakes, and tropical centipedes, as well as localized cutaneous vasculitis of any cause. The iatrogenic perivascular deposition of potentially irritating intravenous medications can produce similar lesions. Differentiation depends upon a history of exposure and the clinical course.

Biopsy site selection

Wedge specimens should be taken from the borders of necrotic ulcers. Specimens sampled should be small, since the inflammation and necrosis produced by the venom inhibit healing of the biopsy site.

Histopathology (Figure 13-11)

The epidermis is usually ulcerated or eroded; superficial exudate may be prominent. Inflammation is diffuse and extends into the panniculus. Necrosis of the dermis may be severe and usually is accompanied by edema, hemorrhage, and sometimes cavitation. Localized vasculopathy of presumed toxic etiology is characterized by swelling of endothelial cells, necrosis, and thrombosis. Inflammatory cells are mixed and include large numbers of neutrophils and macrophages. Eosinophils may not be prominent in comparison with other arthropod-bite reactions. Correlation with the clinical features of a nonhealing ulcer on the face or distal extremity is essential for the diagnosis of spider bite because histopathologic findings are not specifically diagnostic.

Differential diagnoses include pythiosis, deep vessel immune-mediated vasculitis, severe deep bacterial pyoderma, and severe foreign body reactions. Pythiosis is characterized by hemorrhage and vascular necrosis similar to spider bites, but often contains distinctive foci of eosinophilic necrosis. Deep vessel immune-mediated vasculitis may appear similar if significant tissue damage is present. Severe foreign-body reactions or deep bacterial infections may resemble spider bites, but do not have a vascular component.

FELINE EOSINOPHILIC PLAQUE
Clinical features (Figures 13-12 and 13-13)

See Chapter 4.

Biopsy site selection

Well-demarcated, minimally traumatized, erythematous plaques should be selected for biopsy. Ulcers and severely crusted lesions should be avoided.

Histopathology (Figures 13-14 and 13-15)

Epidermal lesions have been described (see Chapter 4), and principally and most characteristically include widespread spongiosis of the epidermis and follicular infundibula. In the dermis, typical eosinophilic plaque is characterized by perivascular to diffuse, moderate to severe infiltrations of eosinophils. Inflammation usually is superficial to middermal but often extends to the deep dermis and upper panniculus in severe lesions. Lymphocytes, mast cells, and macrophages are present in smaller numbers. Neutrophils also

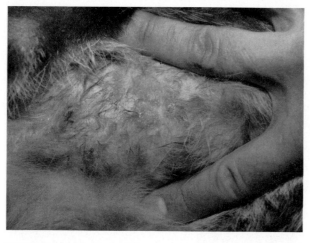

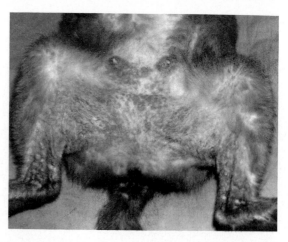

FIGURE 13-12. Early feline eosinophilic plaque. Focal erythematous, erosive, alopecic plaques in a cat with allergic miliary dermatitis. *(Courtesy AH Werner, Los Angeles, California; case material from the University of California, Davis.)*

FIGURE 13-13. Severe feline eosinophilic plaque. Multiple, well-demarcated, erythematous plaques on the ventral abdomen of a cat with allergic miliary dermatitis.

FIGURE 13-14. Feline eosinophilic plaque. Diffuse, severe dermal inflammation is beneath extensive ulceration and exudation. Note spongiosis of the remaining superficial follicular epithelium. (×35.)

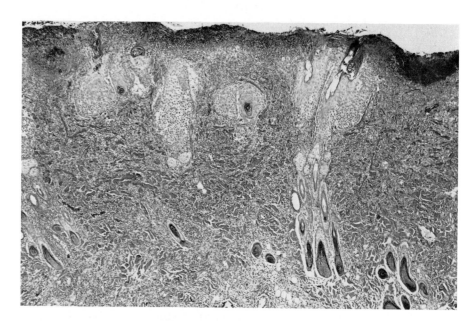

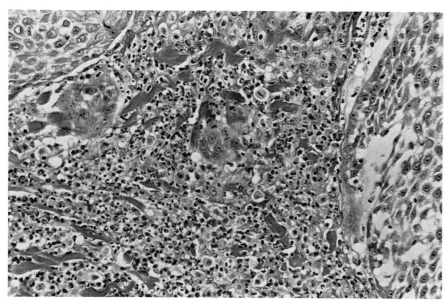

FIGURE 13-15. Feline eosinophilic plaque demonstrating eosinophils and fewer mast cells in the inflammatory infiltrate. The adjacent epithelium is markedly spongiotic. (×220.)

may be prominent beneath areas of severe erosion or ulceration.

The lesions of eosinophilic plaque histopathologically resemble those of allergic miliary dermatitis but are more severely inflamed and include prominent spongiosis. Since eosinophilic plaque and miliary dermatitis both may be manifestations of allergic skin disease in the cat (and can exist concurrently), histopathologic separation of severe lesions of miliary dermatitis from lesions of eosinophilic plaque may not be critical diagnostically. Eosinophilic plaque with deep inflammation may resemble mosquito-bite hypersensitivity; typical spongiosis of eosinophilic plaque, if present, will allow differentiation. In addition, lesions of mosquito-bite hypersensitivity may show collagen degeneration, a feature that is not characteristic of eosinophilic plaque.

FELINE EOSINOPHILIC GRANULOMA (Synonyms: feline collagenolytic granuloma, feline linear granuloma)
Clinical features (Figures 13-16 through 13-18)

Feline eosinophilic granuloma is a common, clinically heterogeneous syndrome unified by a similar histopathologic pattern. An underlying hypersensitivity (atopy, food allergy, flea allergy) often is suggested but rarely is documented. Eosinophilic granulomas have been recently studied by Power in an inbred, closed, specific pathogen–free colony of cats without exposure to ectoparasites or endoparasites and without indications of either atopy or food allergy as documented by intradermal skin testing and elimination diets. This

suggests, at least in this colony, that feline eosinophilic granuloma is an inherited disorder of eosinophil proliferation or function. Elaboration of major basic protein, a collagenolytic product of eosinophils that has been identified in eosinophilic granulomas of human diseases such as Well's syndrome, also may be implicated in the collagen degeneration of eosinophilic granuloma in animals.

Cutaneous and oral forms of eosinophilic granuloma occur in cats. In the typical cutaneous "linear granuloma," linear, well-circumscribed, pinkish-yellow, elevated, firm plaques develop on the caudal thighs. Less commonly, similar lesions may be seen on the forelimbs, neck, and thorax. Firm plaques and nodules may be seen on the pinnae. Asymptomatic pinkish-

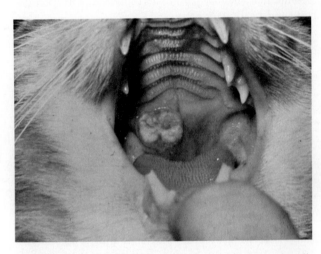

FIGURE 13-17. Feline oral eosinophilic granuloma. A well-demarcated erythematous plaque with caseous, necrotic foci is present on the soft palate. Note the somewhat symmetric, linear ulcers of the hard palate at top.

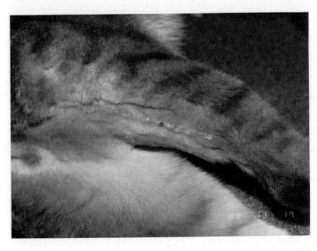

FIGURE 13-16. Feline eosinophilic granuloma (linear granuloma) on the caudal hindlimb. The affected area has been clipped to enhance visualization of the crusted and erythematous linear plaque. *(Courtesy HT Power, Santa Cruz, California; research material from the University of California, Davis).*

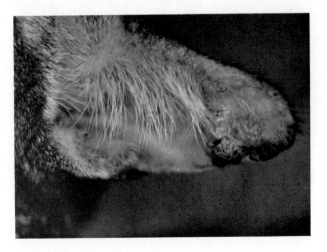

FIGURE 13-18. Feline eosinophilic granuloma of the pinna of the ear. Two crusted, proliferative plaques have coalesced near the margin.

yellow swelling of the lower lip ("pouting cat") and swelling of the chin (chin edema, "fat chin") are additional clinical subtypes of feline eosinophilic granuloma. Pain and pruritus are not observed.

Eosinophilic granuloma of the footpads has also been recognized in cats. Crusting and ulceration of the pad are accompanied by interdigital alopecia and erythema. Lesions may involve several pads concurrently or sequentially. Digital and metacarpal or metatarsal pads may be affected.

Firm, granulomatous nodules involving the tongue, frenulum, or soft palate characterize the oral form of eosinophilic granuloma. If ulceration is present, gritty, pinpoint, white foci may be seen grossly and correspond to the foci of eosinophil degranulation and collagen degeneration seen histopathologically. Oral eosinophilic granulomas may be painful and interfere with prehension and swallowing.

Peripheral lymphadenopathy may be present with any type of collagenolytic granuloma. Concomitant indolent ulcers (eosinophilic ulcers) may occur with eosinophilic granuloma and may represent a variant of the same disorder (see Chapter 5).

Female cats may be predisposed to eosinophilic granuloma. Age or breed predilections have not been documented; however, cats under 2 years of age appear to have an increased incidence of eosinophilic granuloma of the footpads.

Clinical differential diagnoses are few for the visually distinctive cutaneous forms of eosinophilic granuloma. Oral lesions may resemble neoplasms, foreign body reactions, or proliferative traumatic lesions (inflamed granulation tissue). Lesions of the footpads may resemble plasma cell pododermatitis. Histopathology is required for definitive diagnosis.

Biopsy site selection

A deep punch biopsy specimen or wedge specimen should be obtained to establish a diagnosis. If possible, lesions with ulceration should be avoided, since characteristic collagenolytic foci may no longer be present.

Histopathology (Figures 13-19 through 13-21)

The epidermis is normal to moderately acanthotic and occasionally may be eroded, ulcerated, and exudative. The dermis is diffusely inflamed and contains generally large foci of eosinophil degranulation and amorphous degenerating collagen. Foci may be girdled by macrophages and giant cells, often in palisading array. The intervening dermis is diffusely inflamed with eosinophils, macrophages, mast cells, and fewer lymphocytes. Eosinophils are not prominent in chronic lesions, and macrophages and giant cells may predominate around foci of collagen degeneration or interpo-

late between intact collagen fibers. Occasionally, particularly in oral lesions, deeply embedded hair shafts are seen. It has been suggested that hair foreign bodies may have an inciting role in these cases; the authors believe that hairs may elicit or aggravate eosinophil degranulation, but factors initiating the influx of eosinophils are likely to preexist.

Differential diagnoses are few, particularly in mature lesions that have large foci of collagen degeneration. Mild eosinophilic degranulation and collagen degeneration are seen in early indolent ulcers. According to Power, clinically typical indolent ulcers (ulcers that affect the upper lip just lateral to the philtrum) do not show prominent eosinophilic degranulation and collagen degeneration; however, eosinophilic granuloma and indolent ulcer may be manifestations of a common eosinophilic disorder in some cats.

Small foci of eosinophilic degranulation around collagen fibers, sometimes more closely resembling

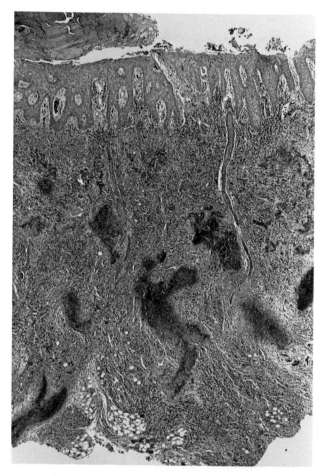

FIGURE 13-19. Feline eosinophilic granuloma of the footpad. Diffusely inflamed tissue contains large, darkly staining zones of eosinophil degranulation and collagen degeneration. (×35.)

FIGURE 13-20. Feline eosino-philic granuloma. Diffuse in-flammation is punctuated by discrete collagenolytic granulo-mas. (×90.)

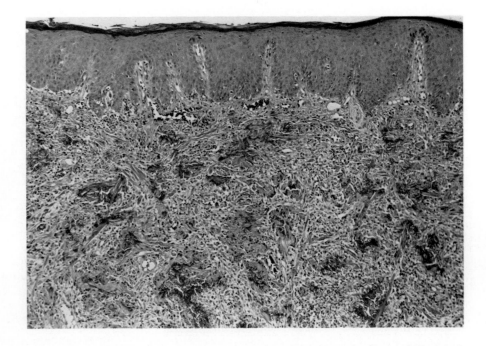

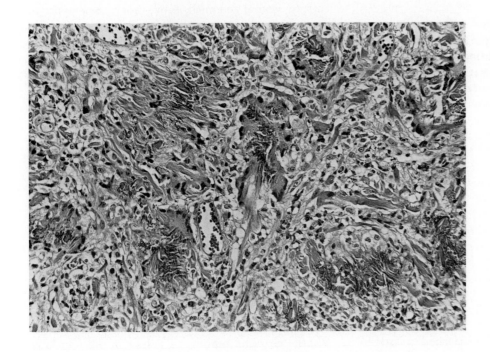

FIGURE 13-21. Higher mag-nification of feline eosinophilic granuloma demonstrating multinucleated giant cells around foci of eosinophilic de-granulation and degenerating collagen. (×220.)

flame figures, may be seen in feline mosquito-bite hy-persensitivity and feline food allergy, as well as in etio-logically unidentified cases of severe eosinophilic der-matitis in cats. It is important to stress that severe eosinophilic inflammation of *many* types (for example, that seen in mast cell tumors) can evoke secondary degranulation and damage to collagen. The diagnosis of eosinophilic granuloma should probably be reserved for those lesions that occur in characteristic clinical sites (lip, chin, oral cavity, and as a linear configuration in the skin) and for which no associated cause can be identified.

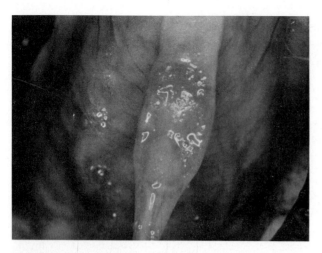

FIGURE 13-22. Canine eosinophilic granuloma on the frenulum of the tongue of a dog. The nodule is ulcerated. *(Courtesy D Carlotti, Carbon Blanc, France.)*

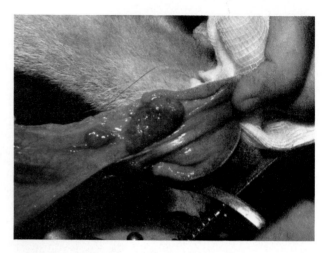

FIGURE 13-23. Canine eosinophilic granuloma on the tongue of a dog. *(Courtesy BR Madewell, Davis, California.)*

CANINE EOSINOPHILIC GRANULOMA (Synonym: canine collagenolytic granuloma)

Clinical features (Figures 13-22 and 13-23)

Canine eosinophilic granuloma is a rare, somewhat heterogeneous group of syndromes unified by their histopathologic pattern. Hypersensitivity or vasculopathy are the proposed pathogenetic mechanisms. Arthropod bites, trauma, or foreign body embedment may be an antecedent event. The authors suspect that focal cutaneous eosinophilic granulomas of dogs often are the direct result of arthropod insult, based on their solitary nature and lack of recurrence following excision. Focal disease of the oral cavity, predominantly in the Siberian Husky, is the most common subgroup, and the marked breed predilection suggests a genetic basis for this type of eosinophilic granuloma. Elaboration of major basic protein, a collagenolytic product of eosinophils that has been identified in eosinophilic granulomas of human diseases such as Well's syndrome, also may be implicated in the collagen degeneration of eosinophilic granuloma in animals.

In the Siberian Husky, well-demarcated, yellowish-brown, vegetative, granulomatous plaques develop on the lateral or ventral surface of the tongue. Ulcers with a slightly elevated border may be present on the soft or hard palate, either coexistent with lingual lesions or alone. Lingual lesions may have a friable surface and bleed readily. The oral cavity has a strong necrotic, fetid odor. Pain is marked, and affected dogs usually are partially anorectic and reluctant to chew dry dog food. Discomfort and odor are not noted in dogs with lesions confined to the palate.

Less commonly, solitary or grouped lesions may be seen at various cutaneous sites, including the pinnae. Erythematous plaques, nodules, or papules form on the muzzle, ventral abdomen, flank, thorax, or prepuce of dogs. Larger lesions may ulcerate. Pain or pruritus are not noted. In rare cases, the authors have observed asymptomatic domed papules and nodules of the tips of the pinnae, clinically reminiscent of granuloma annulare in humans.

Male Siberian Huskies less than 3 years of age are at increased risk for lingual eosinophilic granulomas. Lingual lesions also have been reported in a Bull Mastiff and a mixed-breed dog by Walsh. Ulcerated palatal lesions are most common in Siberian Huskies. This form of eosinophilic granuloma also has been seen in a variety of other breeds, including the Chow Chow and the Malamute. An ulcerative form of oral eosinophilic granuloma has been observed recently in German Wirehaired Pointer mother-daughter cohorts.* Other signalment predilections have not been noted.

Clinical differential diagnoses for eosinophilic granulomas include foreign body reactions and neoplasms. Additionally, the ulcerative oral form must be differentiated from traumatic ulcers. Apart from the visually characteristic lingual lesions in Siberian Huskies, canine eosinophilic granulomas are not clinically distinctive. Consequently, canine eosinophilic granuloma is most often an unexpected histopathologic diagnosis.

Biopsy site selection

Care should be taken in sampling lingual lesions if oral eosinophilic granuloma is suspected, particularly in

---

* Case material courtesy IA Ingram, Phoenix, 1990.

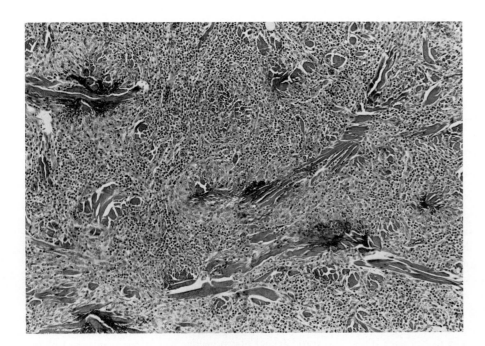

FIGURE 13-24. Canine eosinophilic granuloma. Darkly staining degranulating eosinophils are accumulating along collagen fibers. Large epithelioid macrophages surround these foci to form granulomas. (×90.)

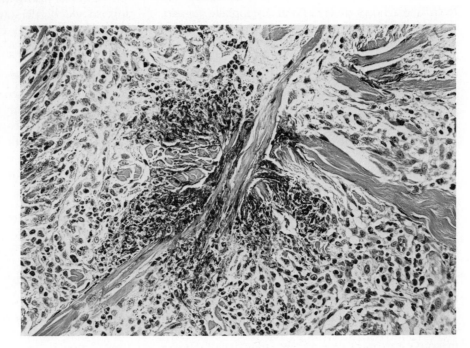

FIGURE 13-25. Canine eosinophilic granuloma. Eosinophils are degranulating along partially degenerated collagen fibers. (×220.)

Siberian Huskies. No attempt should be made to completely excise proliferative lingual lesions, since large specimens are not necessary to establish a diagnosis, deformation may result, and the lesions are readily responsive to glucocorticoids. For solitary skin lesions, the entire mass may be removed using a wedge resection technique.

Histopathology (Figures 13-24 and 13-25)

The epidermis or mucosal epithelium may be acanthotic or ulcerated. The dermis or submucosa have small to large, irregular, brightly eosinophilic foci composed of degranulating eosinophils and amorphous degenerated collagen. Oral eosinophilic granulomas of dogs may have large brightly eosinophilic, amorphous foci of collagen degeneration and eosinophil degranulation, similar to eosinophilic granulomas of cats. Cutaneous eosinophilic granulomas may have smaller degenerative foci that more closely resemble "flame figures." Foci of collagen degeneration may have peripheral, small, radiating projections and are surrounded by eosinophils, macrophages, and sometimes giant cells. Similar inflammation courses among the collagenolytic foci, accompanied by mast cells, lymphocytes, and plasma cells. Fibrosis may be prominent in chronic lesions.

In lesions from canine ear tips, eosinophils are not prominent. Instead, variably sized, pale-staining foci of collagen are surrounded by palisading macrophages (palisading granulomas). In some areas, macrophages have a spindled appearance and are arranged in dense sheets. There may be accompanying vascular abnormalities in aural lesions, including hypertrophy of vessel walls. A single case observed by the authors had a grossly evident blood-filled aneurysm adjacent to the granuloma. Presumably, these lesions are vascular in origin and may be ischemic in their derivation. They bear some resemblance to granuloma annulare in humans, a poorly understood disease of collagen denaturation in which vascular changes occasionally are described (fibrinoid change, endothelial swelling, and occlusion of vascular lumens).

Canine eosinophilic granuloma is distinctive; differential diagnoses are few. Focal eosinophilic granulomas may represent localized reactions to arthropod insult. Eosinophilic furunculosis of the face, also suspected to be arthropod related, also may have foci of eosinophil degranulation and collagen degeneration; typical furunculosis allows differentiation.

FELINE PLASMA CELL PODODERMATITIS
Clinical features (Figure 13-26)

Feline plasma cell pododermatitis is a rare skin disease of cats affecting the footpads. The etiology is unknown, but the marked plasma cell infiltrate coupled with hypergammaglobulinemia suggests an immune-mediated basis.

Spongy swelling of a variable number of footpads occurs on multiple paws. The swelling is uniform such that normal pad symmetry usually is not disturbed. The larger metacarpal and metatarsal pads are most consistently affected. An increased prominence of normal surface architecture caused by stretching of the skin of the pad results in a white, silvery, cross-hatched appearance. Somewhat surprisingly, lesions usually are asymptomatic. If ulceration of more severely affected footpads occurs, hemorrhage may follow and lameness may be seen. Scott (1984, 1987) has reported that a minority of cats have coexistent plasma cell stomatitis, immune-mediated glomerulonephritis, or renal amyloidosis.

Breed, age, or sex predilections have not been noted with feline plasma cell pododermatitis. Feline plasma cell pododermatitis is distinctive, particularly when multiple pads are affected. If only one pad is

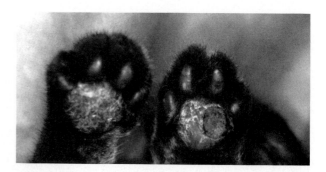

FIGURE 13-26. Feline plasma cell pododermatitis affecting both metacarpal pads. An increased prominence of normal surface architecture results in a white, web-like, cross-hatched appearance. Note the large healing ulcer. *(Courtesy BA Atlee, Davis, California; case material from the University of California, Davis.)*

involved, neoplasia and sterile or infectious granulomas must be ruled out. Exfoliate cytology from aspiration should reveal plasma cells, and hypergammaglobulinemia should be demonstrable on immunoelectrophoresis. Histopathology is necessary to confirm the diagnosis.

Biopsy site selection

A wedge specimen should be obtained from a footpad near the pad margin. Punch-biopsy specimens often are unsuitable because they do not provide a sample of adequate depth. If multiple pads are affected, a moderately rather than severely affected pad should be selected, since severely affected pads may not heal well after biopsy.

Histopathology (Figures 13-27 and 13-28)

The epidermis is acanthotic or eroded, ulcerated, and exudative. The dermis and often the underlying adipose tissue of the pad are diffusely infiltrated with plasma cells, obscuring the normal architecture. Interlobular septal edema of the adipose tissue may be present, and vessels are often prominent and congested. Milder lesions may show dermal inflammation only. Russell body–containing plasma cells (Mott cells) are often conspicuous. Fewer lymphocytes and macrophages are present and are randomly distributed among the plasma cells. Neutrophils vary, depending on the degree of ulceration, but may compose up to 50% of the infiltrate. Eosinophils are observed in small numbers in some cases.

Differential diagnosis is not difficult, particularly when the site of the biopsy is known. The location, type, and distribution of the inflammation are typical. Eosinophilic granuloma of the footpad demonstrates collagen degeneration and eosinophils, features that are absent in feline plasma cell pododermatitis.

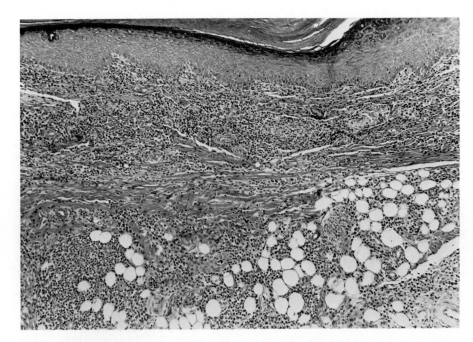

FIGURE 13-27. Feline plasma cell pododermatitis. Diffuse infiltrations of mixed mononuclear cells are partially replacing the adipose tissue of the footpad. (×90.)

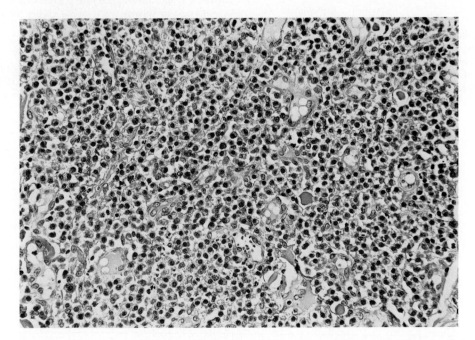

FIGURE 13-28. Feline plasma cell pododermatitis. Note the predominance of plasma cells in the diffuse inflammatory infiltrate. (×220.)

SUGGESTED READINGS

Arthropod-bite granuloma

Ackerman AB: Histologic diagnosis of inflammatory skin diseases, Philadelphia, 1978, Lea and Febiger, pp 295-301.

Doros DL: Hypersensitivity granulomas. In Middleton EM, Reed CE, Ellis EF and others, editors: Allergy: principles and practice, St Louis, 1988, CV Mosby, pp 275-294.

Rees RS and King LE: Arthropod bites and stings. In Fitzpatrick TB, Eisen AZ, Wolff K and others, editors: Dermatology in general medicine, New York, 1987, McGraw-Hill, pp 2495-2506.

Walder EJ and Howard EB: Persistent insect bite granuloma in a dog, Vet Pathol 19:839-841, 1982.

Feline mosquito-bite hypersensitivity

Mason KV and Evans AG: Mosquito bite–caused eosinophilic dermatitis in cats, J Am Vet Med Assoc 198:2086-2088, 1991.

Mason KV and Evans AG: Feline eosinophilic granuloma complex: a further clinical manifestation and etiology. Proceedings of the American Academy of Veterinary Dermatology/American College of Veterinary Dermatology, Washington DC, 4:41, 1988.

Wilkinson GT and Bates MJ: A possible further clinical manifestation of the feline eosinophilic granuloma complex, J Am Anim Hosp Assoc 20:325-331, 1982.

Spider bites

Lever WF and Schaumburg-Lever G: Histopathology of the skin, Philadelphia, 1990, JB Lippincott, p 242.

Meerdink GL: Bites and stings of venomous animals. In Kirk RW, editor: Current veterinary therapy VIII, Philadelphia, 1983, WB Saunders, pp 155-159.

Muller GH, Kirk RW, and Scott DW: Small animal dermatology, ed 4, Philadelphia, 1989, WB Saunders, p 407.

Rees RS and King LE: Arthropod bites and stings. In Fitzpatrick TB, Eisen AZ, Wolff K and others, editors: Dermatology in general medicine, New York, 1987, McGraw-Hill, pp 2497-2499.

Wong RC and others: Spider bites, Arch Dermatol 123:98-104, 1987.

Feline eosinophilic plaque

See Chapter 4.

Feline eosinophilic granuloma

Muller GH, Kirk RW, and Scott DW: Small animal dermatology, ed 4, Philadelphia, 1989, WB Saunders, pp 564-565.

Nutman TB, Ottesen EA, and Cohen SG: Eosinophilia and eosinophil-related disorders. In Middleton EM, Reed CE, Ellis EF and others, editors: Allergy: principles and practice, St Louis, 1988, CV Mosby, pp 861-890.

Power HT: Eosinophilic granuloma in a family of specific pathogen-free cats, Proceedings of the American Academy of Veterinary Dermatology/American College of Veterinary Dermatology, San Francisco 6:45, 1990.

Canine eosinophilic granuloma

Da Silva Curiel JMA and others: Eosinophilic granuloma of the nasal skin in a dog, J Am Vet Med Assoc 193:566-567, 1988.

Guaguere E and Magnol J-P: Granulomes eosinophiliques buccaux chez un Chow-Chow, Pratique Medicale et Chirurgicale de l'Animal de Compagnie 21:309-311, 1986.

Madewell BR and others: Oral eosinophilic granulomas in Siberian Husky Dogs, Am Vet Med Assoc 177:701-703, 1980.

Nutman TB, Ottesen EA, and Cohen SG: Eosinophilia and eosinophil-related disorders. In Middleton EM, Reed CE, Ellis EF and others, editors: Allergy: principles and practice, St Louis, 1988, CV Mosby, pp 861-890.

Potter KA, Tucker RD, and Carpenter JL: Oral eosinophilic granuloma of Siberian Huskies, J Am Anim Hosp Assoc 16:595-600, 1980.

Scott DW: Cutaneous eosinophilic granulomas with collagen degeneration in the dog, J Am Anim Hosp Assoc 19:529-532, 1983.

Turnwald GH, Hoskins JD, and Taylor HW: Cutaneous eosinophilic granuloma in a Labrador Retriever, J Am Vet Med Assoc 179:799-801, 1981.

Walsh KM: Oral eosinophilic granuloma in two dogs, J Am Vet Med Assoc 183:323-324, 1983.

Feline plasma cell pododermatitis

Gruffydd-Jones TJ, Orr CM, and Lucke VM: Foot pad swelling and ulceration in cats: a report of five cases, J Small Anim Pract 21:381-389, 1980.

Medleau L and others: Ulcerative pododermatitis in a cat: Immunofluorescent findings and response to chrysotherapy, J Am Anim Hosp Assoc 18:449-451, 1982.

Scott DW: Feline dermatology 1983-1985: "the secret sits," J Am Anim Hosp Assoc 23:255-274, 1987.

Scott DW: Feline dermatology 1979-1982: introspective retrospections, J Am Anim Hosp Assoc 20:537-564, 1984.

Taylor JE and Schmeitzel LP: Plasma cell pododermatitis with chronic footpad hemorrhage in two cats, J Am Vet Med Assoc 197:375-377, 1990.

Dysplastic and depositional diseases of dermal connective tissue

The depositional diseases are characterized by production or deposition of substances not normally found in the dermis, such as mineral or amyloid, or production of substances in excess of normal, such as mucin. Differentiation among these conditions is accomplished by the identification of specific histomorphologic features of the substances, which is aided by the use of special stains.

The dysplastic diseases are those in which the structure of the dermal collagen is altered through hereditary or acquired (metabolic) stimuli. These diseases result in secondary splitting of the skin through the dermis, a feature that aids in the diagnosis.

CALCINOSIS CUTIS
Clinical features (Figures 14-1 and 14-2)

Calcinosis cutis is an uncommon physiologic process seen in the dog that is characterized by inappropriate deposition of inorganic calcium and phosphate ions in the dermis, epidermis or subcutis. Calcinosis cutis, broadly used, encompasses all forms of calcification, whether dystrophic or metastatic and whether caused by idiopathic, metabolic, traumatic, or other factors. The term calcinosis cutis is used most commonly to denote the specific type of dystrophic calcification seen in association with naturally occurring or iatrogenic hyperglucocorticoidism. In this syndrome, calcium and phosphate ions probably are deposited upon the collagen or elastin matrix of the dermis.

The mechanism of calcium salt deposition in dystrophic calcification is not well understood. Normally, calcium and phosphate ions exist in solution in extracellular fluid in metastable equilibrium. Phase transformation from ions in solution to the solid phase may be induced by changes in collagen fibrils. Phosphate ions may initiate the transformation by the formation of crystal nuclei upon organic matrices.

Calcinosis cutis may be either focal or widespread. Firm, gritty plaques develop from coalescing erythematous papules. Chalky, white-to-pink material with a feathery margin can be seen through the intact epidermis of early nonulcerated lesions and is most easily observed with a hand lens. Ulceration and crusting occur as gritty material is extruded from older lesions and may be aggravated by self-trauma. Calcinosis cutis is seen most commonly in the flexural surfaces of the groin and axillae and on the back of the neck. Chronic, well-established lesions may be pruritic, contrary to popular belief, especially if transepidermal elimination of calcium occurs. Dogs with hyperglucocorti-

223

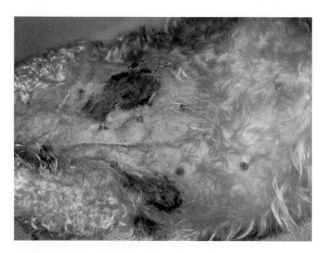

FIGURE 14-1. Calcinosis cutis in an aged Poodle with naturally occurring hyperglucocorticoidism. Somewhat bilaterally symmetric, ulcerated plaques are present in the flexural surfaces of the ventral abdomen.

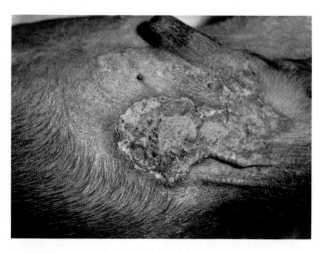

FIGURE 14-2. Chronic calcinosis cutis in an aged Boston Terrier with naturally occurring hyperglucocorticoidism. A well-demarcated plaque is seen in a flexural surface of the ventral abdomen. Peripheral white foci correspond to areas of transepidermal elimination of mineralized debris.

coidism exhibiting calcinosis cutis usually also show other characteristic clinical features of this syndrome (see Chapter 17). Calcinosis cutis may be clinically inapparent in very early cases.

Rarely, widespread idiopathic calcinosis cutis has been seen in dogs without demonstrable metabolic abnormalities. This syndrome is seen most frequently in puppies as a sequela to severe systemic illness. The etiopathogenesis is unknown and lesions usually regress spontaneously.

Calcinosis cutis also has been reported by Schick in association with the percutaneous penetration of calcium chloride powder present in a landscaping product. Lesions were papular to nodular, indurated, ulcerated, and exudative and were widespread in distribution, reflecting sites of contact.

Calcinosis cutis seen in conjunction with naturally occurring canine hyperadrenocorticism will have the age and breed predilections of that syndrome (see

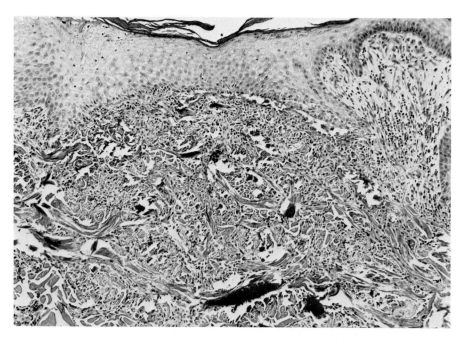

FIGURE 14-3. Calcinosis cutis. Note the partial destruction and fragmentation of dermal collagen by deposition of mineral. (×90.)

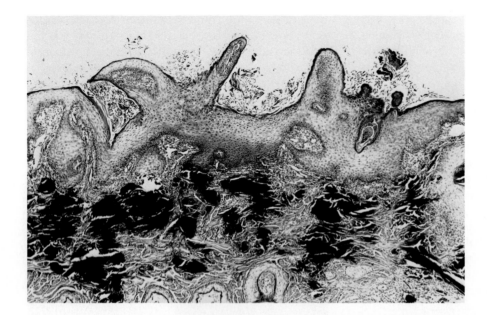

FIGURE 14-4. Severe calcinosis cutis demonstrating replacement of dermal collagen fibers by darkly staining mineral. (×90.)

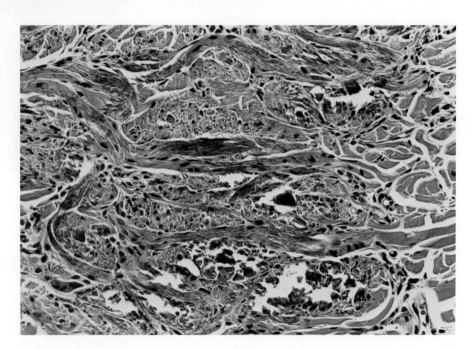

FIGURE 14-5. Higher magnification of calcinosis cutis. Collagen fibers appear fractured because of early mineralization. (×220.)

Chapter 17); sex predilections are not reported. Idiopathic calcinosis cutis following severe illness has been seen to date only in puppies; no breed or sex trends have been observed. Calcinosis cutis caused by contact absorption of calcium-containing material may be more likely in young active dogs because of their propensity for mischief.

Overt calcinosis cutis secondary to hyperglucocorticoidism is clinically distinctive. Erythematous papules of early cases may resemble superficial pyoderma. Calcinosis cutis secondary to percutaneous absorption may resemble severe bacterial or fungal infections.

Biopsy site selection

Areas of affected skin without concurrent self-trauma or ulceration are preferred sites for biopsy. Since the calcium deposits may impede incision by the skin biopsy punch, specimens obtained with smaller punches (4 mm) may be damaged during sampling. Consequently, larger biopsy punches (6 or 8 mm) or the use of the wedge technique is recommended.

Histopathology (Figures 14-3 through 14-5)

The epidermis is often severely acanthotic and may be ulcerated or exudative, depending on the degree of accompanying self-trauma, tissue damage, or pyoderma. Transepidermal or transappendageal elimination of mineral (extrusion of mineral through the epidermis or into hair follicles) is a common feature of calcinosis cutis.

The dermis is characterized by variable mineralization of collagen fibers. Affected collagen will range from slightly hypereosinophilic and mildly fragmented to deeply basophilic and severely disrupted. Macrophages accumulating along slightly fragmented collagen fibers may be the earliest histopathologic feature of calcinosis cutis. Deposition of mineral (dark brown to black) in subtle early lesions will be revealed by von Kossa stain. Frank deposition of small to large foci of dark blue mineral in the superficial and middle dermis is a more common finding; severe mineralization effaces normal dermal collagen. There may be mineralization of the external root sheaths of hair follicles. Macrophages and giant cells accumulate between affected fibers and around larger confluent foci of mineralization. Mixed inflammatory infiltrates of neutrophils, lymphocytes, and plasma cells may be present. Metaplastic bone and severe dermal fibrosis may develop in chronic lesions. Calcinosis cutis caused by percutaneous penetration of calcium chloride–containing substances may be characterized additionally by severe epidermal and dermal necrosis, probably as a direct caustic effect of the contactant.

Differential diagnosis of calcinosis cutis is not difficult if mineralization is obvious in tissue. Mineralization of the external root sheath of hair follicles may occasionally be encountered in older normal dogs, particularly Poodles and Bedlington Terriers.* Although this type of mineralization also may be prominent in hyperadrenocorticism, it is not automatically an indication of glucocorticoid excess if found without other evidence of calcinosis cutis.

CALCINOSIS CIRCUMSCRIPTA
(Synonym: tumoral calcinosis)
Clinical features (Figures 14-6 and 14-7)

Calcinosis circumscripta is a clinical subgroup of calcinosis cutis that is characterized by the deposition of calcium salts in tumor-like nodules, usually in the subcutaneous tissue. The syndrome is uncommon in dogs and very rare in cats. The mechanism of calcium deposition has been termed idiopathic; however, in most circumstances it is probably dystrophic, since lesions occur over pressure points or at sites of previous trauma, such as that incurred during ear cropping. The mechanism of calcium salt deposition in dystrophic

calcification is not completely understood (see discussion above). The tendency for dystrophic mineralization may be enhanced by the active calcium and phosphate metabolism of large, rapidly growing dogs.

Firm, well-circumscribed, domed nodules are noted in the subcutaneous tissue. The overlying skin usually is freely movable. Lesions commonly are solitary. The consistency of the nodules varies from firm to fluctuant. Ulceration is frequent in larger lesions. Gritty, chalky, or pasty material may extrude from ulcerated lesions. Erythema, swelling, and secondary pyoderma may occur. Calcinosis circumscripta is seen most commonly at sites of possible previous trauma such as pressure points or other bony prominences (such as along the spine), in

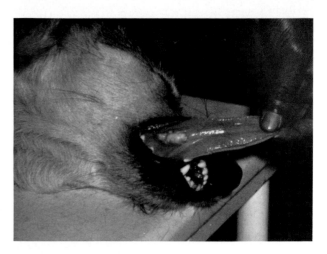

FIGURE 14-6. Calcinosis circumscripta on the tongue of a dog. The lesion is multilobulated. *(Courtesy J-P Magnol, Saint-Germain-Au-Mont-D'Or, France.)*

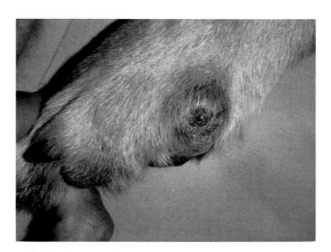

FIGURE 14-7. Calcinosis circumscripta involving a lateral digital pad of a German Shepherd Dog. An ulcer is present in the center of the lesion. *(Courtesy SD White, Fort Collins, Colorado.)*

* Stannard AA: Personal communication, 1990.

the tongue, and at the site of prior ear cropping. One author* observed multiple lesions on the pinnae of a dog that occurred at the sites of previous cat bites. Calcinosis circumscripta of a metacarpal pad in a German Shepherd Dog was reported by Stampley. Cheek lesions have been described by Scott in Boston Terriers. Concurrent disease usually is not a feature of calcinosis circumscripta in domestic animals; however, Scott has reported calcinosis circumscripta with hypertrophic osteodystrophy and polyarthritis in two young dogs.

Rarely, nodular foci of mineralization may arise from degeneration of preexisting cysts of apocrine sweat glands (apocrine cystic calcinosis). These lesions may evolve to nodular foci that are clinically and histopathologically similar to classic calcinosis circumscripta.

Other causes of dystrophic cutaneous mineralization include severe chronic inflammation such as foreign body reaction, otitis externa, interdigital pyoderma, demodicosis, or neoplasia. Lesions may either be multiple, or less commonly, solitary. When these lesions exhibit dystrophic calcification, they have sometimes been identified as calcinosis circumscripta, although they are clinically and histopathologically dissimilar.

Calcinosis circumscripta is seen most frequently in large-breed dogs, particularly the German Shepherd Dog, and in brachycephalic dogs. The syndrome is

* Thelma Lee Gross.

seen more frequently in younger dogs. Apocrine cystic calcinosis may be more common in older dogs. Sex predilection has not been noted.

Calcinosis circumscripta must be differentiated from other nodular, depositional diseases. Metastatic calcification of metabolic origin usually produces multiple lesions. Solitary neoplasms may mimic calcinosis circumscripta. Sectioning of calcinosis circumscripta after surgical removal will show the characteristic pasty or chalky foci of dystrophic calcification.

Biopsy site selection

Solitary lesions should be resected completely using a wedge technique, if this is an appropriate surgical procedure for the site. Removal of lesions from pressure points may be problematic because of poor postoperative healing.

Histopathology (Figure 14-8)

The epidermis or mucosa is normal to slightly acanthotic or severely ulcerated and hyperplastic. Scott reported transepidermal elimination of mineral deposits in late lesions.

In classic calcinosis circumscripta (as typified by focal lesions over pressure points or at sites of ear cropping in young dogs), the deep dermis and subcutis contain large irregular and confluent foci of basophilic granular mineral. Appearance of the mineral varies from lightly basophilic and slightly granular to deeply basophilic and dense. Mineralized foci replace normal

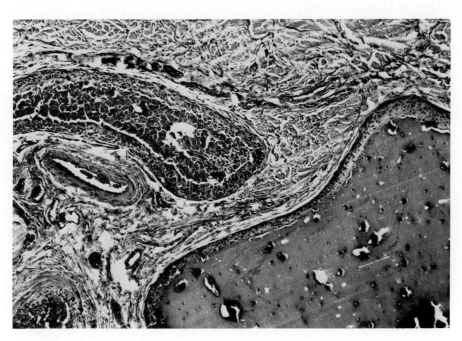

FIGURE 14-8. Calcinosis circumscripta in a dog. Large lakes of darkly staining mineral are surrounded by a thin zone of granulomatous inflammation. (×90.)

tissue and are surrounded by variably intense zones of macrophages and giant cells. Lymphocytes, neutrophils, and plasma cells may be observed between foci. Fibrosis surrounds and separates foci of mineralization and predominates in late lesions. Osseous metaplasia may be seen.

In apocrine cystic calcinosis, a very rare variant of calcinosis cutis, generation of the mineralized lesions from apocrine sweat glands is evident. Recognizable, well-differentiated sweat-gland epithelium may be noted at the margins of mineralized foci. Cystic but nonmineralized apocrine glands are found at the edges of the lesions. Similar lesions have been encountered in conjunction with cystic eccrine glands in humans. Generation of calcinosis cutis from cystic apocrine sweat glands has been overdiagnosed in the past; disordered clusters of cells at the margins of mineralized foci believed to be epithelial in origin were more likely epithelioid macrophages and giant cells.

Typical calcinosis circumscripta is distinctive histopathologically. In other forms of localized dystrophic calcification that accompany cysts or inflammatory foci, large lakes of mineral do not predominate as in typical forms of calcinosis circumscripta or in apocrine cystic calcinosis. Foci of mineralization tend to be smaller, and the contributing process, such as inflammation or neoplasia, is still plainly evident.

CUTANEOUS MUCINOSIS/MYXEDEMA
Clinical features (Figures 14-9 and 14-10)

Cutaneous mucinosis is the excessive accumulation or deposition of mucin in the dermis. Mucin, a jelly-like, clear, viscid glycosaminoglycan, is an acid mucopolysaccharide produced in the skin by dermal fibroblasts. Mucinosis is rare in the dog, with the exception of the Chinese Shar Pei. Abnormal deposition may be focal or diffuse and may vary from mild to severe. Mucinosis may occur as a primary condition, presumably because of congenital or acquired metabolic defects, or mucinosis may be seen in association with other diseases. The term *myxedema* is used more specifically to connote mucinosis seen with hypothyroidism.

Clinically, generalized mucinosis may be manifested as thickened, nonpitting, puffy skin. This is seen most frequently in some so-called normal Chinese Shar Peis. Normal skin integrity is not compromised in mild-to-moderate mucinosis. If generalized mucinosis is severe, skin integrity is compromised and increased skin fragility results. Mucin may exude from abraded areas, leaving a sticky, viscid fluid on the skin surface. Severe focal mucinosis also is most often seen in the Chinese Shar Pei and is associated with some degree of generalized mucinosis. Multiloculated vesicles or bullae have the appearance of bubbles. Rupture of these vesicles yields tenacious, syrupy, viscid fluid. Rarely, focal or multifocal mucinosis, sometimes termed *papular mucinosis,* may be seen in other breeds and is not associated with generalized mucinosis. Solitary or occasionally multiple, white or yellow papules or clear "blisters" are noted as incidental findings and most frequently are localized to the head and neck.

Myxedema is a rare manifestation of canine hypothyroidism. Symmetric thickening of facial skin results in folds that impart the appearance of so-called tragic facies. Recently, Miller reported mucinous vesic-

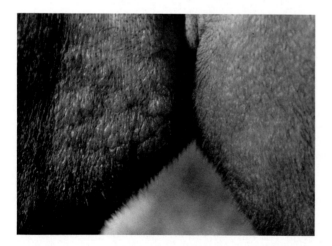

FIGURE 14-9. Cutaneous mucinosis in a Chinese Shar Pei. Multilobulated vesicles and bullae on the caudal thighs have the appearance of bubbles.

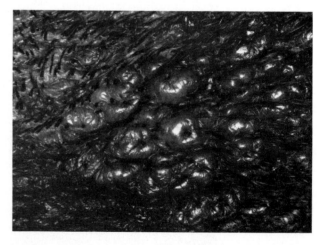

FIGURE 14-10. Closeup of cutaneous mucinosis on the ventral chest of a Chinese Shar Pei. Turgid bullae span multiple hair follicles.

ulation without generalized myxedema as an unusual manifestation of hypothyroidism.

Cutaneous mucinosis is rare in every breed except the Chinese Shar Pei. Age or sex predilections have not been noted. Focal and generalized mucinosis of the Chinese Shar Pei is distinctive clinically, as is myxedema of hypothyroidism. Papular mucinosis may mimic vesicles or cysts of other causes.

Biopsy site selection

Biopsy specimens should be procured from areas of most obvious thickening, since mucinosis may be subtle histopathologically. If focal mucinosis is suspected, wedge biopsy technique is recommended because of the fragility of the lesions. In addition, excisional biopsy of severe lesions may be palliative in the Chinese Shar Pei.

Histopathology (Figure 14-11)

The epidermis is normal in primary mucinosis or will vary based on the underlying disease present. For example, mild or moderate acanthosis usually will be present in hypothyroidism.

The dermis shows widening of spaces between collagen fibers by a pale gray or gray-blue substance in sections stained with hematoxylin and eosin. Mucin is blue or blue-green using Alcian blue stain (pH of 2.5). Deposition of mucin is uniform between collagen fibers of the superficial and deep dermis in generalized mucinosis of the Chinese Shar Pei and in myxedema

and may extend to the subcutis. Papular mucinosis or severe focal mucinosis of the Chinese Shar Pei is characterized by lakes of mucin in the superficial and middle dermis that displace normal dermal collagen. Inflammation is not a feature of uncomplicated mucinosis; however, most specimens obtained from the Chinese Shar Pei have concurrent inflammatory skin disease; mucinosis is rarely the reason for biopsy in this breed unless severe focal mucinosis is present.

Clinically inapparent mucinosis has been reported by Rosenkrantz (1986) as a histopathologic feature of discoid lupus erythematosus. However, the authors have noted microscopic evidence of mucin as an incidental feature of a variety of inflammatory conditions, including severe pyoderma. Visualization of mucin in routine sections stained with hematoxylin and eosin depends on the staining technique used and thus may vary from laboratory to laboratory.

Differentiation of mucinosis or myxedema from urticaria may be necessary when the water content of the dermal mucin is high (resulting in pale staining by hematoxylin and eosin). Mucin stains are helpful; differentiating clinical features also may allow clear separation of these two entities.

CUTANEOUS AMYLOIDOSIS
Clinical features

Cutaneous amyloidosis is a very rare syndrome in the dog and cat that is characterized by an abnormal

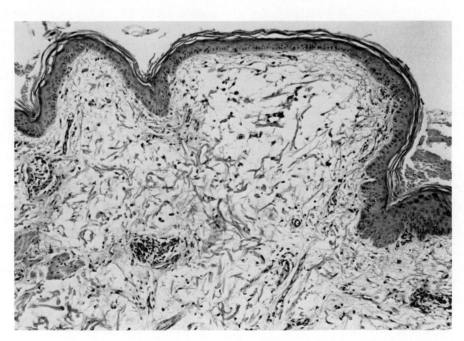

FIGURE 14-11. Focal cutaneous mucinosis in a dog. Note widening of the spaces between collagen fibers by pale staining mucin. (×90.)

accumulation of various proteinaceous deposits. The term *amyloid* refers to a group of protein products that appear hyaline and eosinophilic on hematoxylin and eosin staining and have a high affinity for certain dyes, such as Congo red. Most forms of cutaneous amyloidosis observed to date in dogs and cats probably are caused by immunoglobulin light chains, amyloid AL (referring to light chains). Although amyloid appears hyaline or amorphous microscopically, it is composed of fibrils with distinctive ultrastructural characteristics.

Amyloid deposition may be confined to the skin, or it may be seen in conjunction with systemic amyloidosis. In primary nodular cutaneous amyloidosis, amyloid is deposited in the skin, usually with no evidence of systemic disease. Primary nodular amyloidosis may be the result of abnormal production of amyloidogenic immunoglobulin light chains by locally proliferating plasma cells, as has been shown in humans. Primary nodular cutaneous amyloidosis in humans, dogs, and cats has been associated most often with localized plasma cell proliferation or a discrete cutaneous extramedullary plasmacytoma (see Chapter 31). In contrast, a feline case of cutaneous nodular amyloidosis within an extramedullary plasmacytoma, described by Carothers, also had internal metastases with amyloid deposition and a monoclonal gammopathy (systemic amyloidosis).

Primary systemic amyloidosis affecting the skin most often accompanies multiple myeloma or defects in immunoglobulin metabolism. In cutaneous amyloidosis of this type, deposition of amyloid in the skin is usually diffuse and finely distributed. Immunoglobulin-associated diffuse cutaneous amyloidosis was reported by Schwartzman in a dog with a monoclonal gammopathy; a plasma-cell dyscrasia other than multiple myeloma was probably present because multiple myeloma could not be documented.

Clinically, primary nodular cutaneous amyloidosis is the most frequent type of cutaneous amyloidosis in dogs and cats. Solitary or, rarely, grouped firm nodules are noted in the dermis or subcutis. The nodules are asymptomatic unless larger masses outgrow their blood supply, resulting in necrosis and ulceration. The ear is a common site, but nodules may be seen at any location.

Unexplained purpura is the major cutaneous manifestation of the very rare primary systemic amyloidosis. Hemorrhage may be seen as a sequela to epilation of hair or other minor trauma. Amyloid accumulations often are not visible clinically, since deposits are distributed diffusely in the dermis and dermal blood vessels. Papules and plaques may be observed.

Breed, age, or sex predilections have not been determined for either form of cutaneous amyloidosis. However, because of the association with multiple myeloma and extramedullary plasmacytoma, immuno-globulin-associated amyloidosis should be seen more frequently in older animals.

Clinical differential diagnoses for primary nodular cutaneous amyloidosis should include solitary neoplasms and infectious and noninfectious granulomas and pyogranulomas. Primary systemic amyloidosis affecting the skin should be considered in the differential diagnosis of unexplained cutaneous hemorrhage.

Biopsy site selection

If possible, solitary nodular lesions should be removed by excisional biopsy, which provides a cure as well as a diagnosis. Partially removed masses will not heal well because of the lack of integrity of amyloid-laden tissue, which physically interferes with the healing process. Primary systemic amyloidosis may be confirmed by either punch or wedge biopsy of skin displaying purpura after minimal trauma. Site selection is not critical.

Histopathology (Figures 14-12 through 14-14)

Primary nodular cutaneous amyloidosis may evolve from an amyloid-producing extramedullary plasmacytoma (see Chapter 31). Plasmacytomas of the skin of dogs are common, but amyloid is found only occasionally; thus apparently only a subset of plasma cell tumors possesses the ability to elaborate amyloid. Amyloid can be a minor component of extramedullary plasmacytomas or may predominate in cutaneous nodules. Rowland showed that the plasma cells in amyloid-predominant lesions reacted to a single class of immunoglobulins (IgG), thus indicating probable monoclonality and neoplastic derivation.

Primary nodular cutaneous amyloidosis is characterized by multiple accumulations of amorphous-appearing eosinophilic deposits. Generally well-differentiated but occasionally atypical plasma cells accumulate among foci of amyloid in variable but often sparse numbers. Macrophages and smaller numbers of lymphocytes are seen in association with nodular amyloid, and macrophages frequently surround amyloid deposits.

A single case of primary systemic amyloidosis affecting the skin in a dog was described by Schwartzman. Amyloid was deposited in a laminar fashion in the superficial dermis and around blood vessels of the superficial plexus. Nodular deposition was not present, nor was accompanying plasmacellular infiltrate described.

Amyloid is birefringent and dichroic (orange to apple green) using Congo red stain and a polarizing lens. Application of thioflavine T stain will result in amyloid fluorescence using fluorescent microscopy. Ultrastructurally, amyloid is a highly organized fibrillar structure composed of proteinaceous deposits in cross-beta, antiparallel, beta-pleated sheets.

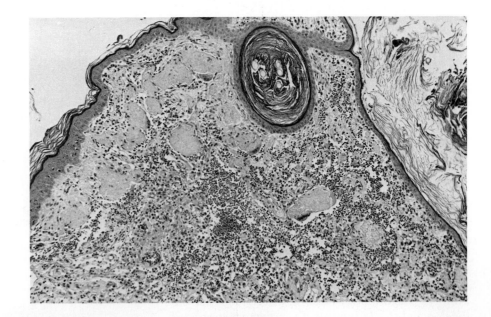

FIGURE 14-12. Cutaneous amyloidosis in a dog. Pale, somewhat nodular deposits of amyloid are distributed throughout the dermis. Note the severe hemorrhage. (×90.)

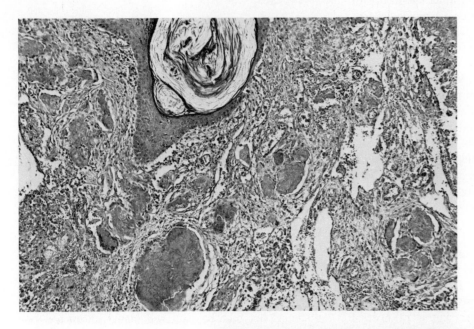

FIGURE 14-13. Cutaneous amyloidosis in a dog. Congo red–positive amyloid is homogeneous and darkly staining. Most of the cellular infiltrate is composed of plasma cells. (Congo red stain; ×90.)

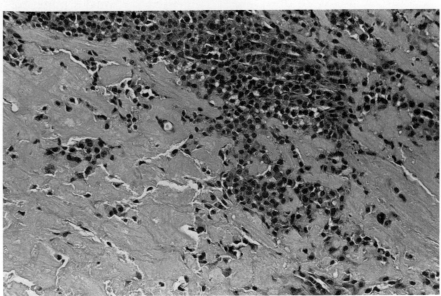

FIGURE 14-14. Cutaneous amyloidosis in a dog. Amyloid is accumulating among monomorphous plasma cells. (×220.)

Amyloid has a distinctive histopathologic appearance, but occasionally may be confused with serum or fibrin in inflammatory lesions. Appropriate staining and polarization will distinguish amyloid. Amorphous-appearing eosinophilic material within an extramedullary plasmacytoma is most likely amyloid.

CUTANEOUS ASTHENIA (Synonyms:
Ehlers-Danlos syndrome, dermatosparaxis)
Clinical features (Figures 14-15 through 14-17)

Cutaneous asthenia is a disease complex that encompasses several heritable congenital defects of dermal connective tissue. Clinically, these diseases are characterized by variable degrees of skin hyperextensibility and fragility. Cutaneous asthenia is rare in both the dog and cat. In humans, 11 distinct subgroups of cutaneous asthenia (usually termed *Ehlers-Danlos syndrome*) have been documented. The biochemical defects delineated in humans include diminished collagen synthesis, intracellular collagen accumulation, improper collagen packing, enzyme deficiencies, procollagen structural mutations, and abnormal fibronectin formation. Dominant cutaneous asthenia caused by improper collagen formation and packing has been documented in the dog and cat by Minor (1980) and Patterson, whereas recessive cutaneous asthenia associated with procollagen peptidase deficiency has been identified in the cat by Counts. Considerable variability in other clinical cases observed suggest that additional specific defects of dermal collagen exist in dogs and cats.

Hyperextensibility and decreased tensile strength of the skin are the unifying clinical features and may be present individually or in concert. Hyperextensibility is characterized clinically by a loose attachment of the skin to subjacent structures. The skin is of normal

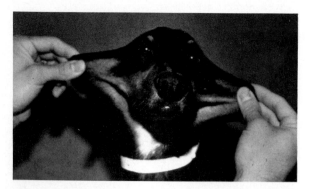

FIGURE 14-16. Cutaneous asthenia in a Dachshund showing severe hyperextensibility of the facial skin. *(Courtesy SI Reinke, Corte Madera, California; case material from the University of California, Davis.)*

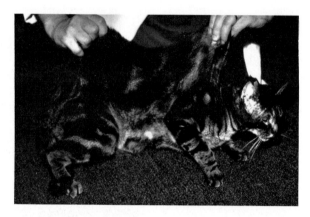

FIGURE 14-17. Cutaneous asthenia in a cat. The skin of the thorax is grossly hyperextensible. *(Courtesy GA Kunkle and J Kunkle, Gainesville, Florida.)*

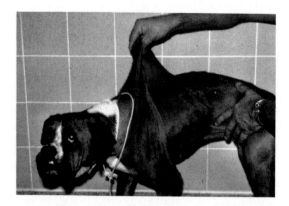

FIGURE 14-15. Cutaneous asthenia in a Boxer. Marked hyperextensibility of the skin is demonstrated. *(Courtesy AA Stannard, Davis, California.)*

thickness but may be stretched many centimeters beyond that possible in normal dogs or cats. Decreased tensile strength leads to lacerations from minimal trauma. Large, gaping wounds have been likened visually to "fish mouths." Surprisingly, little bleeding occurs from these striking lesions. Rapid healing ensues, although the scars that form are thin, abnormally pigmented, and lack normal tensile strength. The term *cigarette paper* has been used to describe these atrophic scars. Subcutaneous hematomas are a less common sequela. Joint hyperextensibility, a common coexistent feature of some subgroups of Ehlers-Danlos syndrome in humans, has been noted rarely in the dog. Stannard has seen a litter of Dachshunds with marked concomitant skin and joint hyperextensibility.*

Cutaneous asthenia has been seen in the Boxer,

* Stannard AA: Personal communication, 1990.

Dachshund, English Springer Spaniel, Greyhound, Beagle, Saint Bernard, mixed-breed dog, domestic short-haired cat, and the Himalayan cat. Sex predilections have not been noted. Signs of cutaneous asthenia generally are noted shortly after birth.

Clinically, cutaneous asthenia is highly characteristic in both dogs and cats. A lifelong history of fragility in skin of apparently normal thickness and hyperextensibility coupled with physical findings of multiple scars or gaping wounds indicate cutaneous asthenia. Definitive diagnosis may require electron microscopy and special biochemical analysis of dermal collagen (not commercially available).

Differential diagnosis is generally not difficult because of the characteristic clinical features of this syndrome. Easily traumatized skin is a feature of feline skin fragility syndrome; markedly thin skin seen in that condition is not a feature of cutaneous asthenia.

Biopsy site selection

Skin specimens adjacent to lesions may be procured by either punch or wedge technique. Care should be taken in choosing sites such that self-trauma or normal activity does not extend the biopsy site to form a new lesion. The dorsal thorax between the scapulae is an ideal site, since the skin is not taut in this region and self-trauma is difficult to accomplish. Areas near pressure points should be avoided.

Histopathology (Figures 14-18 and 14-19)

The epidermis is unremarkable. Dermal collagen may have a normal appearance, and thus a diagnosis of

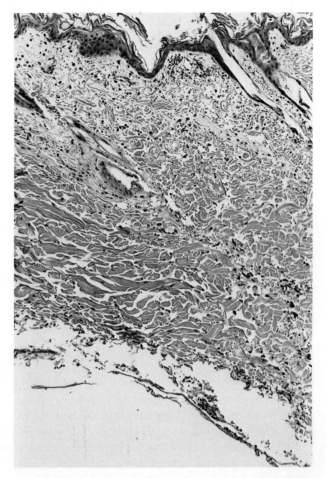

FIGURE 14-18. Cutaneous asthenia in a cat. Note the torn lower edge of the dermis accompanied by mild hemorrhage. (×90.)

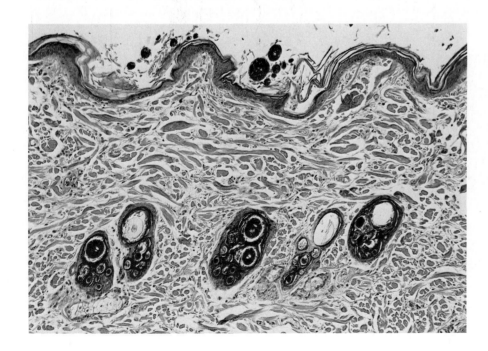

FIGURE 14-19. Cutaneous asthenia in a dog. Dermal collagen fibers are markedly variable in size. *(Case material from E Clark, Saskatoon, Saskatchewan.)* *(×90.)*

cutaneous asthenia frequently cannot be made based on light microscopy alone. Hegreberg reported microscopic fragmentation and disorganization of collagen fibers. Uneven size of dermal collagen bundles has been observed by the authors and others* in some canine cases; fewer large bundles are interwoven with widely spaced, thin, fibrillar bundles. According to Calderwood Mays, marked variation in the size of the dermal collagen bundles may be seen occasionally in normal canine skin, depending on fixation and processing.†

Variability of histopathologic lesions may be caused by the existence of multiple syndromes characterized by separate biochemical defects with variable

---

*Clark E: Personal communication, 1989.
†Calderwood Mays MB: Personal communication, 1989.

---

light microscopic expression. Electron microscopic and biochemical analysis of the dermal collagen are needed for definitive diagnosis.

Biopsy of tears or lacerations may reveal splitting within the dermis. The dermis may end abruptly and granulation tissue may be evident at the deep margin, suggesting a recent tear at that location.

Because of the inconsistent microscopic features of this disease and the often normal appearance of biopsy specimens, histopathologic diagnosis is problematic. Shearing trauma, such as that caused by a degloving injury, might mimic the tears of Ehlers Danlos syndrome. Feline skin fragility syndrome, also characterized by intradermal splitting, is distinct histopathologically in that severe dermal atrophy with marked thinning of collagen fibers is present.

FELINE SKIN FRAGILITY SYNDROME
Clinical features (Figures 14-20 and 14-21)

Feline skin fragility syndrome is a rare disease of multifactorial etiology characterized by markedly fragile, thin skin. The syndrome may be associated with naturally occurring or iatrogenic hyperglucocorticoidism, diabetes mellitus, or with the excessive use of megestrol acetate or other progestational compounds. Diquelou described a cat with skin fragility and hepatic lipidosis and showed ultrastructural alteration of the affected dermal collagen. A small number of cats with this syndrome have had normal serum biochemical profiles and adrenal function tests.

The skin of affected cats becomes markedly thin and is damaged readily by minor trauma. Skin friability

leads to irregular tears such that sheets of skin may be shed. Surgical repair is difficult and often leads to more extensive damage, since the surrounding skin shares the same defect. The combined epidermis and dermis may be so attenuated that the skin acquires a translucent quality. Partial alopecia may be seen.

Breed, age, or sex predilections have not been noted. Clinical differential diagnosis is not difficult. Skin fragility also is seen with cutaneous asthenia, but the unscarred skin is not abnormally thin. Iatrogenic and endogenous endocrinologic causes of feline skin fragility syndrome must be investigated.

Biopsy site selection

If possible, intact skin rather than skin fragments from lacerations or tears should be selected. Because of

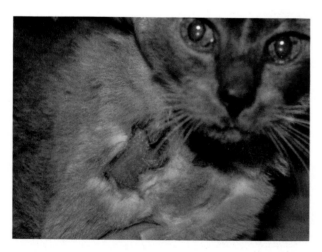

FIGURE 14-20. Feline skin fragility syndrome. Skin friability has led to irregular tears on the neck. *(Courtesy GA Kunkle, Gainesville, Florida.)*

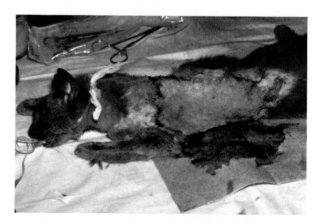

FIGURE 14-21. Feline skin fragility syndrome. Marked skin friability has led to large irregular tears such that sheets of skin have been shed. *(Courtesy MD Song, Phoenix, Arizona; case material from the University of California, Davis.)*

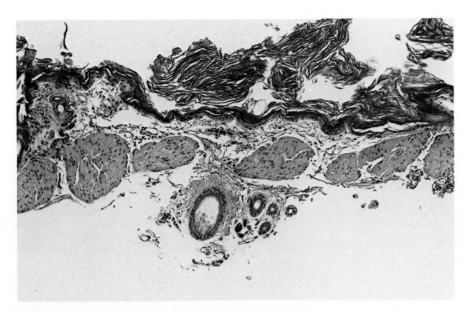

FIGURE 14-22. Feline skin fragility syndrome. The epidermis and dermis are severely atrophic; residual arrector pili muscles are prominent. (×90.)

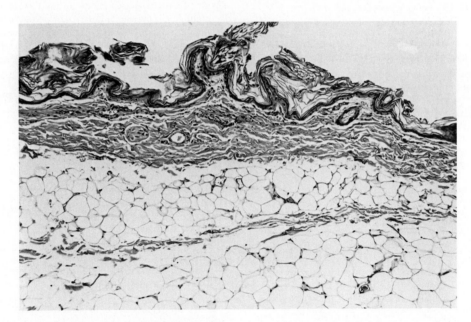

FIGURE 14-23. Feline skin fragility syndrome. The epidermis and dermis are severely atrophic. Note the normal panniculus. (×90.)

the extreme thinness of the skin, skin biopsy is performed with difficulty. The tissue often folds and twists similar to wet tissue paper, which results in inferior specimens for histopathology. Care to include underlying adipose tissue and to maintain its attachment to the overlying dermis by gentle handling is advised. Placement of the specimen on a portion of a wooden applicator or tongue depressor will allow the shape to be retained for optimal tissue processing by the laboratory.

Histopathology (Figures 14-22 and 14-23)

The epidermis is thin and may consist of only a single layer of keratinocytes. The dermis is severely atrophic. Dermal collagen fibers are extremely attenuated and pale staining and often have a wispy appearance. The biopsy specimen may be curled or irregular because of a lack of substantive dermis and twisting of the delicate specimen during fixation and processing. The panniculus usually is not represented in biopsy specimens; the base of the specimen may have strands of collagen fibers that appear torn or stretched because of separation of the dermis from the underlying panniculus during procurement of the specimen. Secondary neutrophilic inflammation and early scarring may be present if older lesions have been selected. Hair follicles may be uniformly small, short, and thin, but dermal atrophy is generally more striking than adnexal atrophy.

The histopathology of feline skin fragility syndrome is distinctive. Cutaneous asthenia, although manifested histopathologically by tears or splits in the dermis, generally has a dermis of normal thickness and lacks severe and diffuse attenuation of dermal collagen.

SUGGESTED READINGS

Calcinosis cutis

Lever WF and Schaumburg-Lever G: Histopathology of the skin, Philadelphia, 1990, JB Lippincott, pp 466-469.

Miller LM and Krane SM: Skin and subcutaneous tissue: calcification, ossification and neoplasms. In Fitzpatrick TB, Eisen AZ, Wolff K and others, editors: Dermatology in general medicine, New York, 1987, McGraw-Hill, pp 1763-1775.

Paradis M and Scott DW: Calcinosis cutis secondary to percutaneous penetration of calcium carbonate in a Dalmatian, Can Vet J 30:57-59, 1989.

Schick MP, Schick RO, and Richardson JA: Calcinosis cutis secondary to percutaneous penetration of calcium chloride, J Am Vet Med Assoc 191:207-211, 1987.

White SD and others: Cutaneous markers of canine hyperadrenocorticism, Comp Small Anim 11:446-463, 1989.

Calcinosis circumscripta

Anderson WI and Scott DW: Calcinosis circumscripta in a domestic short-haired cat, Cornell Vet 77:348-350, 1987.

Christie GS and Jabara AG: Apocrine cystic calcinosis: the sweat gland origin of calcinosis circumscripta in the dog, Res Vet Sci 5:317-322, 1964.

Cordy DR: Apocrine cystic calcinosis in dogs and its relationship to chronic renal disease, Cornell Vet 57:107-118, 1967.

DiGuardo G: Calcinosis circumscripta: speaking out, J Am Anim Hosp Assoc 25:618, 1989.

Flo GL and Tvedten H: Cervical calcinosis circumscripta in three related Great Dane dogs, J Am Anim Hosp Assoc 11:507-510, 1975.

Legendre AM and Dade AW: Calcinosis circumscripta in a dog, J Am Vet Med Assoc 164:1192-1194, 1974.

Lever WF and Schaumburg-Lever G: Histopathology of the skin, Philadelphia, 1990, JB Lippincott, pp 466-469.

Miller LM and Krane SM: Skin and subcutaneous tissue: calcification, ossification and neoplasms. In Fitzpatrick TB, Eisen AZ, Wolff K and others, editors: Dermatology in general medicine, New York, 1987, McGraw-Hill, pp 1763-1775.

Muller GH, Kirk RW, and Scott DW: Small animal dermatology, ed 4, Philadelphia, 1989, WB Saunders, pp 949-952.

Roudebush P, Maslin WR, and Cooper RC: Canine tumoral calcinosis, Comp Cont Ed 10:1162-1165, 1988.

Scott DW and Buerger RG: Idiopathic calcinosis circumscripta in the dog: a retrospective analysis of 130 cases, J Am Anim Hosp Assoc 24:651-658, 1988.

Stampley A and Bellah JR: Calcinosis circumscripta of the metacarpal pad in a dog, J Am Vet Med Assoc 196:113-114, 1990.

Cutaneous mucinosis/myxedema

Beale KM, Calderwood Mays MB, and Buchanan B: Papular and plaque-like mucinosis in a puppy, Vet Dermatol 2(1):29-35, 1991.

Dilberger JE and Altman NJ: Focal mucinosis in dogs: 7 cases and review of cutaneous mucinoses of man and animals, Vet Pathol 23:132-139, 1986.

From L and Assaad D: Neoplasms, pseudoneoplasms, hyperplasias, and mucinoses of supporting tissue origin. In Fitzpatrick TB, Eisen AZ, Wolff K and others, editors: Dermatology in general medicine, New York, 1987, McGraw-Hill, pp 1033-1052.

Miller WH and Buerger RG: Cutaneous mucinous vesiculation in a dog with hypothyroidism, J Am Vet Med Assoc 196:757-759, 1990.

Rosenkrantz WS and others: Idiopathic cutaneous mucinosis in a dog, Comp Anim Pract 1:39-42, 1987.

Rosenkrantz WS and others: Histopathological evaluation of acid mucopolysaccharide (mucin) in canine discoid lupus erythematosus, J Am Anim Hosp Assoc 22:577-584, 1986.

Truhan AP and Roenigk HH: The cutaneous mucinoses, J Am Acad Dermatol 14:1-18, 1986.

Cutaneous amyloidosis

Calkins E: Amyloidosis of the skin. In Fitzpatrick TB, Eisen AZ, Wolff K and others, editors: Dermatology in general medicine, New York, 1987, McGraw-Hill, pp 1655-1666.

Carothers MA and others: Extramedullary plasmacytoma and immunoglobulin-associated amyloidosis in a cat, J Am Vet Med Assoc 195:1593-1597, 1989.

Lever WF and Schaumburg-Lever G: Histopathology of the skin, Philadelphia, 1990, JB Lippincott, pp 452-457.

Rowland PH and others: Cutaneous plasmacytomas with amyloid in six dogs, Vet Pathol 28:125-130, 1991.

Schwartzman RM: Cutaneous amyloidosis associated with a monoclonal gammopathy in a dog, J Am Vet Med Assoc 185:102-104, 1984.

Cutaneous asthenia

Counts DF and others: Dermatosparaxis in a Himalayan cat. I. Biochemical studies of dermal collagen, J Invest Dermatol 74:96-99, 1980.

Hegreberg GA, Padgett GA, and Henson J: A heritable connective tissue disease of dogs and mink resembling the Ehlers-Danlos syndrome of man. III. Histopathologic changes of the skin, Arch Pathol 90:159-166, 1970.

Lever WF and Schaumburg-Lever G: Histopathology of the skin, Philadelphia, 1990, JB Lippincott, pp 87-89.

Minor RR: Animal models of heritable diseases of skin. In Goldsmith LA, editor: Biochemistry and physiology of the skin, New York, 1983, Oxford University Press, pp 1139-1152.

Minor RR: Collagen metabolism: a comparison of diseases of collagen and diseases affecting collagen, Am J Pathol 98:225-280, 1980.

Patterson DF and Minor RR: Hereditary fragility and hyperextensibility of the skin of cats: a defect in collagen fibrillogenesis, Lab Invest 37:170-179, 1977.

Pinnell SR and McKusick VA: Heritable disorders of connective tissue with skin changes. In Fitzpatrick TB, Eisen AZ, Wolff K and others, editors: Dermatology in general medicine, New York, 1987, McGraw-Hill, pp 1780-1786.

Feline skin fragility syndrome

Diquelou A and others: Lipoidose hepatique et syndrome de fragilité cutanée chez un chat, Pratique Medicale et Chirurgicale de l'Animal de Compagne 26:151-158, 1991.

Diseases of the hair follicles

Pustular and nodular diseases without follicular destruction

The diseases of this chapter are characterized by pustular or nodular follicular inflammation without prominent follicular destruction and effacement. Sebaceous adenitis also has been placed in this chapter, although inflammation is adnexal rather than follicular. Clear-cut delineation of this pattern of follicular inflammation from inflammation associated with follicular damage (see Chapter 16) is not always possible, since most follicular inflammation disrupts follicular integrity to some degree. In general, the follicular inflammation of the diseases described in this chapter is less severe and more superficial in location. Histopathologic differentiation among these diseases is generally accomplished by identification of an agent (dermatophytosis), by the recognition of an associated histopathologic feature such as acantholysis (pemphigus foliaceus), or by the predominant cell type (sterile eosinophilic pustulosis).

SUPERFICIAL BACTERIAL FOLLICULITIS (Synonym: superficial pyoderma)

Clinical features (Figures 15-1 and 15-2)

Superficial bacterial folliculitis is a common canine skin disease characterized by superficial follicular pustules. The only canine skin disease seen globally with greater frequency is flea allergy dermatitis. As in other types of canine pyoderma, *Staphylococcus intermedius* is the primary pathogen. Superficial bacterial folliculitis is very rare in cats; concrete data on the clinical presentation are not available.

Most bacterial folliculitis in dogs is seen secondary to coexistent disease or in conjunction with other predisposing factors. Common coexistent diseases or syndromes include seborrhea, atopy, hypothyroidism, and naturally occurring and iatrogenic hyperglucocorticoidism. Other predisposing factors include inflammation or pruritus from any source, defects in the immune response, and poor grooming. The specific initiating factors in the development of pyoderma are not known. Cats that develop superficial folliculitis may be immunosuppressed.

The clinical presentation of canine bacterial folliculitis is highly variable because of differences in breed response, individual host resistance, and intrinsic differences in bacterial virulence. The unifying clinical feature in bacterial folliculitis is the formation of follicular pustules. Pustules vary greatly in size and may be difficult to identify with the naked eye. Intact pustules have an erythematous base and contain white or creamy yellow purulent material. Pustules are transient because of their fragile nature and rupture easily, eventuating in crusted papules. Consequently, crusted papules are the most common lesion seen in superficial bacterial folliculitis. A hand lens may be useful

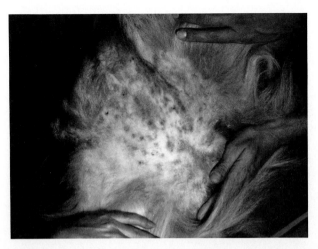

FIGURE 15-1 Superficial bacterial folliculitis on the abdomen of a Keeshond. Pustules, crusted papules, and mottled hyperpigmentation are present.

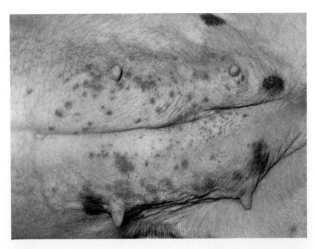

FIGURE 15-2 Superficial bacterial folliculitis on the abdomen of a Bull Terrier. Intact follicular pustules and erythematous papules are seen in a partially intertriginous location.

in determining if intact pustules are follicular rather than between follicles (as seen in pemphigus foliaceus and other superficial pustular diseases of the epidermis; see Chapter 1), since follicular pustules will have central protruding hairs unless the hair has been shed. Erythema and swelling are highly variable. Alopecia also is variable but is a common feature if substantial inflammation is present. Distinct circular patches of transient, nonscarring alopecia may form around previously affected hair follicles and are more obvious in short-coated breeds. These patches of alopecia may be caused by focal, post-inflammatory telogen arrest.

Less commonly, larger, more firm papules, pustules, or nodules are seen in superficial bacterial folliculitis; histopathologically these lesions correspond to superficial perforating folliculitis. In cases of superficial bacterial folliculitis where inflammation is severe, the superficial keratin layer may lift and peel at the margin of the pustule, forming a peripheral collarette. This phenomenon may actually be superficial spreading pyoderma (see Chapter 1) coexisting with folliculitis. Rings of post-inflammatory hyperpigmentation may form within the boundaries of the collarette, or small, hyperpigmented punctate foci may directly mark the sites of more severely affected hair follicles and serve as additional diagnostic clues for superficial folliculitis.

Many cases of canine superficial bacterial folliculitis initially develop in the glabrous inguinal and axillary regions. The dorsal and ventral interdigital webs are additional predisposed sites. Superficial bacterial folliculitis may generalize, especially in dogs with iatrogenic or naturally occurring hyperglucocorticoidism. Pruritus of variable intensity is a common feature. Pru-

ritus and attendant self-trauma may not correlate with the degree of erythema. Regional lymphadenopathy is a common finding.

Breed predilections in dogs probably parallel the predilections for the predisposing or coexisting skin diseases. Age or sex predilections have not been noted.

Differential diagnoses vary with the clinical presentation. Other common causes of follicular pustules include demodicosis and dermatophytosis. Clinically, impetigo, pemphigus foliaceus, subcorneal pustular dermatosis, and sterile eosinophilic pustulosis may resemble superficial bacterial folliculitis. Superficial spreading pyoderma may coexist with superficial folliculitis if the pustules are accompanied by prominent collarette formation. Superficial spreading pyoderma may actually originate from superficial follicular pustules (see Chapter 1), but has more prominent collarette formation and less obvious pustulation than does superficial folliculitis. Differentiation is accomplished by the microscopic examination of smears from pustules, skin scrapings, dermatophyte culture, bacterial culture, and histopathology. If only crusted papules are present, superficial bacterial folliculitis also must be differentiated from predominantly papular dermatoses such as flea allergy dermatitis.

Biopsy site selection

Skin biopsy specimens should be obtained from intact pustules if available. Crusted papules are not ideal because they represent pustules in advanced stages of degeneration. Lesions with excessive crusting should be avoided. Specimens that have been punctured for smears or culture should not be used as specimens for skin biopsy.

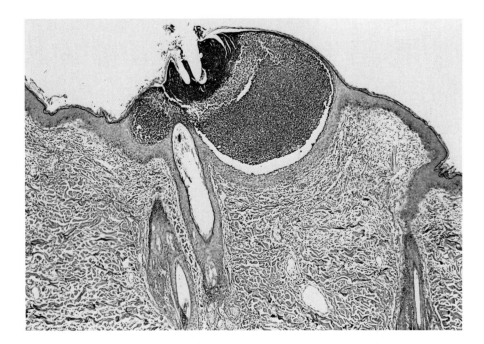

FIGURE 15-3 Superficial bacterial folliculitis in a dog. A pustule distends a follicular ostium. (×35.)

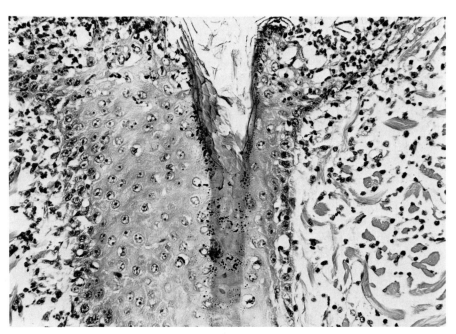

FIGURE 15-4 Superficial folliculitis in a dog. Neutrophils are closely apposed to the outer wall of a superficial follicle. (×220.)

Histopathology (Figures 15-3 and 15-4)

Folliculitis is characterized by the formation of pustules within the infundibulum or ostium of superficial follicles. Pustules are composed of neutrophils and variable eosinophils; in some cases eosinophils may be prominent. Pustules may extend from openings of hair follicles into the adjacent superficial epidermis. As pustules age, superficial follicular or epidermal crusts occur. Neutrophils may closely align themselves along the outer wall of an inflamed superficial follicle; mild exocytosis into the wall may be evident.

The dermis is variably edematous and inflamed. Commonly, loosely organized accumulations of neutrophils, eosinophils, and mixed mononuclear cells surround free keratin in the superficial dermis adjacent to or at the site of previous hair follicles. This pattern of inflammation indicates rupture of an inflamed follicle, with extension of the inflammatory process beyond its confines. Occasionally, actual perforation by a pustule through the wall of a superficial follicle can be observed (superficial perforating folliculitis). Since histopathologic examination includes the lesions at only one level, superficial dermal pustules may be present in the dermis in one section, whereas deeper sections may reveal the affected follicle. Thus folliculitis can be inferred in cases where no actual follicular inflammation is present, particularly if pustules are found in the general vicinity of the hair follicle and if they contain follicular debris.

The superficial dermis in other areas of the specimen may have mild superficial accumulations of neutrophils, plasma cells, macrophages, and lymphocytes. In chronic lesions, perifollicular and perivascular infiltrations of plasma cells, macrophages, and a few neutrophils may predominate, rather than active pustular inflammation. Mild perifollicular fibrosis may be present.

Affected and adjacent hair follicles are often in the telogen phase, possibly as a direct effect of inflammation on the hair growth cycle (telogen arrest). This may explain the transient patchy hair loss seen in dogs with bacterial folliculitis, since dogs normally have a mosaic, asynchronous hair replacement pattern.* However, the presence of telogen hair follicles may also signal the presence of intercurrent endocrine disease (see Chapter 17).

Differential diagnoses in dogs are few if follicular pustules are found. Sterile eosinophilic pustulosis is characterized in part by follicular pustules, but eosinophils predominate. Care should be taken not to rely exclusively on the type of inflammation present, since antibiotic-responsive eosinophilic folliculitis may occasionally be encountered in the dog. Clinical differentiation is required. Superficial spreading pyoderma may generate from superficial follicular pustules of the infundibulum or ostium, but folliculitis is difficult to observe in random biopsy; in contrast, superficial follicular or dermal pustulation (secondary to perforation) is obvious in most biopsy specimens of superficial folliculitis.

* Stannard AA: Personal communication, 1988.

FELINE DERMATOPHYTOSIS

(Synonym: feline ringworm)

Clinical features (Figures 15-5 and 15-6)

Dermatophytosis is one of the most common feline skin diseases. Wide variation in incidence exists globally; warm temperatures and high humidity encourage dermatophyte infection. Greater than 95% of the cases of feline dermatophytosis worldwide probably are caused by *Microsporum canis*. The species designation *Microsporum canis* actually is a misnomer, since the cat is the natural host for this organism. Since this well-adapted dermatophyte induces minimal host response in the cat, inapparent carriers are common. *Trichophyton mentagrophytes*, *M. gypseum*, and various other keratinophilic fungi may, on occasion, cause feline dermatophytosis.

Keratinophilic fungi invade actively growing hair, hair follicles, and, less frequently, the stratum corneum of the epidermis. Transmission is achieved via direct contact or fomites contaminated with hair or scale. Cats with compromised immune systems secondary to naturally occurring or iatrogenic hyperglucocorticoidism, feline leukemia virus infection, or feline immunodeficiency virus infection are at greater risk for the

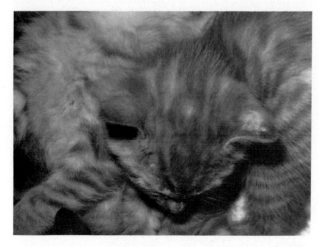

FIGURE 15-5 Feline dermatophytosis affecting multiple kittens in a litter. Patchy alopecia and scaling are present on the pinna, temporal region, and dorsal muzzle of the centrally located kitten.

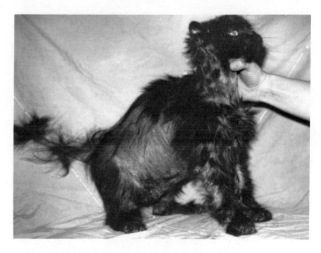

FIGURE 15-6 Generalized dermatophytosis in an adult Persian cat. Extensive alopecia, scaling, and hyperpigmentation are somewhat bilaterally symmetric.

development of generalized dermatophytosis. Feline dermatophytosis is the most common zoonotic skin disease.

Clinical signs of feline dermatophytosis are extremely variable. Inapparent carriage of *M. canis* is observed, particularly in cats from large catteries. Many cases are subtle and consist of irregular, patchy alopecia. Subtle alopecia with minimal other skin changes is seen more frequently in long-haired cats. Affected hairs are shorter than normal and appear mildly disheveled. Less commonly, expanding circular patches of alopecia with central clearing and healing may be present. Hair stubble may appear thickened, and follicular papules may be present. Scaling and crusting can vary from absent to severe. Crusted papules with minimal alopecia also can be a feature of feline dermatophytosis. Feline dermatophytic mycetoma (see Chapter 11) and nail infection (onychomycosis) are rare clinical variants. The face, ears, and forelimbs are the most common initial sites, but infection may generalize. Pruritus is uncommon with feline dermatophytosis.

Long-haired cats such as Persians may be at increased risk for both asymptomatic and symptomatic dermatophytosis. Overt dermatophytosis is seen most commonly in kittens and in adult cats in association with stresses such as queening. Sex predilections are not noted.

Clinical differential diagnoses are contingent upon the clinical presentation. Alopecia without underlying skin changes must be differentiated from pruritus-induced self-traumatic alopecia, psychogenic alopecia, and demodicosis. Severely exfoliative and crusting dermatophytosis may resemble autoimmune skin diseases such as pemphigus foliaceus. Skin scrapings, dermatophyte cultures, and skin biopsy should be performed to differentiate among these diseases.

Biopsy site selection

Biopsy specimens should be obtained from areas exhibiting broken hairs or exfoliation. Sites just within the outer boundaries of expanding foci of alopecia are most beneficial. Centers of alopecic foci may not be as helpful in establishing a diagnosis, since dermatophytes may no longer be present in these healing lesions.

Histopathology (Figures 15-7 and 15-8)

The epidermis may be mildly acanthotic and is often moderately hyperkeratotic. Crusts composed of degenerating neutrophils may be present around protruding hairs or free in superficial keratin.

Hair follicles and superficial vessels may be surrounded by small numbers of lymphocytes and macrophages, with scant or no neutrophils. Neutrophilic folliculitis is rarely evident but when encountered is highly suspicious for dermatophytosis. Surface (protruding) and intrafollicular hairs are colonized by variable numbers of refractile or slightly basophilic dermatophytic spores and hyphae that appear bright magenta with periodic acid–Schiff stain. Organisms may be extremely scant; it is not uncommon for only a single hair to be affected in a given biopsy specimen. Deeper sectioning may be required to locate the organ-

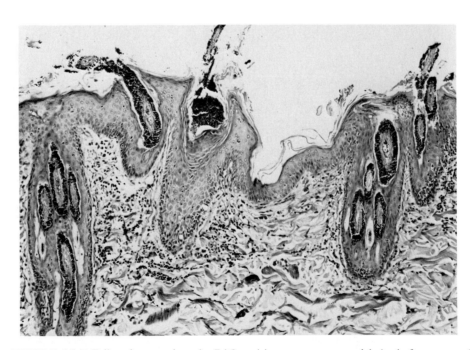

FIGURE 15-7 Feline dermatophytosis. PAS-positive spores surround hair shafts, many of which protrude from follicular ostia. Note the scant inflammation around hair follicles and in the superficial dermis. (Periodic acid-Schiff stain; ×90.)

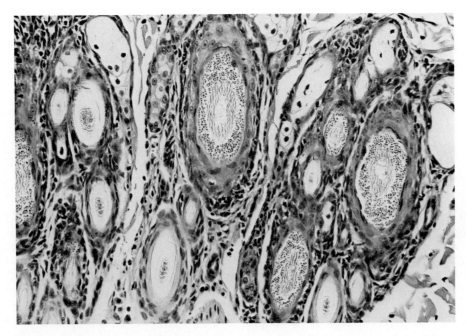

FIGURE 15-8 Feline dermatophytosis. Spores and hyphae heavily colonize hairs. Note the absence of inflammation. (×220.)

isms and provide an etiologic diagnosis in these cases.

In some cases of feline dermatophytosis, epidermal hyperkeratosis is the only histopathologic feature other than the presence of dermatophytes. Dermatophytes may be sparse; a careful search using a periodic acid–Schiff stain, if necessary, should always be made in any uninflamed specimen of skin obtained from a cat, particularly if scaling or alopecia is reported as a gross finding. The principal differential diagnosis in cases where folliculitis is present is demodicosis, which is extremely rare in the cat. Identification of dermatophytes is diagnostic in these cases, but even in the absence of histopathologically identifiable organisms, pustular folliculitis is a strong indication for dermatophytosis and should be pursued via dermatophyte culture. Very rarely, follicular pustules of presumed bacterial origin are observed histopathologically in immunosuppressed cats. Alopecia areata, a rare disease characterized by mild perifollicular lymphocytic inflammation, may resemble dermatophytosis. Inflammation in alopecia areata is centered around the hair bulb, whereas perifollicular inflammation in dermatophytosis is seen primarily in the middle portion of the hair follicle.

CANINE DERMATOPHYTOSIS
(Synonym: canine ringworm)
Clinical features (Figures 15-9 and 15-10)

Canine dermatophytosis is a common skin disease caused by infection with keratinophilic fungi. Wide variation exists globally in the incidence of dermatophytosis in general and in the prevalence of causative species. Warm temperatures and high humidity encourage dermatophyte infection. Canine dermatophytosis is caused most frequently by *Microsporum canis, Trichophyton mentagrophytes,* and *Microsporum gypseum. M. canis* is the most commonly isolated organism. Transmission occurs via direct contact or by fomites contaminated with hair or scale from affected cats or other dogs. Dermatophytes invade actively growing hair, the hair follicle, and less frequently, the stratum corneum of the epidermis. Well-adapted dermatophytes (usually *M. canis*) induce minimal host re-

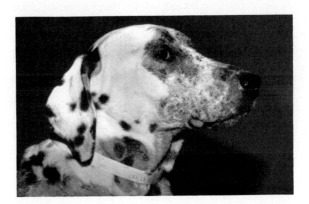

FIGURE 15-9 Dermatophytosis in a Dalmatian. Erythema and crusting are noted in well-demarcated alopecic plaques. *(Courtesy AC Mundell, Seattle, Washington; case material from the University of California, Davis.)*

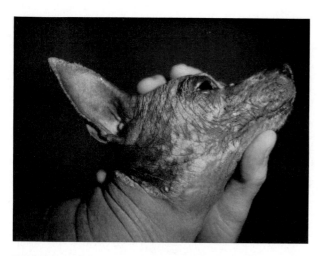

FIGURE 15-10 Dermatophytosis of the head and neck of a blue Toy Manchester Terrier with color-mutant alopecia. Hair regrew on the head following therapy for dermatophytosis.

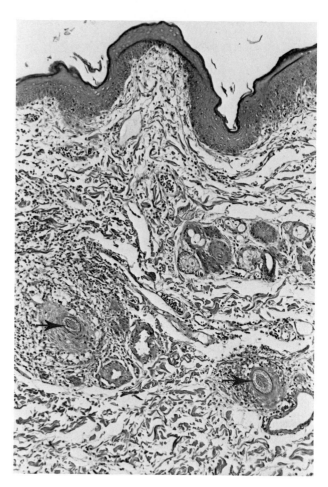

FIGURE 15-11 Canine dermatophytosis. Inflammation surrounds and partially infiltrates follicles. Note colonization of hair shafts by poorly stained hyphae *(arrows)*. (×90.)

sponse, and affected dogs may become inapparent carriers. Infection with *T. mentagrophytes, M. gypseum,* or other dermatophytes that are poorly adapted to the dog elicits a greater inflammatory reaction. Dermatophytosis usually is self-limiting in healthy dogs, since the normal host inflammatory response eliminates infection. Dogs with compromised immune systems are at greater risk for chronic and generalized disease. Canine dermatophytosis is a zoonotic disease.

Dermatophytosis is one of the most pleomorphic canine skin diseases. Classically, dermatophytosis presents as an expanding circular patch of alopecia with an erythematous active border and an area of central clearing and healing. Affected hairs either at the margin of alopecia or remaining within the patch of alopecia are thickened and broken. Follicular papules or frank pustules may be seen. Scaling and crusting vary from minimal to severe. The face and forelimbs are common sites for initial infection, since they interface most prominently with the environment. Somewhat symmetric facial involvement with marked exfoliation and crusting may be seen with *T. mentagrophytes* and *M. gypseum.*

Breed or sex predilections have not been determined statistically. However, the Dalmatian and the Poodle may be at increased risk for generalized disease. Dogs less than a year of age are at greater risk for dermatophytosis. Older dogs with decreased immune function may also be at increased risk for generalized dermatophytosis.

Clinical differential diagnoses are legion for this protean disease. Canine dermatophytosis is greatly overdiagnosed; conversely, bona fide cases are often misdiagnosed. Staphylococcal folliculitis is the major differential diagnosis, since both diseases may present

with rings of alopecia and crusting. Frank pustules and peripheral collarettes are substantially less common with dermatophytosis than with bacterial folliculitis. Seborrheic dermatitis may mimic dermatophytosis; seborrheic dermatitis is seen in breeds affected with primary seborrhea. Severe exfoliative and crusting dermatophytosis (especially facial) may be visually similar to pemphigus foliaceus or pemphigus erythematosus. A differentiating feature from pemphigus is that the planum nasale is rarely violated in facial dermatophytosis. Dermatophyte culture is critical in the differential diagnosis; histopathology also will allow differentiation.

Biopsy site selection

Biopsy specimens should be obtained from areas of broken hairs or exfoliation. Areas just inside the margins of expanding foci of inflammation and alopecia are most beneficial. Centers of alopecic foci may not be as helpful in establishing a diagnosis, since fungal organisms may no longer be present in healing lesions.

Histopathology (Figures 15-11 and 15-12)

The epidermis and follicular infundibula are variably acanthotic and may be hyperkeratotic. In some cases, surface serocellular crusting is evident. Protruding hair shafts may be entrapped by keratin and crusts. Dermatophytes may be seen in or around protruding hairs or occasionally free within epidermal keratin. Rarely, canine dermatophytosis may be characterized by colonization of epidermal keratin exclusively, with no involvement of follicular keratin or hair shafts. This form of dermatophytosis may be missed, since organisms can resemble cellular debris with hematoxylin and eosin staining.

Hair follicles are surrounded by mixtures of lymphocytes, macrophages, and neutrophils. Inflammation may be mild. Mild or moderate neutrophilic folliculitis may be present, and follicular rupture may be encountered. Discrete granulomas at the site of previous follicles surrounding central free hair may be seen in severe lesions. Hair shafts are variably infiltrated and surrounded by dermatophytic spores and hyphae, which are refractile with hematoxylin and eosin. A periodic acid–Schiff stain will accentuate dermatophytes as bright purple or magenta.

Rarely, cases of canine dermatophytosis are characterized by colonization of follicular and epidermal keratin only, without involvement of hair shafts. Two cases seen by one author* were in older dogs that were severely debilitated. Dermatophyte cultures were not obtained.

A superficially diffuse, somewhat lichenoid pattern of dermal inflammation may be encountered in the rare cases of dermatophytosis with colonization of epidermal keratin only. Plasma cells often predominate, but inflammation is mixed and includes neutrophils and macrophages. Basal cells are not obscured or damaged by the inflammation, as seen in many of the lichenoid dermatitides (see Chapter 10).

The folliculocentric inflammation of dermatophytosis may be similar to deep bacterial folliculitis and furunculosis and to demodicosis. Differential diagnosis is facilitated by identification of the offending agent. Generally, location of dermatophytes in tissue is more readily accomplished in the dog than in the cat (see preceding discussion).

PEMPHIGUS FOLIACEUS
Clinical features (Figures 15-13 and 15-14)

See Chapter 1.

Biopsy site selection

Because of the fragile and transient nature of primary lesions in pemphigus foliaceus, early lesions (pustules and vesicopustules) should be obtained promptly.

* Thelma Lee Gross.

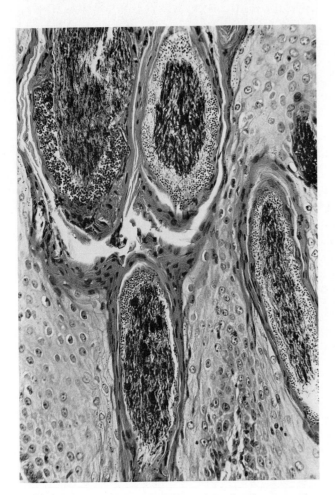

FIGURE 15-12 Canine dermatophytosis demonstrating heavy colonization of hairs by numerous dermatophytic spores and wavy, poorly stained hyphae. (×220.)

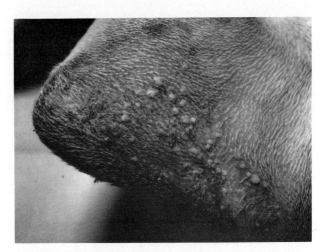

FIGURE 15-13 Pemphigus foliaceus in a dog. Intact pustules span multiple hair follicles on the elbow. Note the asymmetric shape of the pustules.

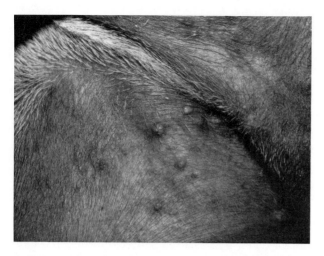

FIGURE 15-14 Pemphigus foliaceus in a dog. Intact and ruptured asymmetric pustules are present on the neck.

Diagnostic histopathology may not be forthcoming from older crusted lesions. If only crusted lesions are available, these should be procured carefully, and the pathology service should be instructed to include any dissociated crusts in the slide preparation. Sites directly adjacent to early pustules should be sampled for direct immunofluorescent testing.

Histopathology (Figures 15-15 and 15-16)

Epidermal features of this disease have been described (see Chapter 1) and principally include subcorneal pustules with acantholysis. In some cases of pemphigus foliaceus, particularly those which are local-

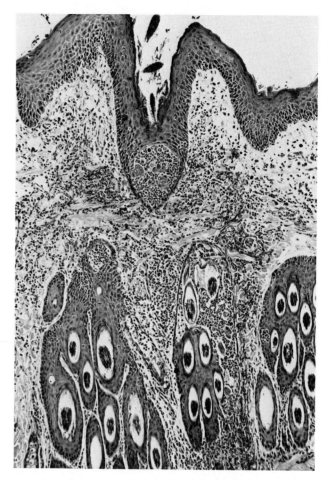

FIGURE 15-15 Follicular pemphigus foliaceus in a dog. Pustules are within the superficial and middle portions of hair follicles; note the acantholytic cells. (×90.)

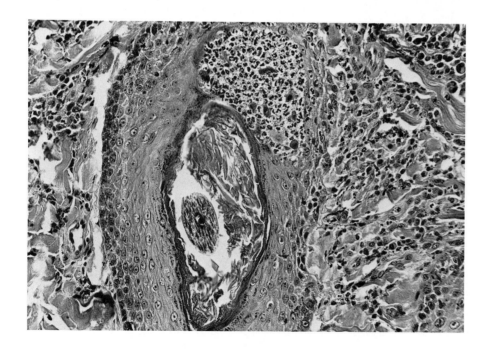

FIGURE 15-16 Follicular pemphigus foliaceus. Note the large "subcorneal" pustule containing acantholytic cells in the follicular wall. (×220.)

ized to the face, pustules with acantholysis also form within follicular infundibula or, less commonly, the isthmus of the hair follicle. These follicular pustules form in a "subcorneal" location; that is, beneath the keratin lining of the outer root sheath, but may extend through the outer wall of the follicle. Occasionally, follicular rupture with release of clusters or "rafts" of acantholytic cells into the surrounding dermis may be present and is associated with severe suppurative and pyogranulomatous dermal inflammation, as seen in deep bacterial folliculitis and furunculosis (see Chapter 16). Furunculosis without evidence of acantholysis has been documented in biopsy specimens from cases of otherwise histopathologically typical pemphigus foliaceus; presumably these cases had concurrent deep pyoderma. Immunofluorescent or immunohistochemical testing may reveal deposition of immunoglobulin in intercellular spaces of the superficial portions of hair follicles in addition to the epidermis.

Differential diagnoses principally include deep bacterial folliculitis and furunculosis and pemphigus vegetans. Active acantholysis is a differential feature of follicular pemphigus foliaceus but may be absent from foci of severe follicular inflammation observed in some isolated lesions. Conversely, secondary acantholysis caused by the proteolytic action of neutrophils may be a feature of bacterial folliculitis, and clinicopathologic correlation is critical. This difficulty may be accentuated by the coexistence of pemphigus foliaceus and bacterial folliculitis and furunculosis is some dogs. Examination of multiple specimens will increase the chances of locating diagnostic histopathologic features of pemphigus foliaceus. A positive result from immunofluorescent or immunohistochemical testing is supportive but is not always forthcoming in random specimens obtained for biopsy. Care also should be taken not to confuse deep follicular pemphigus foliaceus with pemphigus vegetans. The follicular pustules of pemphigus foliaceus may be similar to those of pemphigus vegetans; however, pemphigus vegetans has marked papillomatous hyperplasia, as well as suprabasilar clefting as seen in pemphigus vulgaris.

SEBACEOUS ADENITIS
Clinical features (Figures 15-17 and 15-18)
See Chapter 7.

Biopsy site selection
Multiple specimens are recommended so that more adnexal units may be observed. Subtle early lesions characterized by adherent scale without alopecia are most useful for documenting active sebaceous gland inflammation. Chronic lesions with extensive alopecia

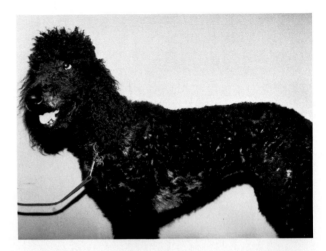

FIGURE 15-17 Sebaceous adenitis in a black Standard Poodle. Matted, whitish keratinaceous debris is present diffusely in a dry, poor-quality haircoat. *(Courtesy HT Power, Santa Cruz, California; case material from the University of California, Davis.)*

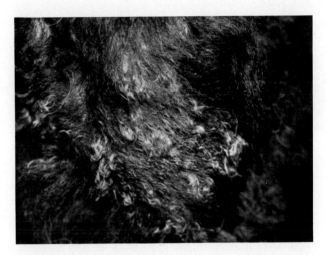

FIGURE 15-18 Closer view of the dog in Figure 15-17. Keratin debris ensheathes hairs. *(Courtesy HT Power, Santa Cruz; case material from the University of California, Davis.)*

commonly show an absence of sebaceous glands without significant inflammation; multiple specimens are then essential to confirm that the absence of sebaceous glands is widespread and therefore diagnostic of sebaceous adenitis.

Histopathology (Figures 15-19 through 15-22)
Lesions of the epidermis have been discussed and consist principally of severe hyperkeratosis, which also fills superficial hair follicles (see Chapter 7). In sebaceous adenitis, periadnexal inflammation is "lopsided," since it parallels the unilateral location of sebaceous

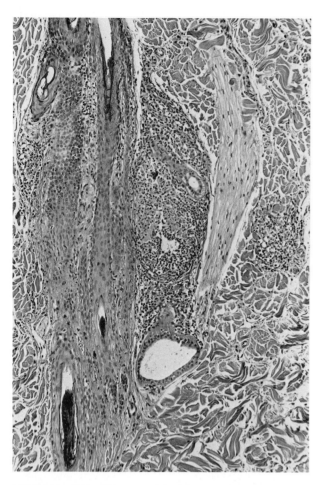

FIGURE 15-19 Sebaceous adenitis in a Standard Poodle. This early lesion demonstrates prominent periadnexal inflammation at the site of previous sebaceous glands. (×90.)

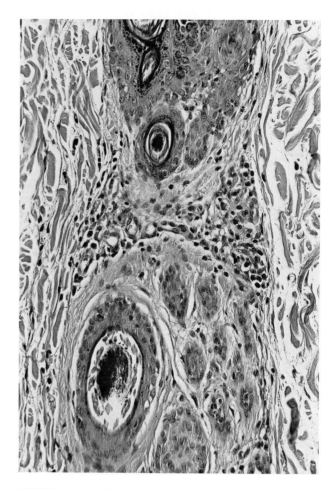

FIGURE 15-20 Sebaceous adenitis demonstrating scant periadnexal, mixed mononuclear inflammation typical of chronic lesions. (×220.)

glands in the pilosebaceous unit. Inflammation varies from scant to severe. Sebaceous glands are diffusely absent from all specimens, particularly in late, relatively uninflamed lesions. The histopathologic finding of severe hyperkeratosis, particularly in a breed known to develop sebaceous adenitis, warrants a careful search for sebaceous glands. The absence of sebaceous glands can be easily overlooked.

Random biopsy specimens from affected Standard Poodles and other breeds often yield scant to no inflammation; a few lymphocytes, histiocytes, and neutrophils may form loose accumulations at the follicular isthmus in the vicinity of previous sebaceous glands. Other breeds, such as Akitas or Samoyeds, may have more obvious inflammation, as will Standard Poodles fortuitously sampled during very early stages of the disease. Inflammation in these cases is centered at the site of previous sebaceous glands and consists of mild to moderate, loosely organized to somewhat nodular accumulations of lymphocytes and histiocytes with

variable neutrophils and rare eosinophils. Late stages of the disease in Standard Poodles or other breeds may be characterized by follicular atrophy or dysplasia. Secondary bacterial folliculitis or furunculosis is common in affected Akitas.

Viszlas with sebaceous adenitis have pronounced and distinctly nodular granulomatous or pyogranulomatous periadnexal inflammation, which is often offset to one side, reflecting the asymmetric distribution of sebaceous glands in the adnexal unit. Inflammation is more severe in this subgroup of sebaceous adenitis and is present at all stages of the disease.

Differential diagnosis for the uninflamed late lesions of sebaceous adenitis is straightforward; absence of sebaceous glands in at least three 6- or 8-mm punch biopsy specimens, accompanied by minimal periadnexal inflammation, is confirmatory. Differential diagnoses for the severely inflamed forms of sebaceous adenitis principally include the sterile histiocytic proliferative disorders (sterile granuloma and pyogranuloma

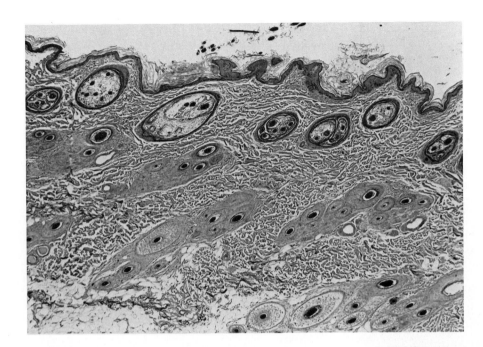

syndrome and cutaneous histiocytosis). In particular, lesions of granulomatous or pyogranulomatous sebaceous adenitis, as seen in Viszlas, should not be confused with the histiocytic proliferative disorders in which sebaceous glands are nonspecifically destroyed as they are swept up by periadnexal infiltrates. Inflammation in granulomatous sebaceous adenitis is more circumscribed and localizes particularly to sebaceous glands. The histiocytic proliferative disorders tend to surround entire adnexal units, including hair follicles and apocrine sweat glands.

Rarely, demodicosis, Vogt-Koyanagi-Harada–like syndrome, or cutaneous leishmaniasis also may be considered. Inflammation of sebaceous glands may be a feature of certain forms of demodicosis, particularly in the Chinese Shar Pei, in which granulomas or pyogranulomas occur in and around sebaceous glands. Identification of mites (which may be scant in this form of demodicosis) may be difficult; step sectioning may be required. The absence of sebaceous glands throughout the specimen supports sebaceous adenitis and is not a feature of granulomatous demodicosis. Nodular periadnexal histiocytic inflammation may be prominent in some cases of Vogt-Koyanagi-Harada–like syndrome and may obscure sebaceous glands; however, the more typical lichenoid band of inflammation is usually also present to allow differentiation from sebaceous adenitis. Sebaceous gland inflammation in cutaneous leishmaniasis, rare in most of the world, might be confused with the more severely inflamed forms of sebaceous adenitis; identification of organisms in tissue allows differentiation of leishmaniasis.

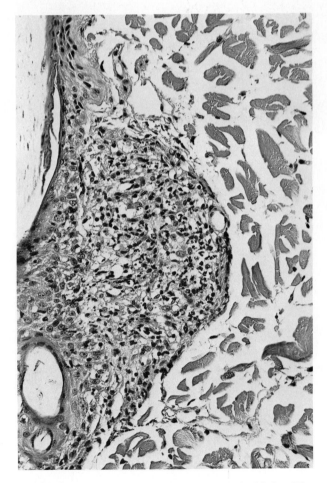

FIGURE 15-22 Granulomatous sebaceous adenitis in a Viszla. A discrete nodule of histiocytes, neutrophils, and lymphocytes is seen at the site of a previous sebaceous gland. (×220.)

STERILE EOSINOPHILIC PUSTULOSIS

Clinical features (Figures 15-23 and 15-24)

Sterile eosinophilic pustulosis, as reported by Scott (1984), is a very rare, idiopathic canine skin disease characterized by sterile eosinophilic pustules and peripheral eosinophilia. Marked tissue and peripheral eosinophilia coupled with a response to immunosuppressive dosages of glucocorticoids suggest an immune dysfunction as a basis for this disease.

Erythematous follicular and nonfollicular pustules and papules develop rapidly. Central healing with hyperpigmentation and the formation of peripheral epidermal collarettes lead to distinctive target lesions. Annular erosions may form within the confines of the collarettes. Pruritus is marked, and self-trauma may lead to excoriations. Reported cases have either involved the ventral abdomen or have been more generalized but have spared the head. Fever, anorexia, depression, and regional lymphadenopathy have been reported by Scott (1984, 1987) as inconsistent findings.

Breed, age, and sex predilections have not been noted. Clinical differential diagnoses should primarily include superficial spreading pyoderma and superficial bacterial folliculitis. Dermatophytosis, demodicosis, pemphigus foliaceus, and subcorneal pustular dermatosis are differential diagnoses of lesser consideration. Smears of pustular contents, bacterial culture from intact pustules, skin scrapings, and dermatophyte cultures should be performed to differentiate among these diseases. Sterile eosinophilic pustulosis must be diagnosed by ruling out the above-mentioned diseases and by supportive histopathology.

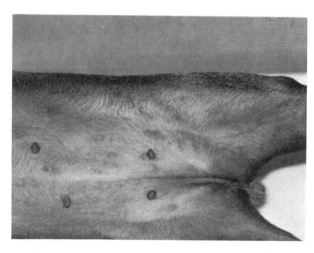

FIGURE 15-23   Sterile eosinophilic pustulosis on the abdomen of a dog. Multiple small intact pustules are seen. (*Courtesy D. Carlotti, Carbon Blanc, France.*)

FIGURE 15-24   Closer view of Figure 15-23. A hair protruding from the central intact pustule indicates the follicular orientation. (*Courtesy D. Carlotti, Carbon Blanc, France.*)

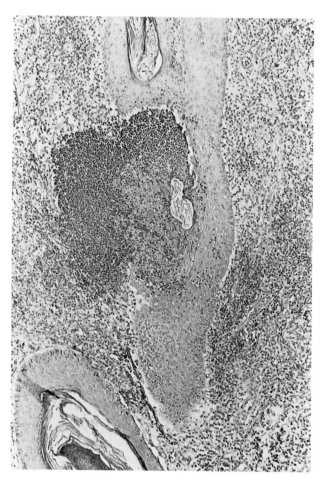

FIGURE 15-25   Sterile eosinophilic pustulosis in a dog. A large eosinophilic pustule has ruptured the affected hair follicle. (×90.)

Biopsy site selection

Skin biopsy specimens should include multiple intact pustules. Care must be taken in sampling not to disrupt fragile pustules.

Histopathology (Figure 15-25)

Acanthosis is mild to moderate. The epidermis has delicate, superficial, often subcorneal pustules that commonly contain exclusively eosinophils. There may be accompanying mild spongiosis.

Similar eosinophilic pustular inflammation also involves superficial and sometimes deep hair follicles and extends into the surrounding dermis. Eosinophils surround affected follicles in a nodular configuration and also may be distributed diffusely throughout the superficial and middle dermis. Mixed infiltrations of neutrophils, lymphocytes, and macrophages also are present. In some cases identified by Scott, eosinophilic furunculosis and eosinophilic degranulation with collagen degeneration were observed.*

Differential diagnoses include eosinophilic furunculosis of the face or superficial bacterial folliculitis in which eosinophils are prominent. Localization of lesions to the face in eosinophilic furunculosis allows separation from sterile eosinophilic pustulosis, which spares the head. Clinical features such as response to appropriate antibiotic therapy may be required to differentiate sterile eosinophilic pustulosis from pyoderma with prominent eosinophils.

* Case material from Scott DW, Ithaca, NY, 1990.

SUGGESTED READINGS

Superficial bacterial folliculitis

Ackerman AB: Histologic diagnosis of inflammatory skin diseases, Philadelphia, 1978, Lea & Febiger, pp 660-672.

Fourrier P, Carlotti D, and Magnol J-P: Les pyodermites superficielles, Pratique Medicale et Chirurgicale de l'Animal de Compagnie 23:473-484, 1988.

Ihrke PJ: Bacterial infections of the skin. In Greene CE, editor: Infectious diseases of the dog and cat, Philadelphia, 1990, WB Saunders, pp 72-79.

Ihrke PJ: The management of canine pyodermas. In Kirk RW, editor: Current veterinary therapy VIII, Philadelphia, 1983, WB Saunders, pp 505-517.

Mason IS: Hypersensitivity and the multiplication of *Staphylococci* on canine skin, doctoral dissertation, London, 1990, University of London Royal Veterinary College, pp 1-172.

Muller GH, Kirk RW, and Scott DW: Small animal dermatology, ed 4, Philadelphia, 1989, WB Saunders, pp 244-285.

White SD and Ihrke PJ: Pyoderma. In Nesbitt GH, editor: Dermatology: contemporary issues in small animal practice, New York, 1987, Churchill Livingstone, pp 112-113.

Feline dermatophytosis

Foil CS: Dermatophytosis. In Greene CE, editor: Infectious diseases of the dog and cat, Philadelphia, 1990, WB Saunders, pp 659-668.

Moriello KA: Management of dermatophyte infections in catteries and multiple-cat households, Vet Clin North Am 20:1457-1474, 1990.

Rebell G and Taplin D: Dermatophytes: their recognition and identification, Coral Gables, FL, 1970, University of Miami Press, pp 1-124.

Thomas ML, Scheidt VJ, and Walker RL: Inapparent carriage of *Microsporum canis* in cats, Comp Cont Ed 11:563-580, 1990.

Canine dermatophytosis

Bourdeau P, Chermette R, and Bussieras J: Quelques formes rares de dermatomycoses des carnivores domestique, Le Point Veterinaire 14:69-72, 1983.

Foil CS: Dermatophytosis. In Greene CE, editor: Infectious diseases of the dog and cat, Philadelphia, 1990, WB Saunders, pp 659-668.

Rebell G and Taplin D: Dermatophytes: their recognition and identification, Coral Gables, FL, 1970, University of Miami Press, pp 1-124.

Pemphigus foliaceus

See Chapter 1.

Sebaceous adenitis

See Chapter 7.

Sterile eosinophilic pustulosis

Carlotti D and others: La maladie D'Ofugi (pustulose eosinophilique sterile), Pratique Medicale et Chirurgicale de l'Animal de Compagnie 24:131-138, 1989.

Scott DW: Sterile eosinophilic pustulosis in dog and man: comparative aspects, J Am Acad Dermatol 16:1022-1026, 1987.

Scott DW: Sterile eosinophilic pustulosis in the dog, J Am Anim Hosp Assoc 20:585-589, 1984.

CHAPTER 16

Pustular and nodular diseases with follicular destruction

The diseases of this chapter are characterized by prominent pustular inflammation of the follicle, leading to follicular rupture and effacement. Subsequent inflammation at the site of a destroyed follicle is often nodular in distribution; a granulomatous infiltrate is common as a foreign body response to released hair and keratin. Most of the diseases have an infectious or parasitic cause that is often apparent in tissue (demodicosis, kerion, rhabditic dermatitis), but sometimes may be relatively inapparent (deep bacterial folliculitis and furunculosis). In several diseases, primary accumulation of keratin in the follicle leads to secondary rupture and pyoderma (callus, acne, actinic comedones).

DEEP BACTERIAL FOLLICULITIS AND FURUNCULOSIS
(Synonym: deep pyoderma)
Clinical features (Figures 16-1 through 16-3)

Deep bacterial folliculitis and furunculosis is a relatively common canine skin disease. It may be seen without evidence of prior superficial pyoderma or as a sequela to superficial bacterial folliculitis. Deep bacterial folliculitis and furunculosis are grouped, since they commonly coexist: deep follicular inflammation leads to follicular rupture, the salient feature of furunculosis. A foreign body response is elicited in furunculosis by released follicular keratin and hair, leading to accentuated inflammation and scarring.

As in other types of canine pyoderma, *Staphylococcus intermedius* is the primary pathogen. However, secondary invaders such as *Proteus* species, *Pseudomonas* species, and *Escherichia coli* are seen more frequently in deeper infections.

Deep pyoderma is common secondary to demodicosis. Other predisposing causes include hyperadrenocorticism, defects in the immune system, and the injudicious use of glucocorticoids (iatrogenic hyperglucocorticoidism). Comedonal diseases such as calluses, actinic comedones, and Schnauzer comedo syndrome also predispose to deep pyoderma. On occasion, follicular trauma is the inciting cause of furunculosis rather than the endstage event. Backcombing, clipping, or other externally induced follicular trauma such as the persistent licking of acral lick dermatitis (see Chapter 6) can induce follicular rupture and inflammation.

Since deep pyoderma may develop from superficial pyoderma, the lesions of superficial pyoderma may precede and coexist with deeper infection (see Chapter 15). The pustules of deep bacterial folliculitis and furunculosis are large and vary in color from white to yellow gray; firm nodules usually are present. Pustules and nodules rupture, forming fistulas and hemorrhagic crusts. Erosions and ulcers develop secondary to inflammation, necrosis, and self-trauma initiated by pain or pruritus. Alopecia is seen as

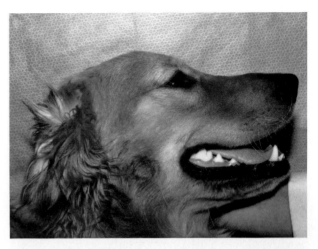

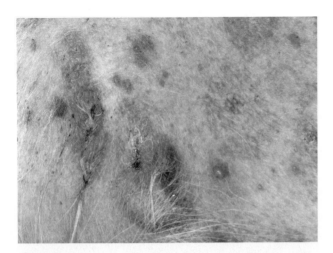

FIGURE 16-1. Deep bacterial folliculitis and furunculosis on the abdomen of a dog. An intact hemorrhagic bulla is surrounded by intact and ulcerated pustules.

FIGURE 16-2. Deep bacterial folliculitis and furunculosis mimicking pyotraumatic dermatitis in a Golden Retriever. A well-demarcated ulcerated plaque is present ventral to the ear.

a sequela to follicular inflammation and destruction. Hyperpigmentation and lichenification also are common sequelae. Commonly affected sites include the intertriginous zones of the groin, axillae, and interdigital webs and pressure points. Lesions may be generalized in some dogs, particularly in the German Shepherd Dog, and less commonly in the Bull Terrier, American Staffordshire Terrier, and the Dalmatian. Regional and generalized lymphadenopathy are common. Constitutional signs may be seen contingent on the severity and distribution of infection.

Hemorrhagic bullae are distinctive clinical features of some cases of canine deep pyoderma. Well-circumscribed, firm nodules exhibit a deep red to dark blue hue. Newer lesions are bright red, signifying fresh hemorrhage. Hemorrhagic rings sometimes are present surrounding the bullae. Hemorrhagic bullae most often are seen in the German Shepherd Dog, but may be present occasionally in the Bull Terrier, American Staffordshire Terrier, Dalmatian, and other breeds. Hemorrhagic bullae may be seen with deep pyoderma secondary to demodicosis and actinic comedones.

An additional subgroup of deep pyoderma clinically closely mimics pyotraumatic dermatitis (see Chapter 5). This syndrome, seen primarily in the Golden Retriever but also in other breeds, including the Saint Bernard, begins with focal areas of deep pyoderma that become secondarily severely traumatized, thus clinically resembling pyotraumatic dermatitis. Deep pyoderma does not occur secondary to pyotraumatic dermatitis in this syndrome.

Breed predilections have been observed for deep bacterial folliculitis and furunculosis. Predisposed long-coated dogs include the German Shepherd Dog,

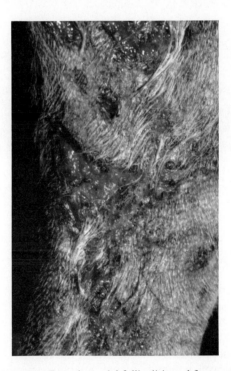

FIGURE 16-3. Deep bacterial folliculitis and furunculosis in a German Shepherd Dog. Visualization has been enhanced by clipping the affected limb. Multifocal exudative ulcers are present. *(Courtesy HT Power, Santa Cruz, California; case material from University of California, Davis.)*

Golden Retriever, and Irish Setter. The Bull Terrier, American Staffordshire Terrier, Dalmatian, Doberman Pinscher, and Great Dane are at apparent increased risk among the short-coated breeds. Deep pyoderma secondary to demodicosis follows the predilections of the

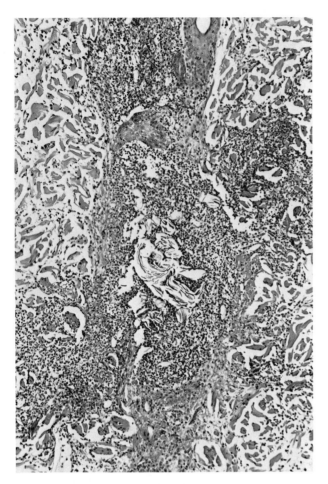

FIGURE 16-4. Furunculosis in a dog. A severely inflamed follicle has ruptured; free follicular keratin is surrounded by extensive pustulation. (×90.)

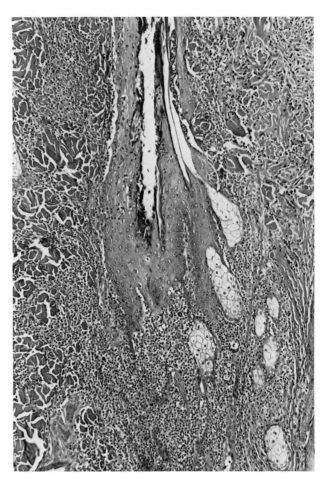

FIGURE 16-5. Furunculosis in a Golden Retriever with pyotraumatic dermatitis. Severe pustular inflammation is replacing most of a deep follicle. (×90.)

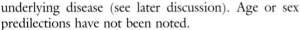

underlying disease (see later discussion). Age or sex predilections have not been noted.

Demodicosis must be ruled out as an underlying cause for any deep pyoderma. Clinical differential diagnoses should include cutaneous infections of systemic fungi, cutaneous infections of opportunistic fungi or algae, opportunistic mycobacterial infection and pythiosis, as well as neoplasia with secondary necrosis and infection. Differentiation is accomplished by skin scrapings, microscopic examination of smears of exudates, bacterial and fungal cultures, and histopathology.

Biopsy site selection

Early intact pustules, nodules, or bullae are recommended lesions for biopsy. Ulcerated or scarred lesions may be less desirable, since they are less likely to yield diagnostic follicular lesions because of loss of normal tissue architecture. If most of the available affected tissue is friable because of severe inflammation or hemorrhage, wedge resection is preferable. Punch biopsy frequently creates traumatic artifacts in fragile tissue.

Histopathology (Figures 16-4 and 16-5)

The epidermis usually is acanthotic and may be ulcerated. Superficial serocellular crusting is common. Features of pyotraumatic dermatitis (see Chapter 5) may be present in breeds prone to produce these lesions (Golden Retriever, Saint Bernard) in the face of deep follicular pyoderma. Epidermal features of acral lick dermatitis may be present (see Chapter 6) if furunculosis is the result of persistent self-trauma, leading to displacement of hairs from follicles or if deep follicular inflammation has induced secondary severe and persistent self-trauma.

Deep folliculitis is characterized by principally neutrophilic inflammation that accumulates within the confines of the follicular wall, generally beneath the level of the isthmus. Superficial folliculitis also may be present (see Chapter 15). Deep folliculitis invariably leads to follicular rupture and the formation of a furuncle as the integrity of the follicular wall breaks down. Follicles may be completely effaced and replaced by severe nodular accumulations of neutrophils, variable eosinophils, macrophages, and plasma cells. Neutrophils and macrophages tend to localize at the center of these inflammatory foci, whereas plasma cells are found at the periphery. Free hairshafts may remain at the center of large furuncles. Granulomas with giant cells may form around fragments of follicular debris (trichogranulomas), which may be displaced below the normal level of adnexa (particularly when traumatic displacement of hair has occurred). Inflammation may become diffuse in the deep dermis as adjacent furuncles coalesce. Extension of inflammation to the panniculus is not uncommon; frank cellulitis occasionally may be observed and is most commonly secondary to demodicosis (see later discussion). Cavitation of severely inflamed tissue and hemorrhage are common accompaniments. Variable fibrosis occurs deep and peripheral to the lesions in the later stages. Milder mixed inflammation extends into the surrounding superficial and deep dermis of less affected areas of skin.

Hemorrhagic bullae consist of large pustules accompanied by severe hemorrhage in the superficial and middle dermis. Typical hemorrhagic bullae tend to exclude follicular involvement and are often localized strikingly in interfollicular spaces. Larger pustules may severely disrupt and replace dermal architecture, often creating "lakes" of neutrophils in the skin. Neutrophils predominate, but small numbers of eosinophils and macrophages may be present within pustules. Scarring and cavitation are seen as in furunculosis.

Differential diagnoses include folliculitis or furunculosis resulting from dermatophytosis or demodicosis. Identification of organisms is required for differentiation. Chronic furunculosis caused by dermatophytosis (kerion) may not have apparent organisms, which makes differentiation difficult on histopathologic grounds alone. Eosinophilic furunculosis of the face is superficially similar, but has a predominance of eosinophils and more striking dermal edema.

CANINE CALLUS AND CALLUS PYODERMA (Synonyms: callus dermatitis, pressure-point granuloma)
Clinical features (Figures 16-6 and 16-7)

A callus is a thickened plaque that develops over bony prominences or pressure points in response to repeated pressure or frictional trauma. Noninfected calluses are a normal protective response to perpetual

environmental trauma, especially from habitual contact with hard, rough surfaces. Callus pyoderma develops as a sequela to repeated callus trauma. Histopathologic evidence indicates that uninflamed calluses frequently contain dilated, keratin-filled hair follicles. Rupture of these dilated hair follicles and traumatic implantation of hairs induces a secondary bacterial furunculosis and a foreign body response to the displaced hairs, creating callus pyoderma.

Thickened plaques with circular or oval smooth borders form over bony prominences or other pressure points. Partial to complete alopecia develops with chronicity. Developing calluses usually are erythematous; noninflamed chronic calluses appear gray or white be-

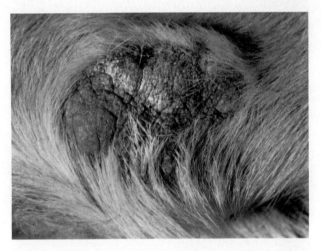

FIGURE 16-6. Lichenified and alopecic callus on the lateral elbow of a Labrador Retriever. Mottled hyperpigmentation is present.

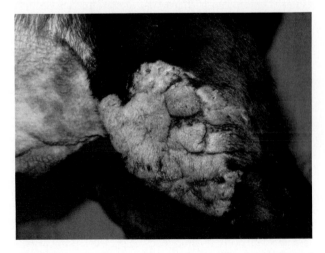

FIGURE 16-7. Severe callus pyoderma affecting the lateral stifle region of a dog. Draining tracts are present within the multilobular callus.

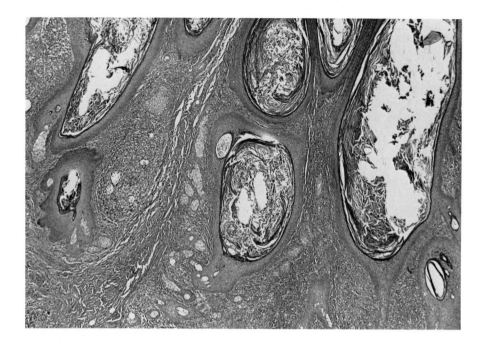

FIGURE 16-8. Canine callus pyoderma. Thickened and keratin-distended follicles are surrounded by severe inflammation. (×35.)

cause of poorly vascularized fibrous tissue. Continuously traumatized calluses often are hyperpigmented. Follicular dilatation and comedo formation are common, and multiple hairs may emanate from abnormally enlarged follicles. Frank pustules or furuncles may be visible but secondary pyoderma may not be obvious clinically. Ulceration may be present in cases of severe callus pyoderma with persistent trauma. The elbow and hock are the most common sites, but calluses may be seen on the sternum, stifle, lateral digits, or bony prominences of the pelvis. Untreated calluses tend to enlarge as the dog ages.

Large-breed dogs such as Doberman Pinschers, Great Danes, Saint Bernards, Newfoundlands, and Irish Wolfhounds are at greater risk. Short-legged dogs with short haircoats such as smooth-coated Dachshunds and Basset Hounds are at increased risk for sternal calluses. Age or sex predilections have not been noted.

Acral lick dermatitis visually may resemble callus pyoderma but has different site predilections. Plaques of coalescing actinic comedones also may resemble calluses but are not associated with pressure points. Histopathology also will allow differentiation.

Biopsy site selection

The risk versus the potential benefit must be weighed when contemplating biopsy of a callus. Classic lesions over bony prominences or pressure points ordinarily should not be sampled, since healing may be difficult at these sites. Surgical removal of an entire callus may be performed, but this procedure is fraught with potential difficulties. Dehiscence is a common se-

quela to elbow callus removal unless special surgical techniques are employed. Wedge biopsy or excisional technique may be performed on sternal calluses and may be curative.

Histopathology (Figures 16-8 and 16-9)

The epidermis is severely acanthotic and hyperplasia extends to follicular infundibula, creating an undulating or papillated surface to the lesion. Variable superficial hyperkeratosis and parakeratosis occur, and crusting or ulceration may be a feature of inflamed lesions.

An uninflamed callus is most specifically characterized by prominent follicular keratosis, often to the degree of follicular cyst formation. Dilated cystic follicles contain fragments of hair in addition to keratin. Rupture of these cysts leads to release of hair and keratin, which provokes severe suppurative and pyogranulomatous inflammation in the dermis and the panniculus (callus pyoderma). Trichogranulomas—the accumulation of macrophages, giant cells, and neutrophils around free hair—may form around deeply embedded hair shafts. Fibrosis may be prominent in severe and chronic lesions.

Histopathologically, lesions bear some resemblance to severely inflamed acral lick dermatitis. Follicular cyst formation is the key differential feature of a callus and is not present in most cases of acral lick dermatitis. Actinic comedones and other comedonal diseases (Schnauzer comedo syndrome, canine acne) also are characterized by prominent follicular keratosis but usually do not have the severe epidermal and follicular infundibular hyperplasia that is seen in callus.

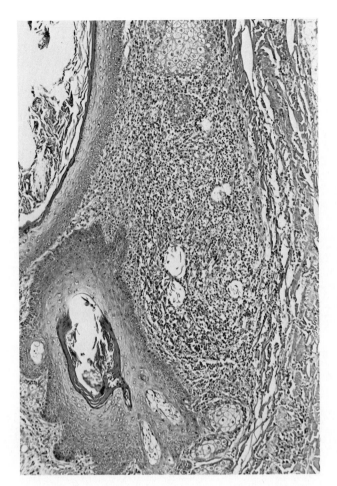

FIGURE 16-9. Higher magnification of callus pyoderma shown in Figure 16-8, demonstrating pustular inflammation surrounding free keratin from a ruptured follicle. (×90.)

initially, accompanied by variable erythema and alopecia. Firm nodules, furuncles, and fistulous tracts may occur as sequelae to follicular rupture, leading to scarring. Comedones containing dark, inspissated material are most prominent centrally on the rostral portion of the chin. Canine acne is seen on the chin and less commonly in the skin surrounding the lower lip. The upper lip and lateral muzzle may be affected in more severe cases. Partial symmetry is common. Pruritus, if present, usually is mild. Pain may be noted in dogs that

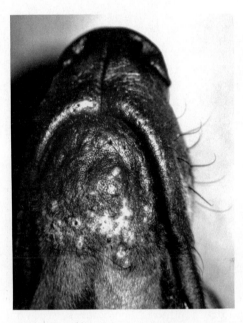

FIGURE 16-10. Canine acne affecting the ventral muzzle of a Doberman Pinscher. Active furuncles are present amid alopecia resulting from previous inflammation.

CANINE ACNE
Clinical features (Figures 16-10 and 16-11)

Canine acne is a common skin disease of young dogs in which comedones (blackheads) form on the chin and lips. Since a temporal association with puberty is seen in dogs, similar to that of humans, it has been speculated by Muller, Kirk, and Scott that the pathogenesis may be similar. In humans, the effect of increased circulatory androgens on sebaceous glands and hair follicles is believed to induce hyperplasia and hypertrophy of sebaceous glands. Increased production of sebum and sebum breakdown to free fatty acids may induce inflammation and comedo formation. An increase in follicular keratinization also is seen. Bacterial involvement, when present, is probably secondary. Since canine acne commonly is a mild and visually distinctive disease, biopsy is performed infrequently.

Comedones, crusted papules, and pustules develop

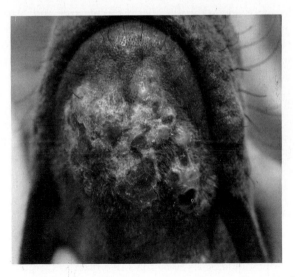

FIGURE 16-11. Severe canine acne affecting the ventral muzzle of a blue Doberman Pinscher. Coalescing nodules are accompanied by ulceration.

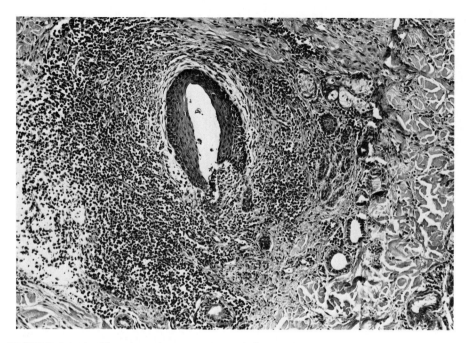

FIGURE 16-12. Chronic canine acne. Severe inflammation is disrupting a hair follicle (furunculosis). (×90.)

are affected with severe secondary deep bacterial folliculitis and furunculosis.

Canine acne is seen most frequently in short-coated breeds such as the Doberman Pinscher, Great Dane, English Bulldog, German Shorthaired Pointer, and Boxer. The onset of the disease usually coincides with puberty and most often occurs between 5 and 12 months of age. Canine acne usually resolves spontaneously after puberty but occasionally persists into adulthood. Sex predilections have not been noted.

Canine acne is visually distinctive. Occasionally, localized demodicosis, dermatophytosis, and early, mild juvenile sterile granulomatous dermatitis and lymphadenitis may mimic canine acne. Negative skin scrapings, dermatophyte culture, and the lack of systemic signs will rule out these diseases.

Biopsy site selection

Punch biopsy specimens should be obtained from characteristic lesions. Cosmetic results are best achieved by sampling the ventral chin. Sampling of larger comedones or furuncles using a 4-mm punch may be curative for individual lesions.

Histopathology (Figure 16-12)

The epidermis is generally moderately acanthotic and may be crusted. Ulceration is rare and limited to severely inflamed lesions that have been aggravated by self-trauma.

The principal feature of canine acne, as in feline acne (see discussion below), is severe follicular keratosis or comedo formation. Early lesions show intact comedones surrounded by mixed inflammatory cells, including neutrophils, macrophages, and plasma cells. Sebaceous glands are large, as is expected for the chin; sebaceous ducts may be dilated. Pustular folliculitis often ensues, and inflamed or uninflamed comedones can rupture, leading to severe furunculosis and its attendant inflammatory and scarring changes (see earlier discussion).

Differential diagnoses include those diseases characterized by comedones, including Schnauzer comedo syndrome, canine callus and callus pyoderma, and actinic comedones. Clinical distribution of the lesions in these diseases is distinctive and allows differentiation; additionally, microscopic identification of the typically large sebaceous glands of the chin indicates acne.

FELINE ACNE
Clinical features (Figures 16-13 and 16-14)

Feline acne is a common skin disease characterized by comedo formation on the chin and lips. The etiopathogenesis of feline acne is not understood. Unlike acne in humans and dogs, feline acne is not associated with puberty, and hence it cannot be linked temporally with the effect of increased circulatory androgens on sebaceous glands and hair follicles. Muller, Kirk, and Scott suggest that improper cleansing of the chin in affected cats may lead to follicular obstruction and sec-

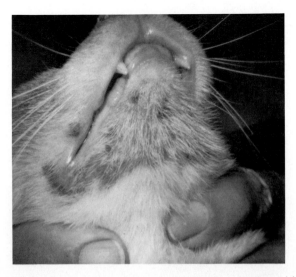

FIGURE 16-13. Severe feline acne. Extensive crusting with alopecia is present on the ventral muzzle. *(Courtesy EM Sleeper, Philadelphia, Pennsylvania.)*

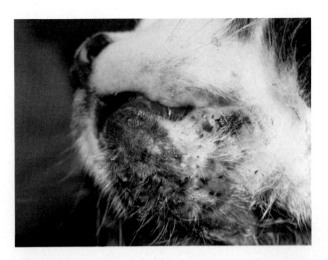

FIGURE 16-14. Severe feline acne with secondary pyoderma. Note the fistulous tracts.

ondary comedo formation. The cyclic or periodic nature of the disease may relate to the inability of the telogen hair to extrude the developing keratosebaceous plug. A localized keratinization defect that is perhaps exacerbated by increased sebum production from the large sebaceous glands in the chin could also explain this process. If present, bacterial involvement is secondary. Feline acne usually is such a mild disease that biopsy is performed infrequently.

Comedones, mildly erythematous crusted papules, and pustules develop on the chin and less commonly on the skin around the lips. Swelling of the chin is variable and may be diffuse. Solitary comedones containing dark, inspissated material are most prominent around the lateral commissures of the mouth and the lower lip. Firm nodules indicative of deep bacterial folliculitis and furunculosis, marked erythema, and alopecia are noted in more severe cases. Partial symmetry is common. Individual lesions may fistulate, leading to focal abscesses and scarring. Feline acne usually is asymptomatic; pruritus or pain are uncommon unless severe pyoderma is present.

Breed or sex predilections have not been noted. Feline acne often commences at less than 1 year of age and remains a lifelong disease, cyclically varying in severity.

Feline acne is visually distinctive. Occasionally, dermatophytosis or feline demodicosis may mimic feline acne. Symmetry and frank comedo formation are helpful differentiating features of feline acne. Skin scrapings, dermatophyte culture, and histopathology will also allow differentiation.

Biopsy site selection

Punch biopsy specimens should be obtained from discrete comedones. Cosmetic results are best achieved by sampling the ventral chin. Sampling of larger comedones using a 4-mm punch may be curative for individual lesions.

Histopathology (Figures 16-15 through 16-17)

The epidermis is acanthotic and occasionally eroded and crusted. Typically, superficial hair follicles are distended with keratin (comedo formation), occasionally to the point of cyst formation. Affected follicles may be uninflamed and are surrounded by large sebaceous glands that identify the skin of the chin. There may be mild to severe pustular folliculitis. Rupture of keratin-filled follicles is common, leading to furunculosis characterized by accumulations of neutrophils and macrophages around keratinaceous debris.

Two cases have been observed by the authors in which keratin-distended follicles contained *Malassezia*. The role that these yeast may play in the development of feline acne is unknown.

In severe longstanding lesions (characterized by diffuse swelling clinically), there is diffuse and severe pyogranulomatous inflammation. The mechanism of generation of these lesions from those more typical of feline acne is not known. Diffuse pyogranulomatous dermatitis of the chin may be a separate syndrome in cats.

Early lesions are diagnostic for feline acne, particularly when the typically prominent sebaceous glands of this area of skin are identified. Diffuse pyogranulomatous lesions may mimic those of fungal granulomas or feline leprosy.

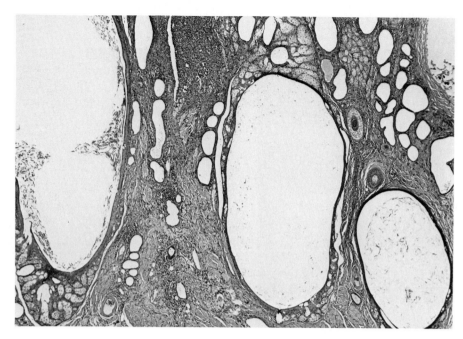

FIGURE 16-15. Feline acne. Distended follicles are interspersed by inflammation. Note the prominent sebaceous glands characteristic of the chin. (×35.)

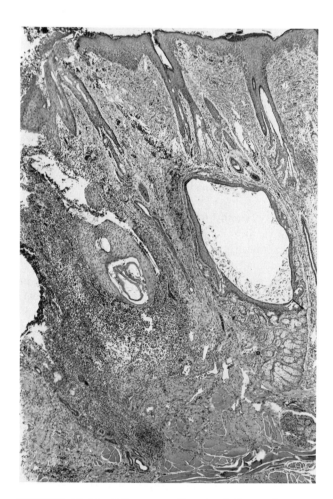

FIGURE 16-16. Feline acne. Pustular inflammation surrounding a ruptured follicle at the left lies adjacent to a dilated follicle. (×35.)

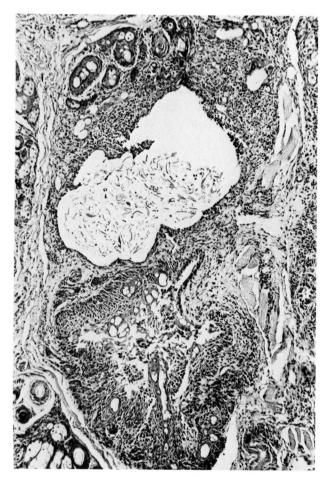

FIGURE 16-17. Feline acne. A keratin-filled follicle has ruptured leading to pustular inflammation (furunculosis). (×90.)

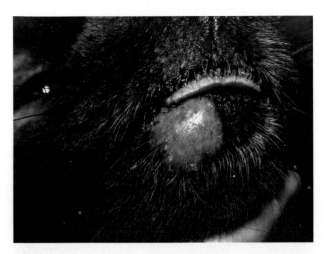

FIGURE 16-18. Kerion caused by *Microsporum canis* on the ventral muzzle of a dog. Note the droplet of exudate at the bottom of the lesion, which originated from a small fistula.

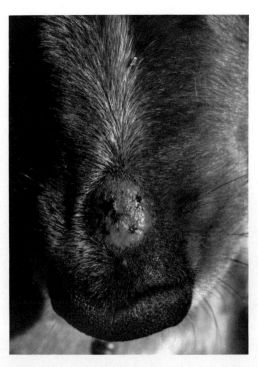

FIGURE 16-19. Kerion on the dorsal muzzle of a dog. Note the foci of hemorrhagic fistulation. The adjacent (non-haired) planum nasale is not affected.

KERION
Clinical features (Figures 16-18 and 16-19)

Kerion is an uncommon variant of canine dermatophytosis characterized by intense focal inflammation. Although kerion may be seen with a variety of dermatophytes, it may occur most commonly in conjunction with *Microsporum gypseum* infection. The mechanism of kerion formation is unknown. Since the kerion type of dermatophytosis often leads to spontaneous resolution, one can speculate that an enhanced host immunologic response may be responsible. The zoonotic potential of kerion seems to be less than for other varieties of canine dermatophytosis; this may be because of the paucity of viable organisms present in most lesions.

Markedly erythematous, exudative, alopecic, usually solitary but occasionally multiple, firm nodules develop acutely. Kerion vary in diameter from 1 to 5 cm. A hand lens may reveal small fistulous tracts on the surface of the nodules. Erosion or ulceration may occur. Peripheral scale is common and crusting may be evident if the lesion is located where the dog cannot remove the exudate. Most kerion develop on the face or forelimbs, but lesions may occur at any site. Regional lymphadenopathy is a common feature. Pruritus or pain are minimal but may occur with larger lesions.

Breed, age, or sex predilections have not been established. However, the Boxer may be at increased risk for solitary lesions, and the Golden Retriever may be at increased risk for widespread, multiple lesions.

Clinical differential diagnoses include neoplasms that may be nodular, erythematous, and alopecic (such as mast cell tumors) and foreign body reactions. Der-

matophyte culture may not be helpful because mature lesions may yield negative culture results. Skin biopsy may be necessary for differentiation.

Biopsy site selection

Since kerion are usually solitary lesions, complete resection is indicated to also obtain a surgical cure. In addition, resection is advisable, since kerion can mimic cutaneous neoplasia clinically.

Histopathology (Figures 16-20 and 16-21)

The epidermis is acanthotic and may be ulcerated or crusted. Severe furunculosis is present throughout the lesion. Hair follicles are ruptured and replaced by tightly oriented, nodular accumulations of macrophages and neutrophils. These discrete, often large pyogranulomas or granulomas containing macrophages, neutrophils, and giant cells may surround hair fragments. Inflammation may become confluent, resulting in a diffuse distribution in the dermis. Variable numbers of eosinophils are often present but can be absent. Remnants of hair shafts at the centers of inflammatory foci may contain dermatophytic spores and hyphae; occasional colonization of superficial hairs also is seen. Dermatophytes may not be evident in severely inflamed lesions, since organisms cannot persist in these conditions.

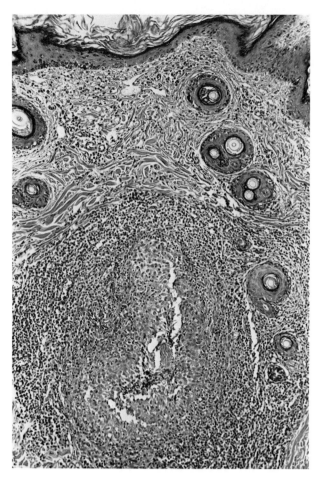

FIGURE 16-20. Kerion in a dog. A large pyogranuloma surrounds a free dermatophyte-colonized hair fragment. (×90.)

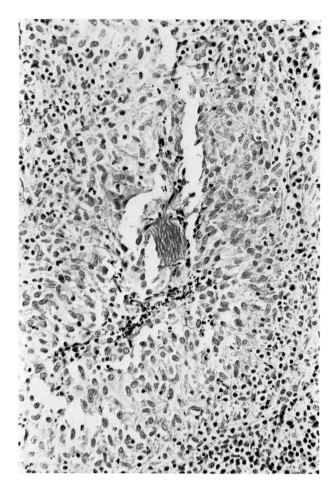

FIGURE 16-21. Higher magnification of the pyogranuloma and free hair shown in Figure 16-20. Note the wavy, pale, dermatophytic hyphae within the hair shaft. (×220.)

Differential diagnosis, if organisms are not located, principally includes deep bacterial folliculitis and furunculosis. However, the often strikingly granulomatous inflammation around free hairs in the kerion is different from most cases of bacterial furunculosis, which tend to be more neutrophilic. The discrete, tightly nodular pattern of inflammation around free hair also allows the differentiation of kerion from bacterial furunculosis in which inflammation is more loosely organized.

DEMODICOSIS (Synonym: demodectic mange)
Clinical features (Figures 16-22 through 16-24)

Demodicosis is a noncontagious, parasitic skin disease caused by an overpopulation of the host-specific follicular mite, *Demodex* species. Canine demodicosis may be divided into juvenile-onset and the less common acquired adult-onset forms; both forms may be

localized or generalized. Localized demodicosis, a mild and benign self-limiting form of the disease, is very common in dogs. Generalized demodicosis, a serious and potentially life-threatening disease that usually evolves from localized demodicosis, is relatively common in the dog. The only forms of demodicosis identified to date in cats are adult-onset localized or generalized; both forms are very rare and comparatively benign in cats. Since demodectic mites are part of the normal fauna, they are present in small numbers in the hair follicles of most healthy animals. Transmission to the newborn is achieved by direct contact with the mother during the first few days after birth.

In demodicosis, a cutaneous environment exists that is somehow ecologically or immunologically favorable for intense colonization by demodectic mites. Alteration in the immune system is probably responsible for the development of demodicosis. However, to date immunologic studies have not documented clear-cut

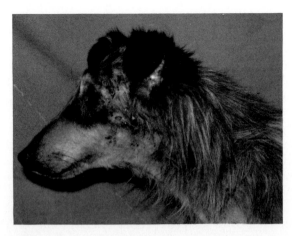

FIGURE 16-22. Juvenile-onset generalized demodicosis in a blue merle Shetland Sheepdog. Note the partial, patchy alopecia. Crusting is visible on the exposed skin.

evidence of a specific immunologic defect. A genetically preprogrammed immunologic defect probably is responsible for the unchecked replication of demodectic mites in dogs exhibiting juvenile-onset demodicosis. This speculation is supported by marked breed predilections and familial involvement. A similar defect may be present in both the localized and generalized forms of juvenile-onset demodicosis, based on the identical breed predilections and the progression from localized to generalized disease in a small number of dogs (<5%). Since ample evidence is available indicating the heritable tendencies of juvenile-onset generalized demodicosis, the American Academy of Veterinary Dermatology adopted a resolution in 1981, sponsored by Kirk,* recommending "neutering all dogs who have had generalized demodicosis so that the incidence of the disease is decreased and not perpetuated."

An immunologic origin of demodicosis also is supported by the frequent association of acquired adult-onset demodicosis with immunosuppressive diseases, such as canine hyperadrenocorticism, feline immunodeficiency virus infection, and neoplasia, and the development of demodicosis as a sequela to immunosuppression induced by antilymphocyte serum, glucocorticoids, or cytotoxic drugs. Immunosuppression or underlying disease is not always documented in adult-onset demodicosis, however.

Marked variation exists in the clinical presentation of demodicosis. Canine localized demodicosis is characterized by the development of patchy, moderately well-circumscribed, alopecic macules. Erythema and

* Courtesy Kirk RW, Ithaca, New York, 1981.

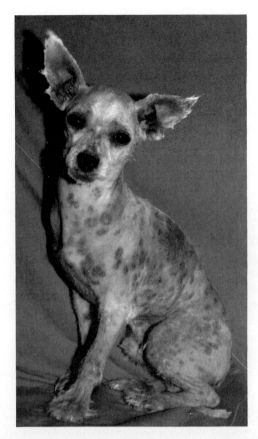

FIGURE 16-23. Juvenile-onset generalized demodicosis in a Shih Tzu. The dog has been clipped to enhance visualization of the lesions. Alopecia was not a feature of the disease in this dog.

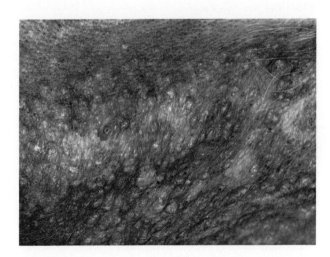

FIGURE 16-24. Generalized demodicosis affecting the ventral abdomen of a German Shepherd Dog. Erythematous nodules and plaques indicate secondary bacterial furunculosis.

mild micaceous scaling are common features. Follicular plugging and comedo formation may be present, particularly in the German Shepherd Dog. The periorbital region, lateral commissures of the mouth, other areas of the face, and forelimbs are the most common sites. Mild pruritus may be present but is not a consistent feature. Regional lymphadenopathy is variable. Rarely, localized demodicosis may be markedly nodular; histopathologically, these nodules are sites of intense, focal granulomatous sebaceous adenitis.

Canine generalized demodicosis usually develops as a sequela to localized demodicosis. The original localized, erythematous, alopecic macules enlarge and coalesce, and multiple new lesions develop on the head, trunk, and limbs. As inflammation becomes more marked, macules evolve into plaques, and hair loss becomes more extensive. Alopecia may be surprisingly minimal in long-coated breeds such as the Maltese, Shih Tzu, and Lhasa Apso, leading to a decreased index of suspicion for demodicosis. Hyperpigmentation and lichenification occur with chronicity. Secondary pyoderma is common and may be characterized by generalized deep folliculitis and furunculosis and even cellulitis. Hemorrhagic bullae may be present. The feet often are severely affected. Tissue devitalization may be marked, and, in severe cases of generalized demodicosis, septicemia may be present. Pruritus, pain, and generalized lymphadenopathy are frequent features.

Severe involvement of the feet (pododemodicosis) may occur alone, in conjunction with generalized demodicosis, or as a sequela to generalized demodicosis after other body sites have responded to miticidal therapy. Erythema, swelling, and secondary deep pyoderma with scarring are seen on the digits, in the interdigital webs, between the pads ventrally, and surrounding the nail beds.

In localized feline demodicosis, patchy alopecia usually is limited to the face and is similar to mild canine localized demodicosis. Feline generalized demodicosis is a less severe disease than the canine counterpart. In most affected cats, the skin disease is largely asymptomatic. Subtle erythema with mild alopecia or hyperpigmentation may occur on the face, trunk, or extremities. Coat coloration changes may be an additional feature. The hair in lesional skin may become darker in breeds in which haircoat pigmentation may be temperature dependent, such as Siamese cats. Secondary pyoderma is rare. Feline generalized demodicosis usually is seen in conjunction with underlying immunosuppressive systemic diseases such as feline immunodeficiency virus infection, diabetes mellitus, hyperadrenocorticism, and feline leukemia virus infection.

Purebred dogs are at greater risk than mixed breed dogs for juvenile-onset demodicosis. Short-haired breeds at increased risk for juvenile onset demodicosis include the Doberman Pinscher, Chinese Shar Pei, American Staffordshire Terrier, Dalmatian, English Bulldog, Great Dane, Boston Terrier, Chihuahua, Boxer, and Pug. Long-haired breeds at increased risk include the Old English Sheepdog, German Shepherd Dog, Collie, and Afghan Hound. Juvenile-onset demodicosis is seen most commonly in dogs between 3 and 12 months of age, before sexual maturity has been reached. Acquired adult-onset demodicosis without demonstrable underlying immunosuppressive disease may be seen more frequently in the Cocker Spaniel. Sex predilections are not noted with canine demodicosis. Breed, age, or sex predilections are not available for feline demodicosis.

Clinical differential diagnoses for juvenile-onset localized demodicosis include dermatophytosis and, less commonly, canine familial dermatomyositis if predisposed breeds (Collie and Shetland Sheepdog) are affected. Skin scrapings should be obtained. The finding of demodectic mites in a Shetland Sheepdog or Collie with facial and pedal alopecia should not preclude skin biopsy, since localized demodicosis and dermatomyositis may coexist (see Chapter 2). Skin scrapings should be obtained to rule out generalized demodicosis in all dogs with unidentified skin diseases, pyoderma, or exfoliative dermatitis. Skin biopsy may be required to diagnose demodicosis in the Chinese Shar Pei and in dogs with pododemodicosis in which the mites may be more deeply located.

Feline demodicosis is a relatively nondescript disease. It may mimic feline psychogenic alopecia or subtle alopecia associated with pruritic allergic skin diseases. Additionally, cats with unidentified skin diseases exhibiting subtle skin or haircoat changes should be scraped for demodicosis.

Biopsy site selection

Generally, clinicians do not submit skin specimens to a pathologist expecting a diagnosis of demodicosis, since the skin scraping is the most efficient diagnostic method. Despite negative skin scrapings, skin biopsy specimens should be taken from alopecic, hyperpigmented plaques of unknown origin in the Chinese Shar Pei. If pododemodicosis is suspected but cannot be confirmed by skin scrapings, multiple specimens should be obtained from maximally affected sites that are normally well haired, such as the dorsum of the digits.

Histopathology (Figures 16-25 an 16-26)

The epidermis is acanthotic, crusted, or ulcerated. Hyperkeratosis may be marked, particularly in cases characterized by granulomatous sebaceous inflammation.

Follicular lesions of canine demodicosis may be

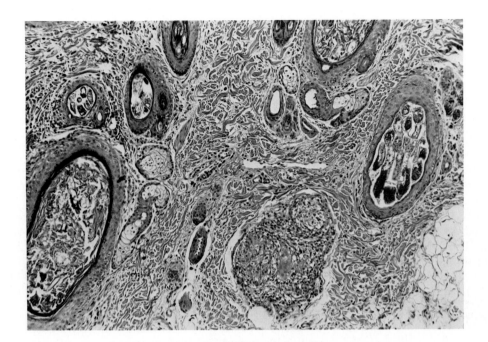

FIGURE 16-25. Demodicosis in a dog. Dilated follicles contain elongated *Demodex* mites; there is scant perifollicular inflammation. Note the large pyogranuloma surrounding adnexal remnants. (×90.)

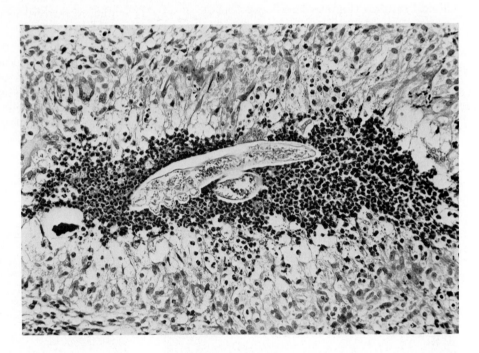

FIGURE 16-26. Canine demodicosis demonstrating an extrafollicular *Demodex* mite within a large pyogranuloma. (×220.)

similar to those of deep folliculitis and furunculosis, since deep pyoderma is a common accompaniment to demodicosis (see earlier discussion). In many cases inflammation may surround rather than invade hair follicles. Plasma cells, macrophages, lymphocytes, and neutrophils are present. Large numbers of plasma cells and lymphocytes surround follicles and apocrine sweat glands in chronic cases. Follicles are colonized by variable numbers of elongated mites (100 to 300 μ in length) with 6 or 8 legs in 2 rows (larva versus adult). In cases of heavy infestation, mites may protrude from

the follicular ostia or may be extruded onto the surface of the specimen. Ruptured hair follicles may result in release of free mites into the dermis, which provokes the formation of discrete pyogranulomas.

In some cases of canine demodicosis (generally nodular localized forms or in the Chinese Shar Pei) small, discrete granulomas or pyogranulomas form within sebaceous glands or as discrete foci immediately adjacent to hair follicles. Mites are often difficult to locate; occasional scattered fragments may be seen within sebaceous gland ducts or associated hair follicles. When inflammatory lesions of this type are found in the skin biopsy, demodicosis should be suspected until proven otherwise, and step sectioning of the specimen should be performed to search for the parasites.

Feline demodicosis is manifested as mild perifollicular inflammation, generally composed of lymphocytes, macrophages, and neutrophils, and occasional pustular folliculitis. The elongated mites generally are located more superficially in the hair follicle than in canine demodicosis and are relatively scant. It has been reported by Conroy that minimal dermal inflammation and acanthosis and hyperkeratosis of the epidermis are histopathologic features of a second form of feline demodicosis caused by a shorter and fatter mite, resembling *Demodex criceti* of hamsters. These mites accumulate in the stratum corneum and are not found within hair follicles.

Differential diagnoses for canine demodicosis include other causes of folliculitis, particularly dermatophytes. However, identification of organisms histopathologically is relatively easy in canine demodicosis, with the exception of the granulomatous form. Granulomatous sebaceous adenitis can resemble the granulomatous form of demodicosis, particularly since inflammation may center on sebaceous glands in both diseases; however, sebaceous adenitis is associated with diffuse loss of sebaceous glands, whereas granulomatous demodicosis is not.

Feline demodicosis is rare, and identification of one organism in tissue section may be an incidental finding. Associated folliculitis and perifolliculitis are supportive. Dermatophytosis should always be considered more strongly than demodicosis in a cat with folliculitis.

RHABDITIC DERMATITIS (Synonym: *Pelodera* dermatitis)

Clinical features (Figures 16-27 and 16-28)

Rhabditic dermatitis is a rare canine skin disease caused by invasion of the skin by larvae from the free-living nematode *Pelodera strongyloides*. The disease has been reported rarely, predominantly from the midwestern United States, but the actual frequency is unknown. As in most parasitic dermatoses, a hypersensitivity to the invading parasite is the presumed mechanism of disease production. The free-living adult nematode is believed to have a direct life cycle and is found most frequently in longstanding, decaying organic debris, especially straw, rice hulls, or hay stored in contact with the ground in damp conditions. Dogs presumably become infected by contact with this contaminated material when it is used as bedding by the animal.

Clinical features include an erythematous, papular rash with crusting. Alopecia is variable but may be profound. Secondary pyoderma may be seen. Affected body sites correlate with contact sites. The ventral paws, limbs, perineum, and comparatively glabrous skin of the ventral abdomen and thorax are most commonly affected. Pruritus usually has been reported as extreme, but Bourdeau described a dog with classic lesions in which pruritus was absent.

Signalment predilections have not been reported.

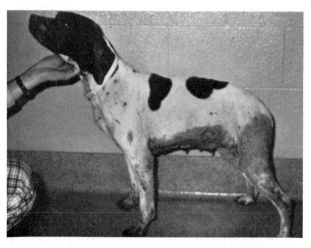

FIGURE 16-27. Rhabditic dermatitis in an English Pointer. Note the ventral, contact distribution pattern affecting the extremities and ventral trunk. *(Courtesy DW Angarano, Auburn, Alabama; CE Griffin, Garden Grove, California; and JM MacDonald, Auburn, Alabama.)*

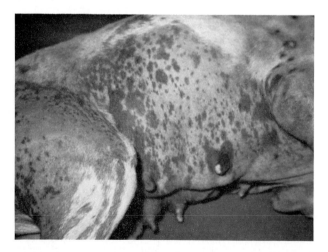

FIGURE 16-28. Closer view of the dog in Figure 16-27. Note the papular rash and extensive alopecia. *(Courtesy DW Angarano, Auburn, Alabama; CE Griffin, Garden Grove, California; and JM MacDonald, Auburn, Alabama.)*

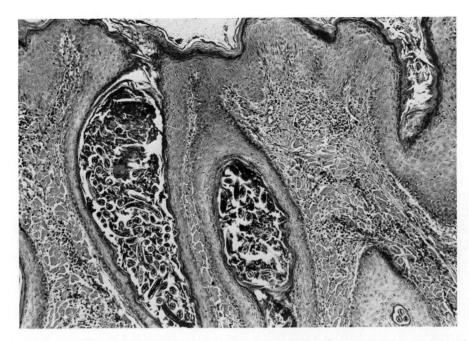

FIGURE 16-29. Rhabditic dermatitis in a dog. Superficial hair follicles are distended with elongated larvae of *Pelodera strongyloides.* (×90.)*(Case material from DW Scott, Ithaca, New York.)*

Clinical differential diagnoses should include sarcoptic acariasis, canine dirofilariasis, hookworm dermatitis, and contact dermatitis. Skin scrapings should readily reveal motile nematode larvae measuring approximately 600 μ in length. Histopathology is diagnostic.

Biopsy site selection

Multiple biopsy specimens should be submitted from new papular lesions. Excoriated skin should be avoided.

Histopathology (Figures 16-29 through 16-32)

The epidermis is severely and irregularly acanthotic. Hyperkeratosis is accompanied by keratin accumulation in follicular infundibula.

Large numbers of elongated nematodes are seen free within superficial keratin and superficial hair follicles. Smaller numbers of mites are found in the deeper follicles. Large and discrete pyogranulomas replace deep follicles and are present subjacent to apparently ruptured follicles. Pyogranulomas frequently contain fragments of nematodes at their neutrophilic centers. Milder folliculitis may be evident. Moderate to large numbers of eosinophils, lymphocytes, macrophages, and mast cells are accumulated around follicles and are present loosely throughout the superficial dermis.

The histopathologic appearance of rhabditic dermatitis is striking and diagnostic. No known differential diagnoses exist.

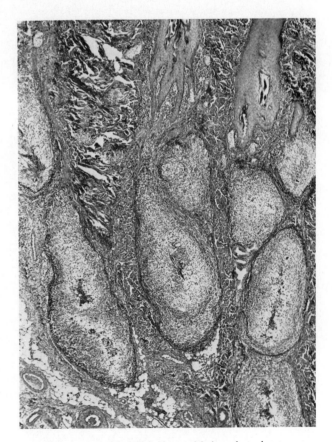

FIGURE 16-30. Rhabditic dermatitis in a dog, demonstrating numerous deep follicular pyogranulomas. (×35.) *(Case material from DW Scott, Ithaca, New York.)*

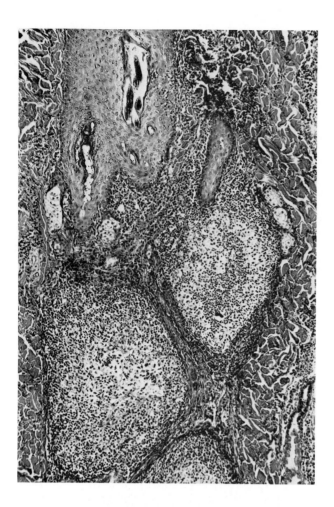

FIGURE 16-31. Higher magnification of the deep follicular pyogranulomas shown in Figure 16-30. Note the nematode larvae within the follicle at the top. (×90.)

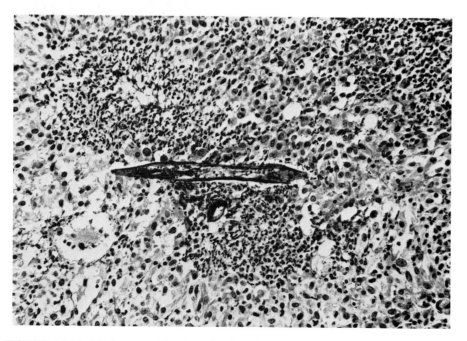

FIGURE 16-32. Higher magnification of a deep follicular pyogranuloma shown in Figure 16-30 that surrounds a fragment of a nematode larva. (×220.)

EOSINOPHILIC FURUNCULOSIS OF THE FACE

Clinical features (Figures 16-33 and 16-34)

Eosinophilic furunculosis is an uncommon canine skin disease characterized by severe, predominantly facial, partially symmetric erosions and ulcers. The striking folliculocentric pattern of eosinophilic inflammation is unexplained. The site, clinical course, and microscopic appearance all suggest hypersensitivity, possibly to insect or other arthropod insult. Recent evidence gathered by one author* suggests the sting of wasps or bees as one likely cause. An increased frequency is seen in the spring and summer. The syndrome bears marked clinical and histopathologic similarities to feline mosquito-bite hypersensitivity (see Chapter 13).

Markedly erythematous or hemorrhagic papules, pustules, and nodules develop acutely and ulcerate to form a hemorrhagic crust. Severe edema may be present. Lesions commonly are localized in a somewhat symmetric pattern to the dorsum of the muzzle and less commonly around the eyes. However, similar lesions have been seen on the axillae, legs, and ventral abdomen. Acute lesions may be exquisitely painful and affected dogs may resist examination. Pruritus is variable but may be severe.

Breed, age, or sex predilections have not been established. However, the syndrome may be more common in young and inquisitive large-breed dogs that have ready access to the outdoors. Clinically, eosinophilic furunculosis must be differentiated from tick-bite hypersensitivity and fulminant facial dermatophytosis. History, dermatophyte culture, and histopathology will aid in differentiation.

Biopsy site selection

Biopsy specimens should be taken from intact papules, pustules, or nodules; areas of frank ulceration should be avoided. If primary lesions are not evident, areas of maximal erythema and swelling should be sampled. General anesthesia is recommended for skin biopsy, since dogs may resist manipulation.

Histopathology (Figures 16-35 and 16-36)

The epidermis is moderately to severely acanthotic and may be covered with a serocellular crust. Erosion or ulceration may be present.

The dermis is characterized by severe, predominantly eosinophilic folliculocentric inflammation. Fewer neutrophils and mixed mononuclear cells may be intermingled. Typically, there are accompanying severe der-

* Thelma Lee Gross.

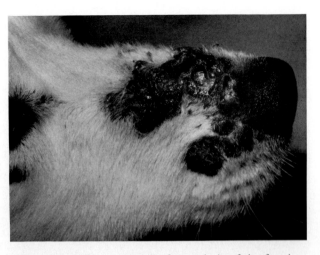

FIGURE 16-33. Eosinophilic furunculosis of the face in a mixed-breed dog. Multiple hemorrhagic nodules have coalesced on the dorsal muzzle.

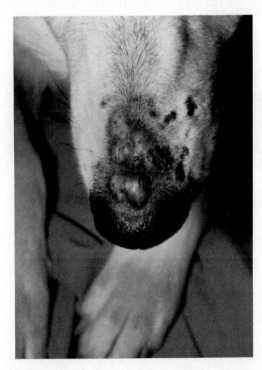

FIGURE 16-34. Eosinophilic furunculosis of the face in a German Shepherd Dog. Ulcerated, coalesced nodules are present on the dorsal muzzle. Lesions are more chronic than those seen in Figure 16-33.

mal edema and mucin deposition. Follicular rupture is characteristic, and large numbers of eosinophils surround free hair shafts. Eosinophils may be degranulated within follicles or around hairs, and smaller foci of eosinophil degranulation and collagen degeneration may be present in the dermis; these features are shared with feline mosquito-bite hypersensitivity (see Chapter

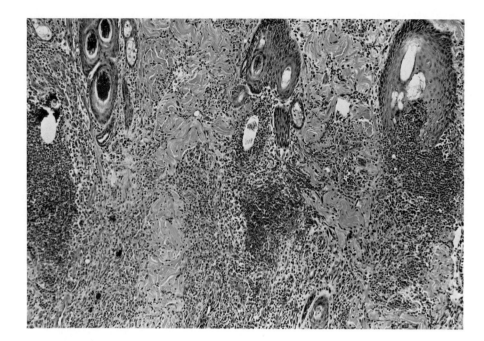

FIGURE 16-35. Eosinophilic furunculosis in a dog. Follicles are partially disrupted and surrounded by darkly staining, intense accumulations of eosinophils. (×90.)

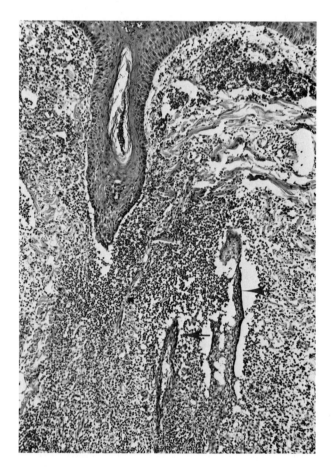

FIGURE 16-36. Eosinophilic furunculosis demonstrating a hair follicle that "exploded" because of severe inflammation. Note residual follicular fragments *(arrows).* (×90.)

13). Hemorrhage is variable. Mixed infiltrations of mononuclear cells, eosinophils, and fewer neutrophils often fill the dermis in later lesions.

Differential diagnoses principally include deep bacterial folliculitis and furunculosis. Although bacterial furunculosis with a predominance of eosinophils can be seen occasionally, neutrophils usually are still a more significant component of the inflammation. Neutrophils are not prominent in eosinophilic furunculosis unless there is secondary bacterial infection. Severe dermal edema and mucin surrounding ruptured follicles are more characteristic features of eosinophilic furunculosis than of bacterial furunculosis. Sterile eosinophilic pustulosis is similar in that eosinophils predominate in both diseases; however, the pustules of sterile eosinophilic pustulosis are usually superficially located. Clinical differentiation may be required.

ACTINIC COMEDONES
Clinical features (Figure 16-37)

Actinic comedones are solar-induced follicular lesions seen uncommonly in the dog. Lesions develop in nonpigmented, lightly haired skin exposed to excessive ultraviolet light. Although ample evidence indicates that solar irradiation induces a continuum of morphologic alteration of the keratinocyte, the mechanisms of actinic comedo formation are not known. Actinic comedones may be seen alone or in conjunction with actinic keratosis (see Chapters 6 and 21) or squamous cell carcinoma (see Chapter 21).

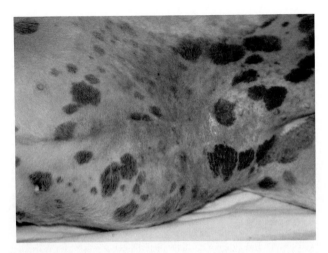

FIGURE 16-37. Widespread actinic damage on the ventrum of a Dalmatian prone to sunbathing. Actinic comedones have become secondarily infected and ruptured, giving rise to hemorrhagic, erythematous nodules.

Actinic comedones (blackheads) are dilated hair follicles filled with darkly colored keratinous material. The lesions usually are multiple and grouped. Actinic comedones may form in otherwise normal-appearing, heavily sun-exposed skin. Alternatively, they may be seen amid scaly, ill-defined erythematous macules and papules or crusted, indurated plaques and nodules characteristic of actinic keratosis or squamous cell carcinoma. The glabrous skin of the ventral and lateral abdomen and inner thighs is most frequently affected. Comedonal rupture commonly leads to deep bacterial furunculosis (see earlier discussion).

Short-coated breeds with lightly pigmented skin, such as Dalmatians, Whippets, white Bull Terriers, and Beagles, are at increased risk for actinic comedones. Lesions occur most commonly in older dogs. Sex predilections have not been noted. Dogs spending substantial time outdoors in areas of the world with increased solar exposure are at greater risk. Many affected dogs are reported to be "sunbathers" and spend long periods in dorsal or lateral recumbency.

Differential diagnoses for actinic comedones include other comedogenic disorders such as demodicosis (especially in the German Shepherd Dog) or hyperglucocorticoidism (especially when iatrogenically induced by topical application of glucocorticoids). The presence of comedones in a lightly pigmented breed with habitual access to sun exposure, with or without evidence of other solar-induced preneoplastic or neoplastic lesions, should increase suspicion for actinic comedones. Prompt skin biopsy of lesions suggestive of actinic comedones is strongly recommended, since awareness of solar damage to the skin may prevent more serious disease.

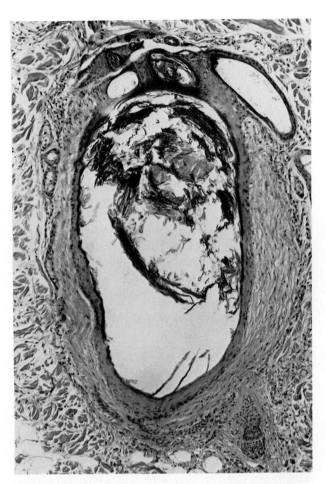

FIGURE 16-38. Actinic comedones. A dilated, keratin-filled follicle is surrounded by concentric layers of pale-staining collagen. (×90.)

Biopsy site selection

Multiple comedones should be surgically excised. If present, erythematous macules, crusted plaques, nodules, or margins of ulcers should be sampled in order to reveal the spectrum of disease present and to uncover possible neoplasia. Solitary lesions suspected of being actinic in origin should be resected in their entirety to prevent possible progression to overt neoplasia.

Histopathology (Figure 16-38)

Features of actinic keratosis may be present or absent (see Chapters 6, 10, and 21). Affected follicles are distended with keratin. Surrounding the follicle are usually concentric layers of very pale eosinophilic or slightly basophilic collagen that appear compressed. Interestingly, elastic stains are negative for solar elastosis in this location.

Rupture of affected follicles leads to severe dermatitis, as seen in deep bacterial furunculosis (see earlier discussion). Severe folliculitis and furunculosis may be seen in specimens obtained from sun-exposed skin of white dogs without histopathologic evidence of comedo formation. Comedones may simply have been destroyed by inflammation in these specimens; alternatively, there may be another solar-related mechanism, other than formation of comedones, which rupture, that induces severe pyoderma in these animals.

Differential diagnoses include those diseases producing comedones, such as acne, Schnauzer comedo syndrome, or hyperglucocorticoidism. The concentric accumulation of pale-staining collagen around the distended follicle suggests actinic comedones but is not always present; correlation with clinical features may be required for definitive diagnosis. The presence of solar elastosis in the superficial dermis also supports an actinic cause for the comedones observed (see Chapter 10).

SUGGESTED READINGS

Deep bacterial folliculitis and furunculosis

Ackerman AB: Histologic diagnosis of inflammatory skin diseases, Philadelphia, 1978, Lea & Febiger, pp 672-693.

Carlotti D, Fourrier P, and Magnol J-P: Les pyodermites profondes, Pratique Medicale et Chirurgicale de l'Animal de Compagnie 23:487-497, 1988.

Ihrke PJ: Bacterial infections of the skin. In Greene CE, editor: Infectious diseases of the dog and cat, Philadelphia, 1990, WB Saunders, pp 72-79.

Krick SA and Scott DW: Bacterial folliculitis, furunculosis and cellulitis in the German Shepherd Dog: a retrospective analysis of 17 cases, J Am Anim Hosp Assoc 25:23-30, 1989.

Muller GH, Kirk RW, and Scott DW: Small animal dermatology, ed 4, Philadelphia, 1989, WB Saunders, pp 244-285.

White SD and Ihrke PJ: Pyoderma. In Nesbitt GH, editor: Dermatology: contemporary issues in small animal practice, New York, 1987, Churchill Livingstone, pp 112-113.

Wisselink MA, Willemse A, and Koeman JP: Deep pyoderma in the German Shepherd Dog, J Am Anim Hosp Assoc 21:773-776, 1985.

Wisselink MA and others: Immunologic aspects of German Shepherd dog pyoderma (GSP), Vet Immunol Immunopathol 19:67-77, 1988.

Canine callus and callus pyoderma

Muller GH, Kirk RW, and Scott DW: Small animal dermatology, ed 4, Philadelphia, 1989, WB Saunders, pp 785-790.

Canine acne

Lever WF and Schaumburg-Lever G: Histopathology of the skin, ed 7, Philadelphia, 1990, JB Lippincott, pp 218-219.

Muller GH, Kirk RW, and Scott DW: Small animal dermatology, ed 4, Philadelphia, 1989, WB Saunders, pp 739-740.

Strauss JS: Sebaceous glands. In Fitzpatrick TB, Eisen AZ, Wolff K and others, editors: Dermatology in general medicine, New York, 1987, McGraw-Hill, pp 666-676.

Feline acne

Muller GH, Kirk RW, and Scott DW: Small animal dermatology, ed 4, Philadelphia, 1989, WB Saunders, pp 740-741.

Strauss JS: Sebaceous glands. In Fitzpatrick TB, Eisen AZ, Wolff K and others, editors: Dermatology in general medicine, New York, 1987, McGraw-Hill, pp 666-676.

Kerion

Foil CS: Dermatophytosis. In Greene CE, editor: Infectious diseases of the dog and cat, Philadelphia, 1990, WB Saunders, pp 661-662.

Lever WF and Schaumburg-Lever G: Histopathology of the skin, ed 7, Philadelphia, 1990, JB Lippincott, pp 364, 851.

Muller GH, Kirk RW, and Scott DW: Small animal dermatology, ed 4, Philadelphia, 1989, WB Saunders, pp 307-308.

Demodicosis

Carlotti D and others: La demodicie feline: a propos de trois cas, Pratique Medicale et Chirurgicale de l'Animal de Compagnie 21:203-208, 1986.

Chalmers S, Schick RO, and Jeffers J: Demodicosis in two cats seropositive for feline immunodeficiency virus, J Am Vet Med Assoc 194:256-257, 1989.

Conroy JD, Healey MC, and Bane AG: New demodex species infesting a cat: a case report, J Am Anim Hosp Assoc 18:405-407, 1982.

Kwochka KW: Canine demodicosis. In Kirk RW, editor: Current veterinary therapy X, Philadelphia, 1986, WB Saunders, pp 531-537.

McDougal WJ and Novak CP: Feline demodicosis caused by an unnamed *Demodex* mite, Comp Small Anim 8:820-822, 1986.

Medleau L and others: Demodicosis in cats, J Am Anim Hosp Assoc 24:85-91, 1988.

Muller GH, Kirk RW, and Scott DW: Small animal dermatology, ed 4, Philadelphia, 1989, WB Saunders, pp 376-395.

White SD and others: Generalized demodicosis associated with diabetes mellitus in two cats, J Am Vet Med Assoc 191:448-450, 1987.

Rhabditic dermatitis

Bourdeau P: Cas de dermatite a rhabditides *(Pelodera strongyloides)* chez un chien, Le Point Veterinaire 16:5-10, 1984.

Horton ML: Rhabditic dermatitis in dogs, Mod Vet Pract pp 158-159, February 1980.

Muller GH, Kirk RW, and Scott DW: Small animal dermatology, ed 4, Philadelphia, 1989, WB Saunders, pp 350-354.

Schwartzman RM: Rhabditic dermatitis in the dog, J Am Vet Med Assoc 145:25-28, 1964.

Willers WB: *Pelodera strongyloides* in association with canine dermatitis in Wisconsin, J Am Vet Med Assoc 156:319-320, 1970.

Eosinophilic furunculosis of the face

No references available.

Actinic comedones

Lever WF and Schaumburg-Lever G: Histopathology of the skin, ed 7, Philadelphia, 1990, JB Lippincott, pp 542-546.

Schwartz RA and Stoll HL: Epithelial precancerous lesions. In Fitzpatrick TB, Eisen AZ, Wolff K and others, editors: Dermatology in general medicine, ed 3, New York, 1987, McGraw-Hill, pp 733-746.

Atrophic diseases of the hair follicle*

Atrophic diseases of the hair follicle principally include those in which the follicle has undergone hair growth cycle arrest, or physiologic "atrophy." In some cases, there may be a metabolic or endocrine stimulus, in others an inflammatory cause. True follicular atrophy (reduction in follicular size over what would be expected for the given stage of the follicular growth cycle) usually is observed in addition to growth cycle arrest, but follicular dysplasia (abnormal development of the hair follicle, resulting in abnormal shape or pigmentation; see Chapter 18) is not present.

Most atrophic diseases of the follicle are characterized by telogen or catagen arrest. The catagen, or regression, phase is characterized by atrophy of the hair bulb, upward migration of the follicle and follicular papilla, and disintegration of the inner root sheath. The outer root sheath continues to keratinize as it regresses; the outer root sheath keratin may merge with the keratin of the hair cortex, resulting in a brush-like mass of brightly eosinophilic keratin. The telogen, or resting, phase of the hair follicle is characterized by a widened infundibulum and narrow base of outer root sheath, which terminates at the level of the sebaceous glands. A thin cord of hair germ cells projects downward from the outer root sheath to end at the follicular papilla.

Exaggerated forms of catagen follicles, in which large spikes of fused keratin appear to protrude through the outer root sheath to the vitreous layer, exist is some disease states; these have been dubbed "flame follicles."† The flame follicle may result from abnormal configuration occurring in the late catagen phase; alternately, a follicle arrested in the catagen phase may develop flame features.

Differentiation among the atrophic follicular diseases on histopathologic grounds alone may be difficult, particularly for the atrophic follicular diseases not characterized by inflammation; the atrophic follicle has limited morphologic variation. Other adjunctive features such as epidermal atrophy, the presence or absence of flame follicles, or the presence of inflammation may be helpful, but clinical data, such as sexual status and endocrine assays, usually are required for definitive diagnosis.

HYPOTHYROIDISM
Clinical features (Figures 17-1 and 17-2)

See Chapter 6.

---

* Dr. Emily J. Walder contributed to this chapter.
† From Dunstan RW: Personal communication, 1984.

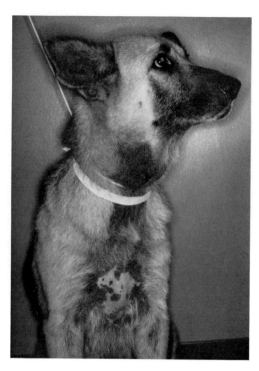

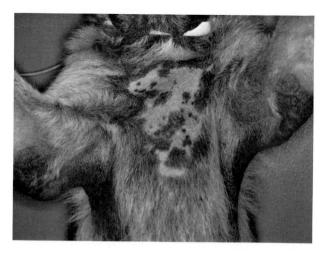

FIGURE 17-2 Closer view of the dog in Figure 17-1. Alopecia, lichenification, and hyperpigmentation are seen on the ventral neck and chest.

FIGURE 17-1 Canine hypothyroidism in a mixed-breed dog demonstrating somewhat symmetric alopecia.

Histopathology (Figures 17-3 and 17-4)

Epidermal and follicular infundibular hyperplasia usually is present, and variable hyperpigmentation may be observed (see Chapter 6). Mild to moderate follicular infundibular and epidermal hyperkeratosis often exist.

Biopsy site selection

Biopsy specimens should be obtained from areas of most advanced hair loss for optimal identification of atrophic follicular changes. Skin from the junctional zone between normally haired areas and areas of alopecia should be strictly avoided, as should lesions with obvious secondary pyoderma.

Hair follicles are in growth cycle arrest (physiologic atrophy) and often are predominantly in telogen phase, although catagen hairs may be prominent in individual cases. Flame follicles have been reported by Scott to be prominent in some cases of hypothyroidism, but this has not been our general experience. Hair follicles are often smaller than normal follicles in

FIGURE 17-3 Canine hypothyroidism. Acanthosis and hyperplasia of follicular infundibula accompany deep follicular atrophy of telogen type. (×35.)

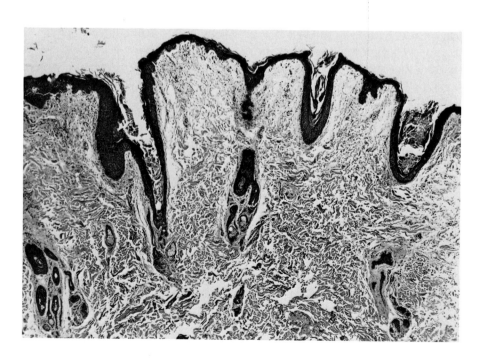

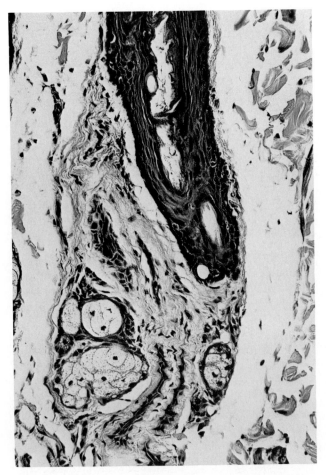

FIGURE 17-4 Canine hypothyroidism demonstrating thin cord-like remnants of telogen follicles beneath hyperplastic superficial follicular epithelium. (×220.)

telogen or catagen phase; therefore, true atrophy is present. The thickened follicular infundibulum often tapers radically to the contracted deep follicle in telogen arrest, creating a V-shaped configuration. Affected dogs frequently have secondary pyoderma, and variable numbers of lymphocytes, macrophages, plasma cells, and neutrophils may be present in the superficial dermis or around hair follicles. Frank folliculitis or superficial epidermal pustulation may be seen.

Differential diagnoses principally include other endocrine alopecias and telogen effluvium. It is not reliable to use the presence and proportion of catagen versus telogen hairs to determine the type of endocrine alopecia present. When hair growth cycle arrest is observed, all other endocrine-related alopecias must be considered, including Sertoli cell tumor, growth hormone/castration-responsive dermatosis, female hyperestrogenism, and hyperadrenocorticism. Acanthosis and hyperplasia of the follicular infundibulum in the face of follicular growth cycle arrest are highly suggestive of hypothyroidism, but Sertoli cell tumor or occa-

sionally canine female hyperestrogenism may have similar changes. Clinical differentiation is required. Telogen effluvium is characterized by telogen arrest, but true follicular atrophy is not present.

CANINE HYPERADRENOCORTICISM

(Synonyms: Cushing's disease, Cushing's syndrome, hyperglucocorticoidism)

Clinical features (Figures 17-5 through 17-8)

Canine hyperadrenocorticism is a relatively common endocrine metabolic disease involving the adrenal-pituitary-hypothalamic axis that produces multiple, characteristic skin lesions. A condition of excessive glucocorticoid production, hyperadrenocorticism is caused by either bilateral adrenocortical hyperplasia as a result of pituitary stimulation (functional tumors of the pituitary gland are not always recognized) or a functional tumor of the adrenal cortex (which induces contralateral adrenocortical atrophy). Similar skin lesions are produced more frequently as a sequela to the injudicious use of exogenous (oral, parenteral, or topical) glucocorticoids. The term iatrogenic hyperglucocorticoidism is preferred to iatrogenic hyperadrenocorticism, since the latter implies overproduction of glucocorticoids by the adrenal gland.

Dermatologic signs include bilaterally symmetric alopecia (often sparing the head and distal extremities), thinning and decreased elasticity of the skin, aberrations in pigmentation (changes in coat color, hyperpigmentation, or depigmentation of the skin), bleeding abnormalities (petechiae, hematomas), delayed wound healing, scaling, comedones (blackheads), phlebectasia, and calcinosis cutis (see Chapter 14). Alopecia often

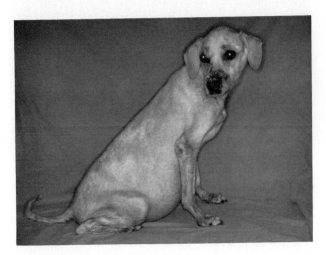

FIGURE 17-5 Severe canine hyperadrenocorticism. Extensive bilaterally symmetric alopecia and thinning of the skin are present. A markedly pendulous abdomen and muscle wasting are obvious, nondermatologic clinical signs.

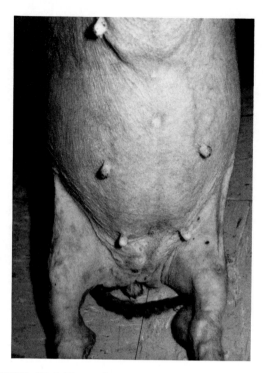

FIGURE 17-6 Hyperadrenocorticism in an aged Dachshund. Increased prominence of subcutaneous blood vessels indicates thinning of the skin. Focal erythematous areas on the groin and legs represent secondary pyoderma.

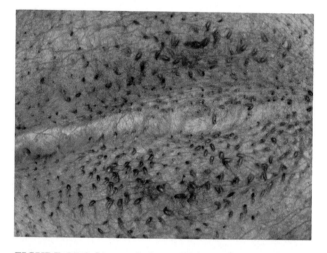

FIGURE 17-7 Iatrogenic hyperglucocorticoidism resulting from the use of topical corticosteroids. Thinning of the skin is obvious at the umbilicus. Characteristic large comedones are present.

begins over bony prominences and other areas of friction such as under collars. Thin, inelastic skin allows visualization of subcutaneous blood vessels. Thinning of the skin may be especially obvious at the umbilicus and at the site of prior ovariohysterectomy surgery. Delayed and inadequate wound healing is manifested

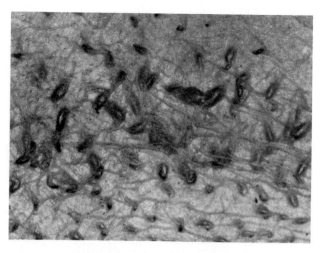

FIGURE 17-8 Closer view of Figure 17-7. Large, visually distinctive comedones typify iatrogenic hyperglucocorticoidism from long-term application of topical corticosteroids.

by the formation of thin scar tissue and striae. Decubital ulcers may be seen in large-breed dogs. Comedones are common and are especially prominent around the nipples and genital region. Large, visually distinctive comedones are seen most frequently with iatrogenic hyperglucocorticoidism resulting from the injudicious use of topical glucocorticoids. On gross examination, phlebectasias, described by Scott, appear as erythematous macules or papules on the trunk. Secondary pyoderma, especially impetigo (see Chapter 1), commonly results from immune suppression. Less commonly, secondary localized or generalized demodicosis may be present.

Polydipsia, polyuria, polyphagia, hematologic abnormalities, muscle weakness and atrophy, lethargy, hepatomegaly, and neurologic abnormalities are common nondermatologic signs of hyperglucocorticoidism. The reader is referred to internal medicine texts for further discussion of the noncutaneous manifestations of this disease.

The Boxer, Boston Terrier, Dachshund, and Poodle are at increased risk for naturally occurring hyperadrenocorticism. Although iatrogenic hyperglucocorticoidism may be seen in any breed, one would expect this syndrome to occur more frequently in breeds predisposed to allergic diseases and hence more likely to receive glucocorticoid therapy. Hyperadrenocorticism is seen more frequently in older dogs. Sex predilections have not been reported for pituitary-dependent hyperadrenocorticism, but females are at increased risk for corticosteroid-producing adrenocortical tumors. Age or sex predilections have not been noted with iatrogenic hyperglucocorticoidism.

Clinical differential diagnoses are contingent upon

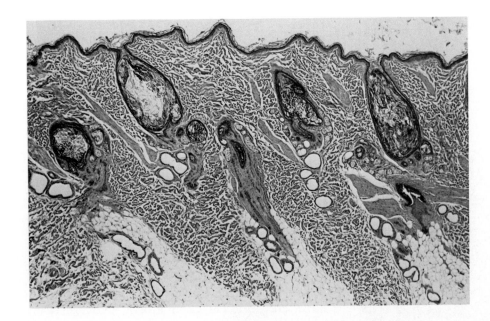

FIGURE 17-9 Canine hyperadrenocorticism. Diffuse follicular keratosis and telogen-type atrophy of hair follicles are present. (×35.)

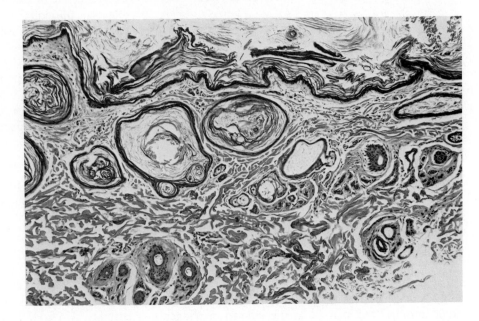

FIGURE 17-10 Canine hyperadrenocorticism demonstrating typical thin-walled follicular comedones and epidermal atrophy. Note the diffuse telogen atrophy of follicles and hyperkeratosis. (×90.)

the presenting clinical signs. If symmetric alopecia is present, other endocrine dermatoses, including hypothyroidism, growth hormone/castration-responsive dermatosis, and sex hormone–related skin disease, must be considered, as well as nonendocrine skin diseases, such as follicular dysplasia and acquired pattern alopecia. Differentiation is accomplished by the presence of nondermatologic signs and laboratory evaluation, including endocrinologic function tests, serum biochemical profiles, and histopathology.

Biopsy site selection

It is important in all cases of suspected endocrine alopecia to obtain skin biopsy specimens from areas of most advanced hair loss for optimal identification of atrophic follicular changes; skin from the junctional zone between normally haired areas and areas of alopecia should be strictly avoided. If firm plaques suggestive of calcinosis cutis are present, they should be sampled, since the presence of this condition usually indicates hyperglucocorticoidism.

Histopathology (Figures 17-9 through 17-11)

The epidermis and the epithelium of the follicular infundibulum frequently are atrophic (fewer than three nucleated cell layers); however, random biopsy specimens from affected animals may show normal epithelial thickness of the epidermis and follicular infun-

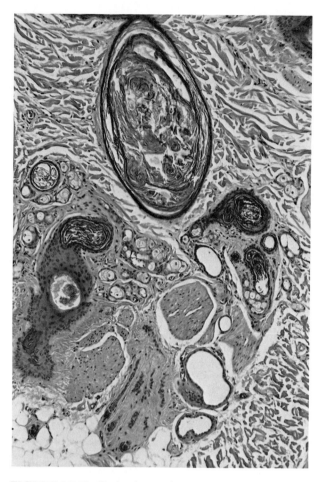

FIGURE 17-11 Canine hyperadrenocorticism. Typical telogen follicle has a markedly dilated infundibulum. (×90.)

dibulum. The exception is in specimens from dogs with calcinosis cutis; the epidermis from affected areas is usually acanthotic and may be exudative (see Chapter 14).

Hair follicles are in growth cycle arrest (physiologic atrophy) and may be in the catagen or telogen phase. The telogen phase usually predominates. Hair follicles are usually smaller than normal follicles in the telogen or catagen phase; therefore, true atrophy is present. Hair follicles from chronic cases may be reduced to an exaggerated state of telogen as a single thin cord of epithelium. Sebaceous glands often are atrophic also. Flame follicles are rare. Although mineralization of the external follicular root sheath is a senile feature found sparingly in normal older dogs (particularly Poodles), hyperadrenocorticism may result in widespread and prominent mineralization of the external root sheath in the absence of calcinosis cutis.

Comedo formation is another variable but characteristic feature of canine hyperadrenocorticism. Come-

dones are characterized by accumulation of keratin within a thin-walled follicular infundibulum. These lesions may approach cystic proportions in some cases and may be most prominent in iatrogenic hyperglucocorticoidism induced by topical application of glucocorticoids.

Phlebectasia was described by Scott in dogs with hyperglucocorticoidism. Superficial vessels are dilated and congested and may proliferate. The epidermis may extend downward and partially enclose the vascular lesion.

Histopathologic differential diagnoses principally include other endocrine alopecias or telogen effluvium. It is not reliable to use the presence and proportion of catagen versus telogen hair follicles present to determine the type of endocrine alopecia present. When hair growth cycle arrest is observed, all other endocrine-related alopecias must be considered. Pronounced follicular and sebaceous gland atrophy accompanied by telogen arrest of the hair follicles and epidermal and follicular infundibular atrophy suggest hyperadrenocorticism. Although follicular keratosis is a nonspecific feature of many atrophic (as well as dysplastic) follicular diseases, comedo or keratin cyst formation within a thin-walled follicular infundibulum is generally restricted to hyperadrenocorticism. Calcinosis cutis, when present, also is diagnostic. Telogen effluvium is characterized by telogen arrest but true follicular atrophy is not present.

CANINE SERTOLI CELL TUMOR
Clinical features (Figures 17-12 through 17-14)
See Chapter 6.

Biopsy site selection

It is important in all cases of suspected endocrine alopecia to obtain skin from areas of most advanced hair loss for optimal identification of atrophic follicular changes; skin from the junctional zone between normal areas and areas of alopecia should be strictly avoided. Multiple specimens, including areas of hyperpigmentation and lichenification, should be taken.

Histopathology (Figures 17-15 and 17-16)

The epidermis is often mildly to moderately acanthotic and hyperpigmented (see Chapter 6). The follicular growth cycle is arrested with telogen hairs or catagen hairs predominating. Flame follicles are rare. Follicles are variably reduced in size. Inflammation may consist of mild to moderate, superficial perivascular or periadnexal infiltrations of lymphocytes, macrophages, plasma cells, and neutrophils and probably reflects secondary chronic pyoderma.

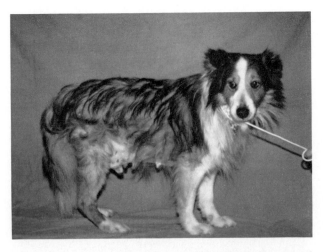

FIGURE 17-12 Skin disease in a Shetland Sheepdog caused by a Sertoli cell tumor. Note the relative lack of hair ventrally.

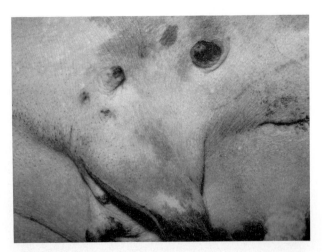

FIGURE 17-14 Ventral abdomen and prepuce of the dog in Figure 17-12. Note the comedones and Griffin's linear preputial erythema.

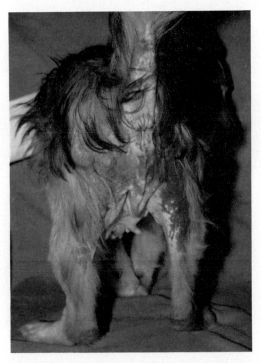

FIGURE 17-13 Caudal view of the dog in Figure 17-12. Bilaterally symmetric alopecia, hyperpigmented macules, and gynecomastia are present.

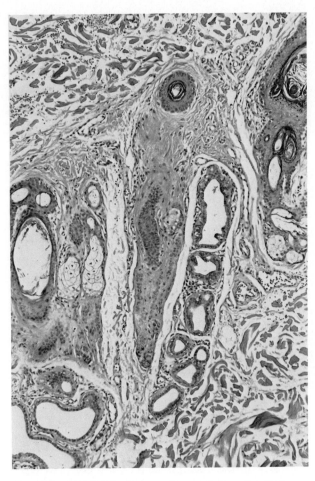

FIGURE 17-15 Skin from a dog with Sertoli cell tumor demonstrating diffuse follicular atrophy. Sebaceous glands are not atrophic. (×90.)

Differential diagnoses principally include the other endocrine alopecias. It is not reliable to use the presence and proportion of catagen versus telogen hairs to determine the type of endocrine alopecia present. When hair growth cycle arrest is observed, all other endocrine-related alopecias must be considered, including hypothyroidism, growth hormone/castration-

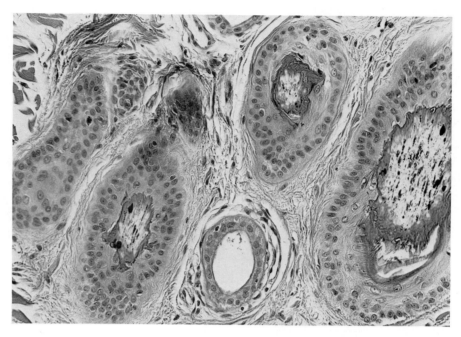

FIGURE 17-16 Skin from a dog with a Sertoli cell tumor. Hair follicles are in the catagen phase. Note the prominent tricholemmal keratin. (×220.)

responsive dermatosis, female hyperestrogenism, and hyperadrenocorticism. In particular, the common features of epidermal acanthosis and follicular atrophy may make distinguishing Sertoli cell tumor from hypothyroidism difficult. Canine hypothyroidism is more common and therefore a more likely diagnosis; however, Sertoli cell tumor should be suggested by these histopathologic changes in intact male dogs, particularly those with gross physical signs of feminization or other characteristic clinical signs.

CANINE FEMALE HYPERESTROGENISM (Synonym: ovarian imbalance type I)

Clinical features (Figures 17-17 through 17-19)

Canine female hyperestrogenism is a rare endocrine skin disease resulting from excess estrogen levels. Hyperestrogenism is a naturally occurring disease in intact bitches with cystic ovaries or, even more rarely, in conjunction with functional ovarian neoplasms. A physiologically identical disease may be induced by estrogen supplementation used in the therapy of urinary incontinence. Both naturally occurring and iatrogenic forms of hyperestrogenism share many features with the skin disease seen in male dogs with estrogen-producing Sertoli cell tumors (see Chapter 6).

Bilaterally symmetric alopecia characteristically be-

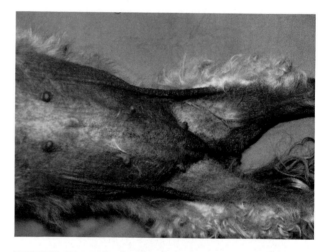

FIGURE 17-17 Canine female hyperestrogenism in a sexually intact adult dog. Bilaterally symmetric alopecia, hyperpigmentation, and lichenification are present in the perineal-genital region and on the abdomen.

gins in the perineal-genital region and may progress to the abdomen, caudal and medial thighs, chest, flanks, and neck. Hyperpigmentation in the areas of alopecia may be seen in advanced cases (especially in naturally occurring disease) and may be accompanied by lichenification and greasy, keratinous deposits. Macular hyperpigmentation is seen with both naturally occurring

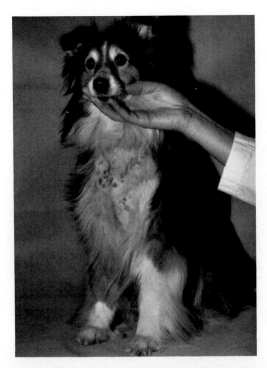

FIGURE 17-18 Iatrogenic hyperestrogenism in a spayed female Shetland Sheepdog caused by administration of diethylstilbestrol. Note the hyperpigmented macules in an area of bilaterally symmetric alopecia on the neck and chest.

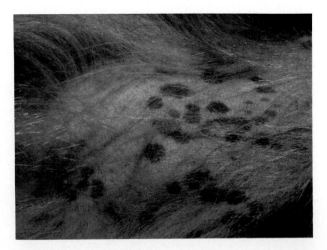

FIGURE 17-19 Lateral thorax of the dog in Figure 17-18. Symmetric alopecia and hyperpigmented macules are the only skin changes noted.

and iatrogenic disease but may be more common in iatrogenic hyperestrogenism. Gynecomastia and vulvar enlargement are common additional features. Abnormal estrous cycles are seen in naturally occurring canine female hyperestrogenism.

Naturally occurring hyperestrogenism may be seen more frequently in English and French Bulldogs. This syndrome occurs more commonly in older female dogs.

Clinical differential diagnoses should include other endocrinopathies, such as hypothyroidism and hyperadrenocorticism. Diagnosis is based on history, clinical findings, laboratory evaluations, histopathology, and on response to ovariohysterectomy or withdrawal of estrogen supplementation.

Biopsy site selection

It is important in all cases of suspected endocrine skin disease to obtain skin from areas of most advanced hair loss for optimal identification of atrophic follicular changes; skin from the junctional zone between normally haired areas and areas of alopecia should be strictly avoided. Multiple specimens should be taken and should include areas of lichenification or hyperpigmentation if present.

Histopathology (Figures 17-20 an 17-21)

The epidermis and superficial follicular epithelial thickness varies from acanthotic to slightly atrophic but is often normal. Acanthosis may be a more prominent feature of naturally occurring hyperestrogenism. Hyperpigmentation may be present.

Follicles are in growth cycle arrest; telogen hairs often predominate, although catagen hairs are present in variable proportions. Follicles are variably reduced in size. Flame follicles are rare.

Differentiation of female hyperestrogenism from other endocrine alopecias, particularly hypothyroidism, is problematic. It is not reliable to use the presence and proportion of catagen versus telogen hairs to determine the type of endocrine alopecia present. Female hyperestrogenism is rare but should be considered as a possible diagnosis in intact females or those receiving estrogen supplementation if endocrine-type follicular atrophy is present.

GROWTH HORMONE/CASTRATION-RESPONSIVE DERMATOSIS (Synonym: hyposomatotropism in the mature dog)
Clinical features (Figures 17-22 and 17-23)

Growth hormone/castration-responsive dermatosis is an uncommon canine endocrinopathy characterized clinically by symmetric alopecia with hyperpigmentation. Strong breed predilections suggest heritability. The clinical response to growth hormone supplementation coupled with abnormal growth hormone response test results have led to the use of the term

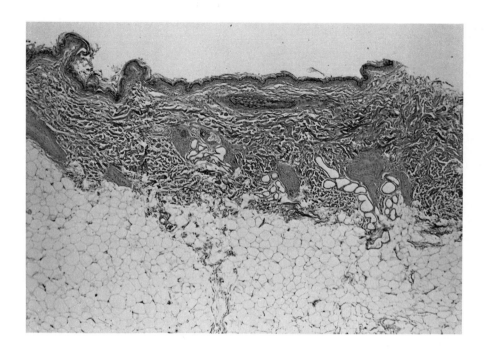

FIGURE 17-20 Canine female hyperestrogenism. Diffuse follicular atrophy of catagen type is present. Note the normal thickness of the epidermis. (×35.)

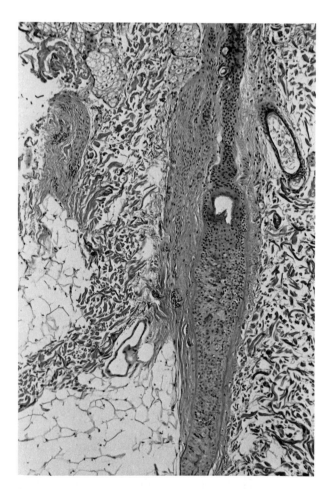

FIGURE 17-21 Canine female hyperestrogenism demonstrating catagen-type follicular atrophy. (×90.)

hyposomatotropism. However, occasional anomalous growth hormone response test results (normal growth hormone response tests in dogs that respond to growth hormone therapy), lack of response to growth hormone, and response to castration indicate that true hyposomatotropism is probably not present. Furthermore, some dogs that have initially responded to growth hormone therapy have recrudesced and then responded to castration.

Recent studies by Schmeitzel and Lothrop indicate that the syndrome, at least in Pomeranians, may be caused by disregulation of adrenal hormone synthesis resulting in adrenal hyperprogestinism and hyperandrogenism, similar to congenital adrenal hyperplasia in humans. The affected Pomeranians may have a nonclassic, late-onset 21-hydroxylase deficiency, leading to progestin and androgen excess at the onset of puberty. Interestingly, clinically unaffected Pomeranians have similar hormonal abnormalities; Schmeitzel and Lothrop speculate that unaffected Pomeranians have a cryptic form of the same enzyme deficiency. In humans, nonclassic late-onset 21-hydroxylase deficiency and the cryptic form of the enzyme deficiency also are biochemically indistinguishable despite clinical differentiating features. Since clinical signs of this syndrome are seen more commonly in Pomeranians bred by successful breeders emphasizing "plush-coated" dogs, current breeding plans dictated by success in showing actually may be accentuating the problem genetically.*

Bilaterally symmetric alopecia originates com-

* Schmeitzel LP: Personal communication, 1990.

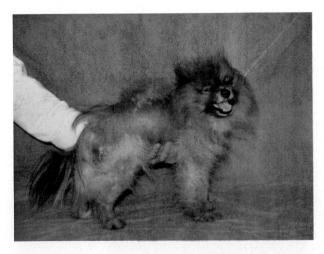

FIGURE 17-22 Growth hormone/castration-responsive dermatosis in a male Pomeranian. Note the bilaterally symmetric alopecia with hyperpigmentation that spares the head and distal extremities.

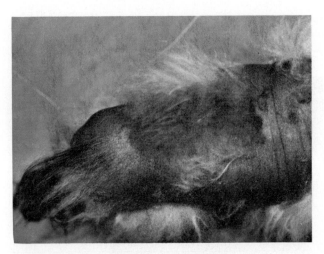

FIGURE 17-23 Closer view of the dog in Figure 17-22. Note the "islands" of normally haired skin.

monly in frictional areas under a collar, on the caudal thighs, or in the perineum. Both primary and secondary hairs are lost, most commonly resulting in nearly total alopecia in affected areas. Occasionally, a sparse, wooly coat may remain. Hyperpigmentation usually develops concomitantly with alopecia in the affected areas but may be absent, especially in white Poodles. Lack of hair regrowth after clipping may be noted even before frank alopecia develops. Hair may regrow focally at the sites of skin scrapings or biopsy. The syndrome progresses gradually to involve the entire thorax, neck, proximal limbs, proximal tail, and, less commonly, the pinnae. The head, distal limbs, and distal tail usually are spared. Islands of apparently normal haircoat and underlying skin occasionally may be present on the thorax. Other clinical abnormalities have not been noted.

Breed predilections have been noted for the Pomeranian, Keeshond, Chow Chow, Miniature Poodle, and Samoyed. Related crossbreeds also may be affected. The syndrome is seen primarily in male dogs. Most affected dogs develop the syndrome between 9 months and 2 years of age near the onset of puberty. However, dogs as old as 12 years of age at initial onset of alopecia have been seen.

Clinical differential diagnoses should include other endocrinopathies such as hypothyroidism, hyperadrenocorticism, and Sertoli cell tumor, as well as canine follicular dysplasia. Endocrinologic function tests, serum biochemical profiles, the history, the clinical course of the alopecia, and histopathology may be helpful in differentiating among these diseases. Definitive diagnosis sometimes is proven only by the response to therapy.

Biopsy site selection

It is important in all cases of suspected endocrine disease to obtain skin from areas of most advanced hair loss, since the type of follicular atrophy may help to distinguish among the various endocrine-related alopecias. Skin from the junctional zone between normally haired areas and areas of alopecia should be strictly avoided. Multiple specimens should be obtained.

Histopathology (Figures 17-24 and 17-25)

The epidermis and superficial follicular epithelium generally are of normal thickness; slight atrophy or slight acanthosis may be present. Epidermal hyperpigmentation usually is evident and is characterized by accumulation of pigment in all viable layers of the epidermis.

Hair follicles are diffusely in hair growth cycle arrest, and the catagen stage predominates. Flame follicles predominate in most cases of growth hormone/castration-responsive dermatosis. Hair follicles are generally reduced in size, particularly in later stages of the disease; thus true follicular atrophy also may be present.

Differential diagnoses principally include other endocrine alopecias. It is not reliable to use the presence and proportion of catagen versus telogen hairs to determine the type of endocrine alopecia present. When hair growth cycle arrest is observed, all other endocrine-related alopecias must be considered. Among the endocrine alopecias, prominent flame follicle production is most compatible with growth hormone/castration-responsive dermatosis. However, recent observations by the authors indicate that the

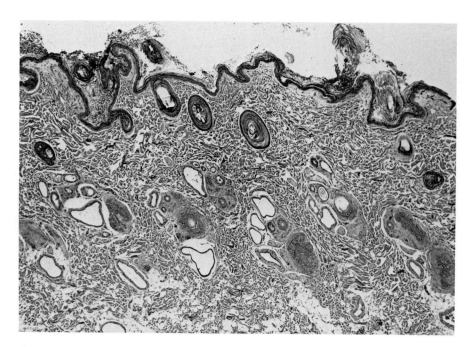

FIGURE 17-24 Growth hormone/castration-responsive dermatosis. Diffuse follicular atrophy of catagen type predominates. Note the flame follicles. (×35.)

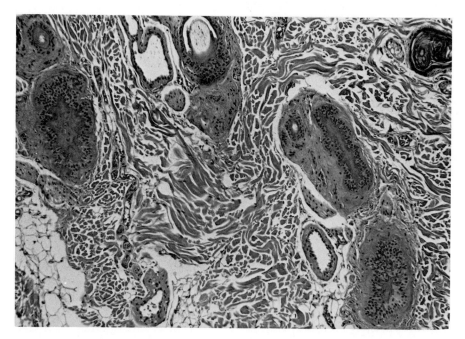

FIGURE 17-25 Higher magnification of the hair follicles shown in Figure 17-24. Flame follicles have spikes of keratin that project through the outer follicular wall. (×90.)

tendency to form flame follicles may be breed dependent; dogs such as the Chow Chow or Pomeranian may develop flame follicles as a result of other atrophic influences on the hair follicle, such as those induced by hyperestrogenism or hyperadrenocorticism.

Other differential diagnoses include nonendocrine follicular disorders in which flame follicles also are prominently observed, principally (1) post-clipping alopecia and (2) follicular dysplasia of the Siberian Husky. Definitive diagnosis of growth hormone/castration-responsive dermatosis is usually made by clinical features and breed type.

POST-CLIPPING ALOPECIA
Clinical features (Figure 17-26)

Post-clipping alopecia is a relatively common syndrome seen secondary to the clipping of hair in dogs. Marked breed predilections (sled-dog breeds) suggest a genetic predisposition for development of hair growth cycle arrest in the catagen phase following clipping. The mechanism responsible for the induction of catagen hair cycle arrest is not known. Decreased perfusion of hair follicles secondary to localized vasoconstriction in skin no longer insulated by the haircoat may lead to premature termination of the anagen phase and subsequent catagen arrest. The almost exclusive limitation of this syndrome to sled-dog breeds suggests that decreased vascular perfusion secondary to haircoat removal might be an adaptive trait that would be beneficial in avoiding heat loss in breeds developed to endure severe winter weather. Alternatively, the natural skin temperature of these breeds may simply be higher because of the insulating properties of their coats, thus the loss of coat may produce enough of a temperature drop to affect vasculature. The significance of altered perfusion as a cause of post-clipping alopecia is supported by the clinical observation that hair regrowth in affected dogs may occur secondary to biopsy, trauma, or vigorous brushing of the affected site, all of which increase perfusion to the skin.

Typically in post-clipping alopecia, hair does not regrow after close clipping for venipuncture, surgery, or wound management. Alopecia usually is complete, but some primary hairs (guard hairs) may regrow. Secondary hair (undercoat) regrowth is not seen. Mild scaling may be an additional clinical feature. Post-clipping alopecia is seen most commonly on the dorsal forelimb secondary to clipping performed to facilitate cephalic venipuncture. Less commonly, post-clipping alopecia may be seen on the trunk, head, or extremities secondary to clipping performed for wound management or surgery. Hair regrowth may not occur for as long as 6 to 12 months after initial hair removal. Newly regrown hair may be darker in "pointed" haircoat breeds (acromelanism) such as the Siberian Husky and the Alaskan Malamute.

Post-clipping alopecia is seen primarily in Siberian Huskies, Alaskan Malamutes, and Samoyeds. The syndrome is seen occasionally in the Chow Chow and Keeshond. Age or sex predilections have not been noted.

Clinical differential diagnoses should include failure of hair regrowth after clipping secondary to iatrogenic or endogenous hyperglucocorticoidism, therapy with cytotoxic drugs, hypothyroidism, and growth hormone/castration-responsive dermatosis. Differentiation is based on history, breed affected, supporting

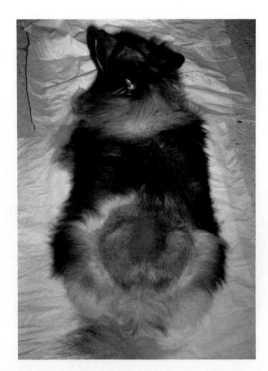

FIGURE 17-26 Post-clipping alopecia in a Keeshond. Hair regrowth has not commenced 4 months after the dorsal lumbosacral area was clipped.

clinical or biochemical evidence of the above-mentioned diseases, and histopathology.

Biopsy site selection

An area of complete alopecia should be selected for skin biopsy. Adjacent normal skin should not be included, since this may confuse interpretation of the biopsy results.

Histopathology (Figures 17-27 and 17-28)

The epidermis and dermis are usually normal; mild hyperkeratosis may be present. Hair follicles are of normal size but are in diffuse catagen and sometimes telogen arrest. Flame follicles may be observed in some cases and can be prominent. Small bulb-like structures may be present at the base of some of the follicles, possibly representing an early phase of recovery to anagen.

Hair follicles in the catagen phase and occurrence of flame follicles may be seen in growth hormone/castration-responsive dermatosis and sporadically in other forms of endocrine alopecia. Specimens from cases of growth hormone/castration-responsive dermatosis may have true follicular atrophy; post-clipping alopecia usually is characterized by hair follicles of normal size for catagen phase. Clinical lesions and the history should help to delineate this disorder from growth hormone–responsive disease; however, early

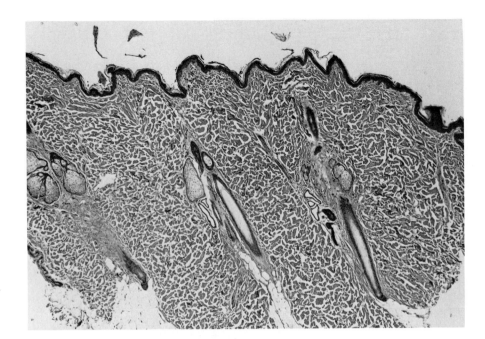

FIGURE 17-27 Post-clipping alopecia in a dog. Hair follicles are in catagen arrest. Note the rudimentary deep hair bulbs at the base of some follicles. (×35.)

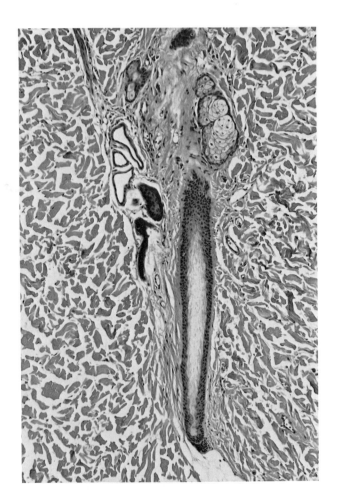

FIGURE 17-28 Higher magnification of Figure 17-27 demonstrating a catagen hair follicle. (×90.)

signs of the latter may include poor hair regrowth after clipping.

TELOGEN EFFLUVIUM (Synonym: telogen defluxion)
Clinical features (Figures 17-29 and 17-30)

Telogen effluvium is a rare syndrome in dogs and cats characterized by widespread alopecia in response to metabolic stress. Serious illness, high fever, pregnancy, lactation, and shock are all potential inducers of telogen effluvium. Rapid, premature cessation of anagen growth leads to synchronization of the follicular cycle such that hair follicles proceed in unison through the catagen and telogen phases. This leads to dramatic hair loss when old telogen hairs are forced out by new, synchronous anagen hairs. Hair loss occurs up to a month after the insult and the syndrome resolves spontaneously as new anagen hairs grow.

Rapid, progressive alopecia develops over a period of several days to a week over most of the body, partially sparing the face. Abnormalities are not noted in the newly exposed skin. Systemic signs, if present, reflect the preexistent or coexistent metabolic stress.

Breed, age, or sex predilections are not noted. The major differential diagnosis is anagen effluvium, a very rare syndrome characterized by shedding during anagen arrest secondary to catastrophic disease or cytotoxic therapy. Microscopic examination of hair and histopathology aid in the differentiation between anagen and telogen effluvium.

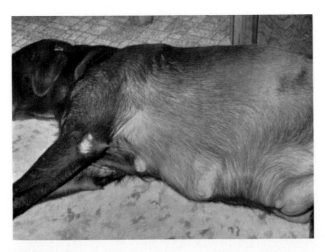

FIGURE 17-29 Telogen effluvium caused by pregnancy and parturition in a Labrador Retriever. *(Courtesy PB Vasseur, Davis, California.)*

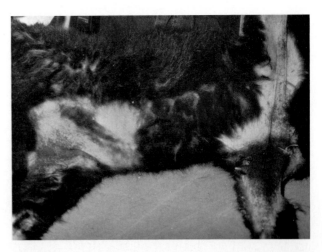

FIGURE 17-30 Telogen effluvium associated with pancreatic adenocarcinoma in a cat. Note the extensive ventral alopecia. *(Courtesy GA Kunkle, Gainesville, Florida.)*

Biopsy site selection

It is essential to perform a skin biopsy as soon as possible after the hair loss has occurred. If specimens are taken later in the course of the syndrome, histopathology may demonstrate normal anagen hair follicles indicative of the recovery phase.

Histopathology (Figure 17-31)

The epidermis and dermis are normal. Hair follicles are diffusely in the telogen phase. Other than physiologic growth arrest, there is no overall diminution in follicular size. In the later stages of the disease, histopathology may reveal a predominance of anagen hairs as the recovery phase begins.

Differential diagnoses include endocrine alopecia with telogen predominance, such as most cases of canine hypothyroidism or canine hyperadrenocorticism. In endocrine alopecia, true follicular atrophy often occurs; the telogen hair follicles are reduced in size over what is expected for the telogen phase. In telogen effluvium, the telogen follicle is of normal size for that phase of the growth cycle.

POST-RABIES VACCINATION ALOPECIA
Clinical features (Figure 17-32)

Post-rabies vaccination alopecia is an uncommon syndrome resulting from a reaction to the subcutaneous deposition of rabies vaccine in dogs. The lesions are presumed to be due to an idiosyncratic hypersensi-

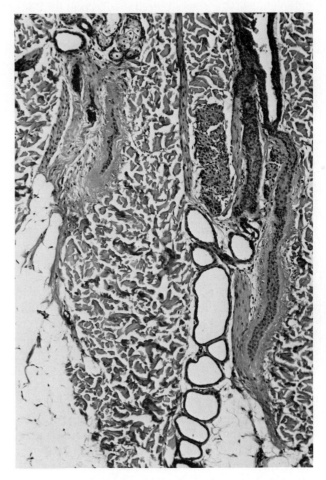

FIGURE 17-31 Telogen effluvium. Elongated cords of follicular epithelium characterize the telogen phase. (×90.)

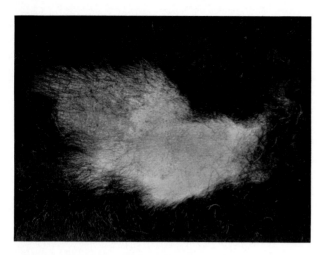

FIGURE 17-32 Post-rabies vaccination alopecia on the shoulder of a black miniature Poodle.

tivity reaction. Wilcock and Yager observed rabies-specific immunofluorescence in the walls of dermal blood vessels and in the epithelium of hair follicles within lesions. The marked breed predilection for Poodles indicates probable enhanced genetic susceptibility for this syndrome.

An alopecic macule or, less commonly, a plaque develops at the site of prior vaccination. The size of the lesion is variable, but most lesions vary between 2 and 10 cm in diameter. The time interval between vaccination and observation of the lesion usually ranges from 2 to 3 months. Although most hair follicles are affected, a few hairs may remain within the boundaries of the lesion. Erythema is minimal or absent. Hyperpigmentation may be an occasional sequela, especially in black Poodles. The lesions are asymptomatic.

Post-rabies vaccination alopecia appears to be a disease of toy or small-breed dogs. Poodles are at markedly increased risk (13 of 17 published cases). Although those previously published reports did not note the size of Poodle affected, all affected Poodles seen by the authors have been either miniature or toy. The syndrome also has been seen in the Bichon Frise, Shih Tzu, Chihuahua, Yorkshire Terrier, Manchester Terrier, American Eskimo, and a Poodle–Cocker Spaniel crossbreed. The authors have observed only a single case of post-rabies vaccination alopecia in a large-breed dog, a Samoyed. Age or sex predilections have not been noted.

Other causes of focal, visually noninflammatory alopecia must be considered in the differential diagnosis of post-rabies vaccination alopecia. Skin scrapings and dermatophyte culture should be performed to rule out demodicosis and dermatophytosis, which occasionally may not exhibit visible inflammation clinically.

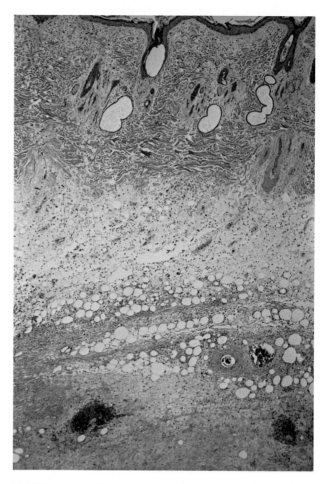

FIGURE 17-33 Post-rabies vaccination alopecia. Diffuse atrophy of hair follicles is accompanied by edema and homogenization of collagenous tissue of the dermis and subcutis; note the nodular lymphocytic panniculitis. ($\times 35$.)

Other atrophic or dysplastic diseases of the hair follicle, such as alopecia areata, cicatricial alopecia, canine traction alopecia, and canine follicular dysplasia, must be ruled out by history, clinical presentation, and histopathology.

Biopsy site selection

Biopsy specimens should be obtained from affected skin just within the outer margin of the plaque or macule. Specimens from near the margin may show more diagnostic histopathologic changes than the central chronic area where typical inflammation may be scant.

Histopathology (Figures 17-33 and 17-34)

The epidermis usually is normal but may be mildly acanthotic. The dermis may be diffusely edematous, and lymphocytes and macrophages may be loosely scattered in the superficial or deep dermis or in small numbers around residual hair follicles. Dermal and subcutaneous connective tissue may appear homogenized or "smudged" and pale.

Hair follicles are severely atrophic. Follicles are small, short, and thin and are in exaggerated telogen phase. Mild vacuolar degeneration may be present in the outer root sheath and in the overlying basilar epidermis. Pigmentary incontinence around hair bulbs and diffuse distribution of melanophages in the surrounding dermis are other possible findings.

The panniculus is characterized by mild or moderate to severe inflammation, which is often nodular and perivascular, and may be accompanied by subtle vascular changes (see Chapter 20). Sometimes, pannicular inflammation may be sparse, most often in advanced lesions. Immunofluorescent testing by Wilcock and Yager with antibody to rabies viral antigen revealed deposition in the epithelium of hair follicles and in the walls of blood vessels.

Follicular atrophy similar to the type observed in post-rabies vaccination alopecia occasionally has been observed overlying subcutaneous injection reactions from other types of vaccines, including canine distemper, and occasionally overlying other chronic lesions of the panniculus. Inflammation of the panniculus that interferes with vascular integrity, through immunologic or other mechanisms, may produce similar follicular atrophy through an ischemic mechanism that interferes with normal hair growth in the overlying dermis.

Lesions of post-rabies vaccination alopecia may resemble canine familial dermatomyositis, lupus erythematosus, or alopecia areata. Canine familial dermatomyositis is not characterized by significant inflammation of the panniculus; however, clinical differentiation may be required if lesions of post-rabies vaccination alopecia are chronic and show minimal pannicular inflammation. Systemic lupus erythematosus may be similar, especially when basal cell vacuolation is prominent; in addition, the lymphocytic panniculitis of post-rabies vaccination alopecia may be confused with lupus panniculitis (see Chapter 10). Lesions of post-rabies vaccination alopecia with minimal panniculitis may resemble alopecia areata. Vacuolar degeneration of follicular epithelium is not prominent in alopecia areata, however.

CANINE FAMILIAL DERMATOMYOSITIS
Clinical features (Figures 17-35 and 17-36)
See Chapter 2.

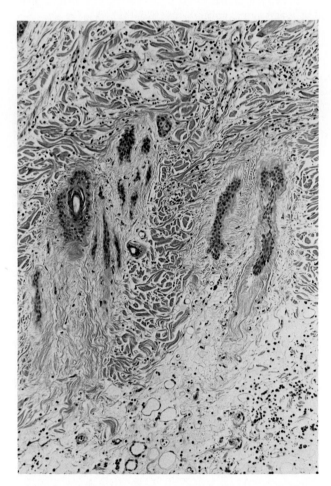

FIGURE 17-34 Post-rabies vaccination alopecia. Diffusely atrophic follicles are surrounded by diffuse mild inflammation. Note the edema and smudging of the collagen around follicles and in the underlying inflamed panniculus. (×90.)

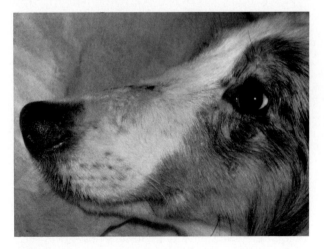

FIGURE 17-35 Canine familial dermatomyositis in a Shetland Sheepdog. Alopecia and scaling are present on the dorsal muzzle and periorbitally over bony prominences.

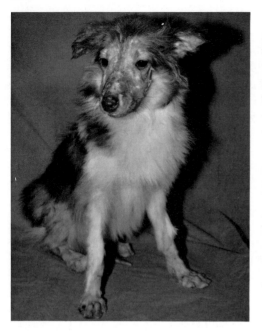

FIGURE 17-36 Severe canine familial dermatomyositis in a Shetland Sheepdog. Note the extensive alopecia on the face and over bony prominences of the distal extremities.

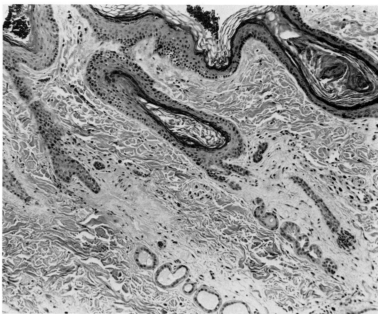

FIGURE 7-37 Canine familial dermatomyositis. Diffuse follicular atrophy is accompanied by scant dermal inflammation. (×100.)

Biopsy site selection

Lesions showing erythema and alopecia are preferred sites for biopsy. Secondarily infected or scarred lesions are not optimal for demonstration of typical histopathology.

Histopathology (Figures 17-37 and 17-38)

Epidermal and dermal lesions have been described in detail (see Chapter 2) and include basal cell degeneration and dermal-epidermal vesiculation. However, typical follicular lesions may be present more reliably in specimens obtained from dogs in random stages of disease. Hair follicles from foci of alopecia are moderately to severely atrophic. Secondary hairs are often absent. Primary hairs are devoid of hair shafts and are narrow and short. Distortion of the hair follicle to a "wavy" configuration may be seen. In some cases, only a thin shaft of external root sheath remains at the site of a previous follicle. Peripheral cells of the outer root sheath have scattered vacuolation and individual necrosis as seen in the overlying epidermis. Sometimes, hair follicles are completely surrounded or replaced by fibrosis (cicatricial alopecia; see also later discussion).

Differential diagnoses for the follicular changes of canine familial dermatomyositis are few as they are unique and characteristic. Lesions of post-rabies vaccination alopecia or alopecia areata may be similar to dermatomyositis. Most cases of post-rabies vaccination alopecia also have prominent pannicular inflammation. Perifollicular inflammation is generally more prominent in alopecia areata than in dermatomyositis, and

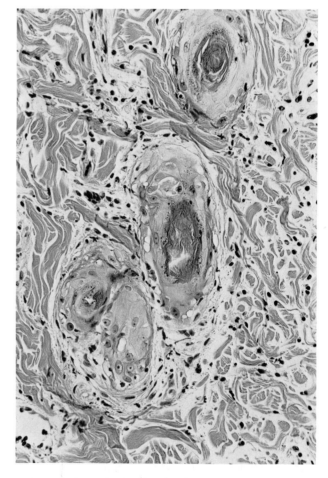

FIGURE 17-38 Canine familial dermatomyositis. Atrophic follicles are surrounded by lymphocytes and macrophages. Note the vacuolar degeneration and necrosis of individual outer root sheath cells. (×250.)

vacuolar degeneration of peripheral cells of the outer root sheath is not observed in alopecia areata. Degeneration of the peripheral cells of the outer root sheath also may be seen in erythema multiforme and ulcerative dermatosis of the Shetland Sheepdog and Collie; however, follicular atrophy is not commonly observed in these diseases.

ALOPECIA AREATA
Clinical features (Figures 17-39 and 17-40)

Alopecia areata, seen very rarely in the dog and cat, is characterized clinically by hair loss without apparent inflammatory changes. In humans, alopecia areata is believed to be an autoimmune disease, since helper T cells predominate in the perifollicular lymphocytic infiltrate and Langerhans cells are present in an abnormal location in the intrabulbar portion of the follicular epithelium. Morphologic changes in follicular melanocytes (indicating that melanocytes may be the target of immunoreactivity) have been reported recently by Fenton in acute alopecia areata. This may explain the dramatic selective loss of pigmented hairs in the rare form of this disease in humans where "hair turns white overnight" and the occasional restriction of the disease to hair of one coat color in dogs.

Focal or multifocal areas of well-circumscribed alopecia develop without visible inflammatory changes in the exposed skin. Areas of alopecia may expand gradually as waves of follicular damage move centrifugally. Hyperpigmentation of exposed skin may occur in chronic cases. Short, stubby "exclamation-mark" hairs with dystrophic proximal tapered portions and frayed damaged distal portions have been described in humans with alopecia areata. One author* has seen hairs

* Peter J. Ihrke.

matching this description in a dog. The head and neck are the most frequent sites of involvement. In multicolored breeds, alopecia areata may be restricted to hair of one color. In breeds such as the German Shepherd Dog or Dachshund with symmetric facial bicolor patterns, restriction of the disease to facial hair of one color may create dramatic patterns of hair loss.

Breed, age, or sex predilections have not been documented. However, the possibility of certain breeds being at elevated risk exists, since alopecia areata in humans is believed to be heritable.

Alopecia areata can mimic any disease with visually noninflammatory alopecia. Skin scrapings and dermatophyte culture should be performed to rule out demodicosis and dermatophytosis, which occasionally may not exhibit visible inflammation clinically. Other atrophic or dysplastic diseases of the hair follicle such as post-rabies vaccination alopecia, cicatricial alopecia, canine traction alopecia, acquired pattern alopecia, and canine follicular dysplasia must be ruled out by history, clinical presentation, and histopathology.

Biopsy site selection

Multiple specimens should be obtained from sites located sequentially along the radius from the center toward the advancing margin of alopecia. In human dermatology, a biopsy specimen from the outer margin of alopecia is less useful than a specimen obtained slightly more centrally. The outer, or advancing, margin may demonstrate abnormal anagen hairs but with only minimally evident follicular insult. Specimens should include only abnormal tissue, particularly if a biopsy punch is used.

Histopathology (Figure 17-41)

The epidermis is normal in lesions of alopecia areata. Hair follicles are small, short, and sometimes

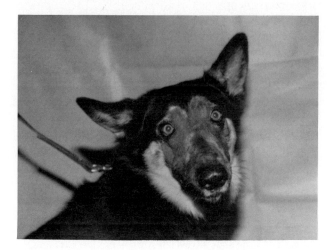

FIGURE 17-39 Alopecia areata in a mixed-breed dog. Hair loss is confined to one coat color and is strikingly bilaterally symmetric.

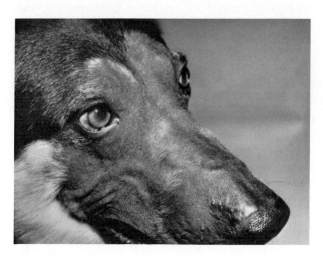

FIGURE 17-40 Closer view of the dog in Figure 17-39. The affected area is almost totally alopecic.

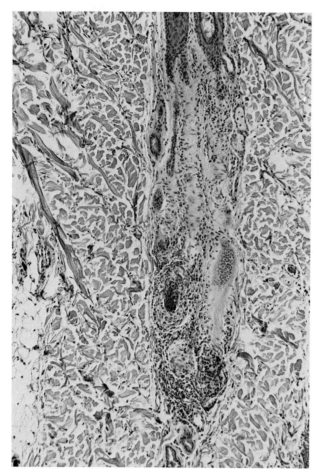

FIGURE 17-41 Alopecia areata in a dog. An atrophic folli-cle is surrounded by mixed mononuclear inflammation, which is most intense around the hair bulb. (×90.)

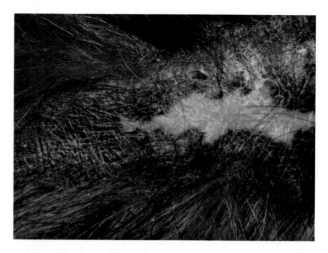

FIGURE 17-42 Cicatricial alopecia in a dog caused by a heating pad burn. Note the lack of a normal follicular archi-tecture and the presence of striae.

distorted in contour and have an overall telogen con-figuration. Lymphocytes, macrophages, and occasional neutrophils encircle and are generally oriented around the lower two thirds of the hair follicle; less commonly, lesions that more closely resemble those of humans are characterized by a tight "swarm of bees" accumulation of lymphocytes around the hair bulbs only. In older lesions, inflammation may be scant.

Differential diagnoses for alopecia areata include those atrophic follicular diseases that are accompanied by inflammation, principally canine familial dermato-myositis and post-rabies vaccination alopecia. Vacuolar degeneration and necrosis of the peripheral cells of the outer root sheath are present in dermatomyositis and may be present in post-rabies vaccination alopecia as well, but are not seen in alopecia areata. Most cases of post-rabies vaccination alopecia have panniculitis, in contradistinction to alopecia areata.

CICATRICIAL ALOPECIA (Synonym: scarring alopecia)
Clinical features (Figure 17-42)

Cicatricial alopecia is a clinical syndrome character-ized by permanent damage to hair follicles such that hair regrowth does not occur. The causes of cicatricial alopecia include physical, chemical, or thermal injury; severe furunculosis (pyoderma, dermatophytosis, de-modicosis); neoplasia; and other diseases, such as sys-temic or discoid lupus erythematosus and canine famil-ial dermatomyositis. In these varied diseases, perma-nent alopecia results from irreversible injury to and ablation of adnexal units with replacement by scar tis-sue. The documentation of cicatricial alopecia is impor-tant clinically, since it proves conclusively that the hair loss is permanent.

Permanent hair loss is the unifying clinical feature. Loss of the normal surface architecture, including fol-licular ostial openings, may be seen with physical, chemical, or thermal injury. Visualization of such ab-normal surface follicular architecture is aided by the use of a hand lens. Striae may be visible if surface scarring is marked. Hyperpigmentation or hypopigmentation may be present. Cicatricial alopecia not caused by in-jury does not have specific visual features. Other skin changes present are contingent on the specific disease creating the cicatricial alopecia.

Breed, age, or sex predilections are not seen with injury-related cicatricial alopecia. Signalment predilec-tions for the other causes of cicatricial alopecia follow those of the specific underlying disease.

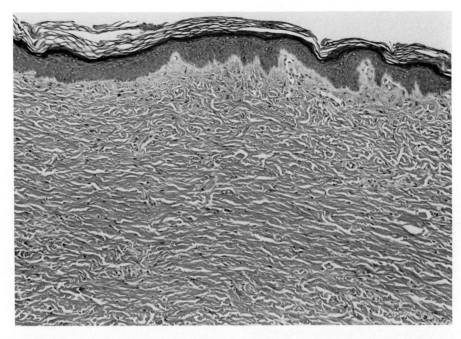

FIGURE 17-43 Cicatricial alopecia in a dog. The entire dermis, including hair follicles, has been replaced by horizontally laminar collagen. (×90.)

Cicatricial alopecia can mimic any disease with visually noninflammatory alopecia. Suspicion of cicatricial alopecia is aided by a history of physical, chemical, or thermal insult or preexisting skin disease. Injury-related cicatricial alopecia generally is focal, and symmetry is lacking. If scarring is not evident, skin scrapings and dermatophyte culture should be performed to rule out demodicosis and dermatophytosis. Other atrophic or dysplastic diseases of the hair follicle such as post-rabies vaccination alopecia, canine familial dermatomyositis, alopecia areata, and canine traction alopecia must be ruled out by history, clinical presentation, and histopathology. Both dermatomyositis and traction alopecia may have components of cicatricial alopecia in severe or chronic cases. Histopathology is the single most valuable tool in differentiating cicatricial alopecia from nonscarring hair loss and in differentiating the multiple causes of cicatricial alopecia.

Biopsy site selection

Specimens from areas of most complete alopecia should be obtained in order to sample the most advanced follicular changes present in the skin. Chronic lesions may be preferred to document fibrous tissue replacement of normal hair follicles. The skin biopsy is a prognostic tool in this regard because it can predict whether hair loss will be permanent.

Histopathology (Figure 17-43)

Scarring alopecia may be seen focally in many diseases, both inflammatory and traumatic. In general, the epidermis is acanthotic or ulcerated, depending on the stage and severity of the insult. Dermal inflammation is variable also, based on the origin of the process that is inducing the dermal damage and the loss of hair follicles.

Hair follicles are replaced by fibrous connective tissue. Collagen may be laminar in distribution and will extend to a variable depth of the dermis, depending on the severity of the previous tissue damage. Rudimentary persistent follicles may be entrapped by scar tissue, thus effectively preventing regrowth of hair. In late-stage lesions, a more normal meshwork pattern of dermal collagen may be present, accompanied by complete absence of adnexal tissue.

Differential diagnoses include canine familial dermatomyositis and traction alopecia, since both of these diseases may have components of dermal scarring. In cases of severe traction-induced damage, differentiation may be difficult. Complete absence of follicles is less common in traction alopecia than in cicatricial alopecia, and laminar deposition of collagen is not a typical feature of traction alopecia. Dermatomyositis may occasionally be characterized by prominent perifollicular fibrosis and severe diminution of follicles; however, again, laminar deposition of collagen is absent and follicles are only rarely completely effaced.

CANINE TRACTION ALOPECIA
Clinical features (Figure 17-44)

Canine traction alopecia is a rare syndrome associated with styling devices such as barrettes or rubber bands. A clinically similar syndrome in humans is believed to be due to interference with the blood supply of the hair root. Traction alopecia in humans usually is reversible. Hair regrowth was not seen in dogs with traction alopecia in a study by Rosenkrantz. This permanent hair loss is similar to that found in cicatricial alopecia. Rosenkrantz theorized that the difference in prognosis may be associated with anatomic differences in the perifollicular vascular bed, leading to greater ischemia, coupled with more prolonged and more severe trauma, since dogs cannot communicate that undue hair tension is inducing pain.

Complete or almost complete alopecia is seen in the affected area. Hair follicle ostia dilated with keratotic debris may be noted with a hand lens. Mild scaling may be present. The pattern of alopecia is contingent on the device used to apply tension to the hair. Rings of alopecia can surround centrally placed rubber bands, and linear bands of alopecia can reflect barrette placement. Canine traction alopecia is seen primarily on the head where devices are used either to keep hair out of the eyes or as decoration.

Breed predilections correlate with dog breeds in which rubber bands and barrettes commonly are used. The syndrome has been seen in the Poodle, Maltese, Yorkshire Terrier, and Shih Tzu. Age or sex predilections have not been seen and would not be expected.

The syndrome is visually distinctive. Usually there is historical correlation by the pet owner with the previous use of a barrette or rubber band. If historical information is not available, cicatricial alopecia, alopecia areata, and other atrophic or dysplastic diseases could possibly mimic traction alopecia. Histopathology is useful both to confirm the diagnosis and to offer a prognosis for hair regrowth.

Biopsy site selection

Skin biopsy specimens should be obtained from areas of most pronounced and complete hair loss. Multiple specimens may be of prognostic and diagnostic value.

Histopathology (Figure 17-45)

The epidermis is normal. Superficial follicular keratosis is present. Hair follicles are typified by extreme diminution in size and are in an exaggerated telogen phase, characterized by reduction to a single cord of epithelium. There may be follicular dropout; a thin

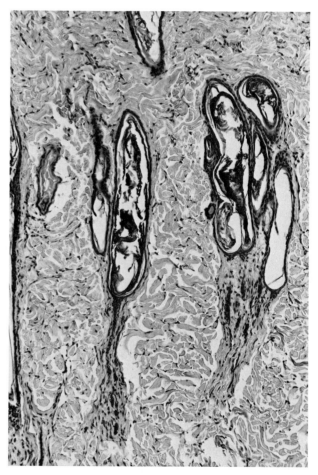

FIGURE 17-45 Canine traction alopecia. Severe follicular attenuation has reduced deep follicles to a single cord of epithelium. Note the mild follicular keratosis. ($\times$90.)

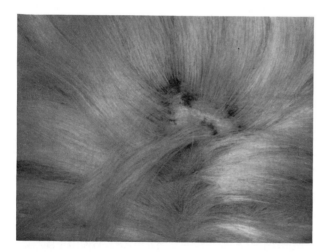

FIGURE 17-44 Canine traction alopecia on the temporal region of a Shih Tzu caused by chronic tension from a tightly applied barrette. (*Courtesy AM Hargis, Seattle, Washington; case material from University of California, Davis*).

cord of connective tissue may be all that remains to mark the location of a previous follicle. Mild mixed mononuclear inflammation may be seen, and melanophages may be present at the site of a previous follicle. Increased, dense fibrous connective tissue is present around and between atrophic follicles; in some cases cicatricial alopecia is present, characterized by laminar bands of connective tissue that replace all normal dermal structures (see preceding discussion).

Occasionally, more severe chronic inflammation is present, composed primarily of macrophages and fewer lymphocytes and neutrophils. Macrophages may have a foamy appearance, suggesting entrapment and destruction of sebaceous and apocrine glands by the hair-retaining device at these sites.

Differential diagnoses principally include cicatricial alopecia. In fact, differentiation between these two entities may be moot, since severe forms of traction alopecia are cicatricial. Cicatricial alopecia from non-traction causes may be characterized by more severe and complete replacement of the normal dermis by fibrosis than is seen in most cases of traction alopecia; in addition, marked diminution of follicles in the midst of increased dermal fibrosis is more suggestive of traction alopecia.

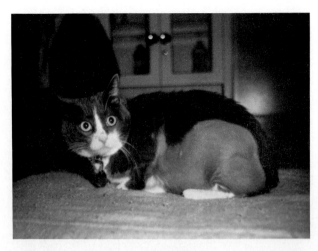

FIGURE 17-46 Feline psychogenic alopecia. Well-demarcated alopecia is present on the trunk. A short stubble is visible. Lesions were strikingly bilaterally symmetric.

FELINE PSYCHOGENIC ALOPECIA
(Synonym: self-induced psychogenic feline hair loss)
Clinical features (Figure 17-46)

Feline psychogenic alopecia is a relatively uncommon feline skin disease in which hair removal is not associated with identifiable underlying causes. It is believed to be an anxiety neurosis associated with displacement phenomena in nervous cats. Incriminated precipitating events include a new environment, changes in animal "pecking order," a new baby or pet in the household, or loss of a favorite owner or other pet. Loss of hair results from excessive grooming or chewing; the underlying skin remains intact. Since cats may be secretive in this endeavor, owners may be unaware of excessive grooming and resist accepting this diagnosis.

Well-demarcated, partial or almost complete alopecia is noted in the affected areas. Partial bilateral symmetry is a common feature. Lesions are not noted in the exposed skin. A short stubble may be visible with a hand lens, giving the visual impression of expertly performed clipping or shaving. Commonly affected sites include the lateral trunk, caudal and medial thighs, abdomen, and limbs. Some hair regrowth may occur if the cat focuses its attention on other previously unaffected body regions. In Siamese cats, new hair growth may be darker, since heat-labile enzymes that enhance

melanization in cool body regions are activated (acromelanism).

Breed predilections have been noted in Siamese and Abyssinian cats but the syndrome may be seen in any breed. Age or sex predilections have not been reported.

A diagnosis of feline psychogenic alopecia should not be made until all possible pruritic and nonpruritic causes of alopecia have been eliminated from consideration. Alopecia secondary to excessive grooming (because of pruritic or psychogenic causes) is best demonstrated by applying an Elizabethan collar; hair will regrow if excessive grooming is prevented by the collar. Underlying pruritic causes of excessive grooming include flea allergy dermatitis, atopy, and food allergy. Intradermal skin testing, in vitro allergy testing, and elimination diets are useful in documenting a pruritic cause for feline self-induced hair loss. Feline demodicosis is an additional rare, usually nonpruritic, cause of alopecia in cats; skin scrapings allow differentiation. Histopathology is required to substantiate feline psychogenic alopecia.

Biopsy site selection

Specimens for biopsy should be obtained from an area of most complete hair loss. Any foci of erythema or crusting also should be obtained to rule out the presence of allergy-induced hair removal by the cat.

Histopathology (Figure 17-47)

Notable histopathologic findings usually are not present in feline psychogenic alopecia. Hair follicles are normal. Occasionally the number of mast cells or mac-

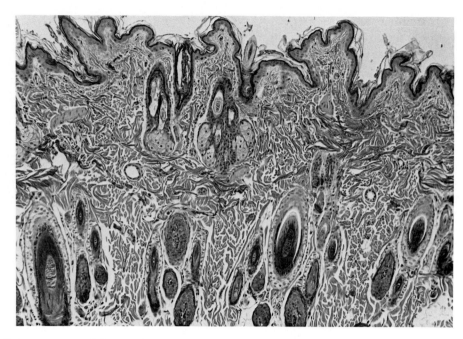

FIGURE 17-47 Feline psychogenic alopecia. All skin components, including hair follicles, are normal. (×90.)

rophages is slightly increased in the superficial dermis. It is important to distinguish mild allergy that is producing excessive grooming from true psychogenic alopecia. The presence of even minimal numbers of eosinophils is presumptive histopathologic evidence for allergic dermatitis.

Rarely, small numbers of lymphocytes or macrophages have been seen encircling the middle portion of hair follicles in cats whose dermatophyte culture was negative and who had symptoms otherwise clinically compatible with psychogenic alopecia. However, the possibility that these cases represent a separate syndrome of inflammatory-mediated alopecia has not been discounted.

Differential diagnoses include very mild allergic dermatitis or alopecia areata. Even rare eosinophils may indicate allergy-induced excessive grooming in the cat. Alopecia areata is rare and is characterized by lymphocytic inflammation encircling the deep, bulb portion of hair follicles; inflammation is diffuse and more intense than the occasional perifollicular inflammation seen in cats with suspected psychogenic alopecia. True endocrine alopecia is very rare in the cat and should be characterized by atrophy and growth cycle arrest of the hair follicles.

SUGGESTED READINGS

Canine hypothyroidism
See Chapter 6.

Canine hyperadrenocorticism

Feldman EC: Adrenal gland disease. In Ettinger SJ, editor: Textbook of veterinary internal medicine, ed 3, Philadelphia, 1989, WB Saunders, pp 1721-1774.

Gross TL and Ihrke PJ: The histologic analysis of endocrine-related alopecia in the dog. In Von Tscharner C and Halliwell REW, editors: Advances in veterinary dermatology, vol 1, London, 1990, Baillière Tindall, pp 77-88.

Muller GH, Kirk RW, and Scott DW: Small animal dermatology, ed 4, Philadelphia, 1989, WB Saunders, pp 595-610.

Scott DW: Cutaneous phlebectasias in cushingoid dogs, J Am Anim Hosp Assoc 21:351-354, 1985.

White SD and others: Cutaneous markers of canine hyperadrenocorticism, Comp Small Anim 11:446-463, 1989.

Canine Sertoli cell tumor
See Chapter 6.

Canine female hyperestrogenism

Barsanti JA, Medleau L, and Latimer K: Diethylstilbestrol-induced alopecia in a dog, J Am Vet Med Assoc 182:63-64, 1983.

Gross TL and Ihrke PJ: The histologic analysis of endocrine-related alopecia in the dog. In Von Tscharner C and Halliwell REW, editors: Advances in veterinary dermatology, vol 1, London, 1990, Baillière Tindall, pp 77-88.

Muller GH, Kirk RW, and Scott DW: Small animal dermatology, ed 4, Philadelphia, 1989, WB Saunders, pp 622-625.

Scott DW: Histopathologic findings in endocrine skin disorders of the dog, J Am Anim Hosp Assoc 18:173-183, 1982.

Watson ADJ: Oestrogen-induced alopecia in a bitch, J Small Anim Pract 26:17-21, 1985.

Growth hormone/castration-responsive dermatosis

Gross TL and Ihrke PJ: The histologic analysis of endocrine-related alopecia in the dog. In Von Tscharner C and Halliwell REW, editors: Advances in veterinary dermatology, vol 1, London, 1990, Baillière Tindall, pp 77-88.

Lothrop CD: Pathophysiology of growth hormone responsive dermatosis, Comp Cont Ed 10:1346-1352, 1988.

Parker WM and Scott DW: Growth hormone responsive alopecia in the mature dog: a discussion of 13 cases, J Am Anim Hosp Assoc 16:824-828, 1980.

Ponec M: Hormone receptors in the skin. In Fitzpatrick TB, Eisen AZ, Wolff K and others editors: Dermatology in general medicine, ed 3, New York, 1987, McGraw-Hill, pp 367-375.

Schmeitzel LP: Sex hormone-related and growth hormone-related alopecias, Vet Clin North Am 20:1579-1601, 1990.

Schmeitzel LP and Lothrop CD: Hormonal abnormalities in Pomeranians with normal coat and in Pomeranians with growth hormone-responsive dermatosis, J Am Vet Med Assoc 197:1333-1341, 1990.

Scott DW: Excessive trichilemmal keratinisation (flame follicles) in endocrine skin disorders of the dog, Vet Dermatol 1:37-40, 1989.

Scott DW and Walton DK: Hyposomatotropism in the mature dog: a discussion of 22 cases, J Am Anim Hosp Assoc 22:467-473, 1986.

White PC, New MI, and Dupont B: Congenital adrenal hyperplasia, N Engl J Med 316:1519-1524, 1987.

Post-clipping alopecia

No references available.

Telogen effluvium

Bertolino AP and Freedberg IM: Hair. In Fitzpatrick TB, Eisen AZ, Wolff K and others, editors: Dermatology in general medicine, ed 3, New York, 1987, McGraw-Hill, pp 640-641.

Muller GH, Kirk RW, and Scott DW: Small animal dermatology, ed 4, Philadelphia, 1989, WB Saunders, pp 699-701.

Post-rabies vaccination alopecia

Schmeitzel LP, Loeffler D, and Bass MC: Focal cutaneous reactions at vaccination sites in a cat and four dogs, Proceedings of the American Academy of Veterinary Dermatology/American College of Veterinary Dermatology, New Orleans 2:39, 1986.

Wilcock BP and Yager JA: Focal cutaneous vasculitis and alopecia at sites of rabies vaccination in dogs, J Am Vet Med Assoc 188:1174-1177, 1986.

Canine familial dermatomyositis

See Chapter 2.

Alopecia areata

Bertolino AP and Freedberg IM: Hair. In Fitzpatrick TB, Eisen AZ, Wolff K and others, editors: Dermatology in general medicine, ed 3, New York, 1987, McGraw-Hill, pp 639-640.

Conroy JD: An overview of immune-mediated mucocutaneous diseases in the dog and cat, Am J Dermatopathol 5:595-599, 1983.

Fenton DA and others: Ultrastructural observations on hair bulb melanocytes in acute alopecia areata, Proc Am Soc Dermatopathol 27:148, 1989.

Guernsey GE: Alopecia areata in a dog, Can Vet J 26:403, 1985.

Lever WF and Schaumburg-Lever G: Histopathology of the skin, ed 7, Philadelphia, 1990, JB Lippincott, pp 223-224.

Messenger AG, Slater DN, and Bleehen SS: Alopecia areata: alterations in the hair growth cycle and correlation with the follicular pathology, Br J Dermatol 114:337-347, 1986.

Muller GH, Kirk RW, and Scott DW: Small animal dermatology, ed 4, Philadelphia, 1989, WB Saunders, pp 559-560.

Nelson DA and Spielvogel RL: Alopecia areata, Int J Dermatol 24:26-33, 1985.

Cicatricial alopecia

Bertolino AP and Freedberg IM: Hair. In Fitzpatrick TB, Eisen AZ, Wolff K and others, editors: Dermatology in general medicine, ed 3, New York, 1987, McGraw-Hill, pp 632-634.

Canine traction alopecia

Bertolino AP and Freedberg IM: Hair. In Fitzpatrick TB, Eisen AZ, Wolff K and others, editors: Dermatology in general medicine, ed 3, New York, 1987, McGraw-Hill, pp 643.

Rosenkrantz WS, Griffin CE, and Walder EJ: Traction alopecia in the canine: four case reports, Proceedings of the American Academy of Veterinary Dermatology/American College of Veterinary Dermatology, St. Louis 5:63, 1989.

Feline psychogenic alopecia

Kunkle GA: Feline dermatology, Vet Clin North Am 14(5): 1065-1087, 1984.

Miller WH: Symmetrical truncal hair loss in cats, Comp Cont Ed 12:461-470, 1990.

Muller GH, Kirk RW, and Scott DW: Small animal dermatology, ed 4, Philadelphia, 1989, WB Saunders, pp 757-760.

CHAPTER 18

Dysplastic diseases of the hair follicle

Dysplastic diseases of the hair follicle are characterized, most broadly, by abnormal growth and development of the follicle and hair. Considered literally, dysplastic diseases may be acquired; for example, the physiologic atrophy of the hair follicle in endocrine alopecia is a type of abnormal growth, and solar irradiation induces dysplastic changes in the follicular infundibulum. By convention with current veterinary dermatology and dermatopathology, the authors consider the dysplastic follicular diseases as those of suspected hereditary cause. Thus the dysplastic follicular diseases are breed specific; they are manifested usually by permanent and often progressive alteration in follicular structure.

Canine hereditary follicular dysplasias have a varied gross and histopathologic appearance, reflecting the diversity of canine breeds. Recognition of individual diseases is often based more on characteristic clinical features than diagnostic histopathology; however, some distinctive microscopic findings recently have been identified. Investigation of this area of dermatology and dermatopathology is in its infancy; the authors recognize that the information available may be incomplete and that much further study is needed and anticipated.

COLOR-MUTANT ALOPECIA (Synonym: color-dilution alopecia; blue dog disease)

Clinical features (Figures 18-1 through 18-3)

Color-mutant alopecia is a relatively uncommon hereditary canine skin disease seen in "blue" and other color-diluted dogs. This condition is characterized by variable alopecia and poor coat quality. The syndrome is associated with a color-dilution gene. It is not known if the color-dilution gene is directly responsible for initiating the skin disease or if a linked gene codes for the associated follicular changes. Brignac has speculated that color-mutant alopecia may reflect a generalized defect in epithelialization that is most severely manifested in the color-dilution coat color areas or, alternatively, may represent a multifactorial epithelial maturation defect. Attempts to breed for color dilution without expression of the skin disease have not been successful.

The initial clinical sign of color-mutant alopecia is the gradual onset of a dry, dull, brittle, poor-quality hair coat. Hair shafts fragment and hair regrowth is poor, resulting in a progressive, partial, patchy (moth-eaten) alopecia. Follicular papules develop and may progress to frank comedones. Hair loss and comedo formation usually are most severe on the trunk. Hyperpigmentation may occur with chronicity. The skin disease is limited to the color-diluted (usually blue) hair with sparing of the tan points. Secondary

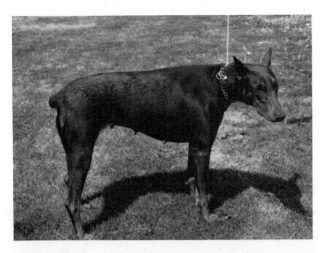

FIGURE 18-1. Color-mutant alopecia in a dark blue Doberman Pinscher. There is diffuse partial loss of hair, especially noticeable on the dorsal trunk.

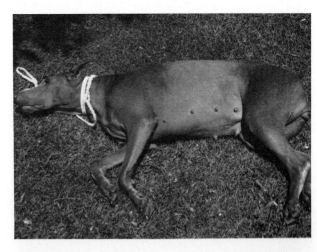

FIGURE 18-2. Color-mutant alopecia in a light blue Doberman Pinscher. Hair loss is more extensive than in the dark blue dog in Figure 18-1.

pyoderma is common in severely affected dogs and may be initiated by comedo rupture. The syndrome varies in severity; lighter colored dogs are more severely affected. Truncal alopecia may be almost complete in lighter colored dogs by 6 years of age.

Color-mutant alopecia is seen most frequently in the blue Doberman Pinscher, hence the original name, *blue Doberman syndrome*. The syndrome also is seen in other breeds with blue color dilution, including the Dachshund, Great Dane, Whippet, Italian Greyhound, Chow Chow, Standard Poodle, Yorkshire Terrier, Miniature Pinscher, Chihuahua, Bernese Mountain Dog, Shetland Sheepdog, and Schipperke. In addition, color-mutant alopecia has been seen in the fawn Doberman Pinscher, fawn Irish Setter, and the red Doberman Pinscher. Most affected dogs develop the syndrome between 4 months and 3 years of age. However, the authors have seen the syndrome develop as late as 5 to 6 years of age. Sex predilections have not been noted.

Clinical differential diagnoses should include other generalized atrophic or dysplastic diseases affecting the hair follicle. Hypothyroidism, hyperadrenocorticism, canine follicular dysplasia, and acquired pattern alopecia are the most likely differential diagnoses. Breed predilections increase clinical suspicion. Differentiation is accomplished by the clinical history and signs, thyroid and adrenal hormone function tests, and histopathology. Color-mutant alopecia shares certain clinical and histopathologic features with black hair follicular dysplasia. The latter condition may represent a more localized expression of a similar color-related defect (see following discussion).

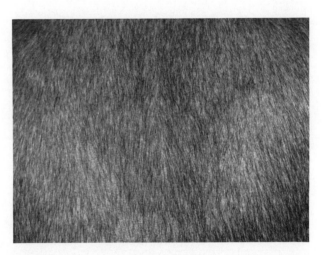

FIGURE 18-3. Closer view of the dog in Figure 18-2. Extensive partial alopecia allows visualization of the underlying skin.

Biopsy site selection

Specimens should be selected from maximally affected areas with complete alopecia. Papules or pustules, usually indicative of a secondary pyoderma, also may be sampled.

Histopathology (Figures 18-4 through 18-6)

The epidermis is usually normal but may be acanthotic if secondary pyoderma is present. Characteristic clumping of melanin in the epidermis indicates color dilution. Mild epidermal hyperkeratosis may be present.

Hair follicles are characterized by atrophy, distor-

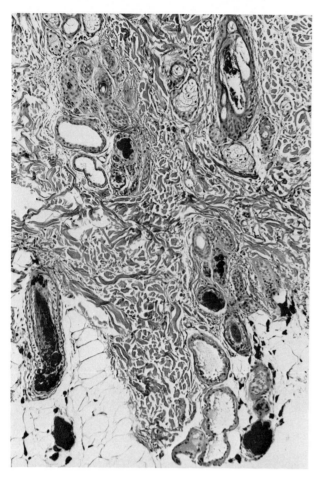

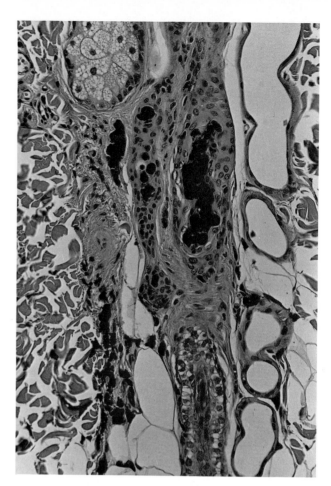

FIGURE 18-4. Color-mutant alopecia. Follicular atrophy is accompanied by marked clumping of melanin at all levels of the hair follicle. (×90.)

FIGURE 18-6. Color-mutant alopecia showing heavily clumped melanin within distorted hair follicles. Note the perifollicular melanin deposition. (×220.)

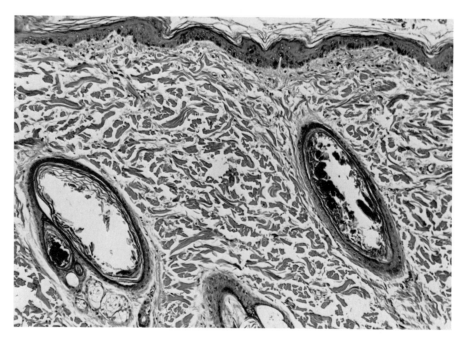

FIGURE 18-5. Color-mutant alopecia demonstrating superficial distension of follicles by keratin and clumped melanin. Hair shafts are absent. Note the characteristic epidermal melanin clumping seen with color dilution. (×90.)

tion, and abnormal melanin pigmentation. Follicles have keratin-plugged infundibula and may be shortened, thin, and have an irregular, misshapen contour. Hair shafts are often absent or markedly thinned. Melanin pigment accumulation can be massive and is present at all levels of the hair follicle. Heavily clumped melanin is present in the dermis around the base of hair follicles, within follicular epithelium, within residual hair shafts, and within follicular keratin. Extrusion of pigment from the follicular infundibulum to the surface keratin may be observed. Secondary inflammation, as in chronic pyoderma, consists of neutrophils and plasma cells that surround superficial vessels and hair follicles. Bacterial folliculitis or furunculosis may be present.

The primary differential diagnosis for color-mutant alopecia is black-hair follicular dysplasia, which is virtually identical histopathologically and may represent localized, "spotty" expression of the color-dilution defect. Clinical differentiation is required. Perifollicular clumping of melanin also can be a nonspecific finding in inflammatory and other dysplastic follicular diseases that involve the hair bulb. Distribution of clumped melanin *within* the follicle is the differentiating feature of color-mutant alopecia from inflammatory follicular diseases with perifollicular melanin deposition.

BLACK-HAIR FOLLICULAR DYSPLASIA (Synonym: canine hereditary black-hair follicular dysplasia)
Clinical features (Figures 18-7 and 18-8)

Black-hair follicular dysplasia is a rare canine hereditary skin disease characterized by poor coat quality and alopecia restricted to the dark-haired areas of white dogs with dark spots. Selmanowitz (1972) speculated that melanocytes (neural crest origin) in the areas of pigmented hair exhibiting follicular dysplasia might be involved in faulty morphogenetic induction of the follicular appendages. Breeding studies by Selmanowitz (1977) suggest that the syndrome is caused by an autosomal gene with an as yet undetermined dominant or recessive characteristic.

Affected dogs are normal at birth. Extensive alopecia develops tardively in the affected dark-haired spots. Darkly haired areas often appear washed out or gray in affected dogs. Most hairs are lost from affected areas, leaving broken stubble and markedly abnormal remaining hairs with fractured dry, dull shafts. The alopecic areas become dry and scaly. Secondary pyoderma is common in the affected alopecic areas. Adjacent white-haired areas are normal.

Black-hair follicular dysplasia was first documented in mongrels but the syndrome also has been seen in purebred dogs with spots, such as the Beagle and Bassett Hound. Skin lesions usually develop within the

first few weeks after birth. Sex predilections have not been noted.

Black-hair follicular dysplasia is a visually striking disease. Observation of lesions restricted to the black-haired areas of white dogs with dark spots is highly suggestive of black-hair follicular dysplasia. Definitive diagnosis is based upon compatible clinical findings and histopathology.

Color-mutant alopecia shares certain clinical and histopathologic features with black-hair follicular dysplasia and probably represents a more localized expression of the same genetic defect. Black-hair follicular dysplasia may be viewed simply as localized color-mutant alopecia restricted to discrete body regions.

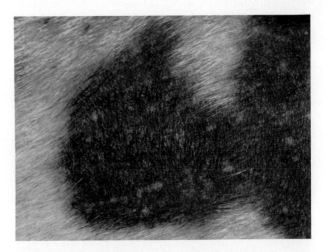

FIGURE 18-7. Black-hair follicular dysplasia in a dog. Hair loss is confined to the darker pigmented area. Secondary pyoderma is confined to this alopecic focus.

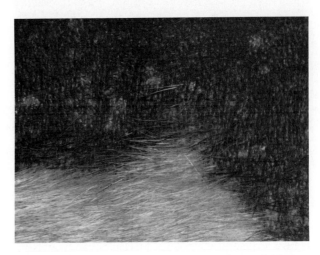

FIGURE 18-8. Closer view of the dog in Figure 18-7. Several white hairs are visible within the margins of the alopecic area.

Biopsy site selection

Specimens should be obtained from maximally affected areas with complete alopecia. Papules or pustules, usually indicative of a secondary pyoderma, also may be sampled.

Histopathology (Figures 18-9 and 18-10)

Histopathologic features of black-hair follicular dysplasia are essentially identical to those of color-mutant alopecia (see preceding discussion). It is this close microscopic resemblance that first suggested the similarity of these two alopecic syndromes.

Abnormal clumping of melanin may be less severe in black-hair follicular dysplasia than in color-mutant alopecia but is similarly distributed throughout the deep perifollicular dermis, the hair follicle, and the overlying stratum corneum. Secondary pyoderma is less common.

Differential diagnoses are similar to those of color-mutant alopecia. Clinical differentiation is required to

distinguish black-hair follicular dysplasia from color-mutant alopecia.

CANINE FOLLICULAR DYSPLASIA
(Synonym: hair follicle dysplasia)
Clinical features (Figures 18-11 through 18-15)

Canine follicular dysplasia is an uncommon canine skin disease characterized clinically by altered coat quality and alopecia. Breed specificity of expression and anecdotal information from dog breeders indicate the likelihood of a hereditary cause. However, genetic studies have not been performed.

The clinical features of canine follicular dysplasia vary with the breed affected. Poor coat quality, coat color change, selective loss of primary (guard) hairs, or complete alopecia may be seen in affected dogs. Lesions may be widespread on the trunk or focal and somewhat bilaterally symmetric. The syndrome tends to spare the face and distal extremities. Occasionally, a

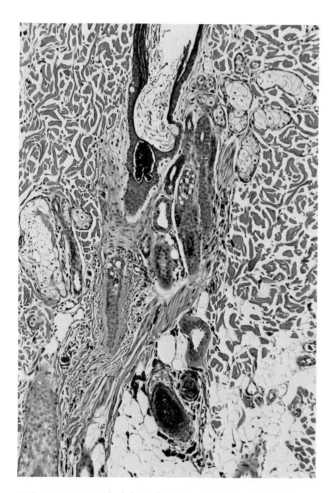

FIGURE 18-9. Black-hair follicular dysplasia. Follicular atrophy is accompanied by clumped melanin deposition. Note the similarity of these features to color-mutant alopecia (Figure 18-4). (×90.)

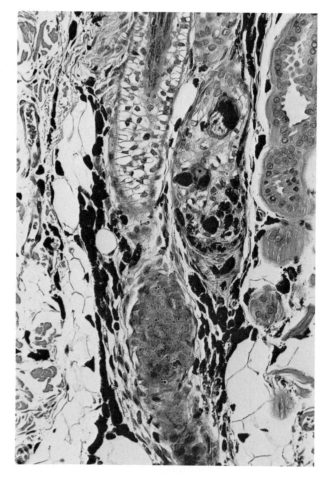

FIGURE 18-10. Black-hair follicular dysplasia. Clumped pigment is distributed in and around deep follicles. (×220.)

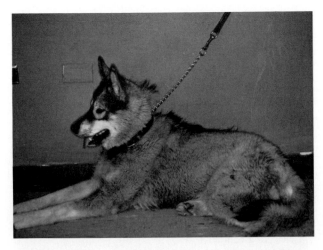

FIGURE 18-11. Follicular dysplasia in a Siberian Husky. Most primary hairs are lost from the trunk. Secondary hairs appear "woolly" and are reddish brown or "rusty." *(Courtesy AM Hargis, Seattle, Washington; case material from the University of California, Davis).*

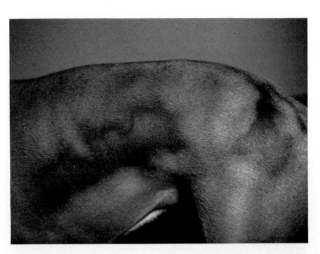

FIGURE 18-14. Follicular dysplasia in a Boxer. Primary and secondary hairs are lost from partially symmetric patches on the lateral trunk.

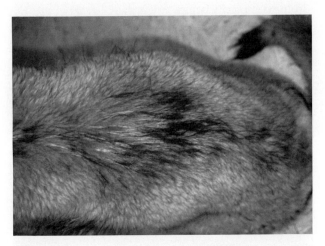

FIGURE 18-12. Closer view of the dorsum of the dog in Figure 18-11. A band of primary hairs surrounded by "woolly" secondary hairs remain along the midline. *(Courtesy AM Hargis, Seattle, Washington; case material from the University of California, Davis).*

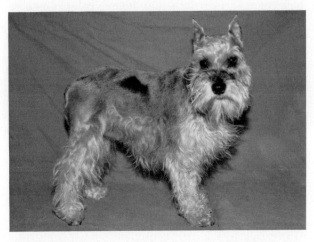

FIGURE 18-15. Follicular dysplasia in a Miniature Schnauzer. Partially symmetric patches of complete alopecia are present on the lateral trunk.

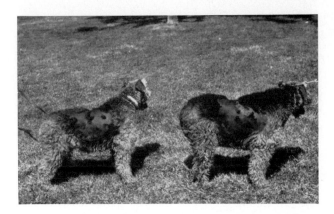

FIGURE 18-13. Follicular dysplasia in two Airedale Terrier male and female littermates. Both dogs have lost primary and secondary hairs in a partially symmetric, saddle-like pattern. *(Courtesy AC Mundell, Seattle, Washington; case material from the University of California, Davis).*

partial regrowth of primary or secondary hairs may be noted transiently, giving false hope for recovery; however, the syndrome usually is progressive. Focal areas of follicular dysplasia may show cyclic improvement and recrudescence. Clinical findings are further categorized by the breeds affected.

Siberian Husky. The syndrome in the Siberian Husky is characterized by loss of primary hairs and a color change in the remaining secondary hairs (undercoat) to a reddish-brown or "rusty" color. Secondary hairs are dry, disheveled, and "woolly." Patches of more complete alopecia may be evident in wear areas such as pressure points and under collars. A visually similar syndrome that has not been documented by histopathology has been seen clinically in an Alaskan Malamute by the authors and in English Springer Spaniels by Post.

Irish Water Spaniel, Portuguese Water Dog, and Curly-Coated Retriever. Similar clinical signs have been seen in these three breeds. Variable numbers of primary hairs are lost, and the remaining undercoat hair color changes to a dull, lighter color. Some remaining primary hairs on the trunk may be abnormally long. Affected Irish Water Spaniels exhibit a coat color change from reddish brown to grayish brown. The coat color of Portuguese Water Dogs changes from black to reddish brown.

Airedale Terrier. A distinctive clinical pattern has been seen in the Airedale Terrier. Hair loss is partially symmetric and is restricted predominantly to the dorsal and lateral thorax in a saddle-like pattern. The alopecic areas are hyperpigmented. Both primary and secondary hairs are lost, creating areas of total alopecia, with the exception of occasional, visually striking, well-demarcated islands of normal hair on the thorax similar to those seen with growth hormone/castration-responsive dermatosis. Cyclical hair regrowth followed by recrudescence is seen. Seasonality has not been noted.

Boxer, English Bulldog, French Bulldog, and Miniature Schnauzer. A localized form of follicular dysplasia (sometimes termed *cyclic flank alopecia*) is seen predominantly on the flanks and lateral trunk. This syndrome is seen most frequently in the Boxer. Primary and secondary hairs are lost from partially bilaterally symmetric patches, commonly beginning in the paralumbar fossa. Most lesions are less than 15 cm in diameter. Partial hair regrowth with poor-quality hairs may occur cyclically.

Follicular dysplasia has been seen in other breeds, including the German Shorthaired Pointer, German Wirehaired Pointer, and Chesapeake Bay Retriever. Secondary and primary hairs were lost from affected areas.

The age of onset is variable. However, the syndrome commonly begins at less than 3 years of age. Sex predilections have not been noted.

Clinical differential diagnoses should include endocrinopathies such as hypothyroidism, hyperadrenocorticism, and sex-hormone alterations. The marked breed predilections of the follicular dysplasias, endocrinologic evaluation, and histopathology will aid in differentiation.

Biopsy site selection

Specimens should be taken from areas of maximal alopecia or haircoat change. It is critical that normally haired skin be obtained for comparison. If normally

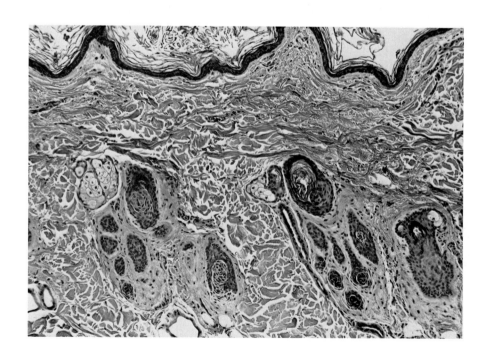

FIGURE 18-16. Canine follicular dysplasia in a Boxer. Hair follicles are truncated and misshapen; note the abnormal hair bulbs. (×90.)

haired areas are not available from the affected animal, then control specimens should be obtained from an age-matched dog of the same breed, preferably from the same site as the abnormal specimen. This comparison sampling is vitally important, particularly when attempting to characterize new forms of hereditary alopecia in individual breeds of dogs.

Histopathology (Figures 18-16 through 18-18)

The canine follicular dysplasias are as yet incompletely characterized. Further histopathologic distinctions among the various follicular dysplasias will hopefully emerge through systematic study of large groups of affected animals. Knowledge of the breed affected and the distribution of hair loss are currently crucial in the diagnosis of the dysplastic follicular diseases.

The epidermis and dermis are usually normal, although variable hyperkeratosis may be present. Follicular infundibular hyperkeratosis is a common feature, as it is in many diseases of abnormal hair growth. Pigmentary incontinence around deep portions of hair follicles may be evident. Histologic findings are further categorized by the breeds affected.

Siberian Husky. Affected hair follicles are predominantly in the catagen stage, as described by Post. The follicular appearance is often that of an exaggerated catagen hair, or "flame follicle," and is characterized by a pronounced glassy membrane and abundant tricholemmal keratin, which may project through the follicular sheath in the configuration of a flame. Thus the follicular morphology of follicular dysplasia of Siberian Huskies may be indistinguishable from growth hormone/castration responsive alopecia of other breeds (see Chapter 17). Knowledge of the breed affected and

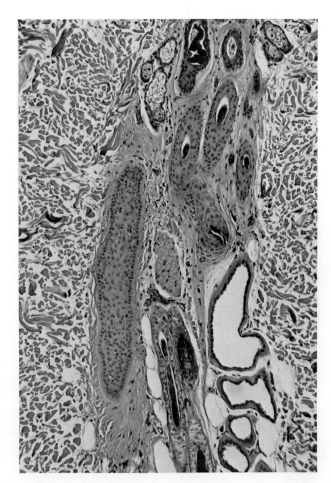

FIGURE 18-17. Canine follicular dysplasia in a Portuguese Water Dog. Follicles are mildly distorted and contain clumped pigment superficially. (×90.)

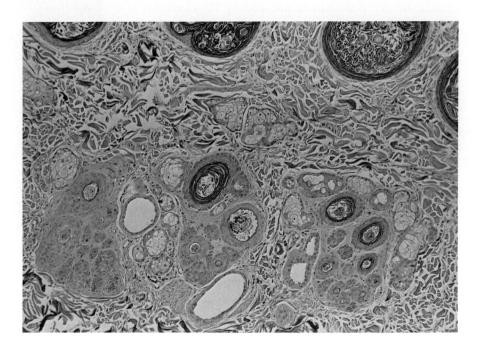

FIGURE 18-18. Canine follicular dysplasia in an Irish Water Spaniel showing hairs in the catagen phase that are mildly distorted. (×90.)

the age of the dog may be invaluable in the diagnosis.

Irish Water Spaniel, Portuguese Water Dog, and Curly-Coated Retriever. These dogs have occasionally been grouped because of their similar hair coats and breeding backgrounds. However, recent examination of cases of follicular dysplasia in the Portuguese Water Dog by one author* has revealed features of color-mutant alopecia (see earlier discussion). Clumping of pigment is present but is less exaggerated than that seen in typical color-mutant alopecia. Lesions in the few Irish Water Spaniels examined to date have been subtle and include lack of normal cycling of the follicle and mild distortion. Insufficient data are available to completely characterize the disease in the Irish Water Spaniel or in the Curly-Coated Retriever.

Airedale Terrier. Interestingly, in the few Airedale Terriers examined by one author* to date, hair follicles are often similar to those described for the Siberian Husky, thus resembling growth hormone/castration-responsive alopecia (see Chapter 17). Other hair follicles may be small or distorted.

Boxer and English Bulldog. Difficulty in histopathologic diagnosis arises from the cyclic nature of some of the follicular dysplasias, particularly those of Boxers and English Bulldogs. Thus, depending on the stage in which biopsy specimens are obtained, hair follicles may have a relatively normal appearance and anagen hairs may be prominent.

The epidermis may show hypermelanosis. In typically diagnostic lesions, both primary and secondary hair follicles are distorted and narrowed, particularly at the base. Often, a normal-sized, keratin-filled follicular infundibulum is perched on a truncated follicle with an atrophic base, creating a "dwarfed" appearance. Anagen hair bulbs, if present, are often greatly misshapen and may be seen at the base of shortened and distorted hairs. Often follicles have a marked wavy or undulating outline. Hair shafts are generally absent. A predominance of normal anagen hairs and more normally contoured hair follicles within a specimen may herald a return to a cycle of regrowth in affected dogs. Similar histopathologic lesions have been recognized in the German Wirehaired and German Shorthaired Pointers.

ACQUIRED PATTERN ALOPECIA
(Synonym: pattern baldness)
Clinical features (Figures 18-19 and 18-20)

Acquired pattern alopecia is a relatively common canine skin disease characterized by somewhat bilaterally symmetric gradual hair loss on the pinnae and elsewhere. The marked breed predilection for Dachs-

* Thelma Lee Gross.

hunds coupled with clinical and histopathologic similarities to pattern baldness in humans suggests a genetic basis.

Slowly progressive thinning of the haircoat with a conversion to diminutive vellus hairs is the principal clinical feature of acquired pattern alopecia. Evidence of inflammation is not seen. Hyperpigmentation and mild scaling may be present, especially in long-standing cases. The pinnae are affected most frequently, but

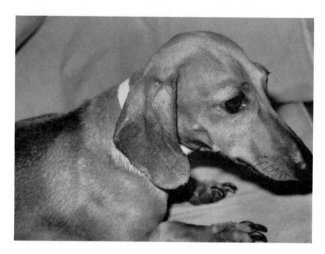

FIGURE 18-19. Acquired pattern alopecia in a Dachshund. Note that the pinnae are almost completely alopecic.

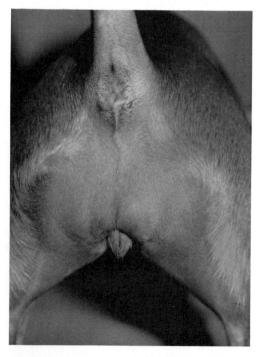

FIGURE 18-20. Perianal area of the dog in Figure 18-19. Hair has been lost in a partially symmetric pattern.

similar hair loss also may be noted behind the ears; on the ventral aspect of the neck, chest, and abdomen; perianally; and on the caudal aspect of the thighs.

Acquired pattern alopecia is seen primarily in Dachshunds, but the syndrome also has been seen in the Boston Terrier, Chihuahua, Whippet, Manchester Terrier, and Italian Greyhound. The syndrome is uncommon in dogs less than 1 year of age. Sex predilections have not been noted.

Acquired pattern alopecia must be differentiated from hair loss secondary to endocrinopathies such as hypothyroidism, hyperadrenocorticism, and sex hormone alterations. Differentiation is accomplished by specific endocrinologic testing and histopathology. Pinnal hair loss also is seen in Dachshunds with ear-margin seborrhea. However, scaling and crusting are the predominant clinical features of ear-margin seborrhea.

Biopsy site selection

Areas of complete alopecia should be selected for biopsy, and an additional specimen should be obtained from as normal an area as possible for comparison. This selection technique will allow detection of potentially subtle follicular changes in size and density by comparison with a normal control.

Histopathology (Figures 18-21)

The epidermis and dermis are normal. Hair follicles are characterized by moderate to severe diminution in size; overall numbers of adnexal units are not reduced. Follicles are both shorter and thinner than normal, and residual hair shafts are extremely fine. Follicular distortion or irregularity of contour is not found. Small rudimentary hair bulbs are present and hair follicles continue to cycle.

The characteristic histopathologic changes of acquired pattern baldness should not be confused with endocrine alopecia. Hair follicles are small in acquired pattern alopecia but are not predominantly in the telogen or catagen phase (growth cycle arrest), as seen in endocrine alopecia. Diminutive hair bulbs are not a feature of endocrine alopecia.

CONGENITAL HYPOTRICHOSIS
(Synonym: congenital alopecia)
Clinical features (Figures 18-22)

Congenital hypotrichosis is a rare disease that occurs both in the dog and cat and is characterized by varying degrees of alopecia present from birth. Affected animals are born with a diminished number of adnexal structures in affected areas. Congenital hypotrichosis may be the only abnormality noted, or it may be seen concomitantly with other ectodermal defects such as abnormal dentition and abnormal tear production. A new classification scheme proposed by Foil encompassing all ectodermal dysplasias is useful. Male sex-linked inheritance is suspected for most affected dogs.

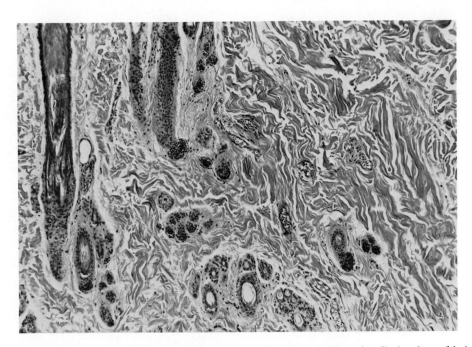

FIGURE 18-21. Acquired pattern alopecia in a Dachshund. Note the diminution of hair follicles and petite hair bulbs. (×90.)

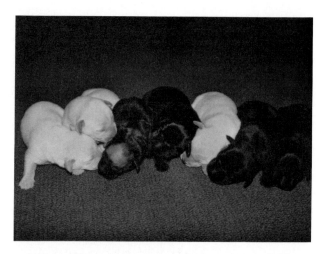

FIGURE 18-22. Congenital hypotrichosis in several members of a litter of Labrador Retrievers. Complete hair loss is seen on the forehead of one puppy. *(Courtesy GA Kunkle, Gainesville, Florida).*

The characteristic clinical feature of congenital hypotrichosis is lack of hair in well-delineated areas. The extent of alopecia may vary from partial to complete. Marked bilateral symmetry may be noted. The head, pinnae, dorsal or ventral thorax, and tail are the areas most frequently affected. Initially, the exposed skin appears normal in hairless areas, but subsequently, hyperpigmentation and scaling may be noted.

All reported cases have been in males except for a female Labrador Retriever reported by Kunkle. Congenital hypotrichosis has been reported convincingly in the Poodle, Basset Hound, Beagle, Labrador Retriever, and Bichon Frise. Recently, one author* has seen this syndrome in a female Rottweiler. The disease is evident at birth.

Congenital hypotrichosis must be differentiated from other hypoplastic or degenerative follicular diseases. For definitive diagnosis, the affected animal must have a history of alopecia present since birth, and the syndrome must not be progressive. Progression should not be confused with natural enlargement of the area of alopecia as the animal grows. If confirmatory history denoting these criteria is lacking, congenital hypotrichosis must be differentiated from other follicular dysplasias or endocrinopathies. Histopathology is required to confirm the diagnosis.

Biopsy site selection

An area of complete alopecia should be selected for biopsy, and a second specimen should be obtained from as normal an area as possible for comparison. This selection technique will allow detection of potentially subtle follicular changes by comparing follicular size and density with that of a normal control.

Histopathology (Figures 18-23)

The epidermis and dermis are normal in congenital hypotrichosis. Follicular changes reported by others and observed by the authors principally include an overall decrease in the density of hair follicles per unit area of dermis. Follicles may also be small but are not

* Peter J. Ihrke.

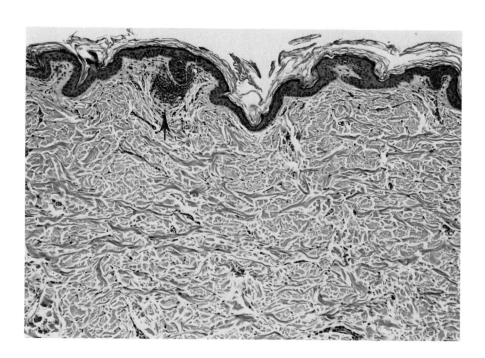

FIGURE 18-23. Congenital hypotrichosis in a dog, demonstrating nearly complete loss of follicles. A rudimentary follicular remnant remains near the epidermis *(arrow)* (×90.)

distorted. Residual hair shafts are thin. Follicular keratosis may be present. Complete absence of hair follicles and adnexal glands has been observed and has also been reported by Selmanowitz, representing a more extensive ectodermal defect of the skin.

Differential diagnosis may include acquired pattern alopecia; however, the overall density of hair follicles is normal in pattern alopecia and is usually decreased in hypotrichosis. It may be critical to obtain areas of normally haired skin (either from the patient or from an age-matched, site-matched, breed-matched control) for comparison of the density and overall size of hair follicles and hair shafts in cases of suspected hypotrichosis.

SUGGESTED READINGS

Color-mutant alopecia

Briggs OM and Botha WS: Color mutant alopecia in a blue Italian Greyhound, J Am Anim Hosp Assoc 22:611-614, 1986.

Brignac MM and others: Microscopy of color mutant alopecia, Proceedings of the American Academy of Veterinary Dermatology/American College of Veterinary Dermatology, Washington DC, 4:14-15, 1988.

Carlotti D: Canine hereditary black hair follicular dysplasia and color mutant alopecia. In Von Tscharner C and Halliwell REW, editors: Advances in veterinary dermatology, vol 1, London, 1990, Baillière Tindall, pp 43-46.

Foil CS: The skin. In Hoskins JD, editor: Veterinary pediatrics: dogs and cats from birth to six months, Philadelphia, 1990, WB Saunders, pp 359-403.

Miller WH: Alopecia associated with coat color dilution in two Yorkshire Terriers, one Saluki, and one mix-breed dog, J Am Anim Hosp Assoc 27:39-43, 1991.

Miller WH: Colour dilution alopecia in Doberman Pinschers with blue or fawn coat colours: a study on the incidence and histopathology of this disorder, Vet Dermatol 1:113-122, 1990.

Muller GH, Kirk RW, and Scott DW: Small animal dermatology, ed 4, Philadelphia, 1989, WB Saunders, pp 677-680.

O'Neill CS: Hereditary skin diseases in the dog, Comp Cont Ed 3:791-800, 1981.

Black-hair follicular dysplasia

Carlotti D: Canine hereditary black hair follicular dysplasia and color mutant alopecia. In Von Tscharner C and Halliwell REW, editors: Advances in veterinary dermatology, vol 1, London, 1990, Baillière Tindall, pp 43-46.

Foil CS: The skin. In Hoskins JD, editor: Veterinary pediatrics: dogs and cats from birth to six months, Philadelphia, 1990, WB Saunders, pp 359-403.

Selmanowitz VJ, Kramer KM, and Orentreich N: Canine hereditary black-hair follicular dysplasia, J Hered 63:43-44, 1972.

Selmanowitz VJ, Markofsky J, and Orentreich N: Black-hair follicular dysplasia in dogs, J Am Vet Med Assoc 171:1079-1081, 1977.

Canine follicular dysplasia

Miller WH: Follicular dysplasia in adult black and red Doberman Pinschers, Vet Dermatol 1:181-187, 1990.

Post K, Dignean MA, and Clark EG: Hair follicle dysplasia in a Siberian Husky, J Am Anim Hosp Assoc 24:659-662, 1988.

Scott DW: Seasonal flank alopecia in ovariohysterectomized dogs, Cornell Vet 80:187-195, 1990.

Acquired pattern alopecia

Muller GH, Kirk RW, and Scott DW: Small animal dermatology, ed 4, Philadelphia, 1989, WB Saunders, pp 698-699.

Congenital hypotrichosis

Chastain CB and Swayne DE: Congenital hypotrichosis in male Basset Hound littermates, J Am Vet Med Assoc 187:845-846, 1985.

Foil CS: The skin. In Hoskins JD, editor: Veterinary pediatrics: dogs and cats from birth to six months, Philadelphia, 1990, WB Saunders, pp 359-403.

Grieshaber TL: Congenital alopecia in a Bichon Frise, J Am Vet Med Assoc 188:1053-1054, 1986.

Kunkle GA: Congenital hypotrichosis in two dogs, J Am Vet Med Assoc 185:84-85, 1984.

Selmanowitz VJ, Kramer KM, and Orentreich N: Congenital ectodermal defect in poodles, J Hered 61:196-199, 1970.

Diseases of the panniculus

An overview of panniculitis

The term *panniculitis* encompasses a group of diseases of multifactorial etiology unified by the localization of the major focus of inflammation to the subcutaneous fat. Panniculitis is one of the most unexplored groups of skin diseases in dogs and cats. Many distinct clinical and histopathologic subgroups have been described in people; thus much comparative information is available from the human literature. Identification of individual types of panniculitis is just beginning in animals; hopefully, new diseases will emerge as data about predisposing conditions and follow-up response to therapy are gathered. An overview of the pathogenesis and diagnosis of panniculitis is provided here; a more detailed description of the recognized entities in dogs and cats is given elsewhere in the text (see Chapter 20).

PANNICULITIS
Clinical features (Figures 19-1 and 19-2)

The lipocytes, fibrous trabeculae or septa, and the blood vessels are the major components of the panniculus. Panniculitis results from direct or indirect damage to lipocytes. A wide variety of pathologic processes affect the subcutaneous fat (see accompanying box). Panniculitis from any cause is enhanced by lipid release from damaged lipocytes, since lipids are vigorous stimulators of inflammation. Panniculitis may be localized or generalized.

As documented by Scott, localized panniculitis is relatively common in the dog and cat. Localized panniculitis may result from trauma; reaction to foreign material, such as injected medicaments or deeply displaced hairs; ischemia; infection, especially from traumatically implanted organisms; or the extension of inflammation from adjacent structures such as the dermis.

Multifocal or generalized panniculitis is rare in the dog and very rare in the cat. Generalized panniculitis may result from nutritional deficiency, autoimmune disease, or pancreatic disease, including pancreatitis and pancreatic carcinoma. However, many cases of multifocal or generalized panniculitis in domestic animals and humans are idiopathic. Immunologically mediated reactions to various antigenic stimuli (infectious agents, malignancies, drugs) have been hypothesized as the underlying pathogenesis for idiopathic panniculitis.

Clinical evaluation of panniculitis is compromised by poor visualization, since the focus of disease is beneath both the epidermis and the dermis. Subcutaneous nodules (1 to 5 cm in diameter) may be palpated. Nodules vary in texture from soft and fluctuant to firm. The color also varies. Lesions may be the same color as adjacent skin, or they may be pale yellow, yellowish brown, or reddish brown.

In localized panniculitis and in early multifocal or generalized panniculitis, intact

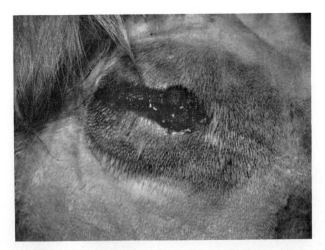

FIGURE 19-1. Focal panniculitis in the dog resulting from injection of a medicament. A well-demarcated area of swelling with a central area of necrosis and hemorrhage is present.

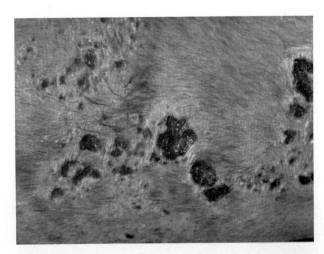

FIGURE 19-2. Idiopathic sterile nodular panniculitis in a Collie. Note the areas of full-thickness dermal necrosis indicative of liquefying panniculitis.

Causes of panniculitis recognized in the dog and cat

Physical or chemical
Trauma, foreign body (post-injection panniculitis)

Infectious
Bacterial, fungal

Immune-mediated
Systemic lupus erythematosus, erythema nodosum–like panniculitis, post-rabies vaccination alopecia, visceral malignancy, drugs

Nutritional
Pansteatitis of vitamin E deficiency in cats

Visceral
Pancreatitis, pancreatic carcinoma

Idiopathic
Idiopathic sterile nodular panniculitis, sterile pedal panniculitis

---

nodules generally are freely movable under the skin. The lesions of localized panniculitis commonly are asymptomatic. In multifocal or generalized panniculitis, larger lesions may cavitate and ulcerate or fistulate. Hemorrhage may occur but usually is minimal. Less commonly, fat necrosis is accompanied by copious drainage of an oily, yellowish-brown liquid and extensive necrosis of the overlying skin. This phenomenon is termed *liquefying panniculitis* in human medicine.

Depressed and sometimes hyperpigmented scars are a common sequela to healing panniculitis. Scarring may be prominent in chronic lesions and may fix the subcutaneous lesion to the overlying dermis. Permanent alopecia may occur if ischemia has led to follicular atrophy. Pruritus is uncommon but pain may be a feature, especially if ulceration or fistulation is present. Fever and malaise may be seen with generalized disease.

Breed, age, or sex predilections have not been noted for panniculitis in general. However, predilections have been noted for various specific syndromes, such as panniculitis seen in conjunction with systemic lupus erythematosus (see Chapter 10). Localized panniculitis must be differentiated from other nodular diseases affecting the subcutaneous tissue, such as neoplasms and cysts. Differential diagnoses for clinically distinct subgroups of panniculitis can be found in Chapter 20.

Biopsy site selection

Punch biopsy is not recommended if panniculitis is suspected. Large, deep, biopsy specimens should be obtained by wedge section to ensure that the sample includes epidermis, dermis, and subcutaneous tissue. Multiple specimens are desirable. Cavitated, ulcerated, or necrotic lesions should be avoided if other earlier lesions are present.

Histopathology (Figures 19-3 through 19-5)

The epidermis and dermis may be variably affected, depending upon the severity and chronicity of the underlying pannicular disease. Any significant inflammation of the panniculus will decrease circulation

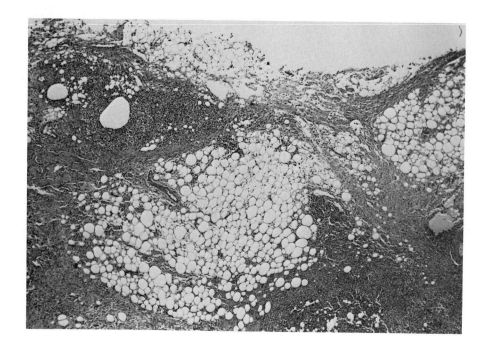

FIGURE 19-3. Lobular panniculitis in a dog. Note the sparing of lobules at the center and right. (×35.)

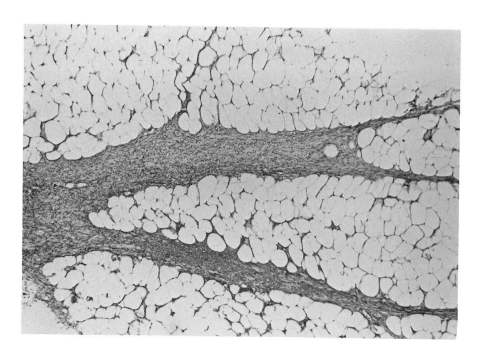

FIGURE 19-4. Septal panniculitis in a dog demonstrating fibrosis and inflammation confined to interlobular septa. (×35.)

to the overlying skin. Ulceration or cavitation may be present; secondary acute and chronic inflammation of the dermis follows. Scarring may be prominent in chronic lesions.

In many cases the damage to the underlying adipose tissue is not severe enough to induce complete scarring of the dermis and epidermis. Follicular atrophy, characterized by telogen arrest and severe diminution of the hair follicles, is prominent in these cases; the presence of this type of atrophy is a marker for chronic lesions of panniculitis, or it may indicate that past circulatory damage to the panniculus has occurred at that site.

Inflammation of the panniculus may be septal and principally involve the interlobular septa that are composed of collagen and vessels, or the inflammation may be lobular and principally affect the adipocytes. These two patterns may overlap; late-stage lesions may show diffuse involvement of the panniculus.

Lobular panniculitis. Lobular panniculitis is the most common histopathologic subtype of panniculitis observed in the dog and cat. The most common causes

FIGURE 19-5. Diffuse panniculitis in a cat. Note the complete replacement of adipose tissue of the panniculus by inflammatory cells. A few lipid vacuoles remain. (×90.)

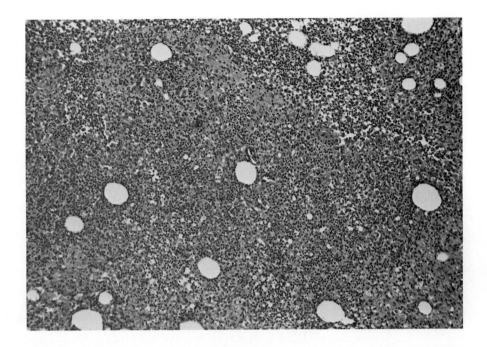

in dogs and cats include trauma, injection of foreign substances (usually vaccines), or idiopathic factors (sterile nodular panniculitis). Infections, usually as extensions from the overlying dermis, also may produce lobular panniculitis, usually with rapid progression to diffuse inflammation. Lobular panniculitis is characterized by mixed inflammation accompanied by degeneration of adipocytes. Early lesions usually demonstrate variable necrosis of adipocytes. Inflammation ranges from neutrophilic to pyogranulomatous; in later lesions, infiltrations of plasma cells and lymphocytes are observed. Most cases of lobular panniculitis progress to diffuse inflammation. Lesions heal through fibrosis.

Septal panniculitis. Bondi has subdivided human septal panniculitis according to presence or absence of vasculitis. Most cases without overt vasculitis have an immunologic basis; it is believed that the pannicular damage is induced by an immunologic reaction relating to concurrent infectious disease, drugs, or malignancies. Although vasculitis is often absent histopathologically, vascular damage is inferred by the presence of endothelial cell swelling, edema, and hemorrhage. Immunoglobulin deposition is often demonstrated in the walls of septal vessels. Septal panniculitis with vasculitis has a poorly understood pathogenesis but may be associated with underlying malignancies; a hypercoagulable state may be present in these cases.

Septal panniculitis has been observed in the dog and cat and is considered to be very rare in both species. Septal panniculitis without vasculitis in dogs and cats is characterized by severe septal inflammation ac-

companied by hemorrhage, edema, and variable vascular endothelial swelling. Scott has described septal panniculitis with vasculitis and thrombosis in two dogs and a cat.

SUGGESTED READINGS

Ackerman AB: Histologic diagnosis of inflammatory skin diseases, Philadelphia, 1978, Lea & Febiger, pp 779-825.

Ackerman LJ: Canine nodular panniculitis, Comp Cont Ed 6:818-824, 1984.

Baker BB and Stannard AA: Nodular panniculitis in the dog, J Am Vet Med Assoc 167:752-755, 1975.

Bondi EE and Lazarus GS: Disorders of subcutaneous tissue. In Fitzpatrick TB, Eisen AZ, Wolff D, and others, editors: Dermatology in general medicine, ed 3, New York, 1987, McGraw-Hill, pp 1131-1148.

Buerger RG and others: Subcutaneous fat sclerosis in a cat, Comp Small Anim 9:1198-1201, 1987.

Cockerell CJ: Biology and pathophysiology of the panniculus. In Soter NA and Baden HP, editors: Pathophysiology of dermatologic diseases, New York, 1991, McGraw-Hill, pp 379-391.

Edgar TP and Furrow RD: Idiopathic nodular panniculitis in a German Shepherd, J Am Anim Hosp Assoc 20:603-606, 1984.

Guaguere E and others: Panniculite nodulaire sterile: a propos d'un cas, Pratique Medicale et Chirurgicale de l'Animal de Compagnie 1:27-33, 1988.

Lever WF and Schaumburg-Lever G: Histopathology of the skin, ed 7, Philadelphia, 1990, JB Lippincott, pp 269-283.

Mason KV: Disseminated necrotizing panniculitis associated with pancreatic carcinoma in a dog. Proceedings of the American Academy of Veterinary Dermatology/American College of Veterinary Dermatology, St Louis, 5:61, 1989.

Shanley KJ and Miller WH: Panniculitis in the dog: a report of five cases, J Am Anim Hosp Assoc 21:545-550, 1985.

Scott DW and Anderson WI: Panniculitis in dogs and cats: a retrospective analysis of 78 cases, J Am Anim Hosp Assoc 24:551-559, 1988.

CHAPTER 20

Diseases of the panniculus

POST-RABIES VACCINATION ALOPECIA
Clinical features (Figure 20-1)

See Chapter 17.

Biopsy site selection

Biopsy specimens should be obtained from the affected skin and subcutis just within the outer margin of the plaque or macule. Specimens from near the margin may show more diagnostic histopathologic changes than the central chronic area where typical inflammation may be scant.

Histopathology (Figures 20-2 and 20-3)

The lesions of the dermis and hair follicles have been discussed and principally include follicular atrophy and dermal edema (see Chapter 17). The panniculus is characterized by diffuse edema, or "smudging," of the collagenous tissue. Moderate to severe, nodular accumulations of lymphocytes, fewer macrophages, and occasional plasma cells are present and often tightly surround vessels. Although vasculitis is not obvious, some vessels have swollen endothelia and thickened walls or are obscured by inflammation. Immunofluorescent testing with antibody to rabies viral antigen may reveal deposition in and around vessels, as reported by Wilcock.

Lesions of post-rabies vaccination alopecia may resemble those of other injection reactions. Eosinophils and the basophilic granular debris seen within lesions of post-injection panniculitis are absent in post-rabies vaccination alopecia.

POST-INJECTION PANNICULITIS
Clinical features (Figure 20-4)

Post-injection panniculitis is diagnosed uncommonly in the cat and rarely in the dog. This syndrome probably is underdiagnosed, since lesions may be deemed inconsequential or may not be obvious clinically. Although the etiology has not been proven, the histopathologic pattern suggests a combined foreign body reaction and hypersensitivity. The syndrome may be caused by vaccines or other injected medications, including antibiotics. This type of reaction pattern has been hypothesized by Hendrick to be associated with previous rabies vaccination in cats and dogs. Post-injection panniculitis due to rabies vaccine is distinct from post-rabies vaccination alopecia (see Chapter 17).

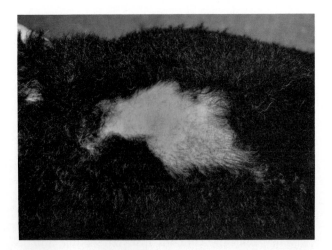

FIGURE 20-1. Post-rabies vaccination alopecia in a black miniature Poodle. The affected area is nearly totally alopecic.

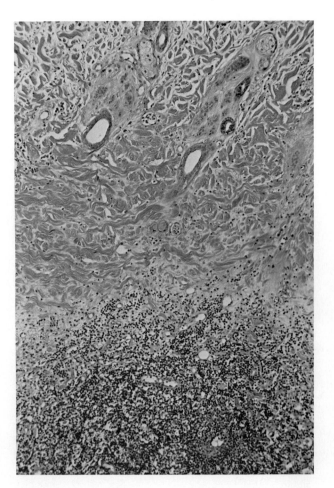

The authors believe that post-injection panniculitis may be difficult to ascribe to rabies vaccine alone, since multivalent vaccines are used commonly.

A solitary subcutaneous nodule, varying from 5 mm to 1 cm in diameter, is noted at the site of a previous subcutaneously administered vaccine or medication. Nodules may be either freely movable or fixed to the overlying dermis and vary in texture from soft and fluctuant to firm. The overlying skin is normal, but some alopecia may be an occasional feature. Rarely, pain can be elicited on palpation. Systemic signs have not been reported. Recently, Hendrick reported the

FIGURE 20-2. Post-rabies vaccination alopecia. Atrophic follicles overlie densed mixed mononuclear inflammation in the panniculus. (×90.)

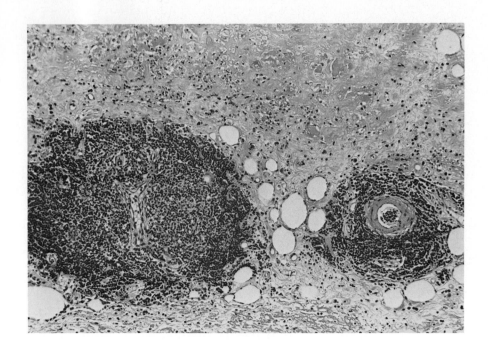

FIGURE 20-3. Post-rabies vaccination alopecia. Nodular accumulations of lymphocytes surround vessels of the panniculus. Note the homogenization and pale staining of the surrounding loose connective tissue. (×90.)

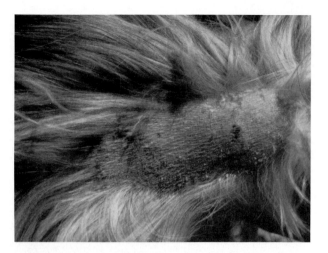

FIGURE 20-4. Post-injection panniculitis in a dog. A solitary subcutaneous nodule is faintly visible to the right of center in the clipped region.

occurrence of fibrosarcoma at the site of previous subcutaneous rabies vaccination in cats.

Breed, age, or sex predilections have not been noted. Post-injection panniculitis must be differentiated from other nodular diseases affecting the subcutaneous tissue, such as neoplasms and cysts. The diagnosis of post-injection panniculitis commonly is made histopathologically after the removal of a suspected tumor.

Biopsy site selection

Excisional biopsy of the entire nodule is preferred if post-injection panniculitis is suspected because surgical excision also is curative. Since cutaneous neoplasia is the most commonly anticipated diagnosis, wide excision usually is performed.

Histopathology (Figures 20-5 and 20-6)

The epidermis and dermis are usually normal. Inflammation may encroach on the deep dermis, depending upon the exact site of injection. Follicular atrophy, as seen in post-rabies vaccination reactions, may be observed; however, specimens obtained for histopathology often exclude the overlying skin.

The panniculus contains a discrete nodule that often has a necrotic center. The necrotic center is amorphous and stains lightly eosinophilic or amphophilic. Granular to elongated flecks of basophilic debris are present in this central zone. Surrounding the core is a layer of macrophages and often giant cells. A zone of intense lymphocytic and eosinophilic inflammation composes the outer layer; merging of the granulomatous and lymphocytic zones is common. Lymphocytes may be arranged in prominent follicular aggregates along the perimeter of the lesion. The inflammatory pattern suggests a combination of foreign body (granulomatous with giant cells) and hypersensitivity (lymphocytic and eosinophilic) reactions to the deposited vaccine or medication.

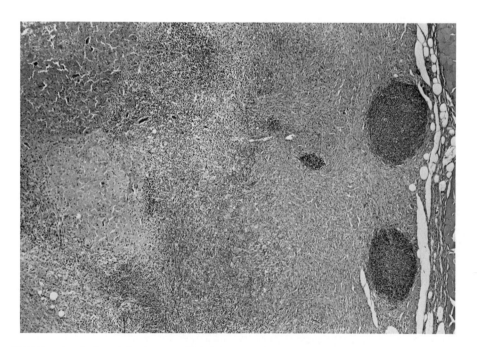

FIGURE 20-5. Post-injection panniculitis in a cat. A central amorphous and necrotic zone is at the left. Note the large peripheral lymphoid nodules at the right. ($\times 35$.)

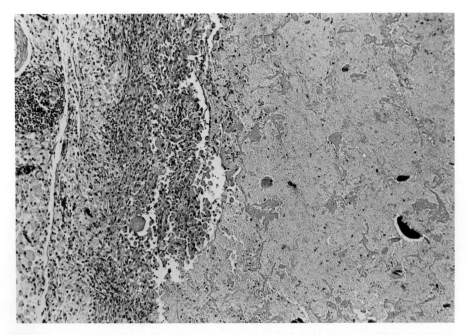

FIGURE 20-6. Post-injection panniculitis in a cat, demonstrating the necrotic central zone containing characteristic darkly staining, floccular foreign deposits (at right). Note the pale foamy macrophages and the lymphoid nodule in the outer zone of inflammation at the left. (×90.).

Differential diagnoses are few, since the reaction pattern of post-injection panniculitis is characteristic. Location of flocculent, basophilic foreign debris at the center of the lesions is essentially diagnostic for post-injection panniculitis. Post-rabies vaccination alopecia reactions are not as discrete and concentrically layered as post-injection panniculitis, basophilic foreign material is not found, and eosinophils are not usually present. Traumatic panniculitis has necrosis but lacks lymphocytic and eosinophilic inflammation.

TRAUMATIC PANNICULITIS
Clinical features

Traumatic panniculitis is a relatively common lesion of cats and dogs. Causes to consider include focal ischemia caused by blunt trauma, chronic pressure, or decreased blood supply. The latter may be more common in obese cats in which excessive fat deposition is accompanied by relatively reduced vascularity, predisposing to ischemia from slight insult. Similar lesions are observed in the internal fat of heavily fatted dairy cows.

Animals usually have a focal firm subcutaneous nodule that most frequently is located on the trunk. The overlying skin is normal. The dorsum over the spine and the ventral sternum are common sites. Lesions also may be seen over the wing of the ilium and lumbar eminences in dogs. No attendant signs are present, nor do the lesions appear to be painful.

Breed, age, and sex predilections have not been noted. Obese animals may be predisposed.

Clinical differential diagnoses include neoplasms, organizing hematomas or seromas, or possibly foreign body reactions or infectious granulomas. Histopathology allows differentiation; however, many infectious lesions are multicentric and foreign body reactions often drain to the surface of the skin.

Biopsy site selection

Wedge removal of the entire nodule usually is performed because of the potential of neoplasia. Occasionally, the ischemic process extends beyond the site of the palpable lesion; local recurrence may be prevented by obtaining reasonable margins of normal tissue during procurement.

Histopathology (Figures 20-7 and 20-8)

The epidermis and dermis are normal, but often are excluded from the specimen submitted for histopathology. The adipose tissue of the panniculus contains a large central focus of lobular fat necrosis. Adipocytes lack nuclei but retain their normal shape, creating "ghosts" or "shells" of fat cells. Ruptured adipocytes form large, cystic spaces. Interspersed and surrounding the devitalized fat cells are foamy macrophages contain-

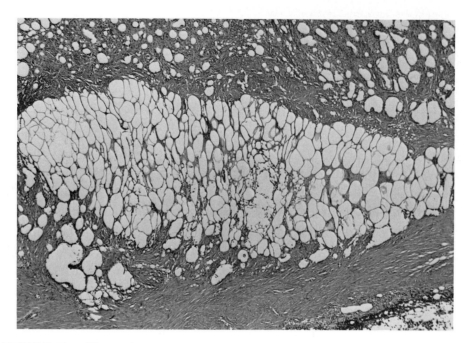

FIGURE 20-7. Traumatic panniculitis. The large central focus of necrotic adipose tissue is surrounded by a dense zone of fibrosis. (×35.)

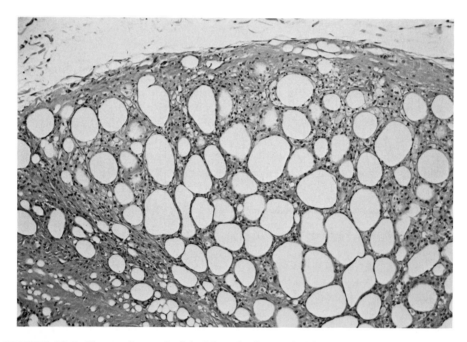

FIGURE 20-8. Traumatic panniculitis. Note the foamy, lipid-bearing macrophages among ruptured adipocytes. (×90.)

ing lipid debris. Other types of inflammatory cells are rare. Cholesterol clefts may occasionally be observed. Hemorrhage or hemosiderosis may accompany these findings. Frequently, marginal fibrosis encroaches upon and interposes among devitalized adipocytes; older lesions may be predominantly fibrotic and fibrocytes may be markedly proliferative (fibrosing steatitis).

Differential diagnoses are few. The extensive necrosis and scant inflammation of affected adipose tissue confirm the diagnosis of traumatic panniculitis. Late stage lesions with predominant fibrosis may resemble chronic scarring panniculitis of any cause.

IDIOPATHIC STERILE NODULAR PANNICULITIS
Clinical features (Figures 20-9 through 20-11)

In its broadest sense the term *idiopathic sterile nodular panniculitis* encompasses all of the sterile inflammatory diseases of the panniculus of unknown etiology. However, current usage has narrowed the meaning of this term to reflect a more specific disease subgroup (or subgroups) seen rarely in the dog and even more rarely in the cat. A marked breed predilection for the Dachshund suggests genetic factors. The syndrome bears some resemblance to a disease in humans termed *idiopathic lobular panniculitis*.

Lesions with clinical and histopathologic similarity to sterile nodular panniculitis have been reported by Mason in a dog with pancreatic carcinoma. Similar lesions have been observed by Walder in a dog with pancreatic carcinoma and acute necrotizing pancreatitis and in a cat with chronic pancreatitis.

Multiple firm to fluctuant nodules develop in the subcutaneous tissue. Larger nodules ulcerate or fistulate, draining an oily, clear to yellowish-brown liquid. Well-demarcated ulcers and fistulas less than 1 cm in diameter typify the disease in Dachshunds. An additional subgroup seen most typically in the Collie has a greater propensity toward coalescing ulcerations with extensive drainage and resembles liquefying panniculitis of humans. Fistulation or ulceration is accompanied by scarring that fixes the subcutaneous lesion to the overlying dermis. Variable hyperpigmentation is seen with healing. Chronic lesions are irregularly firm and nodular to palpation. Systemic signs include fever, anorexia, and general malaise.

The Dachshund is at increased risk for idiopathic sterile nodular panniculitis. The Miniature Poodle and the Collie probably also are overrepresented. Published cases, plus the authors' data, indicate that the syndrome is seen more frequently in dogs less than 6 months of age and in older adult dogs. The syndrome has been seen only in adult cats. Sex predilections have not been noted.

Clinical differential diagnoses should include infectious diseases with cutaneous and subcutaneous involvement such as opportunistic mycobacterial infections, cutaneous and subcutaneous infections of both systemic and other opportunistic fungi, deep bacterial folliculitis and furunculosis, neoplasms, and lupus panniculitis. Clinically, infections of the panniculus are more likely to be focal or grouped in contrast to the multifocal distribution of sterile nodular panniculitis. Aerobic and anaerobic bacterial cultures, fungal cultures, and histopathology should be performed to rule

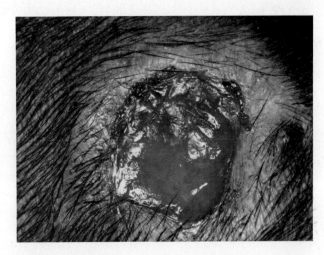

FIGURE 20-10. Closer view of the dog in Figure 20-9. A well-demarcated ulcer is seen on the shoulder.

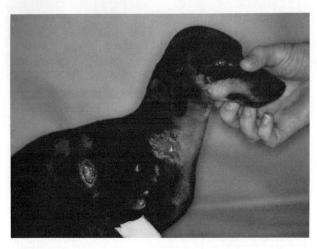

FIGURE 20-9. Idiopathic sterile nodular panniculitis in a Manchester Terrier. Multiple nodules have ulcerated.

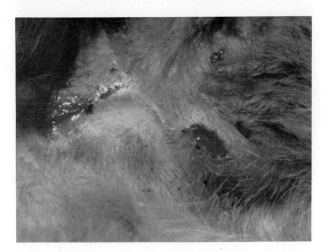

FIGURE 20-11. Idiopathic sterile nodular panniculitis in a cat. Multiple ulcerated nodules are accompanied by scarring.

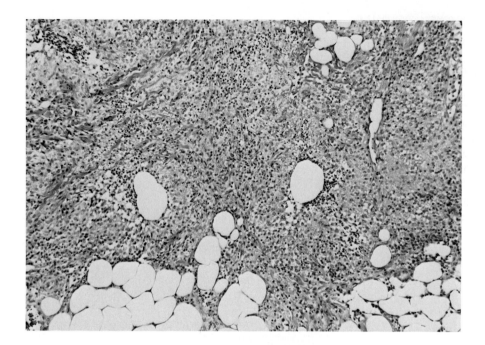

FIGURE 20-12. Idiopathic sterile nodular panniculitis in a Poodle. Confluent pyogranulomas replace adipose tissue of the panniculus. (×90.)

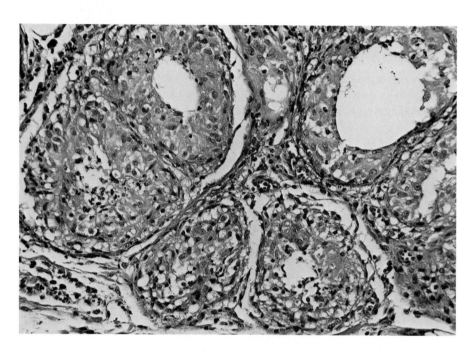

FIGURE 20-13. Idiopathic sterile nodular panniculitis in a Dachshund demonstrating discrete pyogranulomas. (×220.)

out infectious causes before considering a diagnosis of idiopathic sterile nodular panniculitis.

Biopsy site selection

Punch biopsy is not recommended if idiopathic sterile nodular panniculitis is suspected. Large, deep, biopsy specimens should be obtained by wedge section to ensure that the sample includes epidermis, dermis, and subcutaneous tissue. Multiple specimens are desirable. Lesions that are cavitated, ulcerated, or necrotic should be avoided if other, earlier lesions are present.

Histopathology (Figures 20-12 and 20-13)

The epidermis is normal to acanthotic and may be ulcerated if secondary necrosis and exudation to the surface have occurred. The deep dermis may be inflamed as lesions expand and progress from the underlying panniculus.

Inflammation of the panniculus is principally lobular in the early stages, but progresses to diffuse involvement. Neutrophils and macrophages predominate in initial lesions and discrete pyogranulomas may be present. Adipocytes may appear necrotic, as ghosts, or they may be infiltrated with foamy macrophages. Diffuse inflammation is generally mixed and includes macrophages, neutrophils, lymphocytes, and plasma cells in varying distribution. Special stains for fungi and acid-fast bacteria are negative. Chronic lesions have scant neutrophils and variable fibrosis, which replaces the panniculus and often extends to the overlying epidermis.

Differential diagnoses for idiopathic sterile nodular panniculitis include infectious panniculitis, particularly with opportunistic mycobacteria, and juvenile sterile granulomatous dermatitis and lymphadenitis. Because the organisms in some mycobacterial infections may be scant, careful searching using Fite's modification of an acid-fast stain is warranted. Clinical differentiation may be required; opportunistic mycobacterial infections are usually solitary or focally grouped. Juvenile sterile granulomatous dermatitis may have accompanying panniculitis that is indistinguishable from idiopathic sterile nodular panniculitis; however, characteristic periadnexal pyogranulomatous inflammation is also present. It is of interest that the Dachshund may be predisposed to both diseases.

ERYTHEMA NODOSUM–LIKE PANNICULITIS

Clinical features

Erythema nodosum–like panniculitis, a septal panniculitis with vascular damage, is a very rare canine skin disease believed to be associated with a systemic hypersensitivity reaction. Vascular disease, which in humans has been shown to be immune mediated, and associated inflammation are centered in the interlobular septa rather than primarily within the fat lobules. Erythema nodosum, classified as a septal panniculitis without inflammatory vascular disease (true vasculitis) by Bondi, is a similar disease of humans that can be seen concomitantly with infection or drug reaction. Lesions also may be idiopathic. Infections, such as bacterial endocarditis and coccidioidomycosis, and drug reactions are reported by Muller, Kirk, and Scott as possible causes in the dog. One author* has seen erythema nodosum–like panniculitis in conjunction with visceral malignancy in one dog and with putative drug reactions in others. The authors also have seen additional cases without demonstrable underlying cause.

Clinical presentation is similar to other forms of panniculitis in that multiple firm to fluctuant nodules develop in the subcutaneous tissue. Lesions may be hemorrhagic. Larger nodules fistulate and drain. Scarring may fix the subcutaneous lesion to the overlying dermis. Variable hyperpigmentation is seen with healing. Areas of previous disease feel irregularly firm and nodular. Fever, joint pain, and general malaise may accompany skin changes.

Breed, age, or sex predilections have not been noted. Clinical differential diagnoses should include infectious diseases with cutaneous and subcutaneous involvement such as opportunistic mycobacterial infection, cutaneous and subcutaneous infections of both pathogenic and opportunistic fungi, deep bacterial folliculitis and furunculosis, neoplasms, lupus panniculitis, and other forms of panniculitis. Aerobic and anaerobic bacterial cultures, fungal cultures, and histopathology should be performed to help rule out infection and other diseases. If erythema nodosum–like panniculitis is documented histopathologically, the possibility of underlying systemic infection, infection at other sites, neoplasia, or drug reactions must be evaluated. Erythema nodosum–like panniculitis must not be deemed idiopathic unless all likely possible causes are investigated.

Biopsy site selection

Punch biopsy is not recommended if erythema nodosum–like panniculitis is suspected. Wedge section should be used to ensure that the specimen includes epidermis, dermis, and subcutaneous tissue. Multiple specimens are desirable. Cavitated, ulcerated, or necrotic lesions should be avoided if earlier lesions are present.

Histopathology

The epidermis and dermis are normal unless full-thickness necrosis and ulceration have occurred. Septal hemorrhage and fibrin exudation may be prominent; vessels may show endothelial swelling, mild fibrinoid change, and occasional thrombosis, but overt inflammation of the vessel walls (true vasculitis) is absent. The panniculus shows diffuse septal inflammation with neutrophils and mixed mononuclear cells. Inflammation may spread to the surrounding lobules, resulting in a diffuse pattern, and may be predominantly granulomatous in late stages. Fibrosis occurs in chronic lesions.

Differential diagnoses of early lesions are limited if vascular changes are visualized. Chronic lesions may resemble those of chronic idiopathic sterile nodular panniculitis if fibrosis and diffuse inflammation of the panniculus predominate.

FELINE PANSTEATITIS (Synonyms: feline vitamin E deficiency, vitamin E deficiency steatitis)

Clinical features

Feline pansteatitis is a nutritional skin disease caused by a severe deficiency of vitamin E. The syn-

---

* Peter J. Ihrke.

drome is worldwide in distribution, but the frequency is contingent upon feeding practices. Feline pansteatitis is uncommon in North America and Europe. Vitamin E deficiency may be caused by the feeding of food deficient in vitamin E or food with excess highly unsaturated fatty acids, which destroy vitamin E. A ration may be deficient in vitamin E either through formulation or as the result of oxidation of fat from improper storage. The most commonly reported causes of feline pansteatitis are the feeding of canned red tuna as an exclusive diet or excessive cod liver oil supplementation.

Multiple, irregularly firm nodules of variable density develop diffusely in the subcutis and the abdominal mesenteric fat. Abnormalities are not seen in the overlying skin unless nodules fistulate. Fistulation is rare. Systemic signs of fever, malaise, pain (elicited by palpation), anorexia, lethargy (sometimes alternating with hyperexcitability), and depression may precede or occur simultaneously with the development of subcutaneous and visceral nodules. Death is a frequent sequela.

As would be expected, breed, age, or sex predilections have not been noted. Feline pansteatitis is a highly characteristic disease clinically. However, clinical differential diagnoses could include other causes of panniculitis and neoplasia.

Biopsy site selection

An intact nodule should be removed by wedge section to ensure that the specimen includes epidermis, dermis, and subcutaneous tissue. The index of suspicion for feline pansteatitis is enhanced if yellow, discolored fat is seen during surgical biopsy.

Histopathology

The epidermis and dermis are normal. The pattern of pannicular inflammation is lobular to diffuse. The subcutaneous fat principally demonstrates deposition of yellow or yellow-brown, acid-fast ceroid pigment between adipocytes. Deposits approach the size of a normal fat cell, and similar pigment may also be found within macrophages and giant cells. Giant cells may be of the Langhans' type (containing a peripheral ring of nuclei). Early stages of the disease show neutrophil infiltration, but granulomatous inflammation soon predominates. Adipocytes may be necrotic, and there may be saponification and cholesterol cleft formation in some cases.

Differential diagnosis is not difficult, since typical ceroid pigment deposition identifies pansteatitis. Traumatic panniculitis has histiocytic infiltrates, but these contain foamy debris of fat degeneration and not pale brown ceroid. Acid-fast stains may be applied to differentiate ceroid from the iron pigment of hemosiderin seen in some lesions of traumatic panniculitis.

STERILE PEDAL PANNICULITIS OF THE GERMAN SHEPHERD DOG
Clinical features (Figures 20-14 through 20-16)

Sterile pedal panniculitis is a very rare canine skin disease of unknown etiology characterized by well-demarcated, frequently symmetric, deep fistulous tracts located dorsal to the midline of single or multiple footpads. The strong breed predilection for the German Shepherd Dog suggests heritability.

Deep fistulous tracts with well-demarcated, slightly swollen, erythematous borders sparingly exude a serous to milky, viscid fluid. The most common site is dorsal to the midline of the tarsal or carpal pad, but lesions may be seen dorsal to other footpads on the hindlimbs or the forelimbs. Lesions may be either single or mul-

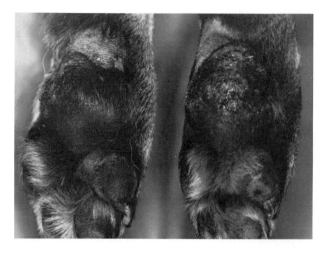

FIGURE 20-14. Sterile pedal panniculitis in a German Shepherd Dog. Fistulous tracts are present dorsal to both carpal pads.

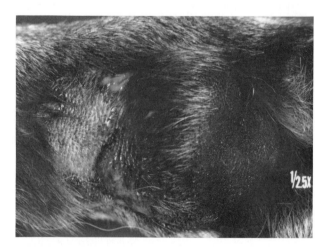

FIGURE 20-15. Closer view of the dog in Figure 20-14. Fistulous tracts exude a milky fluid.

tiple. Deep palpation elicits pain. Secondary bacterial infection is common. Lymphadenopathy is variable but usually is mild unless secondary bacterial infection is marked. Scarring is seen with chronicity.

The syndrome is seen primarily in German Shepherd Dogs and related mixed-breed dogs. Age or sex predilections have not been noted.

Clinically, this syndrome is quite distinctive. Fistulous tracts initiated by foreign bodies should be considered; however, sites caudal to the footpads, particularly the large tarsal or carpal pads, would be atypical for foreign body penetration.

Biopsy site selection

Specimen collection is difficult. The tissue needed is the deep dermis and subcutis directly dorsal to a footpad. Wedge technique performed under general anesthesia is recommended, since local anesthesia is difficult and hemostasis may be problematic. At least part of the fistula should be included in the specimen.

Histopathology (Figures 20-17 and 20-18)

The epidermis is severely ulcerated and the superficial dermis may be cavitated. Intact marginal epidermis is severely acanthotic.

The dermis and the underlying panniculus are severely inflamed; inflammation replaces all normal tissues. In earlier lesions, neutrophils and macrophages predominate, and discrete pyogranulomas may be observed. However, most specimens are obtained from advanced lesions that contain diffuse infiltrations of neutrophils, macrophages, plasma cells, and lymphocytes. Inflammation grades into areas of variable fibrosis, depending on the stage of the lesions. Fibrosis is generally striking and deep and borders the edge of a

fistula, which penetrates well into the panniculus. Fibrous connective tissue emanates outward from the edge of the deep cavity and extends into adjacent tissue, where it is accompanied by chronic inflammation, consisting primarily of plasma cells.

Differential diagnosis based on histopathology alone is difficult because the microscopic lesions of sterile pedal panniculitis are not distinctive. Knowledge of the breed affected and the site of the lesion is required for definitive diagnosis of this syndrome. Any foreign body reaction or puncture-induced traumatic lesion that extends to the panniculus may appear similar, as may deep bacterial or fungal infections.

SUGGESTED READINGS

Post-rabies vaccination alopecia
See Chapter 17.

Post-injection panniculitis
Hendrick MJ and Dunagan CA: Focal necrotizing granulomatous panniculitis associated with subcutaneous injection of rabies vac-

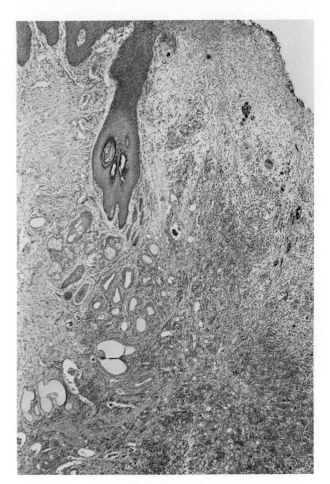

FIGURE 20-17. Sterile pedal panniculitis in a German Shepherd Dog. Severe ulceration at the opening of a fistula overlies severe deep inflammation and fibrosis. (×35.)

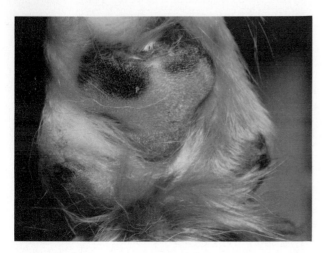

FIGURE 20-16. Chronic sterile pedal panniculitis in a German Shepherd Dog. Scar tissue deforms the dorsal aspect of the carpal pad.

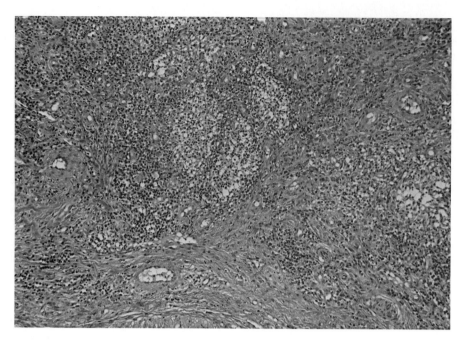

FIGURE 20-18. Sterile pedal panniculitis in a German Shepherd Dog. Mixed inflammation and fibrosis are evident. (×90.)

cine in cats and dogs: 10 cases (1988-1989), J Am Vet Med Assoc 198:304-305, 1991.

Hendrick MJ and Goldschmidt MH: Do injection site reactions induce fibrosarcomas in cats? J Am Vet Med Assoc 199:968, 1991.

Schmeitzel LP, Loeffler D, and Bass MC: Focal cutaneous reactions at vaccination sites in a cat and four dogs. Proceedings of the American Academy of Veterinary Dermatology/American College of Veterinary Dermatology, New Orleans 2:39, 1986.

Traumatic panniculitis

No references available.

Idiopathic sterile nodular panniculitis

Ackerman LJ: Canine nodular panniculitis, Comp Cont Ed 6:818-824, 1984.

Baker BB and Stannard AA: Nodular panniculitis in the dog, J Am Vet Med Assoc 167:752-755, 1975.

Bondi EE and Lazarus GS: Disorders of subcutaneous tissue. In Fitzpatrick TB, Eisen AZ, Wolff K and others, editors: Dermatology in general medicine, ed 3, New York, 1987, McGraw-Hill, pp 1131-1148.

Edgar TP and Furrow RD: Idiopathic nodular panniculitis in a German Shepherd, J Am Anim Hosp Assoc 20:603-606, 1984.

Guaguere E and others: Panniculite nodulaire sterile: a propos d'un cas, Pratique Medicale et Chirurgicale de l'Animal de Compagnie 1:27-33, 1988.

Lever WF and Schaumburg-Lever G: Histopathology of the skin, ed 7, Philadelphia, 1990, JB Lippincott, pp 269-283.

Mason KV: Disseminated necrotizing panniculitis associated with pancreatic carcinoma in a dog. Proceedings of the American Acad-

emy of Veterinary Dermatology/American College of Veterinary Dermatology, St Louis 5:61, 1989.

Muller GH, Kirk RW, and Scott DW: Small animal dermatology, ed 4, Philadelphia, 1989, WB Saunders, pp 831-838.

Shanley KJ and Miller WH: Panniculitis in the dog: a report of five cases, J Am Anim Hosp Assoc 21:545-550, 1985.

Scott DW and Anderson WI: Panniculitis in dogs and cats: a retrospective analysis of 78 cases, J Am Anim Hosp Assoc 24:551-559, 1988.

Erythema nodosum–like panniculitis

Bondi EE and Lazarus GS: Disorders of subcutaneous tissue. In Fitzpatrick TB, Eisen AZ, Wolff K and others, editors: Dermatology in general medicine, ed 3, New York, 1987, McGraw-Hill, pp 1131-1148.

Lever WF and Schaumburg-Lever G: Histopathology of the skin, ed 7, Philadelphia, 1990, JB Lippincott, pp 270-272.

Muller GH, Kirk RW, and Scott DW: Small animal dermatology, ed 4, Philadelphia, 1989, WB Saunders, pp 831-837.

Feline pansteatitis

Holzworth J: Diseases of the cat: medicine and surgery, Philadelphia, 1987, WB Saunders, pp 27-28.

Jones TC and Hunt RD: Veterinary pathology, Philadelphia, 1983, Lea & Febiger, pp 1044-1048.

White SD: The skin as a sensor of internal medical disorders. In Ettinger SJ, editor: Textbook of veterinary internal medicine, ed 3, Philadelphia, 1989, WB Saunders, pp 5-10.

Sterile pedal panniculitis of the German Shepherd Dog

References not available.

NEOPLASTIC DISEASES OF THE SKIN

EMILY J. WALDER
THELMA LEE GROSS

INTRODUCTION

Solitary or multiple cutaneous masses are a frequent presenting sign for the veterinary dermatologist. Differentiation among nonneoplastic nodular lesions, benign neoplasms, and malignant neoplasms is often not possible on a clinical basis; incisional or excisional biopsy and histopathologic examination are required for definitive diagnosis in most instances.

Classification systems for cutaneous tumors in the veterinary literature were established early in the history of veterinary pathology. Over the years, newer entities were added sporadically, but little in the way of major revision has been done. As veterinary pathology becomes more sophisticated in its understanding of cutaneous embryology and structure and function, the precision with which neoplastic lesions are categorized as to cell of origin and path of differentiation should increase. Some of the information presented in this section will be such an attempt and hopefully will generate a more meaningful and consistent nomenclature. However, the fact remains that nomenclature is made by humans and neoplasms are biologic aberrations; some lesions will always defy neat classification.

GENERAL REFERENCES

Carpenter JL, Andrew LK, and Holzworth J: Tumors and tumor-like lesions. In Holzworth J, editor: Diseases of the cat, Philadelphia, 1987, WB Saunders, pp 406-596.

Conroy JD: Canine skin tumors, J Am Anim Hosp Assoc 19:91-114, 1983.

Lever WF and Schaumburg-Lever G: Histopathology of the skin, ed 7, Philadelphia, 1990, JB Lippincott, pp 523-846.

Macy DW and Reynolds, HA: The incidence, characteristics and clinical management of skin tumors of cats, J Am Anim Hosp Assoc 17:1026-1034, 1981.

Mehregan AH: Pinkus' guide to dermatohistopathology, ed 4, Norwalk, Conn, 1986, Appleton-Century-Crofts, pp 385-594.

Muller GH, Kirk RW, and Scott DW: Small animal dermatology, ed 4, Philadelphia, 1989, WB Saunders, pp 844-958.

Nielsen SW: Classification of tumors in dogs and cats, J Am Anim Hosp Assoc 19:13-60, 1981.

Pulley LT and Stannard AA: Tumors of the skin and soft tissues. In Moulton J, editor: Tumors in domestic animals, ed 3, Berkeley, Calif, 1990, University of California Press, pp 23-87.

Scott DW: Feline dermatology, 1900-1978: a monograph, J Am Anim Hosp Assoc 16:331-425, 1980.

Theilen GH and Madewell BR, editors: Veterinary cancer medicine, ed 2, Philadelphia, 1987, Lea & Febiger, pp 233-325.

Weiss E: Tumours of the soft (mesenchymal) tissues, Bull World Health Organ 50:101-110, 1974.

Weiss E and Frese K: Tumours of the skin, Bull World Health Organ 50:79-100, 1974.

Epithelial tumors

Epidermal tumors

ACTINIC KERATOSIS

Clinical features (see Figures 6-19, 6-20, and 10-30)

The term *keratosis* refers to a small, reactive proliferation of keratinocytes. The only commonly occurring keratosis in dogs and cats is the actinic keratosis. The incidence varies markedly with geographic location and climate. In the Beagle colony in Colorado in which this syndrome was first described by Hargis in 1977, approximately 25% of the animals were affected. As the name implies, actinic keratoses develop as a result of chronic solar damage and frequently coexist with frank squamous cell carcinoma. Ultraviolet radiation causes dimerization and protein cross-links in DNA molecules. In addition, ultraviolet light induces formation of a carcinogen, cholesterol alpha-oxide, from natural sterols in unpigmented skin.

Actinic keratoses are single or more often multiple, plaque-like or papillated lesions, ranging from several millimeters to several centimeters in diameter. Lesions have prominent, adherent scale; hyperkeratosis may be so dramatic that the lesion appears clinically as a cutaneous horn (see later discussion). Actinic keratoses occur most commonly on the pinnae, nose, and eyelids of white-faced cats. In dogs they are found primarily on the ventral abdomen and medial thighs of short-coated, white-haired breeds.

Dalmatians, American Staffordshire Terriers, Beagles, Bassett Hounds, and other dogs with similar coat coloration have an increased incidence of actinic keratoses and other solar-induced neoplasias. Actinic keratoses can continue to proliferate and become invasive into the dermis as frank squamous cell carcinoma. They should therefore be regarded as one form of squamous cell carcinoma in situ. (See also Chapters 6 and 10 for further clinical discussion of actinic keratoses.)

Histopathology (see Figures 6-21, 6-22, and 10-31 through 10-33)

The epidermis in actinic keratosis shows irregular hyperplasia, diffuse dysplasia, and marked hyperkeratosis or parakeratosis. Mild-to-moderate architectural distortion results from loss of polarity of variable numbers of keratinocytes in the basal and spinous layers. Rete ridge formation may be present, but the basement membrane zone is intact; there is no dermal invasion by atypical squamous epithelial cells. Mild-to-moderate nuclear atypia, characterized by nuclear enlargement, nucleolar prominence and hyperchromatism, is observed. Mitotic activity is slightly increased, and mitotic figures can occur at all levels of the epidermis. Small numbers of giant cells with single or multiple nuclei may be observed. Scattered, brightly eosinophilic, dyskeratotic cells may be present. Cells of the stratum spinosum may be vacuolated. Hyperplasia and dysplasia can also affect the superficial hair follicles. Dermal inflammation and degenerative changes are as previously described (see Chapter 10).

An acantholytic variant of actinic keratosis, which also occurs in humans, is occasionally observed in cats and dogs. Clefts or lacunae develop above dysplastic basal epithelial cells. The clefts contain groups of individualized keratinocytes exhibiting round, brightly eosinophilic cytoplasm and pleomorphic, hyperchromatic nuclei.

Actinic keratosis is differentiated from frank squamous cell carcinoma by the absence of dermal invasion. Serial sections may be helpful in ruling out a diagnosis of squamous cell carcinoma. Actinic keratosis is distinguished from Bowen's disease (multicentric squamous cell carcinoma in situ) primarily on clinical grounds. Actinic keratoses affect only sun-exposed, sparsely haired, lightly pigmented areas of the skin and are often solitary; lesions of Bowen's disease occur in haired, pigmented skin and are often multicentric in dogs and cats. Acantholytic actinic keratosis is differentiated from autoimmune acantholytic disorders by the presence of dyskeratotic acantholytic cells, as well as other features of dysplasia.

PIGMENTED EPIDERMAL NEVUS
Clinical features

A nevus may be defined as a stable malformation of skin of presumed congenital origin and thus may affect any tissue component of the skin. *Pigmented epidermal nevus* is the term chosen to describe a rare, benign, nonneoplastic lesion of dogs. The canine lesion has several clinical and histopathologic features in common with verrucous or linear epidermal nevus in humans, which may exhibit pigmentation. The authors believe that the lesions described as lentigines (see Chapter 29) in the Pug by Briggs and also Muller, Kirk, and Scott are probably pigmented epidermal nevi rather than primary melanocytic proliferations. Epidermal nevi are described in the Schnauzer by Muller, Kirk, and Scott. The epidermal proliferative features of the canine lesions the authors have designated as pigmented epidermal nevi are not consistent with any type of lentigo.*

Pigmented epidermal nevi usually appear as multiple, deeply pigmented, ovoid or circular plaques that are less than 1 cm in diameter. Lesions may be numerous or, occasionally, are solitary. The nevi have scaly, irregular, slightly papillated surfaces. The lesions occur most often on the ventral abdomen, ventral thorax, and medial limbs. Involvement may be bilateral or unilateral. Distal limbs may also be involved.

_____
* Barr RJ: Personal communication, 1990.

Affected animals are usually young adults. There is a strong breed predilection for Pugs and Schnauzers, supporting a hereditary pathogenesis. The nevi develop progressively over a period of time and then become stable.

Histopathology (Figures 21-1 and 21-2)

Pigmented epidermal nevi are discrete plaques of mild-to-moderate acanthosis and hyperkeratosis. The epidermis usually has a papillated or digitated configuration, resulting in the roughened surface observed clinically. The lower layers of the epidermis have moderate-to-marked hyperpigmentation, but melanocytic proliferation is not present. Melanin pigment may extend into the upper cell layers of the epidermis and into the stratum corneum. The epidermal granular cell layer contains enlarged keratohyalin granules, and some cells may demonstrate cytoplasmic vacuolation. This may be a mild manifestation of epidermolytic hyperkeratosis, which is sometimes observed in human epidermal nevi. (Epidermolytic hyperkeratosis is a specific degenerative pattern observed in several human nonneoplastic and neoplastic dermatologic lesions. It is a keratinocyte maturation defect that results in giant keratohyalin granules, vacuolation of granular and spinous cell layers, and loss of discrete cytoplasmic margins.) The underlying dermis may contain increased numbers of melanophages, particularly in heavily pigmented nevi.

The differential diagnosis for pigmented epidermal nevus is lentigo simplex. Simple lentigines are flat or slightly elevated lesions, whereas epidermal nevi are papillated or scaly clinically. Lentigines contain increased numbers of deeply pigmented melanocytes in the basal cell layer. Lentigines do not exhibit papillomatous epidermal hyperplasia, hypergranulosis, or hyperkeratosis.

CUTANEOUS HORN OF FELINE FOOTPAD
Clinical features

Cutaneous horn is a general clinical term describing a circumscribed, conical, or cylindric keratotic mass in which the height is generally greater than the diameter. Cutaneous horns in dogs and cats may arise from actinic keratoses (see previous discussion) or papillomas (see following discussion) or from dilated pores or infundibular keratinizing acanthomas (see Chapter 22).

Cutaneous horn of footpads in cats is a rare disorder that was first described by Scott. Affected cats tested positive for the feline leukemia virus, and the virus was isolated on a culture of the cutaneous horns.

The lesions are single or multiple, conical or cylin-

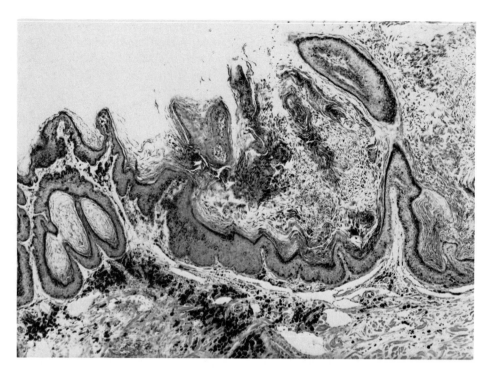

FIGURE 21-1. Pigmented epidermal nevus in a dog. The epidermis shows hyperpigmentation, papillomatous hyperplasia, and marked hyperkeratosis. Note the melanophages in the superficial dermis. (×50.)

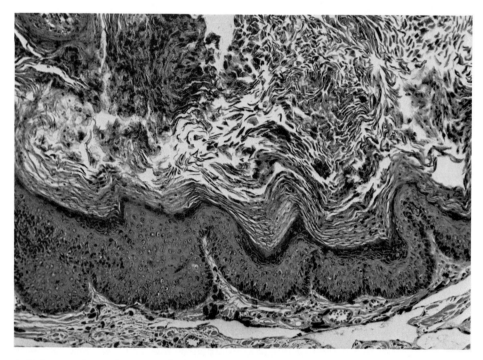

FIGURE 21-2. Higher magnification of the pigmented epidermal nevus in Figure 21-1 showing an increase in the number and size of keratohyalin granules in the superficial epidermis. The melanocytes are not increased in number. (×150.)

FIGURE 21-3. Cutaneous horn of feline footpad. A column of pale, compact keratin arises from moderately hyperplastic epidermis. (×55.)

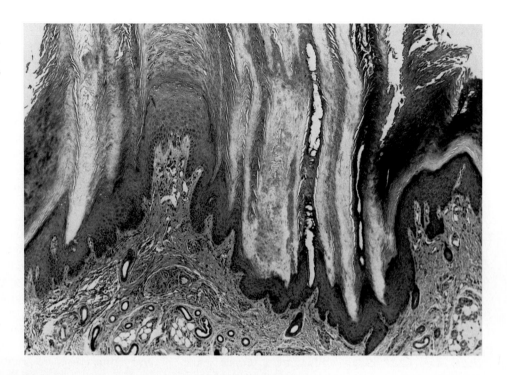

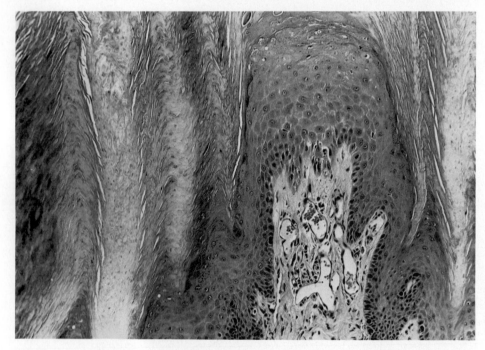

FIGURE 21-4. Higher magnification of the cutaneous horn in Figure 21-3 showing papillomatous hyperplasia of the epidermis and mild vacuolation of the stratum granulosum. (×120.)

dric masses of hard keratin measuring several millimeters in diameter and 1 to 2 cm in height. The viral-associated cutaneous horns occur on the footpads only. There is no known age or breed predisposition.

Histopathology (Figures 21-3 and 21-4)

Cutaneous horn of feline footpad is characterized by a well-demarcated zone of moderate-to-marked pap-

illomatous hyperplasia of the epidermis from which emanates a column of compact keratin. The shape and homogeneous quality of the keratin column resemble a toenail. Parakeratotic cells may also be present within the keratin column. Epidermal stratification of the underlying hyperplastic epidermis is well maintained, but scattered dyskeratotic epithelial cells are observed. Occasional multinucleated or vacuolated keratinocytes may be present. Cutaneous horn of feline footpad is clinically and histopathologically unique; there are no known differential diagnoses.

VIRAL SQUAMOUS PAPILLOMA

(Synonyms: wart, verruca)

Clinical features

Squamous papillomas induced by the prototypic canine papillomavirus occur uncommonly in dogs. The reported incidence ranges from 1% to 2.5% of all canine skin tumors.

Classic, fully developed, exophytic warts are papillated masses that vary from several millimeters to several centimeters in diameter; most lesions are less than 1 cm. Viral papillomas appear as single or multiple lesions, occurring most commonly on the face and oral mucosa. Isolated lesions can also occur on other parts of the body. Viral papillomas often spontaneously regress over a period of weeks to months.

Verruca plana, or flat warts, occasionally occur in dogs. Two cases in cats, caused by a unique feline papillomavirus, have recently been reported by Carney. These have a plaque-like or papular appearance and are usually less than 5 mm in diameter. Site predilections are similar to those for exophytic papilloma. Verruca plana may represent a regression phase of exophytic papillomas.

Another uncommon variant of viral wart is cutaneous inverted papilloma, which was originally described by Campbell. These usually appear as multiple, raised, firm masses that are usually less than 1 cm in diameter and have a small central pore. Most cutaneous inverted papillomas arise on the ventral abdomen. Cutaneous horn may occasionally be the clinical presenting sign for any type of papilloma.

Viral papillomas generally affect dogs less than 3 years of age. There is no known breed predisposition for any of the viral papillomas.

Histopathology

Exophytic papilloma (Figure 21-5). Typical viral papillomas comprise finger-like projections of mature squamous epithelium. The peripheral papillary structures are angled inward at their base; this is referred to as a "toed-in" configuration. The epithelial fronds are heavily keratinized, and the keratin is arranged in peaks and spires. Mild-to-moderate inflammation is generally present in the connective tissue cores of the papillae, and serous crusts are present at their tips.

The cytopathic effects of the papillomavirus are manifested by giant keratohyalin granules and koilocytosis. Koilocytes are altered keratinocytes described in papillomavirus-induced lesions in humans and animals. They are characterized by clear or gray cytoplasm and small smudged or vesicular nuclei. Occasionally, baso-

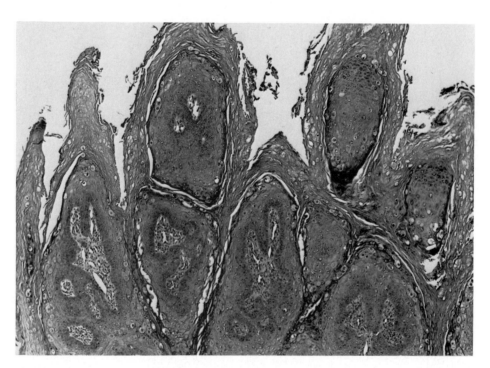

FIGURE 21-5. Exophytic viral squamous papilloma in a dog. Hyperplastic, hyperkeratotic epithelium covers closely grouped papillary projections. Note the prominent keratohyalin granules and large, pale, vacuolated cells (koilocytes) in the stratum granulosum. (×50.)

philic intranuclear inclusions can be found at the junction of keratinized and nonkeratinized epithelium.

Verruca plana. Flat warts are plaque-like, rather than papillated, lesions characterized by epidermal hyperplasia and hyperkeratosis. The epithelium demonstrates similar cytopathic changes to exophytic warts. Enlarged keratohyalin granules and scattered koilocytes are present. The feline lesions also had amphophilic, nonviral, cytoplasmic inclusion bodies. The flat wart may represent a regression phase or *forme fruste* of exophytic viral papilloma.

Inverted papilloma (Figures 21-6 and 21-7). Cutaneous inverted papilloma is the endophytic variant of viral papilloma in dogs. These are cup-shaped lesions with a central core of keratin leading to an umbilicated surface. The cup is lined by mature squamous epithelium with centripetal papillary projections. Koilocytosis and intranuclear inclusions are present. Papillomavirus was detected in these lesions by both electron microscopy and immunohistochemistry by Campbell.

Exophytic viral papillomas and verruca plana are distinctive diseases and have no known differential diagnoses. Inverted papilloma must be differentiated from infundibular keratinizing acanthoma, which is also a cup-shaped, keratin-filled, squamous epithelial mass. Infundibular keratinizing acanthoma has small cysts and anastomosing trabeculae of keratinocytes comprising its epithelial wall, in comparison to the papillary structures of an endophytic wart. Koilocytosis and viral inclusions are not present in infundibular acanthoma.

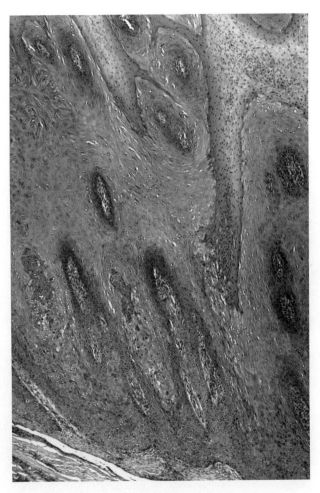

FIGURE 21-6. Inverted viral squamous papilloma in a dog. Papillary structures project into a keratin core from a peripheral wall of mature squamous epithelium. (×50.)

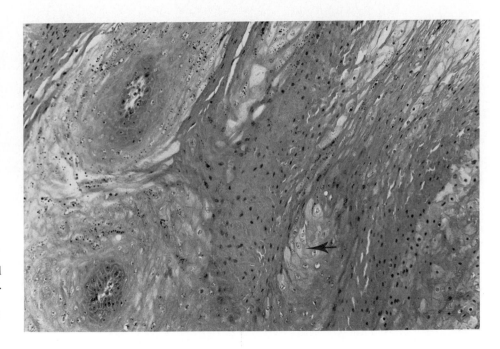

FIGURE 21-7. Inverted viral squamous papilloma in a dog. Note the giant keratohyalin granules and pale koilocytotic cells *(arrow)*. (×120.)

IDIOPATHIC SQUAMOUS PAPILLOMA (Synonym: wart)

Clinical features

Papillomas in which viral cytopathic effects are not evident occur uncommonly in dogs and rarely in cats. It remains to be definitively shown whether or not these lesions have a viral etiology. Idiopathic papillomas are delicate, papillated masses that may be pedunculated. Idiopathic papillomas are generally smaller than viral warts; they are usually 1 to 5 mm in diameter. Lesions are most often observed on the face, eyelids, conjunctiva, and footpads. There is no known age or breed predisposition.

Histopathology (Figure 21-8)

The overall architecture of idiopathic papilloma is similar to viral papilloma, but the epithelium covering the papillary projections is not as hyperplastic or hyperkeratotic. The collagenous cores of the finger-like projections usually have less inflammation than in viral papilloma. Giant keratohyalin granules, koilocytosis, and inclusion bodies are not evident.

Lesions referred to as *fibropapillomas*—masses containing abundant fibrous tissue covered by papillated squamous epithelium—are probably reactive rather than neoplastic (see fibropruritic nodule, Chapter 6). The term fibropapilloma is probably best reserved for the lesion caused by bovine papillomavirus on the penis of bulls.

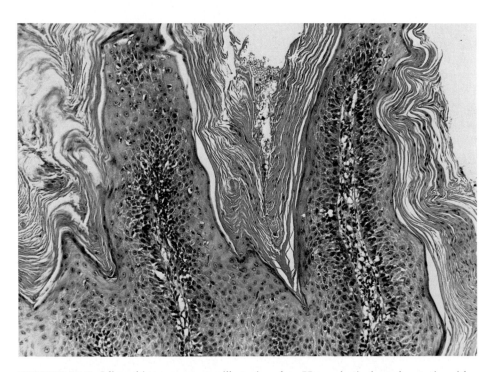

FIGURE 21-8. Idiopathic squamous papilloma in a dog. Hyperplastic, hyperkeratotic epithelium covers papillary projections. Hypergranulosis and koilocytosis are not present. (×120.)

SQUAMOUS CELL CARCINOMA

Clinical features

Squamous cell carcinoma is the most common malignant neoplasm of the skin in cats and the second most common in dogs, following mast cell tumor. The reported incidence in cats ranges from 17% to 25%, and in dogs, from 3% to 20%. Squamous cell carcinoma occurs most frequently in sun-damaged skin and may be preceded by actinic keratosis; the incidence therefore partially depends upon geography and climate. Thermal injury may also be a predisposing factor.

Squamous cell carcinomas appear as plaque-like, crateriform, papillary or nodular masses that vary from several millimeters to several centimeters in diameter. Alopecia, erythema, ulceration, and crusting are present. Lesions may be single or multiple. There is usually a temporal progression from small plaques to larger ulcerative or exophytic lesions. Nasal planum, pinnae, and eyelids are the most common sites in cats.

In dogs the most frequently affected areas are the ventral abdomen and medial stifles. The lateral elbow is a less common preferential site in dogs; the acantholytic variant of squamous cell carcinoma in dogs appears to occur more commonly on the lateral elbow than at sun-exposed sites.

White cats and short-coated dogs with white or piebald ventral coat color have the highest incidence of squamous cell carcinoma. Dalmatians, American Staffordshire Terriers, Bull Terriers, and Beagles are typical high-risk breeds. Affected cats are usually 5 years of age or older. Dogs may develop squamous cell carcinoma as early as 3 years of age.

Tumors in cats may be highly destructive with a gradual loss of tissue of the pinna or nose. The majority of squamous cell carcinomas in dogs and cats are of the well-differentiated histopathologic subtype, and the metastatic incidence is low. Poorly differentiated, acantholytic, and spindle-celled variants also occur; these may have a higher rate of metastasis, but specific data are not reported. Metastasis is often limited to regional lymph nodes, but more widespread dissemination may occur. In humans, the metastatic incidence of squamous cell carcinoma is also low, ranging from 6% to 10%, and depends upon the degree of histopathologic differentiation.

Histopathology

Well-differentiated squamous cell carcinoma (Figure 21-9). Well-differentiated tumors are erosive, plaque-like lesions comprising islands and trabeculae of squamous cells that originate from the epidermis and extend into the dermis. There is fairly orderly progression from polyhedral, nonkeratinized cells at the periphery of the neoplastic epithelial structures to large, polygonal, keratinized cells at the centers. Central accumulations of compact laminated keratin, or keratin pearls, are present in variable numbers. Keratinization progresses through a granular cell layer as in normal epidermis or follicular infundibulum. The keratinized centers of the lobules often undergo necrosis and become infiltrated by neutrophils.

Nuclei are large and vesicular and have prominent nucleoli. Mitotic activity is moderate to high. Some degree of stromal collagen production is always present, and the stroma often contains small clusters of partially-keratinized tumor cells. Stromal infiltration by a variety of inflammatory cells is generally present. One of the authors* has seen occasional examples of well-differentiated squamous cell carcinoma arising from

---

* Thelma Lee Gross.

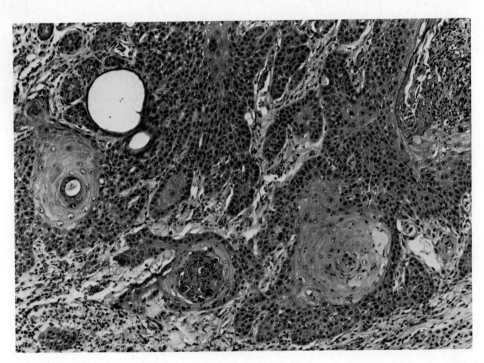

FIGURE 21-9. Well-differentiated squamous cell carcinoma in a cat. Islands and trabeculae of squamous epithelium show orderly differentiation from nonkeratinized to keratinized cells. Note the central keratin pearls infiltrated by neutrophils. (×120.)

superficial hair follicles without involvement of the epidermis.

Poorly differentiated squamous cell carcinoma (Figure 21-10). This is a less common subgroup with similar overall architecture to well-differentiated squamous cell carcinoma. Epithelial structures tend to be smaller; cords and nests rather than large islands of squamous epithelial cells often predominate. Stromal collagen production is generally less prominent. The neoplastic cells exhibit basophilic cytoplasm, hyperchromatic nuclei, and prominent nucleoli, which may be multiple. Other characteristics include high mitotic activity and frequent mitotic atypia. Keratin pearls are not observed, but individual dyskeratotic

cells or clusters of partially keratinized cells may be present. Identification of intercellular bridges may be helpful in the diagnosis of very anaplastic lesions. Contiguity of neoplastic tissue with intact epidermis also supports a diagnosis of squamous cell carcinoma. Immunohistochemical detection of high–molecular weight cytokeratins may be required to differentiate some squamous cell carcinomas from other anaplastic carcinomas.

Acantholytic squamous cell carcinoma (Figures 21-11 and 21-12). Acantholytic, or pseudoglandular, squamous cell carcinoma is an uncommon variant of squamous cell carcinoma. The pseudoglandular structures are formed by drop out of partially keratinized

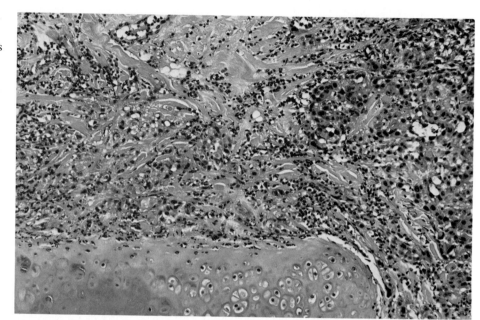

FIGURE 21-10. Poorly differentiated squamous cell carcinoma in a cat. Islands and nests of pleomorphic epithelial cells infiltrate an inflammatory stroma. Nasal cartilage is at the bottom. (×120.)

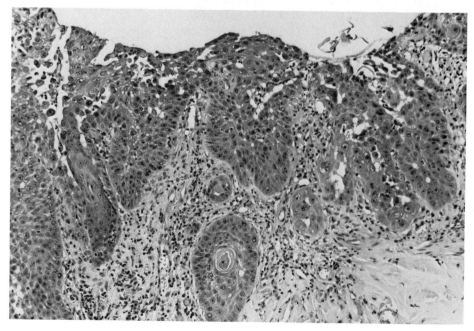

FIGURE 21-11. Acantholytic squamous cell carcinoma in a cat. Individualized keratinocytes are present within clefts in the superficial aspects of this plaque-like neoplasm. Note the reactive collagenous stroma with mixed inflammatory cells in the superficial dermis. (×120.)

FIGURE 21-12. Acantholytic squamous cell carcinoma in a dog. Pseudoglandular structures contain individualized keratinocytes within their lumens. Note that occasional acantholytic cells are still connected by attenuated cytoplasmic bridges *(arrow)*. (×240.)

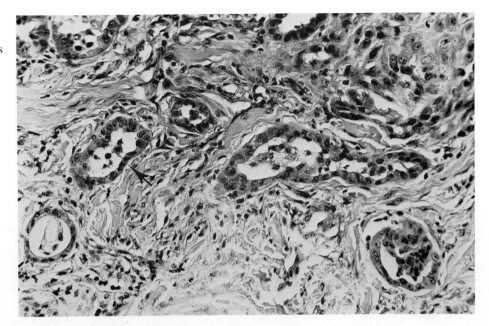

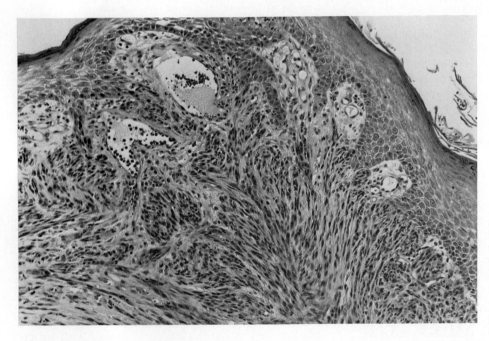

FIGURE 21-13. Spindle-celled squamous cell carcinoma in a cat. Pleomorphic spindle and polygonal cells are arranged in loose bundles and nests. Note the small areas of contiguity with hyperplastic and dysplastic foci of the epidermis. (×120.)

cells from the centers of epithelial islands and trabeculae. Residual keratinized cells float in the pseudolumens or are attached to the peripheral cell layer by elongated intercellular bridges. Foci of well-differentiated squamous cell carcinoma are often identifiable in the more superficial aspects of the neoplasm.

Differentiation of the acantholytic squamous cell carcinoma from apocrine or other glandular neoplasms is sometimes required. The absence of classic apocrine decapitation secretion and the absence of accumulations of secretory protein may be useful features for differentiation. Immunoperoxidase studies are also of diagnostic value; acantholytic squamous cell carcino-

mas are generally negative for carcinoembryonic antigen, whereas adenocarcinomas are positive.

Spindle-celled squamous cell carcinoma (Figures 21-13 and 21-14). This is a rare variant of poorly differentiated squamous cell carcinoma that is found most often on the pinnae of cats. This tumor comprises a large, pleomorphic spindle and polygonal cells that have abundant, pale or amphophilic cytoplasm. Areas of malignant transformation of the epidermis have loss of a distinct basement membrane zone, and atypical spindle cells appear to stream downward into the dermis. Foci of partial keratinization characterized by polygonal cells with moderate, glassy,

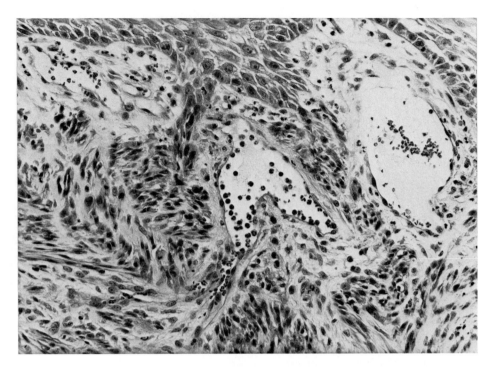

FIGURE 21-14. Higher magnification of the spindle-celled squamous cell carcinoma in Figure 21-13. The spindle cells appear to stream downward from a focus of malignant transformation of keratinocytes. (×240.)

eosinophilic cytoplasm may be present in some areas of the mass. Nuclei are large and vesicular and have prominent nucleoli. The mitotic index is high.

Differentiation of spindle-celled squamous cell carcinoma from fibrosarcoma and other mesenchymal malignancies is problematic unless contiguity with the overlying epidermis can be established. Serial sectioning to establish epidermal connection may be helpful. Definitive diagnosis may require immunohistochemical studies, using cytokeratins to identify squamous cell carcinoma and vimentin to rule out neoplasia of mesenchymal origin.

MULTICENTRIC SQUAMOUS CELL CARCINOMA IN SITU (Synonym: Bowen's disease)

Clinical features

Multicentric squamous cell carcinoma in situ, or Bowen's disease, is a form of carcinoma in situ first recognized in humans in 1912. This condition has been documented only recently in veterinary medicine and is considered to be rare in cats and very rare in dogs. The cause is not known, but association with other forms of neoplasia has been suggested in humans and reported in the dog.

Lesions of Bowen's disease appear as multifocal, heavily crusted plaques and verrucous lesions occurring in any location on the body. They often involve darkly pigmented or non-sun–exposed haired skin. Mucous membranes of the mouth and genitalia may be affected in dogs.

Multicentric squamous cell carcinoma in situ usually affects older cats. There is no known breed predilection. Lesions may occasionally become locally invasive, but the majority remain as in situ carcinomas. Metastasis has not been observed.

Histopathology (Figure 21-15)

The lesions of multicentric squamous cell carcinoma in situ are characterized by irregular epidermal hyperplasia with formation of broad rete ridges. Marked hyperkeratosis and parakeratosis with hyperpigmentation of the stratum corneum are often present. Full-thickness dysplasia is manifested by marked disruption of normal epithelial stratification in a pattern classically described as a "windblown" appearance. Keratinocyte size and appearance are highly variable and range from small with ovoid, hyperchromatic nuclei to large with pale, glycogenated cytoplasm and atypical, multilobular nuclei. Mitotic figures are present in all cell layers. Dysplastic epithelium frequently descends around follicular infundibula as an irregularly contoured cuff. The basement membrane zone is intact until late in the course of the disease when invasive squamous cell carcinoma may develop. The underlying

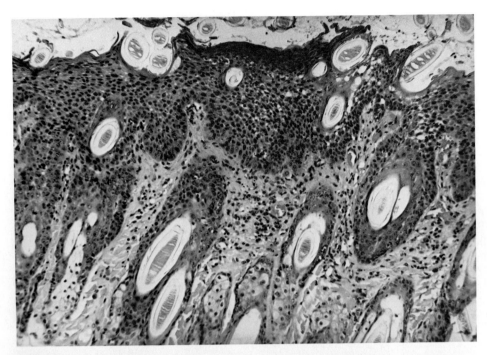

FIGURE 21-15. Multicentric squamous cell carcinoma in situ (Bowen's disease) in a cat. Irregularly thickened epidermis and superficial hair follicles have full-thickness disruption of stratified squamous epithelial architecture. Note the enlarged nuclei with loss of polarity and paler cytoplasm. (×120.)

dermis exhibits vascular dilatation and perivascular mixed mononuclear cell inflammation.

"Bowenoid" epithelial changes (windblown appearance, large pale keratinocytes) can also be observed in solitary actinic keratoses or in early squamous cell carcinoma, especially on the nasal planum of cats. Bowenoid actinic keratoses have also been described in humans. Multicentric squamous cell carcinoma in situ is distinguished from actinic keratosis primarily on clinical grounds. Actinic keratosis affects only sun-exposed, sparsely haired, lightly pigmented areas of the skin.

BENIGN FELINE BASAL CELL TUMOR

The name *basal cell tumor* has been used in the veterinary literature since 1932 to classify a large group of commonly occurring neoplasms of dogs and cats presumed to be derived from basal epithelial cells of both epidermal and adnexal origin. Numerous histopathologic subclassifications have been applied to these neoplasms: medusa head, garland, trabecular, solid, cystic, basosquamous, adenoid, and granular cell. Most veterinary basal cell tumors are benign and are not contiguous with the basal cell layer of the epidermis (medusa head, garland, trabecular, adenoid, and gran-

ular cell types); these lesions generally show differentiation toward follicular structures and thus have been reclassified (see Chapter 22). The subclassifications solid basal cell tumor and basosquamous basal cell tumor are reported to be biologically aggressive in some instances; most of these lesions are probably true basal cell carcinomas (see following discussion).

The term *basal cell tumor,* borrowed from human dermatopathology, is now considered in that discipline to be synonymous with the low-grade malignancy, basal cell carcinoma. Some authors prefer the terms *basal cell epithelioma* or *basalioma,* both of which connote the relatively good prognosis of this neoplasm.

In conclusion, the name *basal cell tumor* appears to have limited usage in veterinary pathology. The authors have recognized a true basal cell tumor in cats that does not have obvious adnexal features. Retention of the name basal cell tumor for this neoplasm thus seems appropriate until additional clinical or histochemical data indicate otherwise.

Clinical features

Basal cell tumor is an uncommon, benign cutaneous neoplasm found in cats only. The entire basal cell tumor category accounted for 11% to 28% of all feline skin tumors in multiple surveys. It is therefore not possible to determine what proportion of the incidence represents benign feline basal cell tumors.

Benign feline basal cell tumors are solitary, dome-shaped masses that are usually 1 to 2 cm in diameter. The neoplasms are usually nonpigmented, but may have a gray or blue tint if melanization is present. The epidermis is partially alopecic and frequently ulcerated. Lesions most commonly involve the dorsal trunk and head. There is no known age or breed predilection.

Histopathology (Figures 21-16 and 21-17)

Benign feline basal cell tumor is a well-circumscribed dermal nodule that generally has a fairly broad zone of connection to the overlying epidermis. Ulceration is common. Benign basal cell tumor commonly has a lima bean–shaped silhouette, with the central indentation at the tumor surface. The neoplasm is composed of small basaloid epithelial cells arranged in

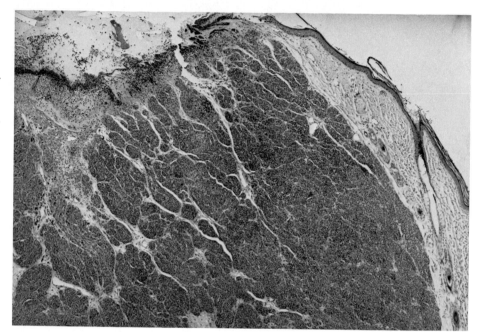

FIGURE 21-16. Benign feline basal cell tumor. Aggregates of small basaloid epithelial cells form a well-circumscribed nodule with a broad zone of epidermal contiguity and ulceration. Note the sparse stroma, which does not extend beyond the epithelial margins. (×50.)

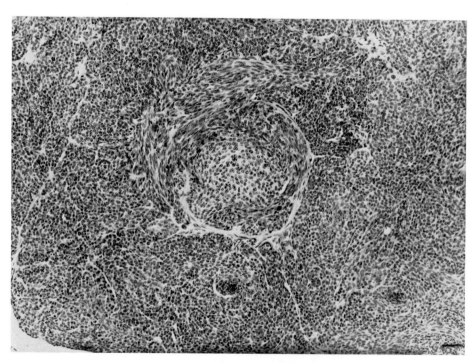

FIGURE 21-17. Higher magnification of the benign feline basal cell tumor in Figure 21-16 showing basaloid epithelial cells with scant, pale cytoplasm and ovoid nuclei. Note the mild melanization, absence of peripheral palisading, and central zone of spindling of the basaloid cells. (×120.)

tightly packed lobules and trabeculae without prominent peripheral palisading. The sparse collagenous stroma does not extend beyond the boundaries of the neoplastic epithelial structures. Stromal mucin is often present at the center of the neoplasm.

The epithelial cells are characterized by scant, pale cytoplasm and bland, ovoid nuclei. Nucleoli are inconspicuous, and mitotic activity is low. Frequently there are zones of spindling characterized by elongation of the nuclei and a swirled configuration of the entire epithelial cell aggregation. Squamous differentiation or keratinization is not observed. Stromal melanophages may be present, and there may be mild-to-moderate melanization of the epithelial cells.

Differential diagnoses for benign feline basal cell tumor include basal cell carcinoma and trabecular trichoblastoma. Basal cell carcinoma has an asymmetric, irregular silhouette and more abundant, reactive stroma, which separates the epithelial aggregates and generally extends beyond the boundaries of the epithelial component. Areas of epithelial cell spindling are infrequently observed. Mitotic activity is usually higher, and atypical mitoses are present. Trabecular trichoblastoma is distinguished from benign feline basal cell tumor by a distinct trabecular pattern, prominent peripheral palisading, and more abundant stroma.

BASAL CELL CARCINOMA (Synonyms:
basal cell epithelioma, basalioma)
Clinical features

Basal cell carcinoma is a low-grade malignancy arising from small, pluripotential epithelial cells within the basal cell layers of the epidermis and adnexa. It is the most common cutaneous epithelial malignancy in humans. Human ultrastructural studies, cited by Lever and also Mehregan, indicate a close relationship between basal cell carcinoma and primary epithelial germ, the embryonic cells giving rise to folliculosebaceous units. Subsets of undifferentiated cells that retain these embryonic features must therefore exist in adult epidermis. The pluripotentiality of the basaloid epithelial cells is manifested by limited differentiation toward hair follicles, sebaceous glands, and sweat glands occurring in some basal cell carcinomas.

The authors believe that basal cell carcinomas are common in cats and uncommon in dogs. Numeric incidence data are difficult to provide, since these neoplasms have been traditionally included in the very broad category of basal cell tumor (see discussion above). Most reviews of canine and feline cutaneous neoplasia do not describe a specific malignant variant of basal cell tumor, although basosquamous basal cell tumor is cited as a locally aggressive subtype. Conroy

described basosquamous carcinoma as a distinct clinicopathologic entity in dogs. The authors recognize three major histopathologic variants of basal cell carcinoma in dogs and cats: solid, keratinizing (basosquamous), and clear cell. Solid basal cell carcinoma is the most common variant in cats, and several subcategories are created by secondary features such as melanization and cystification. The keratinizing basal cell carcinoma is the most common variant in dogs.

A causal relationship between solar radiation and basal cell carcinoma is well established in humans. Basal cell carcinomas in cats occasionally coexist with actinic keratoses and squamous cell carcinomas, but the majority arise in non-sun–exposed locations.

Basal cell carcinoma usually appears as a solitary, firm, nodular, plaque-like or cystic mass measuring several millimeters to several centimeters in diameter. Lesions in cats are usually considerably smaller than those in dogs. The epidermis overlying a basal cell carcinoma is commonly alopecic and ulcerated. The skin may have a black or blue tint because of melanin pigment within the neoplasm. Basal cell carcinomas occur most commonly on haired skin of the head, neck, and thorax. Lesions in cats occasionally arise on the nasal planum or eyelids.

Basal cell carcinomas occasionally may be multiple, either synchronously or metachronously. Multicentric basal cell tumors consistent with basal cell carcinoma in cats were reported by Fehrer and have been observed by the authors. One of the authors* has seen 6 basal cell carcinomas which were removed from one dog over a 2-year period.

The average age of cats with basal cell tumors was 7 to 10 years in several surveys. The age prevalence in dogs is unknown. Siamese cats and long-haired cats have a higher incidence of basal cell tumors, according to reviews by Carpenter and Diters, respectively. There is no known breed predisposition in dogs.

The incidence of recurrence and metastasis of basal cell carcinoma in dogs and cats is very low. Carpenter reported one instance of lymph node metastasis out of 97 feline basal cell tumors. Recurrence and regional lymph node metastasis occurred in two digital basal cell carcinomas in cats seen by one of the authors,* suggesting that anatomic location may influence biologic behavior. Conroy reported that basosquamous carcinoma in dogs is locally aggressive and has a metastatic capacity approaching that of squamous cell carcinoma; specific numeric data were not given. Basosquamous basal cell carcinomas are more likely to recur and metastasize than other histopathologic subtypes in humans, but the overall metastatic rate is very low. The appellation *basal cell epithelioma* has been chosen for

* Emily J. Walder.

human basal cell carcinoma by several authors because of its limited metastatic potential. The designation *epithelioma* is well accepted in veterinary pathology for small-cell epithelial neoplasms of low-grade malignancy, such as sebaceous epithelioma. Further study to compile accurate data on the biologic behavior of basal cell carcinoma in animals may indicate that the term basal cell epithelioma is preferable because of its clinical implications of locally aggressive behavior and rare metastasis.

Histopathology

Solid basal cell carcinoma (Figures 21-18 through 21-23). Solid basal cell carcinoma is the most common histopathologic subtype in cats. It also occurs occasionally in dogs. Most solid basal cell carcinomas are circumscribed, irregular dermal masses comprising multiple epithelial cell aggregates of varying size and shape. The epithelial structures may have smooth or spikey margins. Variable palisading of cells occurs around the periphery of the epithelial aggregates.

FIGURE 21-18. Solid basal cell carcinoma in a cat. Aggregates of small epithelial cells form a poorly circumscribed mass with multifocal epidermal contiguity. Note the variability in the size and shape of the epithelial aggregates. (×50.)

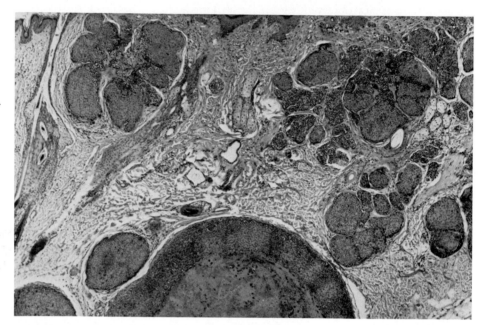

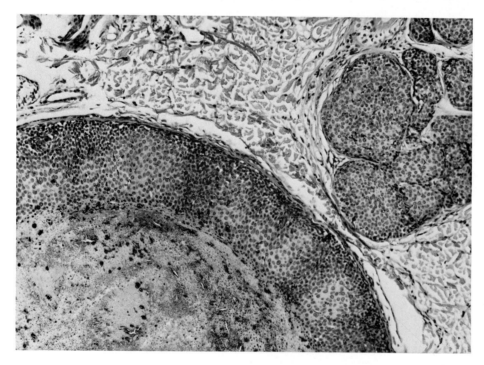

FIGURE 21-19. Higher magnification of the solid basal cell carcinoma in Figure 21-18 showing moderate melanization and central necrosis of a large epithelial aggregate. Note the clumps of melanin in the necrotic zone. (×120.)

FIGURE 21-20. Solid basal cell carcinoma in a cat. The small epithelial cells have scant, pale cytoplasm and round-to-ovoid nuclei. Note the patchy peripheral palisading and small central focus of necrosis. (×240.)

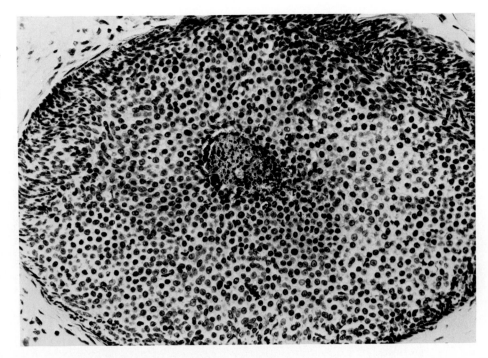

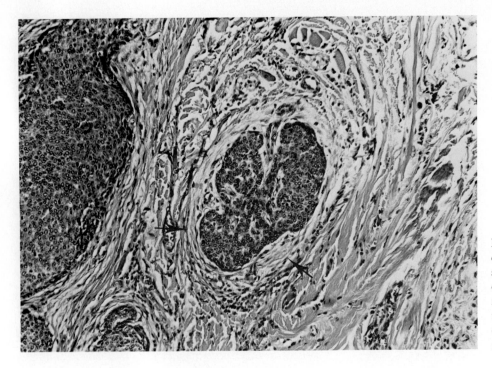

FIGURE 21-21. Solid basal cell carcinoma in a dog. A small, irregular aggregate of epithelial cells invades the dermis at the tumor margin. Note the cuff of collagenous stroma extending beyond the epithelial margins *(arrows)*. (×120.)

Poor peripheral palisading and a predominance of spikey epithelial aggregates were reported by Dixon to be predictive of increased recurrence in humans. Caseation necrosis is often present in the centers of the epithelial islands. There is focal or multifocal contiguity with epidermis, which is generally eroded or ulcerated.

The epithelial aggregates are embedded in a mod-erate stroma of fibrous tissue that has moderate cellularity. The stroma generally extends beyond the boundaries of the epithelial component of the neoplasm and is not well demarcated from the adjacent dermis. The stroma frequently contains infiltrates of lymphocytes and plasma cells. Small solid basal cell carcinomas, particularly those which occur in conjunction with actinic

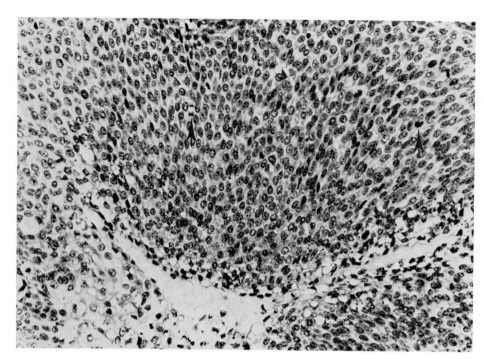

FIGURE 21-22. Higher magnification of solid basal cell carcinoma showing small epithelial cells with scant, pale cytoplasm and ovoid nuclei. Note the scattered atypical mitotic figures *(arrows).* (×240.)

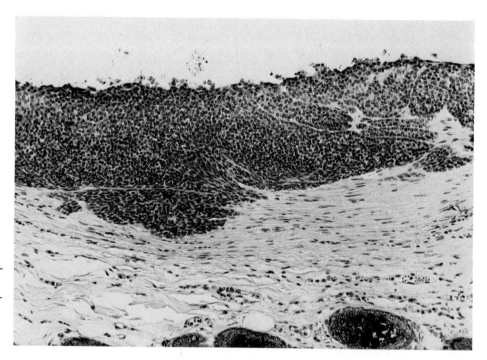

FIGURE 21-23. Solid basal cell carcinoma in a cat. Extensive necrosis has left a large central cystic cavity *(top).* Note the invasive tumor margins and collagenous stroma extending beyond the epithelial aggregates. (×120.)

keratosis, may be single plaque-like aggregates of epithelial cells that are limited to the superficial dermis. Stromal features are similar to the multilobular lesions.

The epithelial cells of basal cell carcinoma produce small amounts of mucin, and occasional neoplasms show small pools of mucin that accumulate between cords of epithelial cells. Mucin production may result in artifactual cleft formation between the stroma and the epithelial structures (a classic feature of human

basal cell carcinoma). However, this does not appear to be a consistent phenomenon in dogs or cats.

The basaloid epithelial cells of all subtypes of basal cell carcinoma are small and polyhedral and lack obvious intercellular bridges. The epithelial cells have scant, pale cytoplasm and large, ovoid nuclei. The nuclei are usually uniform; nuclear pleomorphism is another feature that is reported by Dixon to indicate more aggressive behavior. Nucleoli are usually small, and mitotic activity varies from low to moderately high. Atypical mitotic figures are commonly detected.

Secondary features occurring in basal cell carcinoma include cystification, melanization, and adnexal differentiation. These features may occur individually or in combination. Cystic change is a common secondary feature of basal cell carcinoma, particularly in cats. Cystic degeneration is most likely secondary to necrosis and liquefaction or resorption of degenerate epithelial cells. The residual epithelium of some cystic basal cell carcinomas may be limited to a narrow band surrounding a single, large cyst cavity.

Melanization of the epithelial cells is another common secondary feature of solid basal cell carcinomas. The stroma of pigmented basal cell carcinomas contains variable numbers of melanophages. If necrosis or cystification is present in a pigmented basal cell carcinoma, clumps of melanin are frequently present in the degenerate areas.

Solid basal cell carcinomas may also have small foci of squamous, sweat gland, or sebaceous gland differentiation. Squamous differentiation is characterized by zones of slightly larger, polygonal cells with eosinophilic cytoplasm; complete keratinization is not observed. Apocrine differentiation is manifested by short, tubular, or cleft-like structures that are lined by one or two layers of small, cuboidal epithelial cells. Sebaceous differentiation is characterized by occasional, individual, lipidized cells resembling mature sebocytes.

Differential diagnoses for solid basal cell carcinoma

include benign feline basal cell tumor, sebaceous epithelioma, feline ductular apocrine adenoma, and trabecular trichoblastoma. Benign feline basal cell tumor has a smooth, symmetric silhouette. Its sparse, noninflammatory stroma does not extend beyond the limits of the epithelial component. Spindling and whorled aggregations of epithelial cells are typical of benign basal cell tumor but are uncommon in basal cell carcinoma. Sebaceous epithelioma contains slightly larger numbers of well-differentiated sebocytes than does basal cell carcinoma exhibiting sebaceous differentiation, and the lipidized cells are often arranged in clusters. Differentiation between these two tumor types is not always possible, but their biologic behavior is identical. Feline ductular apocrine adenoma has more extensive tubular differentiation than does basal cell carcinoma with sweat gland differentiation, and most of the glandular structures are lined with a double layer of cuboidal epithelial cells. Pigmentation, mitotic atypia, and an inflammatory stroma are not observed in feline ductular apocrine adenoma. Trabecular trichoblastoma has a focal or absent epidermal connection and a sparse, well-circumscribed, noninflammatory stroma. The epithelial aggregates have a distinct anastomosing trabecular pattern, and mitotic atypia is not observed.

Keratinizing basal cell carcinoma (basosquamous carcinoma) (Figures 21-24 and 21-25). This is the most common type of basal cell carcinoma in dogs. Keratinizing basal cell carcinoma is an irregular dermal mass comprising epithelial cell aggregates that vary

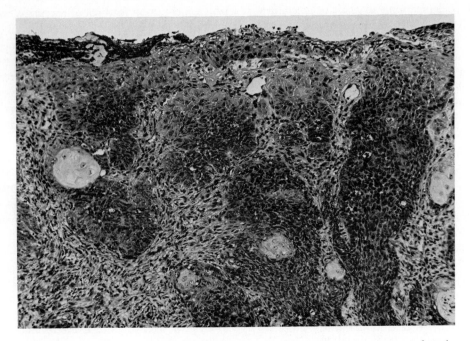

FIGURE 21-24. Keratinizing basal cell carcinoma in a dog. Irregular aggregates of predominantly basaloid epithelial cells have multiple nests of larger, keratinized squamous cells. Note the multifocal epidermal contiguity and highly cellular collagenous stroma. (×120.)

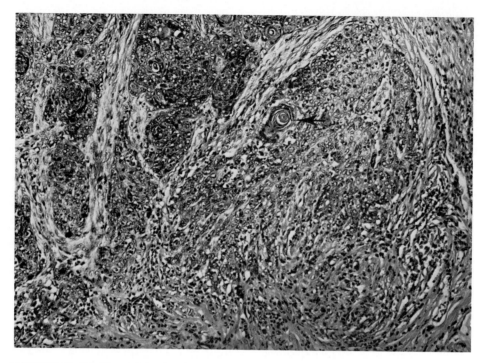

FIGURE 21-25. Keratinizing basal cell carcinoma in a dog. Irregular aggregates of basaloid epithelial cells show multifocal squamous differentiation with formation of keratin pearls *(arrow)*. Note the cellular collagenous stroma. (×120.)

considerably in size and shape. A plaque-like configuration is common. Angular islands and trabeculae predominate in most tumors. The epithelial structures have multifocal contiguity with the epidermis, which is usually ulcerated. Melanization and cystic degeneration are uncommon. There is a moderate-to-abundant collagenous stroma that is poorly demarcated from the surrounding dermis. Stromal infiltrates of lymphocytes and plasma cells are common.

The epithelial aggregates are composed predominantly of small basaloid epithelial cells identical to those of solid basal cell carcinoma. The centers of many of the epithelial islands exhibit abrupt squamous differentiation and keratinization. The keratinizing zones exhibit epidermal/infundibular, isthmus, or, rarely, matrical features. Epidermal/infundibular keratinization occurs through a granular cell layer and produces lamellar keratin. Isthmus-type (tricholemmal) keratinization produces compact keratin, and no keratohyalin granules are present in the squamous cells. Matrical keratinization results in the direct formation of keratinized "shadow" cells, without an intervening zone of viable squamous epithelium. Necrosis is a common secondary feature.

Keratinizing basal cell carcinoma must be differentiated from trichoepithelioma and matrical carcinoma. Keratinizing basal cell carcinomas usually have a plaque-like configuration and irregular margins, whereas trichoepitheliomas are nodular and circumscribed. Multifocal contiguity with the epidermis is not seen in trichoepithelioma. Multiple cystic structures and melanization are common features of trichoepithelioma but are not typical of keratinizing basal cell carcinoma. Necrosis is uncommon in trichoepithelioma and common in basal cell carcinoma. Differentiation between matrical carcinoma and keratinizing basal cell carcinoma is difficult. The absence of connections to the epidermis supports a diagnosis of matrical carcinoma. Keratinizing basal carcinoma can have small foci of matrical differentiation with formation of shadow cells, but large zones of matrical keratinization are typical of matrical carcinoma. Both basal cell carcinoma and matrical carcinoma often show tricholemmal and infundibular differentiation, but inner root sheath keratinization via trichohyalin granules is observed almost exclusively in matrical carcinoma. The authors have observed limited inner root sheath differentiation in occasional basal cell carcinomas, trichoepitheliomas, and hybrid follicular cysts.

Clear-cell basal cell carcinoma (Figure 21-26). This rare variant of basal cell carcinoma occurs more frequently in cats. The overall architecture is identical to that of solid basal cell carcinoma. The stroma of clear-cell basal cell carcinoma is often sparser than in the solid or keratinizing variants. Palisading at the pe-

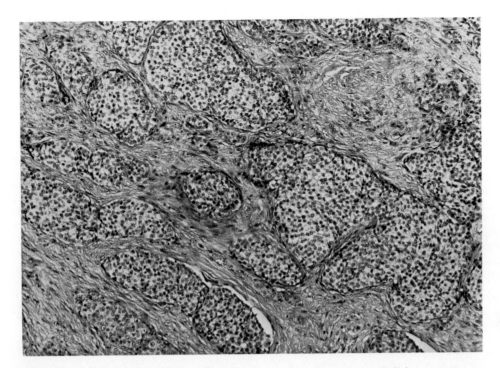

FIGURE 21-26. Clear-cell basal cell carcinoma in a cat. Irregular epithelial aggregates are composed of larger polygonal cells with clear cytoplasm. Note the clefts between the epithelium and stroma at the bottom. (×120.)

riphery of the epithelial aggregates is inconsistently present. Necrosis is a common secondary feature. The epithelial cells of clear-cell basal cell carcinoma are large and polygonal and have water-clear or finely granular cytoplasm. The distinctive cytoplasmic features of clear-cell basal cell carcinoma are a result of degenerative alterations manifested by accumulation of numerous phagolysosomes within the cells. The nuclei are large, ovoid, and fairly uniform. The nucleoli are small, and mitotic activity varies from low to moderate. Atypical mitoses can usually be detected.

Differential diagnoses include sebaceous carcinoma and bulb-type tricholemmoma. Differentiation between clear-cell basal cell carcinoma and sebaceous carcinoma can be difficult. Most sebaceous carcinomas contain cells with multiple round vacuoles or the foamy cytoplasm indicative of lipid content. The nuclei of sebaceous carcinomas usually have more prominent nucleoli and higher mitotic activity than those of basal cell carcinoma. Sebaceous carcinoma does not have multifocal epidermal contiguity. Bulb-type tricholemmoma comprises predominantly clear epithelial cells, but clear-cell basal cell carcinoma generally has larger cells and larger cell aggregates than does tricholemmoma. Bulb-type tricholemmoma does not connect to the epidermis.

SUGGESTED READINGS

Actinic keratosis

Hargis AM, Thomasson RW, and Phemister RD: Chronic dermatosis and cutaneous squamous cell carcinoma in the Beagle dog, Vet Pathol 14:218-228, 1977.

Scott DW: Feline dermatology, 1979-1982: introspective retrospections, J Am Anim Hosp Assoc 20:537-564, 1984.

Pigmented epidermal nevus

Briggs OM: Lentiginosis profusa in the pug: three case reports, J Small Anim Pract 26:675-680, 1985.

Muller GH, Kirk RW, and Scott DW: Small animal dermatology, ed 4, Philadelphia, 1989, Harcourt, Brace, Jovanovich, pp 706-708, 939.

Cutaneous horn of feline footpad

Scott DW: Feline dermatology, 1979-1982: introspective retrospections, J Am Anim Hosp Assoc 20:537-564, 1984.

Viral and idiopathic squamous papilloma

Bevier DF and Goldschmidt MH: Skin tumors in the dog. I. Epithelial tumors and tumor-like lesions, Comp Cont Ed 3:389-398, 1981.

Campbell KL and others: Cutaneous inverted papillomas in dogs, Vet Pathol 25:67-71, 1988.

Carney HC and others: Papillomavirus infection in aged Persian cats, J Vet Diagn Invest 2:294-299, 1990.

Squamous cell carcinoma

Bevier DF and Goldschmidt MH: Skin tumors in the dog. I. Epithelial tumors and tumor-like lesions, Comp Cont Ed 3:389-398, 1981.

Hargis AM, Thomasson RW, and Phemister RD: Chronic dermatosis and cutaneous squamous cell carcinoma in the Beagle dog, Vet Pathol 14:218-228, 1977.

Nappi O, Pettinato G, and Wick MR: Adenoic (acantholytic) squamous cell carcinoma of the skin, J Cutan Pathol 16:114-121, 1989.

Multicentric squamous cell carcinoma in situ

Gross TL and Brimacomb BH: Multifocal intraepidermal carcinoma in a dog histologically resembling Bowen's disease, Am J Dermatopathol 8:509-515, 1986.

Benign feline basal cell tumor

Bevier DF and Goldschmidt MH: Skin tumors in the dog. I. Epithelial tumors and tumor-like lesions, Comp Cont Ed 3:389-398, 1981.

Diters RW and Walsh KM: Feline basal cell tumors: a review of 124 cases, Vet Pathol 21:51-56, 1984.

Fehrer SL and Lin SH: Multicentric basal cell tumors in a cat, J Am Vet Med Assoc 189:1469-1470, 1986.

Basal cell carcinoma

Ackerman AB, Niven J, and Grant-Kels JM: Differential diagnosis in dermatopathology, Philadelphia, 1983, Lea & Febiger, pp 130-133.

Carpenter JL, Andrew LK, and Holzworth J: Tumors and tumor-like lesions. In Holzworth J, editor: Diseases of the cat, Philadelphia, 1987, WB Saunders, pp 407-410.

Conroy JD: Canine skin tumors, J Am Anim Hosp Assoc 19:91-114, 1983.

Diters RW and Walsh KM: Feline basal cell tumors: a review of 124 cases, Vet Pathol 21:51-56, 1984.

Dixon AY, Lee SH, and McGregor DH: Factors predictive of recurrence of basal cell carcinoma, Am J Dermatopathol 11:222-232, 1989.

Fehrer SL and Lin SH: Multicentric basal cell tumors in a cat, J Am Vet Med Assoc 189:1469-1470, 1986.

Lever WF and Schaumburg-Lever G: Histopathology of the skin, ed 7, Philadelphia, 1990, JB Lippincott, pp 633-634.

Mehregan AH: Pinkus' guide to dermatohistopathology, ed 4, Norwalk, Conn, 1986, Appleton-Century-Crofts, pp 509-521.

Oliver GF and Winkelmann RK: Clear-cell, basal cell carcinoma: histopathological, histochemical, and electron microscopic findings, J Cutan Pathol 15:404-408, 1988.

Strafuss AC: Basal cell tumors in dogs, J Am Vet Med Assoc 169:322-324, 1976.

See also General References, pp 327-328.

Follicular tumors

FOLLICULAR CYST (Synonyms: epidermoid cyst, epidermal inclusion cyst)
Clinical features

A cyst may be defined as a nonneoplastic, simple sac-like structure with an epithelial lining. Classification of cysts depends on identification of the lining epithelium or the preexisting structure from which the cyst arose. The majority of cysts in the skin of dogs and cats are of follicular origin and can be further categorized by the level of the follicle from which they develop. Infundibular and isthmus-catagen cysts are common in dogs and relatively common in cats. Exclusively matrical cysts are uncommon in dogs and rare in cats. Hybrid cysts, those which combine two or three types of follicular epithelium, are relatively common in dogs and uncommon in cats.

Follicular cysts usually appear as solitary, firm, intradermal, or, occasionally, subcutaneous nodules less than 2 cm in diameter. Larger lesions occur occasionally. The overlying epidermis is intact unless cyst rupture has occurred. Partial alopecia may be present. The cyst contents have a semisolid, caseous, or doughy consistency; the color may be yellow white, light brown, or gray.

There is no age, breed, or site predisposition for solitary cysts. Follicular cysts can sometimes be multiple and recurrent, suggesting a developmental basis for their formation. Congenital and familial cases of multiple follicular cysts, such as eruptive vellus cysts, occur in humans. Multiple follicular cysts of presumed congenital etiology occur on the dorsal midline of the head in young dogs. Multiple follicular cysts also develop on pressure points in dogs, especially the elbow; these are probably secondary to chronic trauma, dermal fibrosis, and obstruction of follicular ostia (see callus pyoderma, Chapter 15).

Histopathology

Hair follicles are divided longitudinally into three levels. The upper portion, or infundibulum, of the follicle extends from the entrance of the sebaceous duct to the follicular ostium. This segment of the follicle is composed predominantly of outer root sheath epithelium that is continuous with and histopathologically indistinguishable from the epidermis. The middle portion, or isthmus, of the hair follicle extends from the insertion of the arrector pili muscle to the level of the sebaceous duct. The outer root sheath epithelium of the follicular isthmus is made up of smaller keratinocytes, which keratinize without a granular cell layer. This tricholemmal pattern of keratinization produces amorphous keratin, in contrast to the lamellar keratin arising from epithelia that possess a granular cell layer. The keratinocytes of the isthmus have homogeneous, pale-pink cytoplasm. The lower, or inferior, segment of the follicle extends from the follicular papilla to the insertion of the arrector pili muscle. The inferior segment of the follicle during the anagen phase contains the hair bulb, inner root sheath, and outer root sheath. The hair bulb comprises the basaloid matrix cells that give rise to most of the other epithelial components of the follicle. Keratinization of matrix cells leaves the cytoplasmic and nuclear membranes intact, producing sheets of "ghost" or "shadow" cells. The keratinocytes of the inferior outer root sheath have clear cytoplasm during the anagen phase of follicular growth. The isthmus outer root sheath replaces the atrophic inferior segment during the catagen phase and continues to exhibit tricholemmal keratinization. The inner root sheath is composed of small cells with clear cytoplasm, which keratinize through distinctive, bright-red, trichohyalin granules. Inner root sheath epithelium produces large plates of keratin that have a hyaline appearance in tissue sections.

Infundibular cyst (Figures 22-1 and 22-2). Because of the histopathologic similarity between infundibular and epidermal keratinization patterns, these cysts are generally classified as epidermal inclusion cysts in the veterinary literature. This nomenclature suggests that the cysts are formed as a result of traumatic embedding of epidermal fragments or a congenital anomaly of epidermal development, both of which are probably rare phenomena.

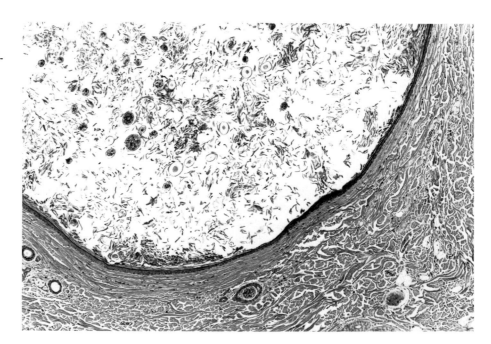

FIGURE 22-1. Infundibular cyst in a dog. The cyst is lined by a thin layer of squamous epithelium. The cyst cavity contains flaky keratin and numerous hair fragments. (×55.)

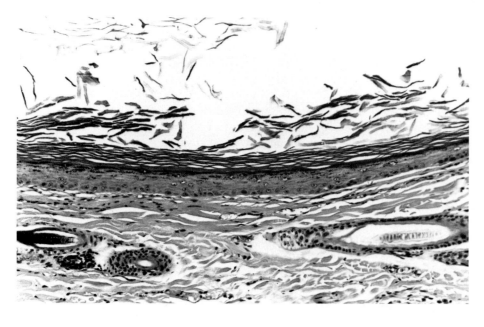

FIGURE 22-2. Infundibular cyst in a cat. The cyst wall has a prominent granular cell layer, and the cyst cavity contains lamellar, flaky keratin. (×120.)

Cysts arising from the infundibulum of the hair follicle are lined by squamous epithelium with an obvious granular cell layer, as in the upper portion of the normal follicle. The keratin contents are lamellar and are often concentrically arranged. The keratin is delicate and may be organized as loose flakes within the cyst lumen. Hair fragments are only rarely present.

Rupture of this or any other type of keratinous cyst results in a marked foreign body–type inflammatory reaction in the dermis. Free keratin fragments are surrounded by macrophages, neutrophils, plasma cells, and multinucleated giant cells. Cholesterol cleft formation is frequently observed. Fibroplasia occurs with eventual encapsulation of the residual cyst wall and keratinous debris.

Isthmus-catagen cyst (tricholemmal cyst) (Figure 22-3). The lining epithelium and keratinization pattern of this type of cyst closely resemble the middle segment of anagen follicles and the lower portion of catagen phase follicles, hence the term *isthmus-catagen cyst*. Cysts arising from the follicular isthmus are lined by epithelium that has a sparse or absent granular cell layer. The keratinocytes have pale-pink, slightly glassy cytoplasm. Tricholemmal keratinization predominates, and the cyst contents are paler and more homogeneous than in infundibular cysts. Occasional hair fragments may be present.

Proliferating isthmus-catagen cyst (Figure 22-4). This cyst is an uncommon variant of the isthmus-catagen cyst in which the epithelium of the

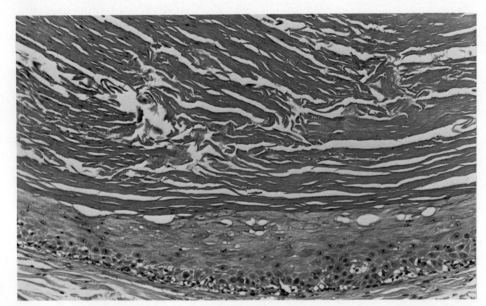

FIGURE 22-3. Isthmus-catagen cyst in a dog. The epithelium lining the cyst does not have a granular cell layer. Note that the keratin contents are paler and more amorphous than in the infundibular cyst in Figure 22-2. (×120.)

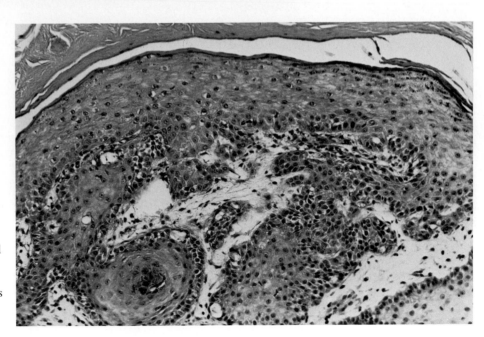

FIGURE 22-4. Proliferating isthmus-catagen cyst in a dog. Short trabeculae and occasional small horn cysts project outward from the cyst wall. Note the sparse keratohyalin granules and amorphous keratin contents. (×120.)

cyst wall develops short trabecular projections into the surrounding dermis. Small secondary cysts filled with subtly laminated keratin eventually form. As proliferation continues and cystic structures increase in number, the lesion begins to resemble infundibular keratinizing acanthoma (see later discussion). Weiss also proposed that follicular "cyst with epithelial proliferation" is an early stage of infundibular keratinizing acanthoma.

Matrical cyst (Figure 22-5). This type of cyst appears to be derived from the matrical or inferior segment of the anagen hair follicle. Matrical cysts are lined by deeply basophilic, basaloid epithelial cells that abruptly keratinize, forming ghost or shadow cells. Keratinized ghost cells are pale and refractile and have

delicate eosinophilic demarcation of cell membranes and nuclear envelopes. The matrical follicular cyst also may be regarded as a unilocular variant of pilomatricoma (see later discussion). Some lesions resembling matrical cysts have several smaller cystic structures adjacent to the primary cyst; these secondary cysts are lined predominantly by basaloid epithelial cells but may also contain isthmus- or infundibular-type epithelium. Tumors of this type may be designated as proliferating matrical cysts and may represent precursors to pilomatricoma or trichoepithelioma (see later discussion).

Hybrid cyst (Figure 22-6). As further evidence for the follicular origin of most cutaneous cysts, two or

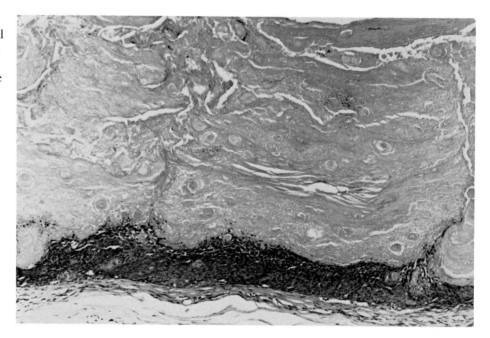

FIGURE 22-5. Matrical follicular cyst in a dog. The cyst wall is composed primarily of small, dark, basaloid epithelial cells. Keratinized shadow cells fill the cyst cavity. (×120.)

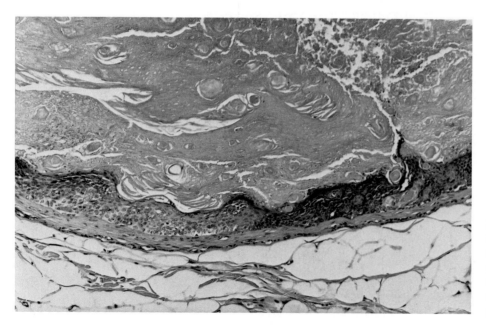

FIGURE 22-6. Hybrid cyst in a dog. The cyst wall is lined by a mixture of basaloid and squamous epithelial zones. The cyst cavity contains some laminated keratin in addition to shadow cells. (×120.)

all three levels of follicular epithelium may be represented in a single lesion. The terms *mixed cyst* or *hybrid cyst* may be used to describe lesions exhibiting multi-level follicular components. Dunstan has applied the term *panfollicular cyst* to lesions with infundibular, isthmus, and matrical areas.* In the transitional zones between matrical and isthmus epithelia in hybrid cysts, small foci of inner root sheath differentiation may be present. The cells in these foci have clear cytoplasm and trichohyalin granules.

DERMOID CYST (Synonym: dermoid sinus)
Clinical Features

Dermoid cysts are observed rarely in dogs and cats. These cysts are developmental anomalies manifested by focal reduplication of the entire skin structure, including epidermis and adnexa. Dermoid cysts may be single or multiple and appear clinically similar to follicular cysts. The cysts are dermal or subcutaneous in location. A small pore often connects the cyst to the skin surface, and hair may protrude through the pore. Lesions occasionally extend into the spinal canal where they are attached to dura mater. As would be predicted by embryology, dermoid cysts often occur along the dorsal midline, which is the site where ectoderm was continuous with neuroectoderm before neural tube closure.

* Dunstan RW: Personal communication, 1987.

However, they may also be found at other anatomic sites.

The propensity of the Rhodesian Ridgeback for development of dorsal midline dermoid cysts is believed to be inherited via a simple recessive gene. Because these are congenital anomalies, affected animals are usually young.

Histopathology (Figure 22-7)

The central cyst is lined by epidermal epithelium, which keratinizes through a granular cell layer. The cyst cavity is often filled with hair, in addition to lamellar keratin, and may also contain sebaceous secretions. Within the dermal collagen surrounding the cyst are well-developed small hair follicles, sebaceous glands, and, occasionally, apocrine sweat glands. The hair follicles are usually compound, and delicate hair shafts are often present. The folliculosebaceous units are sparse or moderate in number and tend to be evenly spaced within the dermal collagen.

A small dermoid cyst may resemble a trichofolliculoma with predominantly mature secondary follicles, particularly if hair shafts and sebaceous glands are present. The follicles that radiate from the central cyst of a trichofolliculoma are more numerous and also show secondary branching. The central cyst of a trichofolliculoma may contain epithelial segments resembling isthmus and/or matrical portions of a hair follicle, whereas the central cyst of a dermoid cyst is lined entirely by epidermal-type squamous epithelium.

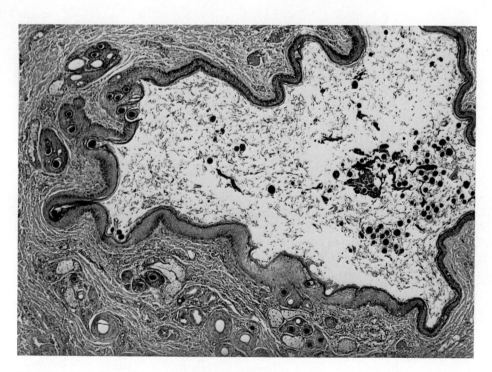

FIGURE 22-7. Dermoid cyst in a dog. Small hair follicles and sebaceous glands project outward from the cyst wall. Note the numerous hair fragments in the cyst lumen. (×50.)

DILATED PORE (Synonym: dilated pore of Winer)

Clinical features

Dilated pore is a variant of infundibular follicular cyst that occurs uncommonly in cats and resembles dilated pore of Winer in humans. It was first described by Scott in 1986. Dilated pore appears as a solitary, firm mass, less than 1 cm in diameter, with a central dome-shaped protrusion of dense keratin. The protruding keratin may occasionally appear as a cutaneous horn. Lesions are often located on the head and neck but may be found at any site. Dilated pore of Winer in humans also has a predilection for the head and neck. There is no known age prevalence.

Histopathology (Figures 22-8 and 22-9)

Dilated pore is a cup-shaped or balloon-shaped, dilated, superficial follicle lined by a hyperplastic layer of squamous epithelium. The cyst cavity is filled with compact, laminated keratin that projects above the skin surface through the central pore. The pore is a greatly distended follicular ostium. In contrast, intact follicular ostia are rarely present in routine follicular infundibular

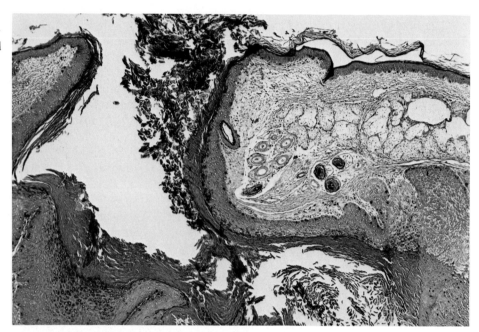

FIGURE 22-8. Dilated pore in a cat. Cystically dilated follicular infundibulum has a keratin-filled central pore that communicates with the skin surface. Note the irregular hyperplasia of the squamous epithelium lining the cyst. (×50.)

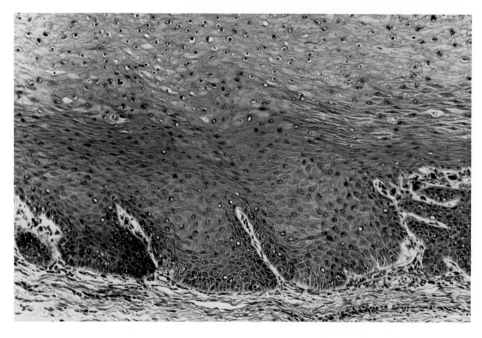

FIGURE 22-9. Dilated pore in a cat. The squamous epithelium at the base of the cyst is markedly thickened, and the peripheral margin has a scalloped configuration. (×120.)

cysts. The epithelium of the cyst wall of a dilated pore has a prominent granular cell layer consistent with an infundibular origin. The outer edge of the cyst wall has irregular hyperplasia, frequently with a scalloped configuration.

FOLLICULAR HAMARTOMA (Synonym: hair follicle nevus)

Clinical features

The concepts of *nevus* and *hamartoma* tend to be elusive and confusing in most pathology texts, but Mehregan's working definition of a nevus as a circumscribed, stable malformation of skin of presumed congenital origin creates a category that has applications in veterinary dermatopathology. In contrast to a nevus, a hamartoma also has a presumed congenital basis but tends to deviate more from the normal histologic structure and may show more expansive growth. The terms nevus and hamartoma are used almost interchangeably and are often selected more by convention than by strict adherence to definition. Although the underlying tissue abnormality in any type of nevus or hamartoma is theoretically present at birth, lesions may not become clinically apparent until later in life. Late recognition of nevi and hamartomas is particularly common in animals, and this may be sometimes explained by the fact that thick pelage makes early small or nonelevated lesions difficult to detect. In other instances, however, nevoid and hamartomatous lesions occurring in adult animals may be acquired rather than congenital.

Follicular hamartoma is an uncommon, nonneoplastic lesion in dogs that usually appears as multiple, grouped, nonalopecic, firm nodules and plaques. The affected skin has an irregularly thickened texture. Hairs arising from the hamartoma are thick and brush-like. The number of nodules gradually increases, and the lesion expands over time. Most lesions are several centimeters in size; some may be as large as 6 cm. Less commonly, the hamartoma appears as a single nodule measuring 0.5 to 1 cm in diameter. There is no known age, breed, or site predilection.

Histopathology (Figure 22-10)

Follicular hamartoma contains one or more clusters of architecturally normal anagen hair follicles that are larger and extend more deeply than adjacent normal follicles. All follicles within a cluster are uniform and have the appearance of primary follicles. Follicular bulbs are often located in the hypodermal fat. Hair shafts are proportionately enlarged. Follicular infundibular hyperkeratosis, as would be expected in reactive hyperplasia of hair follicles, is not observed. The sebaceous glands within the lesions are slightly enlarged, are increased in number, and frequently extend

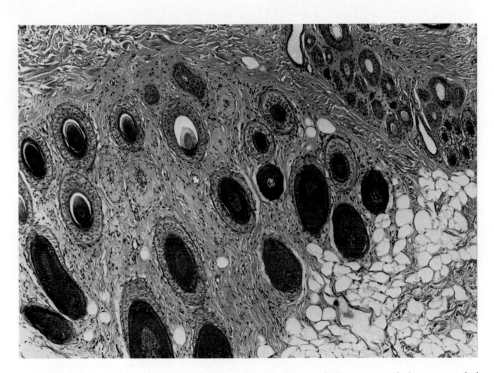

FIGURE 22-10. Follicular hamartoma in a dog. A cluster of giant anagen hairs surrounded by increased collagen encroaches on the panniculus. Note the normal-sized hair follicles at right. (×50.)

proximally and distally beyond their normal location at the follicular isthmus. The follicles are embedded in hyalinized collagen, and a zone of mucin is located peripheral to the vitreous sheaths. The overlying epidermis is mildly hyperplastic and elevated. The zones of dense collagenous stroma and hyperplastic epidermis create the irregular, nodular skin texture observed clinically.

FOCAL ADNEXAL DYSPLASIA
Clinical features

Focal adnexal dysplasia, as coined by Hill,* is a common nonneoplastic lesion of adnexal appendages that occurs in dogs. It has not been previously described as a specific clinicopathologic entity in animals. The etiology of focal adnexal dysplasia is controversial. Scar tissue formation after the resolution of an inflammatory process could result in entrapment and subsequent distortion of folliculosebaceous units. Many of these lesions do have a prominent inflammatory component, and their typical location over pressure points supports this pathogenesis. However, smaller masses frequently have no evidence of inflammation but show marked distortion of adnexal structures. Thus the pos-

sibility also must be considered that some or all of these lesions are hamartomas involving dermal collagen and folliculosebaceous units. In humans similar lesions are diagnosed as folliculosebaceous hamartoma.*

The lesions of focal adnexal dysplasia are solitary, firm, circumscribed, dome-shaped to polypoid masses that range from approximately 1 cm to greater than 4 cm in diameter. Smaller lesions have partial alopecia. Larger lesions frequently exhibit alopecia and ulceration. Adnexal dysplasia occurs most commonly on the distal limbs; pressure points and interdigital areas are frequently affected. Lesions may also occur on other parts of the body. Animals are generally middle aged or older, and there is no known breed predilection.

Histopathology (Figure 22-11)

Focal adnexal dysplasia is a circumscribed nodule composed of loosely distributed folliculosebaceous units, abundant collagen, and occasionally apocrine sweat glands. Smaller lesions are confined to the dermis; larger masses extend into the subcutis. Superficial ulceration may be present. Intact epidermis is acanthotic. The hair follicles are thickened, dilated, and tortuous. Orientation of the follicles is severely askew; they often appear to run tangential or parallel to the

* Hill JR: Personal communication, 1982.

*Ackerman AB: Personal communication, 1988.

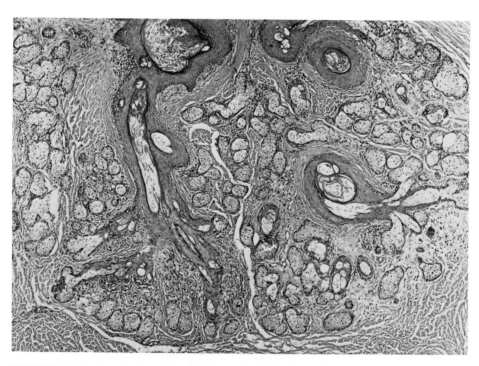

FIGURE 22-11. Focal adnexal dysplasia in a dog. A group of markedly distorted, hyperplastic folliculosebaceous units is surrounded by dense collagen. Note the numerous sebaceous lobules distributed haphazardly around the dilated follicles. (×50.)

skin surface. Follicles are often cystic and contain abundant keratin and occasional hair shafts. Multiple large sebaceous gland lobules are distributed haphazardly around hair follicles, often without obvious ductal connections. When apocrine glands are present, they are dilated and abnormally distributed. The adnexa are surrounded and interspersed with abundant, hyalinized collagen. The stroma is sharply demarcated from the adjacent dermis or subcutis in uninflamed lesions but blends into the reactive fibrous tissue around inflamed nodules. Larger lesions frequently have rupture of cystic hair follicles, resulting in severe suppurative or pyogranulomatous inflammation. Patchy, chronic inflammatory infiltrates of plasma cells and macrophages may also be present around the periphery of these lesions.

TRICHOFOLLICULOMA
Clinical features

Trichofolliculoma is a rare, benign hair follicle tumor of dogs and cats. The analogous tumor in humans is considered by Mehregan to be a type of follicular hamartoma rather than a true neoplasm. Trichofolliculoma appears as a solitary, dome-shaped nodule less than 2 cm in diameter. The overlying epidermis is intact, but there may be a central pore or depression. In human trichofolliculomas, tufts of fluffy hair frequently emerge through the central pore; this does not appear to be a feature of the tumor in dogs or cats. There is no known age, breed, or site predisposition.

Histopathology (Figure 22-12)

Trichofolliculoma is a well-circumscribed, but unencapsulated dermal nodule composed of one or more primary follicular structures that are cystically dilated and keratinize through a granular cell layer. Hair shafts may also be present. The primary follicles may possess infundibular segments that open onto the skin surface, creating the pores observed clinically. Multiple secondary follicular structures radiate outward from the primary follicles in an arborizing pattern. The secondary follicles exhibit various stages of maturation from predominantly basaloid hair germ to small but fully developed follicles containing delicate hair shafts. Sebaceous glands also may be connected to the primary follicles. The glands may be rudimentary or fully developed and probably parallel the degree of differentiation of the secondary follicles. There is a well-demarcated collagenous stroma of low cellularity separating the mass from adjacent dermis.

A trichofolliculoma with predominantly mature secondary follicles may resemble a dermoid cyst, particularly if hair shafts and sebaceous glands are present. The follicles that radiate from the central cyst of a

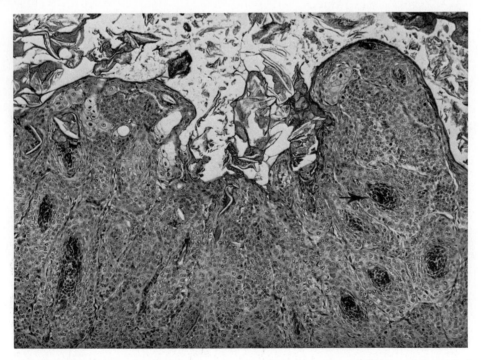

FIGURE 22-12. Trichofolliculoma in a cat. Numerous immature follicles and occasional sebaceous lobules radiate outward from a keratin-filled cyst. Note that several of the hair follicles contain follicular papillae *(arrow).* (×130.)

trichofolliculoma are more numerous and also show secondary branching. The central cyst of a trichofolliculoma may contain epithelial segments resembling isthmus or matrical portions of a hair follicle, whereas the central cyst of a dermoid cyst is lined entirely by epidermal-type squamous epithelium. Differentiation from other follicular neoplasms is not difficult, since the arborizing pattern of the secondary follicular structures is unique to trichofolliculoma.

TRICHOEPITHELIOMA
Clinical features

Trichoepithelioma is an uncommon, benign neoplasm of dogs and cats that differentiates toward all three segments of the hair follicle. The incidence estimates range from 1% to 3% of canine skin tumors and 1.5% to 4% of feline skin tumors, as cited by Bevier and Theilen, respectively.

Trichoepitheliomas are solitary, round to ovoid dermal masses that are usually less than 2 cm in size. Masses up to 8 cm may occur occasionally. There is partial or complete alopecia, and ulceration is common in larger lesions. These tumors have a predilection for the dorsal trunk but may affect other parts of the body. Most affected animals are 5 years of age or older. There is no known breed predisposition.

Histopathology (Figures 22-13 and 22-14)

Trichoepithelioma is a well-circumscribed, but unencapsulated dermal nodule comprising a random admixture of budding epithelial islands and cystic structures of variable size. Neoplastic epithelium may be focally contiguous with the overlying epidermis. The epithelial aggregates are encompassed in a moderate, well-demarcated fibrous or myxoid stroma of low cellularity. The epithelial islands are composed of basaloid epithelial cells that have prominent peripheral palisading and resemble primitive follicular bulbs. The basaloid cells have scant, pale cytoplasm and uniform, ovoid, euchromatic nuclei. Mitotic activity is moderately low. Some of the cystic structures are lined entirely by similar basaloid epithelial cells and exhibit matrical keratinization with formation of shadow cells. The basaloid and shadow cells may be melanized. Other cysts may be lined by squamous epithelium with or without a granular cell layer, resembling infundibular and/or isthmus segments of the hair follicle. The proportion of basaloid and squamous epithelium is highly variable; infundibular- and isthmus-type cysts may be absent or predominant. Cysts with combined epithelial features can be found in most lesions; these resemble hybrid or panfollicular cysts (see earlier discussion).

Trichoepithelioma with prominent squamous dif-

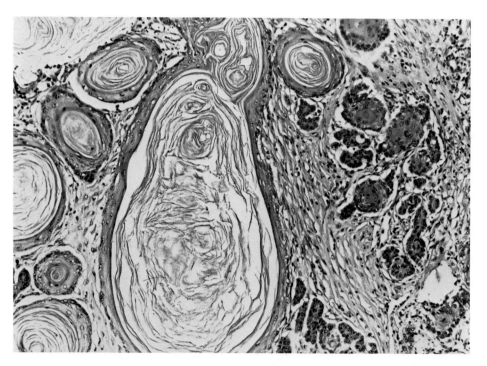

FIGURE 22-13. Trichoepithelioma in a dog. Cystic structures of varying size are lined by squamous epithelium and are filled with laminated keratin. Note the short cords of basaloid epithelial cells at right. (×120.)

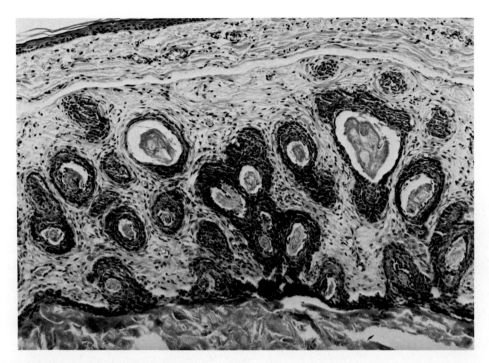

FIGURE 22-14. Trichoepithelioma in a dog. Cystic structures of varying size are lined primarily by basaloid epithelial cells. Cyst lumens contain amorphous keratin and keratinized ghost cells. (×120.)

ferentiation is distinctive; however, differential diagnoses for predominantly basaloid trichoepitheliomas include pilomatricoma and keratinizing basal cell carcinoma. The cystic structures of pilomatricoma are generally large and fewer in overall number than in trichoepithelioma. Calcification and granulomatous inflammation are common in pilomatricoma and rare in trichoepithelioma. In addition, the majority of predominantly basaloid trichoepitheliomas will contain occasional small cysts lined by isthmus- or infundibular-type epithelium, a feature that is absent in pilomatricoma. Keratinizing basal cell carcinomas usually have a plaque-like configuration with diffuse ulceration, and the epithelial aggregates show multifocal contiguity with the epidermis. Discrete cystic structures are not present, and the keratinized foci rarely contain shadow cells. Necrosis is uncommon in trichoepithelioma and common in basal cell carcinoma.

INFUNDIBULAR KERATINIZING ACANTHOMA (Synonyms: intracutaneous cornifying epithelioma, keratoacanthoma)

Clinical features

The authors have coined the term *infundibular keratinizing acanthoma* to describe an uncommon, benign follicular neoplasm of dogs. Infundibular kerati-

nizing acanthomas accounted for 2% to 3% of all canine skin tumors in a large survey by Stannard.

Although the term *intracutaneous cornifying epithelioma* proposed by Weiss in 1974 provides an accurate distillation of the histopathologic features, it gives no indication of the origin of the tumor. In addition, the authors believe that the designation *epithelioma* should be reserved for neoplasms of very low-grade malignancy composed of basaloid cells, such as sebaceous epithelioma (see Chapter 23). The name *keratoacanthoma* is also confusing, because the lesion is significantly different, both biologically and histopathologically, from keratoacanthoma in humans. A follicular origin for the canine neoplasm was first proposed by Seiler in 1981.

Infundibular keratinizing acanthomas appear as solitary or multiple, partially alopecic nodules ranging from 0.5 to 4.0 cm in diameter. The nodules usually have a central pore that is 1 mm to several centimeters in diameter. Larger pores may contain cutaneous horns or club-shaped, protruding masses of keratin and some embedded hairs. Some tumors are more deeply located within the dermis and do not open onto the skin surface. Infundibular keratinizing acanthomas are located primarily on the dorsal neck and trunk.

The average age of affected animals in Stannard's report was 5 years, and the median age was less than 5.

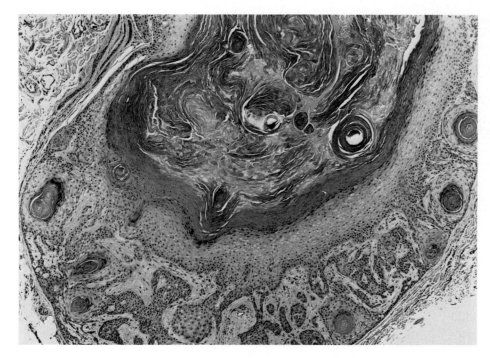

FIGURE 22-15. Early infundibular keratinizing acanthoma in a dog. Small horn cysts and short cords and trabeculae of epithelial cells project outward from a central keratin-filled cyst. Note the well-demarcated tumor margins. (×50.)

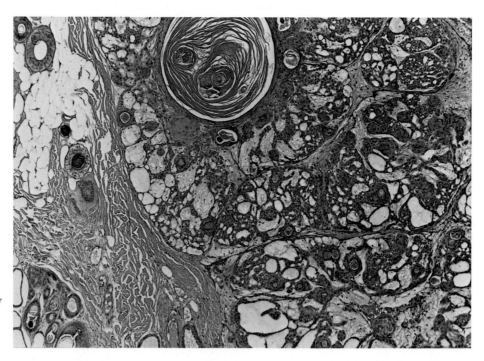

FIGURE 22-16. Mature infundibular keratinizing acanthoma in a dog. Numerous small horn cysts are interconnected by a reticular network of cords of epithelial cells. Note the pale, mucinous stroma. (×50.)

There was a slight male predominance. The Norwegian Elkhound breed has a predisposition to develop infundibular keratinizing acanthomas, and lesions are often multiple in this breed. Purebred dogs in general have a higher incidence of this neoplasm than do mixed breeds.

Histopathology (Figures 22-15 through 22-17)

Infundibular keratinizing acanthoma is a very well-circumscribed dermal nodule which is oriented around a central cyst filled with laminated keratin. The upper portion of the cyst wall is usually open, forming a **C**-shaped or cup-shaped structure that is connected

FIGURE 22-17. Higher magnification of the infundibular keratinizing acanthoma in Figure 22-16 showing a sparse granular cell layer in the horn cysts. The anastomosing cords of small keratinocytes are generally 1 to 2 cells wide. (×120.)

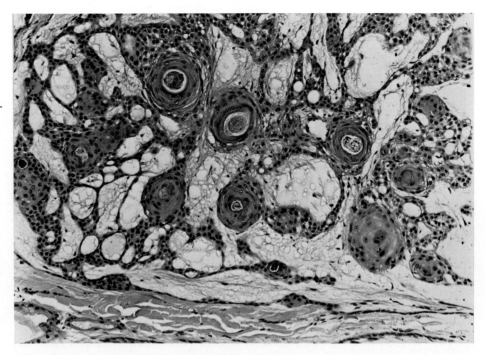

with the epidermis, creating the central pore observed clinically. Serial sectioning may be required to demonstrate the pore in tissue sections. The earliest lesions show broad trabecular projections of epithelium extending outward from the cyst wall. Later lesions develop small keratinous cysts within the trabeculae; the cysts become interconnected by delicate cords of epithelial cells. Mature infundibular keratinizing acanthomas have a complex epithelial wall composed of multiple small horn cysts interconnected by a reticular network of cords and trabeculae. The central cyst and secondary cysts are lined by pale pink, glassy squamous epithelium that keratinizes through a sparse granular cell layer. This morphology is identical to the lower portion of the normal follicular infundibulum where it joins the isthmus. Nuclei are vesicular and uniform with inconspicuous nucleoli and minimal mitotic activity. The cords between the secondary cysts generally comprise two rows of uniform basaloid cells. Broader trabeculae contain basaloid and squamous cells.

A sparse to moderate stroma containing abundant mucin and few mesenchymal cells is present, creating a distinctive pale blue background for the epithelial structures. Adjacent dermal collagen is slightly compressed, forming a pseudocapsule. Rarely, metaplastic bone may be found. Pyogranulomatous inflammation secondary to breakdown of cyst epithelium is not uncommon.

A small percentage of infundibular keratinizing acanthomas show no connection to epidermis, even when serially sectioned, and are frequently located in the deeper dermis. The architecture and morphology of these lesions are virtually identical to the typical superficial tumors, but the central cyst closely resembles an isthmus-catagen follicular cyst. A proliferating follicular cyst (see earlier discussion) probably represents an early form of this deeper type of infundibular keratinizing acanthoma. The apparent progression from isthmus-catagen cyst to proliferating follicular cyst to keratinizing acanthoma lends further support for the follicular origin of both superficial and deep variants of this neoplasm.

There may be a rare variant of infundibular keratinizing acanthoma that has a plaque-like, rather than a cup-shaped, configuration. The single example was a fenestrated plaque with multifocal epidermal contiguity and scattered keratinous cysts. The morphology was identical to that of typical infundibular keratinizing acanthoma, but the architecture was similar to tumor of follicular infundibulum in humans.*

Infundibular keratinizing acanthomas in which a central cyst is not obvious because of tangential sectioning may need to be differentiated from trichoepitheliomas with predominantly squamous epithelium. The salient features of infundibular keratinizing acanthoma are small, fairly uniform cysts, a reticular network of epithelial cords, and a pale-blue, mucinous stroma.

* Case material from Hargis AM, Seattle, Washington, 1991.

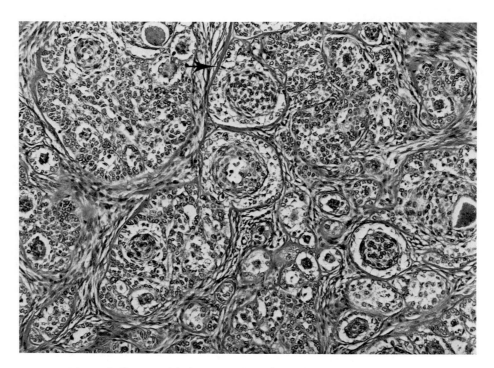

FIGURE 22-18. Bulb-type tricholemmoma in a dog. Islands and nests of small epithelial show peripheral palisading and clear cytoplasm. Note the prominent basement membranes resembling vitreous sheaths around some of the epithelial aggregates *(arrow).* (×120.)

TRICHOLEMMOMA
Clinical features

Tricholemmomas are, by definition, neoplasms of the outer root sheath of the hair follicle. Two types have been observed in dogs. The first type derives from the inferior segment of the tricholemma, or outer root sheath of the hair bulb. These are rare benign neoplasms in dogs. One group of six cases was reported by Diters, and another small series was described by Walsh. These lesions appear as firm, circumscribed nodules, ranging from 1 to 7 cm in diameter, which are mostly located on the head and neck. The overlying epidermis is intact and slightly thickened. The average age is 10 years, and there may be a breed predisposition in Afghan Hounds. This form of canine tricholemmoma (hair bulb type) is similar, but not identical, to tricholemmoma in humans.

The authors recognize a second type of tricholemmoma that resembles the outer root sheath of the isthmus segment of the follicle, particularly as it appears during the catagen phase. This type of tricholemmoma has not been previously reported as a separate entity and has probably been included in the basal cell tumor category. The tumors are rare in dogs and cats. Lesions are dome-shaped alopecic nodules that are usually less than 2 cm in diameter. Larger lesions may be ulcerated. There is no known age, breed, or site predilection.

Histopathology

Bulb type (Figure 22-18). Tricholemmomas of this type are well-circumscribed, unencapsulated dermal nodules made up of lobular groupings of small polyhedral cells. Within each lobule the epithelial cells are arranged in islands, nests, and delicate trabeculae. There is no contiguity with the overlying epidermis. The aggregations of epithelial cells are cuffed by thick, glassy, periodic acid–Schiff–positive basement membrane zones reminiscent of the vitreous sheath of normal hair follicles. There is a sparse stroma of dense collagen with minimal cellularity. The majority of cells have clear cytoplasm, and peripheral palisading is prominent. The small clear cells are analagous to the glycogen-rich, periodic acid–Schiff–positive, outer root sheath cells of the hair bulb. The cells in the centers of the islands may have more abundant, eosinophilic cytoplasm, and there may be small foci of keratinization without formation of keratohyalin or trichohyalin granules. Nuclei are small, ovoid, and euchromatic; nucleoli are inconspicuous, and mitotic activity is low.

Differential diagnoses for bulb-type tricholemmoma are limited, since cutaneous tumors composed predominantly of small clear cells are uncommon. The rare clear-cell variant of basal cell carcinoma generally has larger cells and larger cell aggregates than tricholemmoma. Multifocal connection to the epidermis is present in most basal cell carcinomas. Granular cell

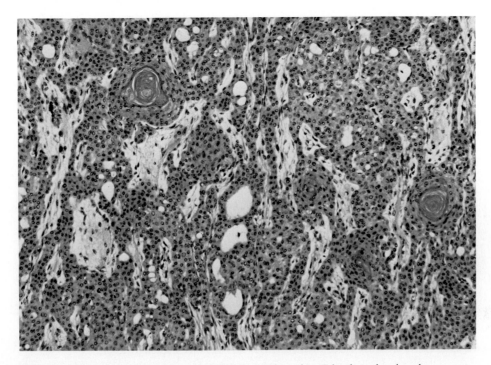

FIGURE 22-19. Isthmus-catagen tricholemmoma in a dog. Islands and trabeculae are composed of small, pale keratinocytes often containing glassy cytoplasm. Cystic structures are filled with amorphous, tricholemmal-type keratin. Note that a granular cell layer is absent. ($\times$130.)

trichoblastoma is architecturally similar to tricholemmoma, and the granular cells may appear almost clear. However, the nuclei of tricholemmoma are not peripherally displaced as they are in granular cell trichoblastoma. Both basal cell carcinoma and granular cell trichoblastoma do not show reduplication of follicular vitreous sheath.

Isthmus-catagen type (Figure 22-19). Tricholemmomas derived from the isthmus segment during the catagen phase are well-circumscribed, unencapsulated dermal nodules composed of epithelial aggregates that vary markedly in size and shape. There is usually focal continuity with the epidermis. The moderate stroma, comprising collagen and small amounts of mucin with low cellularity, is well demarcated from the adjacent dermis. Cords and trabeculae of epithelial cells radiate outward from large epithelial islands and often interconnect adjacent islands. The centers of the islands have small foci of tricholemmal-type keratinization (without formation of keratohyalin or trichohyalin granules). Larger islands may have a cystic appearance because of drop out of central keratin. Scattered dyskeratotic cells may be present. Melanization of the epithelial cells is occasionally observed.

Neoplastic cells are small and have moderate, pale-pink, often glassy cytoplasm. Nuclei are small, ovoid, and euchromatic with inconspicuous nucleoli and low mitotic activity. Peripheral palisading is not prominent.

Differential diagnoses for isthmus-catagen tricholemmoma are limited, since few tumors are composed predominantly of small, pale-pink epithelial cells. Infundibular keratinizing acanthoma has some similar features but is distinguished from isthmus-catagen tricholemmoma by the presence of a well-defined central cyst, multiple secondary cysts, and abundant stromal mucin. Trabecular trichoblastoma may have a similar overall architecture but is differentiated from isthmus-catagen tricholemmoma by the presence of prominent peripheral palisading, the absence of foci of tricholemmal keratinization, and the paucity of glassy, pale-pink, isthmus-type keratinocytes.

PILOMATRICOMA (Synonyms: pilomatrixoma, calcifying epithelioma)
Clinical features

Pilomatricoma is an uncommon, benign neoplasm of dogs that arises from the germinative cells of the follicular matrix, or hair bulb. A single case in a cat was reported in a survey by Carpenter. The reported incidence in dogs in a review by Weiss was 3%.

Lesions usually appear as solitary, firm, well-circumscribed masses. The tumors are dome shaped to plaque-like and vary in size from 2 to 10 cm. Some lesions have a gritty or bony consistency and may be chalky when sectioned. The overlying epidermis is usu-

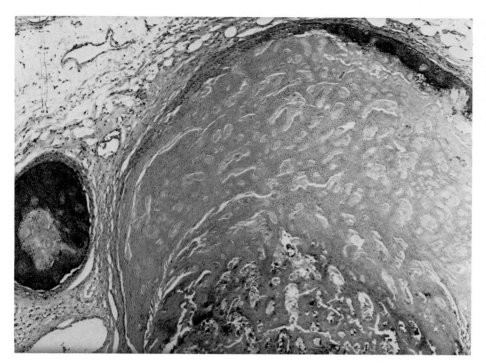

FIGURE 22-20. Pilomatricoma in a dog. Large cystic structures are lined predominantly by dark, basaloid keratinocytes and are filled with keratinized shadow cells. Note the mineralization of cyst contents at the bottom. (×50.)

ally atrophic and alopecic. Pilomatricomas occur most commonly on the dorsal trunk, particularly over the rump and shoulders.

The majority of affected animals are 5 to 10 years of age. Poodles and Kerry Blue Terriers have a predisposition for development of pilomatricoma, and tumors may be multiple in these breeds. Theilen states that Bedlington Terriers and Schnauzers are also overrepresented. These breeds have in common a continuously growing coat, which requires greater numbers of mitotically active anagen follicles. Increased hair matrix cell division may provide a larger cell pool for neoplastic transformation in these breeds.

Histopathology (Figures 22-20 and 22-21)

Pilomatricoma is a well-circumscribed dermal and subcutaneous tumor composed of multiple cystic structures of varying size that are lined predominantly by deeply basophilic, basaloid keratinocytes that resemble the matrix cells of the anagen hair bulb. Small zones of squamous epithelium, with or without a granular cell layer, may also be present. Occasional foci of inner root sheath differentiation may be detected. The tumor is not contiguous with the overlying epidermis. There is a sparse stroma of collagen and mucin, with moderate cellularity. The basaloid epithelial cells have scant cytoplasm and hyperchromatic, large, ovoid nuclei. Nucleoli are small, and mitotic activity is fairly high. Nuclear or mitotic atypia is not present. The neoplastic cells undergo matrical keratinization with formation of large masses of keratinized ghost or shadow cells that fill the cyst lumens.

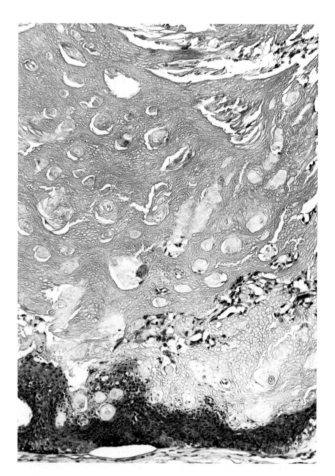

FIGURE 22-21. Higher magnification of pilomatricoma showing abrupt keratinization of the basaloid cells. Note the small number of mononuclear inflammatory cells amongst the shadow cells. (×120.)

Melanization of neoplastic matrix cells and shadow cells may be present. The shadow cells often become calcified, and osseous metaplasia may occur, particularly in later stages. Some tumors of long duration have a predominance of ghost cells and bone, and little residual epithelium can be identified. Cyst rupture and release of keratinized and mineralized material frequently evoke a granulomatous inflammatory response characterized by macrophages, multinucleated giant cells, and frequent formation of cholesterol clefts.

The multilocular architecture of pilomatricoma distinguishes it from simple matrical cyst, which is a unilocular lesion. Proliferating matrical cyst may represent an early form of pilomatricoma, and the division between these two entities is arbitrary. Differentiation of pilomatricoma from variants of trichoepithelioma in which basaloid cells predominate may be difficult. The cystic structures of pilomatricoma are larger than trichoepithelioma, and zones of nonmatrical epithelium are absent or limited. Most trichoepitheliomas have at least occasional cysts that are lined primarily by squamous epithelium. Mineralization of cyst contents in trichoepithelioma is rare. The epithelial cells of matrical carcinoma and keratinizing basal cell carcinoma are cytologically similar to those of pilomatricoma, but the carcinomas contain a much higher proportion of cellular areas in comparison with keratinized zones. In addition, the epithelial aggregates of the carcinomas are more irregular in size and shape.

TRICHOBLASTOMA (Synonym: basal cell tumor)

Clinical features

Trichoblastoma refers to a group of neoplasms derived from or reduplicating primitive hair germ. Primary hair germ is the epithelial anlage of the folliculosebaceous unit. It appears early in embryonic life as a dense ball of basaloid cells with peripheral palisading that projects downward from the epidermis. Secondary hair germ is the column of small adnexal keratinocytes at the base of telogen hair follicles, and this is presumably a direct descendant of primary hair germ. A third type of trichoblastic epithelium, referred to as *epigenic hair germ,* is derived from basal cells of either the epidermis or adnexa, which may under certain circumstances undergo some degree of follicular differentiation.

Classification schemes for neoplasms of trichoblastic epithelium in humans were proposed by Headington in 1962 and 1976. The biologic behavior and histopathologic patterns of these human hair germ tumors conform very closely to many of the common types of basal cell tumors in dogs and cats. The term *trichoblastoma* would thus seem more appropriate and more specific for this group of canine and feline neoplasms, which are presumably (based on comparison with their human counterparts) derived from trichoblastic epithelium.

Trichoblastomas are benign neoplasms that occur commonly in dogs and cats. The incidence in dogs is probably very close to the total incidence of neoplasms in the basal cell tumor category; this ranges from 3% to 12% in several surveys cited by Bevier and Theilen. The incidence in cats is harder to estimate, because cats are afflicted with several different types of neoplasms that are composed predominantly of small basaloid epithelial cells. Tumors that have been included in the feline basal cell tumor group include apocrine ductular sweat gland neoplasms, neoplasms of epidermal basal cell origin, and primitive hair follicle tumors.

In dogs, trichoblastomas appear as solitary, firm, alopecic nodules that are dome shaped or polypoid. Most tumors range from 1 to 2 cm, but much larger lesions may occur on the trunk. The larger masses may be ulcerated. There is a site predilection for the head and neck with the base of the ear being a typical location. Most affected animals are between 6 and 9 years of age. Bevier reported that Poodles, Cocker Spaniels, and mixed-breed dogs appear to have an increased frequency of trichoblastoma.

In cats trichoblastomas are usually solitary, dome-shaped, firm nodules generally less than 2 cm in size. Alopecia and secondary ulceration are common. Tumors occur most often on the cranial half of the trunk. The lesions are often pigmented and may be confused clinically with melanocytic neoplasms. There is no known age or breed predilection.

Histopathology

Ribbon type (Figures 22-22 through 22-24). The classic canine basal cell tumors have been designated as "ribbon," "garland," or "medusa-head" variants. These basal cell tumor types also are mentioned in several surveys of feline skin tumors, but in the authors' experience they are very rare in cats. Most canine tumors contain a mixture of these patterns and are virtually identical to Headington's subtype, trichogenic trichoblastoma. The human and canine ribbon-type trichoblastomas are well-demarcated dermal nodules that do not have contiguity with the epidermis (indicating that they are not of epidermal basal cell origin). They are made up predominantly of undifferentiated, basaloid epithelial cells arranged in branching, winding, and radiating columns, generally two cells in width. Islands of cells with radiating columns at their periphery create the "medusa-head" appearance. Occasional small, but well-organized hair follicles, sometimes containing delicate hair shafts, are detected; these are generally located at the periphery of the neoplasm but do not appear to represent residual follicles that have been entrapped by the mass. The epithelial struc-

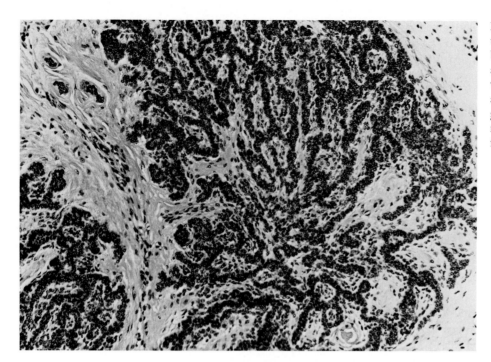

FIGURE 22-22. Ribbon-type trichoblastoma in a dog. Double rows of small, basaloid cells are arranged in branching and winding patterns. Note the abundant stroma of pale collagen containing small mesenchymal cells, resembling primitive follicular papillae. (×120.)

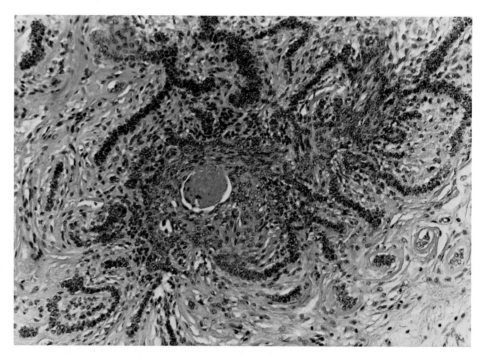

FIGURE 22-23. Ribbon-type trichoblastoma in a dog. Medusoid island is composed of slightly larger keratinocytes. Note the small central cyst exhibiting tricholemmal keratinization. (×130.)

tures are embedded in an abundant collagenous stroma that is usually hyalinized but may contain small numbers of small mesenchymal cells arranged in clusters, resembling primitive dermal hair papillae. The stroma also may contain small amounts of mucin concentrated around the epithelial columns.

Neoplastic cells have scant, pale cytoplasm with uniform, ovoid, euchromatic nuclei. Nuclei are ori-ented perpendicular to the long axis of the columns. Feline ribbon trichoblastomas have spindled cells with elongated nuclei, creating a palisaded apppearance in the cell columns. Mitotic figures are infrequent. The medusoid islands of cells may have slightly more abundant, eosinophilic cytoplasm in their central zones and may occasionally exhibit outer root sheath keratinization.

FIGURE 22-24. Ribbon-type trichoblastoma in a cat. Winding cords of spindled cells with elongated nuclei create a palisaded appearance. (×130)

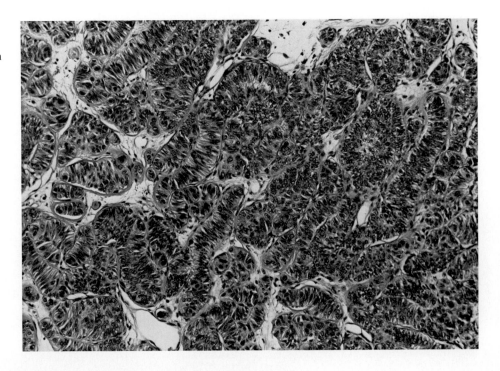

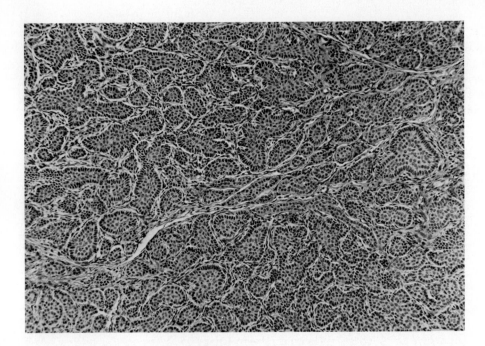

FIGURE 22-25. Trabecular-type trichoblastoma in a cat. Small islands and branching trabeculae are composed of small keratinocytes with prominent peripheral palisading. (×50.)

Trabecular type (Figures 22-25 and 22-26). One of the variants of basal cell tumor in cats appears analogous to Headington's simple trichoblastoma. This type of trichoblastoma also occurs occasionally in dogs. In both humans and animals these are well-circumscribed dermal nodules comprising lobules and broad trabeculae of basaloid epithelial cells with prominent peripheral palisading. Connection to the overlying epidermis is focal or absent. There is a sparse stroma of collagen and mucin with moderate cellularity. The peripheral cell layer of the epithelial structures shows scant, pale cytoplasm with uniform, ovoid, euchromatic nuclei and low mitotic activity. The internal cells have slightly more abundant, eosinophilic cytoplasm, and nuclei are often more elongated. The epithelial cells of trabecular-type trichoblastoma may be lightly melanized. Trabecular trichoblastoma is distinguished from benign feline basal cell tumor by the

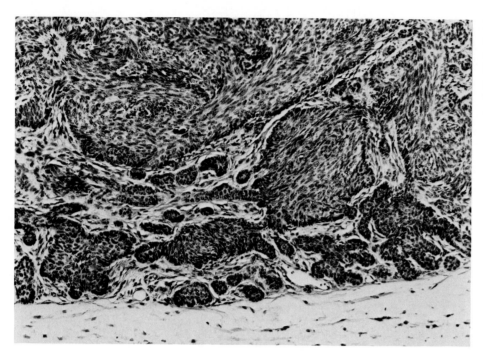

FIGURE 22-26. Trabecular-type trichoblastoma in a cat. Spindling of the epithelial cells is prominent. Note sparse, moderately cellular stroma and well-demarcated tumor margins. (×140.)

presence of a distinct trabecular pattern, prominent peripheral palisading, and a more abundant stroma. Trabecular trichoblastoma is differentiated from isthmus-catagen tricholemmoma by the presence of prominent peripheral palisading, absence of foci of tricholemmal keratinization, and paucity of glassy, pale-pink, isthmus-type keratinocytes.

Granular cell type (Figures 22-27 and 22-28). This rare variant of hair germ tumor in dogs was first reported by Seiler in 1981 as a subtype of basal cell tumor. Histopathologically, the architecture is identical to the canine ribbon-type trichoblastoma described previously, but some of the epithelial aggregations are composed entirely of larger cells with abundant, finely

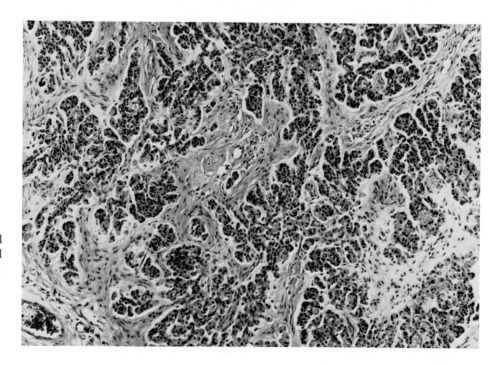

FIGURE 22-27. Granular cell trichoblastoma in a dog. Small polygonal cells are arranged in branching and winding cords similar to ribbon-type trichoblastoma. Note the abundant stroma of collagen and mucin. (×50.)

FIGURE 22-28. Higher magnification of the granular cell trichoblastoma in Figure 22-27 showing granular cytoplasm and eccentric, angular nuclei. (×280.)

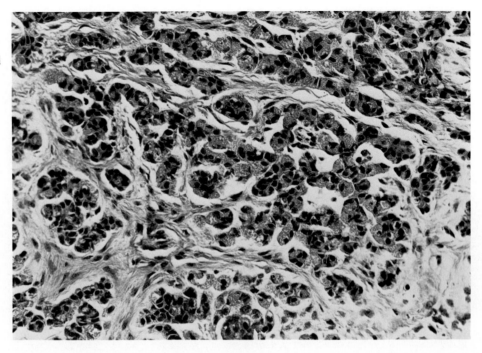

granular or vacuolated cytoplasm. Nuclei of the granular cells are small, angular and eccentric. Other lobules of the neoplasm contain typical basaloid cells.

Ultrastructurally, the granules are lysosomes containing numerous intact and fragmented vesicles of undetermined origin. Similar degenerative changes may also be observed in granular cell schwannoma, granular cell ameloblastoma, and granular cell basal cell carcinoma (the latter two entities are reported in humans only). Granular cell trichoblastoma is distinguished from granular cell basal cell carcinoma by the absence of contiguity with the epidermis and by its delicate ribbon-like architecture.

MATRICAL CARCINOMA (Synonym: malignant pilomatricoma)

Clinical features

Malignant epithelial neoplasms exhibiting hair follicle differentiation are rare in dogs. The first documentation of their occurrence is a case report by Sells in 1976. These neoplasms are of matrical origin but also demonstrate features of the inner root sheath, outer root sheath, and infundibulum.

Matrical carcinomas are large, plaque-like or dome-shaped, alopecic masses that are frequently ulcerated. The tumors reported by Sells and also Johnson occurred on the neck, thorax, and tail. There is no known age or breed predisposition. All of the reported cases described multifocal metastasis to either the lungs or the lymph nodes. Local recurrence also was described.

Histopathology (Figure 22-29)

Matrical carcinomas are poorly circumscribed dermal neoplasms composed primarily of basaloid epithelial cells arranged in large, irregular islands and trabeculae. Some neoplasms have multifocal contiguity with the epidermis. Ulceration is frequently observed, and there are multiple foci of caseation necrosis. A fairly abundant collagenous stroma often contains clusters and cords of infiltrating tumor cells.

The majority of the tumor cells have matrical features characterized by minimal cytoplasm, hyperchromatic, ovoid nuclei, and moderately high mitotic activity. Mitotic atypia is present. Multiple zones of matrical keratinization are manifested by abrupt formation of shadow cells. The basaloid cells also show foci of transition to inner root sheath, outer root sheath, and infundibular types of epithelium. The inner root sheath and infundibular epithelia produce compact, laminated keratin. The outer root sheath epithelium exhibits tricholemmal keratinization. The inner root sheath keratinocytes are slightly larger than the matrical cells and have clear cytoplasm with brightly eosinophilic trichohyalin granules. The infundibular epithelium is composed of typical squamous cells with keratohyalin

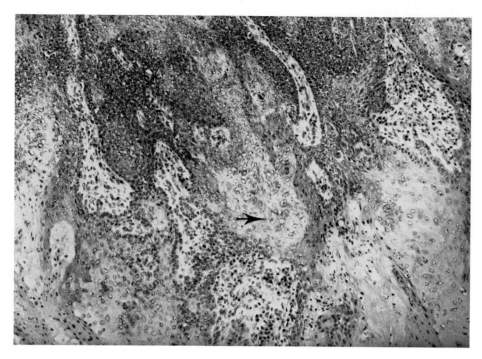

FIGURE 22-29. Matrical carcinoma in a dog. Irregular islands and broad trabeculae are composed of basaloid and squamous epithelial cells in varying proportions. Note the large and pale trichohyalin granules in the central island *(arrow)*. (×120.)

granules. The outer root sheath epithelial cells are slightly smaller and paler and lack a granular layer. The nonmatrical epithelial cells generally do not have cytologic features of malignancy.

Differentiation between matrical carcinoma and keratinizing basal cell carcinoma is problematic. The absence of connections to the epidermis, as confirmed by serial sections, supports a diagnosis of matrical carcinoma. Keratinizing basal carcinoma can have small foci of matrical differentiation with formation of shadow cells; large zones of matrical keratinization are a more typical feature of matrical carcinoma. Basal cell carcinomas may show tricholemmal and infundibular differentiation, but multifocal inner root sheath differentiation appears to occur almost exclusively in matrical carcinoma. Hybrid follicular cysts, trichofolliculomas, and pilomatricomas may have multiple small foci of inner root sheath morphology but have marked architectural differences from matrical carcinoma.

SUGGESTED READINGS

Follicular cyst

Bevier DF and Goldschmidt, MH: Skin tumors in the dog. I. Epithelial tumors and tumor-like lesions, Comp Cont Educ 3:389-398, 1981.

Hashimoto K, Mehregan AH, and Kumakiri M: Tumors of skin appendages, London, 1987, Butterworth, pp 95, 100-105.

Satoh T and others: Follicular cyst derived from hair matrix and outer root sheath, J Cutan Pathol 16:106-108, 1989.

Weiss E and Frese K: Tumours of the skin, Bull World Health Organ 50:79-100, 1974.

Dermoid cyst

Bevier DF and Goldschmidt MH: Skin tumors in the dog. I. Epithelial tumors and tumor-like lesions, Comp Cont Educ 3:389-398, 1981.

Dilated pore

Scott DW: Feline dermatology 1983-1985: "the secret sits," J Am Anim Hosp Assoc 23:255-274, 1986.

Follicular hamartoma

Mehregan AH: Pinkus' guide to dermatohistopathology, ed 4, Norwalk, Conn, 1986, Appleton-Century-Crofts, p 386.

Focal adnexal dysplasia

Kimura T and others: Folliculosebaceous cystic hamartoma: a distinctive malformation of the skin, Am J Dermatopathol 13:213-220, 1991.

Trichofolliculoma

Hashimoto K, Mehregan AH, and Kumakiri M: Tumors of skin appendages, London, 1987, Butterworth, pp 89-90.

Mehregan AH: Pinkus' guide to dermatohistopathology, ed 4, Norwalk, Conn, 1986, Appleton-Century-Crofts, p 470.

Trichoepithelioma

Bevier DF and Goldschmidt MH: Skin tumors in the dog. I. Epithelial tumors and tumor-like lesions, Comp Cont Educ 3:389-398, 1981.

Hashimoto K, Mehregan AH, and Kumakiri M: Tumors of skin appendages, London, 1987, Butterworth, pp 106-110.

Headington JT: Tumors of the hair follicle, Am J Pathol 85:480-514, 1976.

Theilen GH and Madewell BR, editors: Veterinary cancer medicine, ed 2, Philadelphia, 1987, Lea & Febiger, pp 257.

Infundibular keratinizing acanthoma

Bevier DF and Goldschmidt MH: Skin tumors in the dog. I. Epithelial tumors and tumor-like lesions, Comp Cont Educ 3:389-398, 1981.

Hashimoto K, Mehregan AH, and Kumakiri M: Tumors of skin appendages, London, 1987, Butterworth, pp 86-87.

Seiler RJ: Intracutaneous cornifying epithelioma in the dog: evidence for origin of the hair follicle. Proceedings of the Thirty-Second Annual Meeting of the American College of Veterinary Pathologists, Monterey, Calif, 1981.

Stannard AA and Pulley LT: Intracutaneous cutaneous cornifying epithelioma (keratoacanthoma) in the dog: a retrospective of 25 cases, J Am Vet Med Assoc 167:385-388, 1975.

Weiss E and Frese K: Tumours of the skin, Bull World Health Organ 50:79-100, 1974.

Tricholemmoma

Diters RW amd Goldschmidt MH: Hair follicle tumors resembling tricholemmomas in six dogs, Vet Pathol 20:123-125, 1983.

Hashimoto K, Mehregan AH, and Kumakiri M: Tumors of skin appendages, London, 1987, Butterworth, pp 92-93.

Headington JT: Tumors of the hair follicle, Am J Pathol 85:480-514, 1976.

Walsh KM and Corapi WV: Tricholemmoma in three dogs, J Comp Pathol 96:115-117, 1986.

Pilomatricoma

Bevier DF and Goldschmidt, MH: Skin tumors in the dog. I. Epithelial tumors and tumor-like lesions, Comp Cont Educ 3:389-398, 1981.

Carpenter JL, Andrew LK and Holzworth J: Tumors and tumor-like lesions. In Holzworth J, editor: Diseases of the cat, Philadelphia, 1987, WB Saunders, pp 416-417.

Hashimoto K, Mehregan AH, and Kumakiri M: Tumors of skin appendages, London, 1987, Butterworth, pp 114-116.

Theilen GH and Madewell BR, editors: Veterinary cancer medicine, ed 2, Philadelphia, 1987, Lea & Febiger, pp 257.

Weiss E and Frese K: Tumours of the skin, Bull World Health Organ 50:79-100, 1974.

Trichoblastoma

Barr RJ and Graham JH: Granular basal cell carcinoma: a distinct histopathologic entity, Arch Dermatol 115:1064-1067, 1979.

Bevier DF and Goldschmidt, MH: Skin tumors in the dog. I. Epithelial tumors and tumor-like lesions, Comp Cont Educ 3:389-398, 1981.

Blake Gilks C, Clement PB, and Wood WS: Trichoblastic fibroma: a clinicopathologic study of three cases, Am J Dermatopathol 11:397-402, 1989.

Hashimoto K, Mehregan AH, and Kumakiri M: Tumors of skin appendages, London, 1987, Butterworth, pp 111.

Headington JT: Tumors of the hair follicle, Am J Pathol 85:480-514, 1976.

Seiler RJ: Granular basal cell tumor in the skin of three dogs, Vet Pathol 18:23-29, 1981.

Theilen GH and Madewell BR, editors: Veterinary cancer medicine, ed 2, Philadelphia, 1987, Lea & Febiger, pp 255-357.

Matrical carcinoma

Bevier DF and Goldschmidt MH: Skin tumors in the dog. I. Epithelial tumors and tumor-like lesions, Comp Cont Educ 3:389-398, 1981.

Johnson RP and others: Malignant pilomatrixoma in an Old English Sheepdog, Can Vet J 24:392-394, 1983.

Sells DM and Conroy JD: Malignant epithelial neoplasia with hair follicle differentiation in dogs (malignant pilomatrixoma), J Comp Pathol 86:121-129, 1976.

See also General References on pp 327-328.

CHAPTER 23

Sebaceous tumors

SEBACEOUS DUCT CYST
Clinical features

The misnomer "sebaceous cyst" is frequently applied to follicular cysts because of the grumous nature of their keratinaceous contents. Cysts that involve sebaceous structures are extremely rare in dogs and cats. Sebaceous duct cysts appear as solitary, firm dermal nodules that are usually less than 1 cm in size. The cysts contain small amounts of keratin and milky sebum. There is no known age, breed, or site predisposition.

Histopathology (Figure 23-1)

Lined by a thin, undulating layer of squamous epithelium with a sparse granular cell layer, sebaceous cysts are histologically identical to the normal sebaceous duct. Most sebaceous duct cysts have a thin collagenous capsule. Projecting outward from the cyst wall are multiple, atrophic, but architecturally normal sebaceous gland lobules composed of central lipidized cells and a single layer of peripheral basaloid reserve cells. Occasional cysts are accompanied by moderately hyperplastic sebaceous glands. Most of the cyst contents are lost during tissue processing, but some delicate, laminated keratin generally adheres to the cyst lining.

NODULAR SEBACEOUS HYPERPLASIA (Synonym: senile sebaceous hyperplasia)
Clinical features

Nodular sebaceous gland hyperplasia is a common, focal or multicentric, nonneoplastic lesion of dogs. Nodular sebaceous hyperplasia is uncommon in cats. Lesions are yellow-white, alopecic, firm, dome-shaped or papillated nodules that are less than 5 mm in diameter. A waxy or pearly quality clinically differentiates nodular sebaceous hyperplasia from squamous papillomas despite their wart-like configuration. Lesions may arise anywhere on the body but are most common on the head and face.

Nodular sebaceous hyperplasia is most common in older animals. Poodles and Cocker Spaniels may be predisposed.

Histopathology (Figure 23-2)

Nodular sebaceous hyperplasia is characterized by multiple, enlarged, but architecturally normal sebaceous lobules clustered around dilated duct-like structures. The sebaceous lobules have central fully lipidized cells and a single peripheral layer of

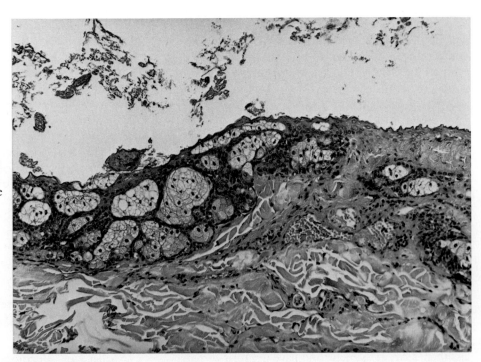

FIGURE 23-1. Sebaceous duct cyst in a dog. Note the delicate undulating epithelium lining the cyst lumen. (×120.)

basaloid reserve cells. The duct-like structures are lined by thickened squamous epithelium that keratinizes through a granular cell layer, and they contain loosely laminated keratin and small amounts of sebum. These structures may represent hyperplastic sebaceous ducts or follicular infundibula. Secondary erosion and inflammation are frequent features of larger lesions.

Nodular sebaceous hyperplasia must be differentiated from sebaceous adenoma. Nodular sebaceous hyperplasia retains the normal orientation of sebaceous glands around ducts or follicular infundibula. Degeneration of large zones of sebocytes and secondary cyst formation are common in simple sebaceous adenoma but are not observed in nodular sebaceous hyperplasia.

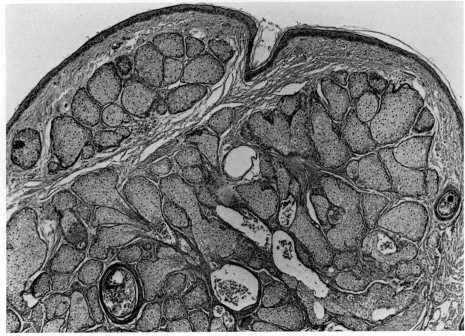

FIGURE 23-2. Nodular sebaceous hyperplasia in a dog. Enlarged sebaceous lobules are grouped around duct-like structures lined by keratinizing squamous epithelium. (×50.)

Nodular sebaceous gland hyperplasia and compound sebaceous adenoma are differentiated by the increased number of basaloid reserve cells and immature sebocytes in the latter. The ductular structures of compound sebaceous adenoma are usually more numerous and more varied in size than those of nodular sebaceous hyperplasia.

SEBACEOUS NEVUS
Clinical Features

In dogs, occasional nonneoplastic cutaneous lesions of adnexal (principally sebaceous gland) origin have been seen that histologically resemble nevus sebaceus of Jadassohn in humans. Nevus sebaceus of Jadassohn arises in childhood and can eventuate in a variety of benign and malignant epithelial neoplasms. However, these lesions in dogs have been observed too infrequently to determine if they evolve similarly or progress to neoplasia.

Sebaceous nevi appear as alopecic, scaly plaques less than 2 cm in diameter and have irregular or papillated surfaces. Most lesions are detected in middle-aged or older animals, but some have been identified in puppies. There is no known breed or site predisposition.

Histopathology (Figure 23-3)

Sebaceous nevus is a plaque-like lesion covered by hyperplastic, hyperkeratotic epidermis that has a papillated configuration. Hair follicles are small and incompletely developed; they have thickened, dilated infundibula but often lack an obvious hair bulb. The sebaceous glands are large, numerous, and randomly distributed through the superficial dermis. Ductal connections may be evident between the sebaceous glands and follicular structures. Sweat glands are generally present and are histologically normal. Some lesions contain increased stromal collagen, which is slightly more cellular than that of the adjacent dermis.

Sebaceous nevus is distinguished from nodular sebaceous hyperplasia by its plaque-like configuration and involvement of multiple folliculosebaceous units. Epidermal hyperplasia may occur in traumatized nodular hyperplasia. However, in sebaceous nevus, epidermal hyperplasia is a consistent feature, regardless of the presence of inflammation.

SEBACEOUS ADENOMA
Clinical features

Sebaceous adenomas are benign cutaneous neoplasms of glandular or combined ductal and glandular origin. Lesions are common in dogs, and they are also seen occasionally in cats. Sebaceous adenomas accounted for approximately 6% of all canine skin and subcutaneous tumors in a survey of 1141 neoplasms by one of the authors.* Histologically identical lesions on

* Emily J. Walder.

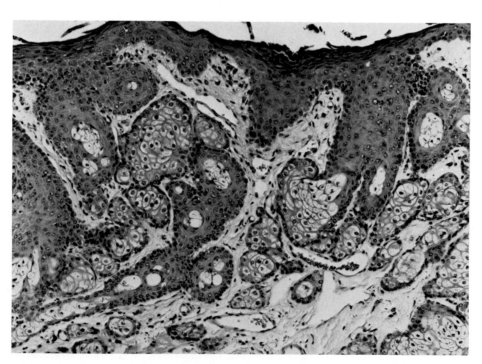

FIGURE 23-3. Sebaceous nevus in a dog. Randomly distributed sebaceous lobules of varying size are associated with abortive hair follicles below a hyperplastic epidermis. (×120.)

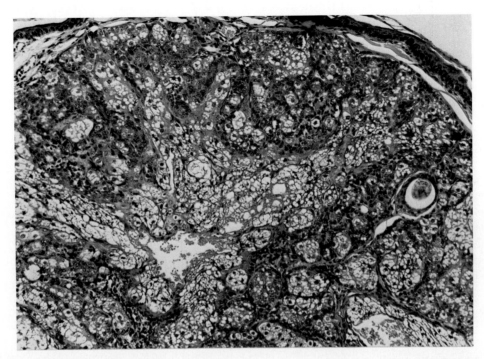

FIGURE 23-4. Simple sebaceous gland adenoma in a dog. Note the cystic degeneration of mature sebocytes in the center of the mass. (×120.)

eyelid margins arise from specialized tarsal sebaceous glands, called meibomian glands, and are thus designated *meibomian gland adenomas.*

Sebaceous adenomas are solitary or multiple, dome-shaped or papillated tumors that usually measure less than 1 cm in diameter. The overlying skin is usually alopecic and sometimes ulcerated. Sebaceous adenomas may occur anywhere on the body but are found commonly on the head.

The average age of affected animals is 10 years. Cocker Spaniels, Poodles, Beagles, Dachshunds, and Boston Terriers are reported to be predisposed. There is a slightly higher incidence in females than in males.

Histopathology

Simple sebaceous adenoma (Figure 23-4). Adenomas typically comprise multiple large lobules of sebaceous cells that show normal maturation from the basaloid peripheral reserve cell layer to the large, pale, lipid-laden central cells. Mitotic activity is low and is confined to the reserve cell layer. Cystic degeneration, characterized by zones of acellular, brightly eosinophilic, lacy material, is frequently present in the centers of the lobules. As would be expected from the high lipid content of the degenerating cells, any accompanying inflammation is predominantly granulomatous. Occasionally, complete degeneration of a sebaceous adenoma leads to the formation of a discrete granuloma composed of distended macrophages containing large

lipid vacuoles; this occurs most often on the eyelids.

In contradistinction to nodular sebaceous hyperplasia, the lobules in simple adenoma are not oriented around ducts or follicular infundibula. Cystic degeneration and lipogranulomatous inflammation are uncommon in nodular sebaceous hyperplasia.

Compound ductular and glandular adenoma (Figure 23-5). An infrequent variant of sebaceous adenoma involves both glandular lobules and ducts. The sebaceous lobules radiate from central ductal structures. The lobular component resembles typical sebaceous adenoma, but reserve cells and partially lipidized cells are more frequent than mature sebocytes. The ductal component is characterized by multiple irregular cysts of varying size that are lined by mature squamous epithelium. The term *sebaceoma* is used by some human dermatopathologists to categorize this variant.

Compound sebaceous adenoma is differentiated from nodular sebaceous hyperplasia by the increased number of basaloid reserve cells and immature sebocytes. The ductular structures of compound sebaceous adenoma are usually more numerous and more varied in size than those of nodular sebaceous hyperplasia.

SEBACEOUS EPITHELIOMA
Clinical features

Sebaceous epitheliomas are relatively common neoplasms of dogs that arise from the basaloid reserve

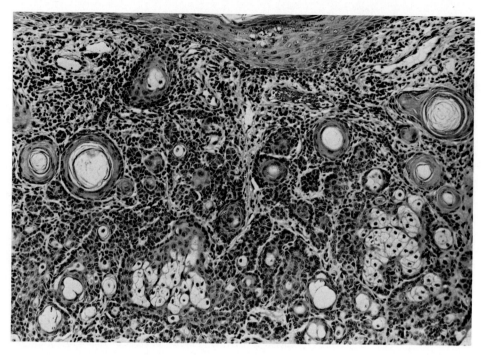

FIGURE 23-5. Compound sebaceous gland adenoma in a dog. Aggregations of sebocytes in various stages of maturation radiate from numerous keratinizing duct-like structures. (× 120.)

cells of sebaceous glands. They are rare in cats. The reported incidence is difficult to ascertain; some authors regard sebaceous epithelioma as a variant of sebaceous adenoma, whereas others include it with sebaceous carcinoma. Analogous neoplasms develop from the specialized sebaceous glands of the eyelid and are designated *meibomian epitheliomas.*

Sebaceous epitheliomas are usually solitary, firm, nodular or plaque-like masses ranging from several millimeters to several centimeters in diameter. The tumors may be multiple, either synchronously or metachronously. Surface ulceration is frequent. Some tumors, especially those on the eyelids, are melanized and may be confused clinically with melanoma. Sebaceous epitheliomas occur most often on the head, dorsal neck, and back.

There is no known age prevalence. Cocker Spaniels and Poodles are reported by several authors to have a higher incidence of sebaceous neoplasms in general.

Sebaceous epitheliomas have similar biologic behavior to basal cell carcinomas; these two entities are both derived from a germinative population of small, mitotically active, theoretically pluripotential epithelial cells. Sebaceous gland epitheliomas can be locally aggressive and may exhibit regional lymph node metastasis in rare cases. The designation "epithelioma" is preferred to adenoma or carcinoma because it implies very low malignant potential.

Histopathology (Figures 23-6 and 23-7)

Sebaceous epitheliomas are composed of multiple lobules of basaloid epithelial cells in a sparse stroma of reactive collagenous tissue with secondary suppurative and plasmacytic inflammation. The margins of the neoplasm are irregular and mildly infiltrative. As in basal cell carcinoma (see Chapter 21), multifocal contiguity with the overlying epidermis is present.

Basaloid cells of the neoplasm resemble the reserve cells at the periphery of normal sebaceous glands. These cells have scant, amphophilic cytoplasm and ovoid, hyperchromatic nuclei. Multiple small foci of distinct sebaceous differentiation are characterized by individual cells or clusters of cells with expanded, foamy cytoplasm. There may also be small foci of squamous metaplasia and formation of small horn cysts. Mitotic activity is fairly high, as would be expected in a normal reserve cell population.

Meibomian epitheliomas have a greater tendency to melanize than do sebaceous epitheliomas in other locations. Pigmented tumors have variable numbers of melanin granules within the basaloid epithelial cells as well as many dendritic melanocytes and melanophages in the stroma.

Sebaceous or meibomian epithelioma with few lipidized cells may be indistinguishable from basal cell carcinoma with sebaceous differentiation. Both tumors are made up of predominantly small, dark epithelial

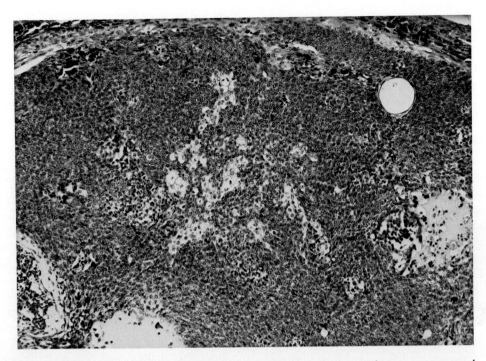

FIGURE 23-6. Meibomian epithelioma in a dog. Clusters of mature sebocytes are scattered among small basaloid epithelial cells. Note the melanization of the epithelial cells and large, dark melanophages in the stroma. (×50.)

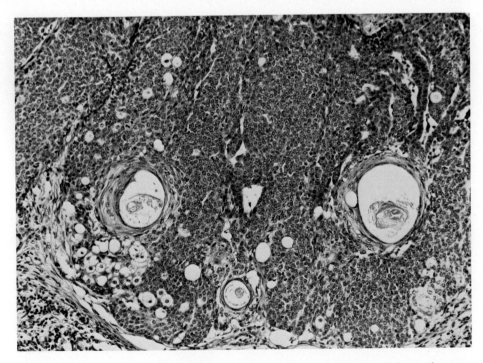

FIGURE 23-7. Sebaceous epithelioma in a dog. Note the individual and clustered mature sebocytes and small horn cysts. (×140.)

cells and have multifocal connection to the epidermis. Sebaceous epithelioma and basal cell carcinoma with sebaceous differentiation represent neighboring entities in a continuum of adnexal neoplasms. Clusters of mature sebocytes support a diagnosis of sebaceous epithelioma, whereas individual sebaceous cells are more consistent with a diagnosis of basal cell carcinoma.

SEBACEOUS CARCINOMA
Clinical features

Sebaceous gland carcinomas are rare malignant neoplasms in cats and dogs. Sebaceous carcinoma was diagnosed in 0.8% of all canine skin and subcutaneous tumors in a large survey by Strafuss. However, histologic description was not provided, and sebaceous epithelioma may have been included in the statistical analysis.

Sebaceous carcinomas are usually solitary, firm nodules less than 4 cm in diameter. Alopecia and ulceration are common. More than half of the cases in the Strafuss survey occurred on the head. The average age of affected animals was 9 years. Cocker Spaniels appear to be predisposed to the development of sebaceous carcinomas. The neoplasms may recur after surgical excision, but reports of distant metastasis are rare in both dogs and cats.

Histopathology (Figures 23-8 and 23-9)

Sebaceous carcinomas are generally irregular, but circumscribed, multilobular dermal neoplasms composed of islands of pleomorphic polygonal cells. The tumor lobules are delineated by a moderate stroma of dense collagen. The majority of cells have abundant, pale, vacuolated cytoplasm. The lipid content of the vacuoles may or may not be obvious, depending on the degree of differentiation. Well-differentiated sebaceous carcinomas have cells with foamy cytoplasmic vacuoles resembling normal sebocytes. Poorly differentiated tumors may have cells with clear cytoplasm only. Nuclei are large and vesicular and have prominent nucleoli. Mitotic activity is moderately high. Areas resembling squamous cell carcinoma or basal cell carcinoma may be present.

Some sebaceous carcinomas have tumor cells arranged in sheets and infiltrative cords with a minimal stromal component. Ulceration is more common in these poorly circumscribed, invasive variants.

Differential diagnoses include clear-cell basal cell carcinoma, balloon cell melanoma, poorly differentiated perianal gland carcinoma, metastatic carcinoma, and liposarcoma. Differentiation between clear-cell basal cell carcinoma and sebaceous carcinoma can be difficult. Most sebaceous carcinomas contain cells with multiple round vacuoles or foamy cytoplasm indicative

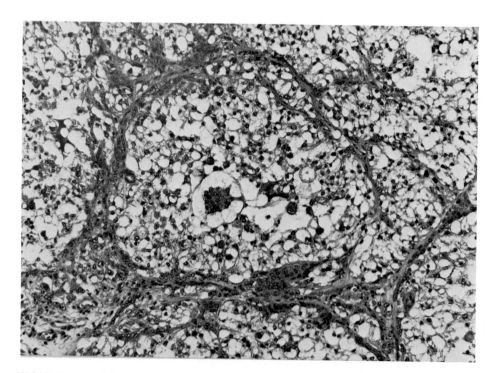

FIGURE 23-8. Sebaceous carcinoma in a dog. Note the lobular architecture and abundant foamy cytoplasm in the majority of the tumor cells. (× 140.)

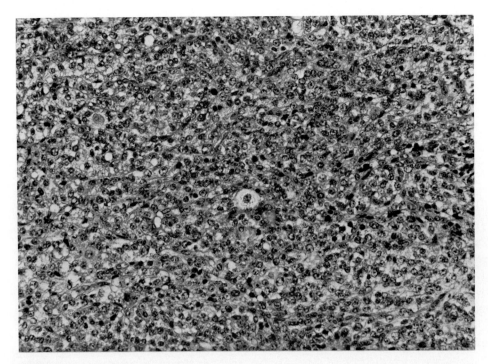

FIGURE 23-9. Poorly differentiated sebaceous carcinoma in a dog. Note the single well-differentiated sebocyte in the center of solid sheets of anaplastic epithelial cells. (×240.)

of lipid content. The nuclei of sebaceous carcinomas usually have more prominent nucleoli and higher mitotic activity than those of basal cell carcinoma. Sebaceous carcinoma does not have multifocal epidermal contiguity as observed in most basal cell carcinomas. Balloon cell melanoma may have minimal pigment and a predominance of cells with abundant, foamy cytoplasm. Most melanomas have bimorphic features, and small areas of spindle cells can usually be detected. Fontana-Masson stain is helpful in identifying melanin pigment. Although both sebaceous carcinomas and liposarcomas have lipid-laden cells, most sebaceous carcinomas have multilobular architecture that is absent in liposarcomas. Differentiation from other poorly differentiated carcinomas may not be possible at the light microscopic level. Electron microscopy or immunohistochemistry may be required for definitive diagnosis of the more anaplastic forms of sebaceous carcinoma.

NODULAR PERIANAL (HEPATOID) GLAND HYPERPLASIA AND PERIANAL (HEPATOID) GLAND ADENOMA

Clinical features

Benign perianal (hepatoid) gland proliferations, including hyperplasia and adenoma, are common lesions in dogs and account for 8% to 18% of all canine

skin tumors as indicated in several surveys. Hepatoid glands in dogs are sebaceous gland derivatives that have been modified by the influence of androgenic hormones. They are located primarily in perianal skin but can also be found circumferentially around the proximal third of the tail, in the dorsal lumbosacral area, lateral to the prepuce, and along the ventral midline as far cranial as the base of the skull. The etiology of perianal gland hyperplasia and neoplasia has not been definitively proven, but gonadal hormones appear to play an important role. A causal relationship is implied by the regression of a high percentage of benign perianal gland tumors following castration alone, as reported by Wilson.

Perianal gland hyperplasia generally has a nodular configuration but may also appear as an annular perianal growth. The size of hyperplastic nodules and benign neoplasms varies from several millimeters to 10 cm. Lesions are often multiple, and ulceration is common in larger masses. The nodules have a rubbery consistency and tan coloration.

Because of the widespread normal distribution of hepatoid glands, hyperplastic and neoplastic lesions are not limited to the classic perianal or ventral tailbase location, but can be found anywhere on the tail or trunk. Other aberrant sites, including the head and feet, also have been observed.

Hepatoid gland lesions occur far more frequently

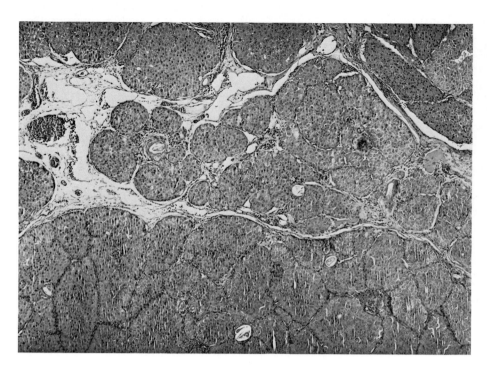

FIGURE 23-10. Nodular perianal gland hyperplasia in a dog. Note that individual lobules of hepatoid glands are still discernible. (×50.)

in intact males than in females or neutered males. Wilson's data indicate that the ratio of males to females with perianal gland neoplasms is 6:1. The ratio of neutered females to intact females is 3:1. Most affected animals are 8 years of age or older. Breed predilections are reported in Cocker Spaniels, Beagles, English Bulldogs, Samoyeds, Dachshunds, and German Shepherd Dogs.

Histopathology

Nodular perianal gland hyperplasia (Figure 23-10). Perianal gland hyperplasia consists of multiple enlarged lobules of well-differentiated hepatoid cells with a narrow peripheral zone of basaloid reserve cells. The overall glandular architecture is well maintained; the groups of lobules are discernible as discrete units frequently centered around small ductal structures. Lobules within a particular lesion are of approximately equal size.

Mature hepatoid cells are characterized by abundant, polygonal, eosinophilic cytoplasm. Nuclei are centrally located, ovoid, and vesicular and have small nucleoli. Mitotic activity is confined to the reserve cell layer. The small interlobular ducts are lined by flattened, keratinizing epithelial cells. Nodular perianal gland hyperplasia is distinguished by the persistence of a uniform lobular architecture instead of the proliferation of trabeculae or islands of hepatoid cells found in perianal gland adenoma.

Perianal gland adenoma (Figures 23-11 and 23-12). Perianal adenoma is a well-circumscribed nodular mass composed of broad, anastomosing trabeculae of well-differentiated hepatoid cells and a peripheral layer of basaloid reserve cells. A thin fibrous capsule may be present. Discrete glandular lobules are not evident within the mass, and adjacent hepatoid glands are frequently compressed. There is a delicate fibrovascular stroma.

Cytologic features are identical to nodular perianal gland hyperplasia. The hepatoid cells have uniform, eosinophilic cytoplasm, vesicular nuclei, and small nucleoli. Mitotic activity is confined to the reserve cell layer. The frequent small foci of squamous metaplasia with keratin pearl formation may represent attempted ductal differentiation.

Some perianal gland adenomas are highly vascular and have dilated sinusoidal blood vessels separating the epithelial trabeculae. This pattern may be referred to as an *angiomatoid variant*. Another variant, which occurs more commonly in female dogs, is characterized by formation of small islands and nests of hepatoid cells rather than trabeculae. This variant occasionally has an abundant stroma composed of adipose tissue.

Ulceration is common in larger perianal gland adenomas, and infarction may also occur. Infarcted perianal gland adenomas have a distinct pattern of inflammation characterized by caseation necrosis, granulomatous inflammation, fibrosis, and cholesterol cleft formation.

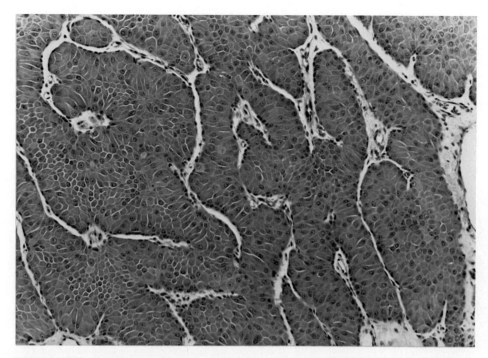

FIGURE 23-11. Perianal gland adenoma in a male dog. Well-differentiated hepatoid cells are arranged in anastomosing trabeculae. (×120.)

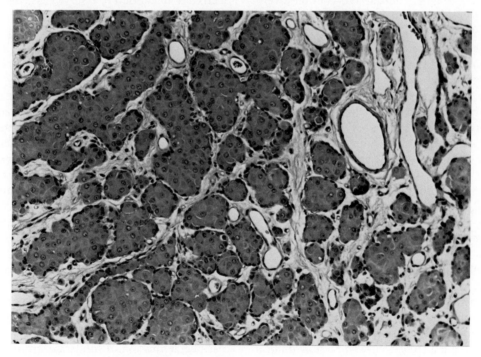

FIGURE 23-12. Perianal gland adenoma in a female dog. Well-differentiated hepatoid cells are arranged in islands and clusters. (×120.)

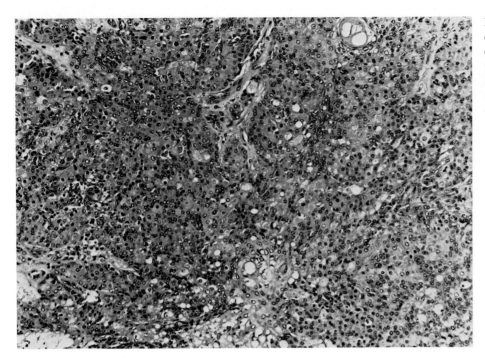

FIGURE 23-13. Well-differentiated perianal gland carcinoma in a dog. Mature hepatoid cells predominate, but maturation patterns are haphazard. Note the scattered sebaceous cells. (×120.)

PERIANAL (HEPATOID) GLAND CARCINOMA

Clinical features

Perianal gland carcinomas are uncommon malignant neoplasms of dogs that appear to occur exclusively in a perianal location. Perianal gland carcinomas accounted for 2.6% of 1141 canine skin and subcutaneous neoplasms in a survey by one of the authors.* According to Wilson's review, perianal gland carcinomas are not influenced by gonadal hormones and do not respond to castration.

Well-differentiated carcinomas are clinically indistinguishable from adenomas. Most carcinomas are at least 2 cm in diameter. Poorly differentiated carcinomas are firmer, uncircumscribed, and usually ulcerated.

The large majority of perianal gland carcinomas occurs in older male dogs. There is no known breed predilection. Regional lymph node metastasis is common in poorly differentiated variants and infrequent in well-differentiated lesions.

Histopathology (Figures 23-13 and 23-14)

Perianal gland carcinomas vary from well differentiated to anaplastic. The majority are of low-grade malignancy. Well-differentiated perianal gland carcinomas have similar architecture and morphology to perianal gland adenomas, but a tendency toward mildly infiltra-

* Emily J. Walder.

tive growth is present at the tumor margins. Fibrous stroma may be more prominent than in adenomas. Nuclei are larger than in benign tumors, are slightly pleomorphic, and have prominent nucleoli. Moderate numbers of mitotic figures are found in the differentiated cells in addition to reserve cells, and mitotic atypia is present. Maturation patterns from reserve cells to hepatoid cells are somewhat haphazard. The hepatoid cells exhibit variable fatty vacuolation reminiscent of their sebaceous gland origin. Small foci of squamous metaplasia may be present.

A second type of low-grade perianal gland carcinoma is composed primarily of basaloid reserve cells arranged in islands and anastomosing trabeculae within a sparse collagenous stroma. The reserve cells have scant, amphophilic cytoplasm and ovoid, hyperchromatic nuclei. Scattered clusters of cells exhibit hepatoid differentiation characterized by abundant, eosinophilic cytoplasm and larger, vesicular nuclei. Moderate mitotic activity is observed. This neoplasm is analogous to sebaceous epithelioma in architecture and clinical behavior and thus also may be designated perianal gland epithelioma to reflect its morphologic features and very low metastatic potential.

Poorly differentiated variants of perianal gland carcinoma are poorly circumscribed tumors composed of trabeculae and cords of anaplastic cells with prominent peripheral invasion. A moderate stroma of reactive collagen is often infiltrated by cords and clusters of neoplastic epithelial cells. The origin of the neoplasm may

FIGURE 23-14. Poorly differentiated perianal gland carcinoma in a dog. Clusters and cords of vacuolated epithelial cells are distributed through a sclerotic collagenous stroma. (×120.)

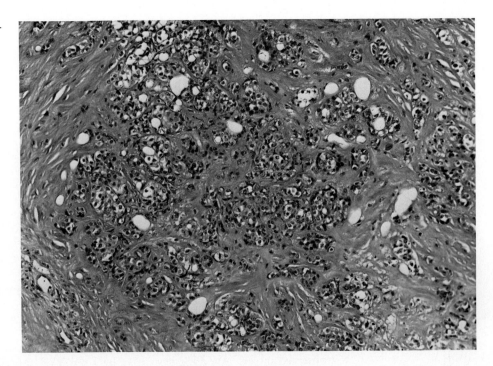

be recognizable only by its location. The cells are polygonal and have eosinophilic or amphophilic cytoplasm with variable vacuolation. Smaller cytoplasmic vacuoles may appear to contain lipid material, whereas larger vacuoles often have a mucinous appearance. Nuclei are large and vesicular with prominent nucleoli. Mitotic activity is high, and mitotic atypia is commonly observed. Intermediate variants also exist, which have zones of discernible hepatoid differentiation and anaplastic zones. Differential diagnosis for the poorly differentiated perianal gland carcinoma includes poorly differentiated variants of squamous cell carcinoma, sebaceous gland carcinoma, and apocrine sweat gland carcinoma. The absence of contiguity with the overlying epidermis is a useful feature in ruling out squamous cell carcinoma. Differentiation from other glandular malignancies may not be possible on a histologic basis.

SUGGESTED READINGS

Sebaceous duct cyst

Hashimoto K, Mehregan AH, and Kumakiri M: Tumors of skin appendages, London, 1987, Butterworth, pp 97-100.

Nodular sebaceous hyperplasia

Bevier DF and Goldschmidt MH: Skin tumors in the dog. I. Epithelial tumors and tumor-like lesions, Comp Cont Ed 3:389-398, 1981.

Hashimoto K, Mehregan AH, and Kumakiri M: Tumors of skin appendages, London, 1987, Butterworth, pp 130-131.

Sebaceous nevus

Hashimoto K, Mehregan AH, and Kumakiri M: Tumors of skin appendages, London, 1987, Butterworth, pp 131-132.

Sebaceous adenoma

Bevier DF and Goldschmidt MH: Skin tumors in the dog. I. Epithelial tumors and tumor-like lesions, Comp Cont Ed 3:389-398, 1981.

Hashimoto K, Mehregan AH, and Kumakiri M: Tumors of skin appendages, London, 1987, Butterworth, pp 132-137.

Sebaceous epithelioma

Hashimoto K, Mehregan AH, and Kumakiri M: Tumors of skin appendages, London, 1987, Butterworth, pp 137-139.

Sebaceous carcinoma

Bevier DF and Goldschmidt MH: Skin tumors in the dog. I. Epithelial tumors and tumor-like lesions, Comp Cont Ed 3:389-398, 1981.

Hashimoto K, Mehregan AH, and Kumakiri M: Tumors of skin appendages, London, 1987, Butterworth, pp 139-141.

Strafuss AC: Sebaceous carcinoma in dogs, J Am Vet Med Assoc 169:325-326, 1976.

Nodular perianal gland hyperplasia and perianal gland adenoma

Bevier DF and Goldschmidt MH: Skin tumors in the dog. I. Epithelial tumors and tumor-like lesions, Comp Cont Ed 3:389-398, 1981.

Wilson GP and Hayes HM: Castration for the treatment of perianal gland neoplasms in the dog, J Am Vet Med Assoc 174: 1301-1303, 1979.

Perianal gland carcinoma

Bevier DF and Goldschmidt MH: Skin tumors in the dog. I. Epithelial tumors and tumor-like lesions, Comp Cont Ed 3:389-398, 1981.

Wilson GP and Hayes HM: Castration for the treatment of perianal gland neoplasms in the dog, J Am Vet Med Assoc 174: 1301-1303, 1979.

See also General References, pp 327-328.

CHAPTER 24

Sweat gland tumors

APOCRINE CYST
Clinical features

Apocrine cysts are common, nonneoplastic lesions in dogs. These cysts are rarely observed in cats. Apocrine cysts may be a result of obstruction of sweat gland ducts. Lesions appear as well-defined, tense nodules ranging from several millimeters to several centimeters. The cysts are usually single but may be multiple. The masses often have a blue tint when viewed through the overlying skin. The overlying epidermis is frequently atrophic and alopecic. Cyst contents are usually clear and watery, but they are occasionally brown and gelatinous because of inspissation. Sweat gland cysts occur most frequently on the head, neck, and dorsal trunk.

Affected animals are usually 6 years of age or older. There is no breed predilection.

Histopathology (Figure 24-1)

Sweat gland cysts are unilocular or multilocular structures lined by a single layer of cuboidal-to-columnar epithelial cells with small, uniform, basally located nuclei. Apocrine decapitation-type secretory activity, manifested by apical blebbing of the cytoplasm, is generally apparent but may be absent if the lining cells have undergone pressure atrophy. Cyst contents are usually not visible in tissue sections, but occasionally cysts will contain inspissated secretory material that stains deep pink.

APOCRINE CYSTOMATOSIS
Clinical features

Apocrine cystomatosis is a rare, nonneoplastic condition in dogs characterized by multiple clusters of cystically dilated sweat glands. The etiology of this condition is unknown. The lesions appear as grouped nodules or vesicles, several millimeters in diameter, that are distributed over the head and neck. Rarely, generalized distribution is present. The overlying skin is generally atrophic and alopecic. The cysts may have a translucent appearance and a slightly blue tint.

Affected animals are usually middle aged or older. There is no known breed predisposition.

Histopathology (Figure 24-2)

Apocrine cystomatosis is characterized by clusters of dilated apocrine glands that are grouped among hair follicles in the middle and deep dermis. The cysts within a given lesion are usually of similar size, but single large cysts with smaller satellite cysts may

FIGURE 24-1. Apocrine cyst in a dog. A single layer of atrophic cuboidal epithelial cells lines the cyst. (×120.)

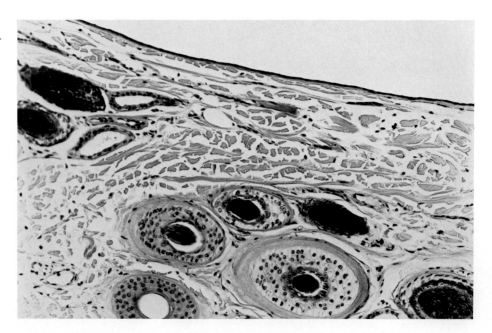

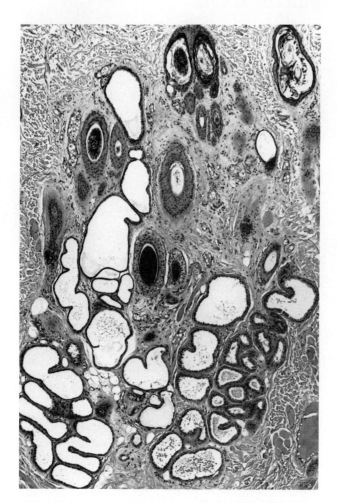

FIGURE 24-2. Apocrine cystomatosis in a dog. Clusters of dilated sweat glands are present among hair follicles. (×60.)

also be observed. The cysts are lined by low cuboidal epithelial cells. Apical blebbing is observed infrequently; this is probably a reflection of mild pressure atrophy of the lining epithelial cells. Adjacent dermal architecture shows minimal perturbation; mild fibrosis may be present.

APOCRINE CYSTADENOMA
Clinical features

Apocrine cystadenoma is an uncommon, benign neoplasm in dogs that is derived from the secretory portion of the sweat gland. Apocrine cystadenomas are rare in cats. All variants of apocrine adenoma accounted for only 1.4% of canine skin tumors in a large survey cited by Bevier.

Apocrine cystadenomas are usually solitary and range from 1 to 4 cm, although some attain sizes of 10 cm or more. The overlying epidermis is generally atrophic and alopecic, and ulceration is uncommon. As in apocrine cysts (see earlier discussion), a blue or purple hue may be observed through the skin surface. The secretory product within the neoplasms is often brown and gelatinous because of inspissation. The head, neck, and dorsal trunk are the most frequent locations.

Affected animals are usually 6 years of age or older. There is no breed predisposition.

Histopathology (Figures 24-3 and 24-4)

Apocrine cystadenoma is a circumscribed, but unencapsulated dermal neoplasm composed of closely packed cystic and glandular structures of varying size

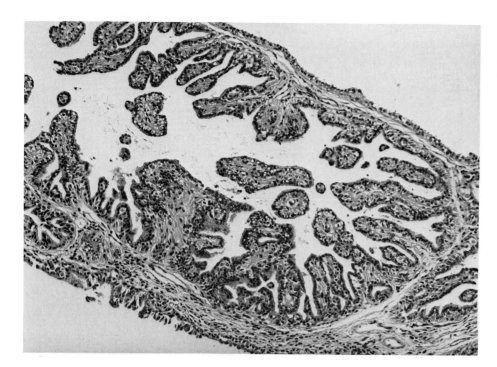

FIGURE 24-3. Apocrine cystadenoma in a dog. Note the small papillary projections covered by uniform cuboidal cells. (×120.)

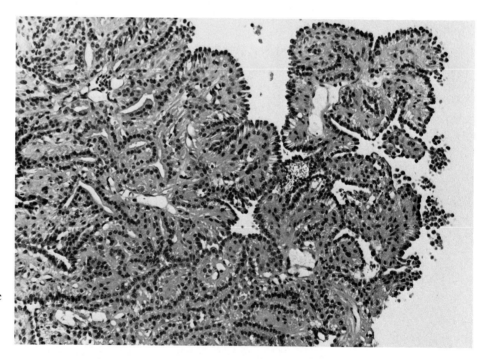

FIGURE 24-4. Larger papillary structure from apocrine cystadenoma in a dog. Note the apical blebbing of cytoplasm, particularly along the top and right margins. (×120.)

lined by a single layer of cuboidal-to-columnar epithelial cells. Cysts may also contain some branching, papillary proliferations lined by a single layer of columnar epithelial cells. The secretory material within cyst lumens frequently stains rose pink in tissue sections. The sparse collagenous stroma and surrounding dermis are frequently infiltrated by macrophages containing light-brown pigment, which most likely represents iron from escaped apocrine secretion.

The epithelial lining cells have abundant, bright-pink cytoplasm with prominent apical blebbing present in most of the glandular and cystic structures. Nuclei may be moderately enlarged and contain small nucleoli, but atypia is not present. Mitotic activity is minimal. Variable numbers of plasma cells and neutrophils are present within the stroma and adjacent dermis, depending upon the presence of ulceration or degeneration of cyst walls.

APOCRINE ADENOMA

Clinical features

Apocrine adenomas are uncommon benign neoplasms of dogs and cats that may arise from the secretory portion (glandular adenoma) or ductal portion (ductular or basaloid adenoma) of apocrine sweat glands. All variants of apocrine adenoma account for fewer than 2% of canine skin neoplasms in most surveys. Ductular apocrine adenomas are not generally reported in the literature as a distinct entity in animals. Spiradenoma, described by Weiss as the canine analogue to the ductular eccrine neoplasm in humans, is probably ductular apocrine adenoma.

The incidence of apocrine adenomas in cats is difficult to estimate, since ductular adenomas have most likely been traditionally included in the basal cell tumor group. Diters reported frequent "tubuloacinar differentiation" in their retrospective survey of feline basal cell tumors; many of these probably represented apocrine ductular adenomas.

Apocrine glandular adenomas of dogs and cats are well-circumscribed, solitary, dermal nodules that usually measure between 1 and 4 cm. The overlying skin is often alopecic, and ulceration is common in larger lesions. Some surveys report a predilection for the head and neck; others indicate no site predilection.

Affected animals are usually 6 years of age or older. There is no known breed predilection.

Apocrine ductular adenomas in dogs are solitary, circumscribed, multinodular, dermal and subcutaneous masses that are usually 2 cm or larger. The epidermis may be partially alopecic, but ulceration is infrequent. Most tumors occur on the trunk. Feline ductular adenomas are usually solitary, firm nodules that are less than 2 cm in diameter. The neoplasms are often alopecic and have a blue-to-brown hue. Lesions generally occur on the head, neck, and shoulders. There are no known age or breed predispositions for the ductular variants in dogs or cats.

Histopathology

Apocrine glandular adenoma (Figure 24-5). Adenomas arising from the secretory portion of sweat glands are well-circumscribed, but unencapsulated, dermal masses exhibiting tubular patterns, papillary patterns, or both. The neoplastic epithelial structures are generally lined by a single layer of cuboidal-to-columnar cells that have moderate-to-abundant eosinophilic cytoplasm. Decapitation secretion is discernible in most lesions, and eosinophilic secretory material is often present in glandular lumens. Nuclei are moderately enlarged and vesicular and have small nucleoli. Mitotic activity is low. Nuclear or mitotic atypia is not observed. Most neoplasms have a sparse collagenous stroma with variable infiltration by plasma cells and pigmented macrophages.

Apocrine glandular adenomas on the ventral abdo-

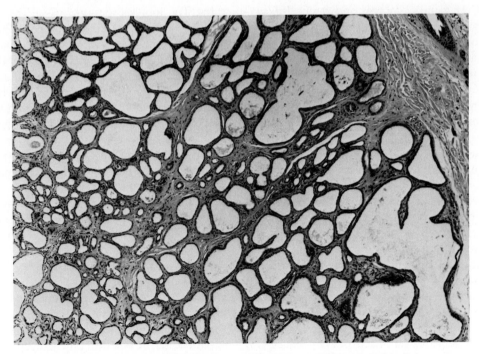

FIGURE 24-5. Apocrine glandular adenoma in a dog. The glandular structures are lined by a single layer of low cuboidal epithelial cells. (×50.)

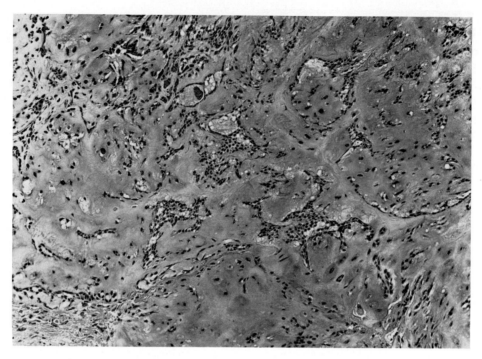

FIGURE 24-6. Mixed (compound) apocrine adenoma in a dog. Small glandular structures are distributed through an abundant, well-differentiated chondroid stroma. (×130.)

men may need to be differentiated from mammary gland adenomas. Mammary adenomas, with the exception of neoplasms arising in major mammary ducts, are subcutaneous and are usually encapsulated. The epithelial cells of mammary adenomas are smaller than those of apocrine sweat gland adenomas and rarely display apical blebbing.

Mixed (compound) apocrine adenoma (Figure 24-6). Some apocrine adenomas have nodular or diffuse zones of myoepithelial proliferation with myxoid and chondroid differentiation. These lesions are analogous to benign mixed mammary tumors. The stroma usually contains multiple nodules of small spindle and stellate cells that have pale cytoplasm and bland, ovoid-to-fusiform nuclei. The mesenchymal cells are separated by a lightly basophilic mucinous stroma or are entrapped in lacunar spaces within a deeply basophilic chondroid matrix. Unlike benign mixed mammary tumors, osseous metaplasia is extremely rare. The epithelial component of mixed sweat gland tumors is identical to that of the glandular adenomas. Differentiation from benign mixed mammary tumors is as described for glandular adenomas.

Canine ductular (basaloid) apocrine adenoma (Figure 24-7). These circumscribed, but unencapsulated, multilobular neoplasms are located in the deep dermis and subcutaneous fat. Each of the lobules is composed of winding trabeculae and tightly packed

tubular structures lined by a double layer of cuboidal cells. The double epithelial layer is structurally consistent with a ductal origin. There are multiple, patchy foci of squamous metaplasia with formation of irregular keratin lakes but without formation of cystic structures. The lobules of tumor tissue are separated by a moderate stroma of dense collagen. The luminal cell layer has scant, clear cytoplasm and small, hyperchromatic nuclei. The outer cell layer has moderate, eosinophilic cytoplasm and slightly larger, euchromatic nuclei. Apocrine secretory activity is not observed. Nucleoli are inconspicuous, but mitotic activity is moderate. (In human sweat gland neoplasms, the mitotic index has been shown not to be an important factor in distinguishing benign from malignant neoplasms.) There is usually a mild stromal infiltrate of plasma cells and histiocytes.

The histologic appearance of this neoplasm is virtually identical to that of basaloid mammary gland adenoma, which is also believed to be of ductal origin. In a ventral abdominal location, ductular apocrine adenoma would be distinguished from basaloid mammary adenoma by the absence of identifiable mammary glands. Differentiation of ductular apocrine adenoma from follicular neoplasms composed predominantly of small basaloid cells, such as trichoblastoma and trichoepithelioma, is based upon the deep location, multilobular configuration, formation of double rows and

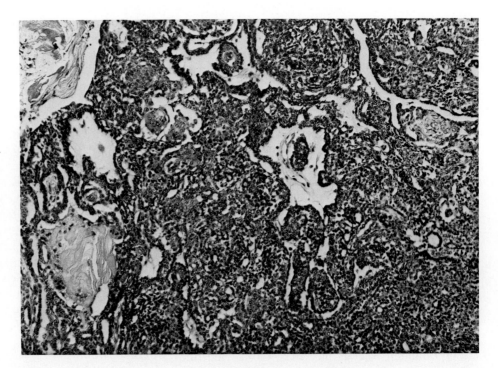

FIGURE 24-7. Canine ductular apocrine adenoma. Double layers of small basaloid epithelial cells line winding tubular structures. Note the keratin lakes at left. (×130.)

tubular structures, and lack of organization of keratinized areas into cystic structures.

Feline ductular (basaloid) apocrine adenoma (Figure 24-8). These tumors are well circumscribed, small, and often multilobular. The centers of the lobules frequently have cystic degeneration; true cyst formation is rarely noted. There may be focal contiguity

with the epidermis. The lobules are separated by a sparse stroma of dense collagen. The tumor is composed primarily of solid sheets of uniform basal cells that have scant, pale cytoplasm and dark, ovoid nuclei. Mitotic activity is low. Distributed through the solid cellular background are multiple, small tubular structures lined by a distinct double-cell layer indicative of

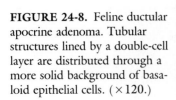

FIGURE 24-8. Feline ductular apocrine adenoma. Tubular structures lined by a double-cell layer are distributed through a more solid background of basaloid epithelial cells. (×120.)

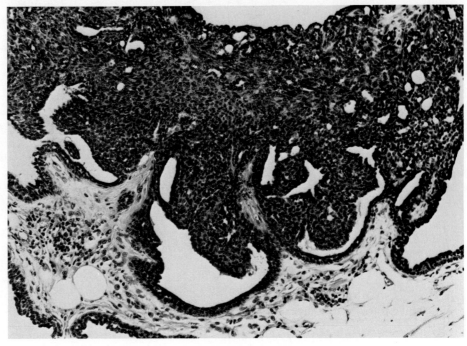

ductal differentiation. As in canine basaloid apocrine adenoma, the luminal cells of the tubules are smaller and have darker nuclei, and the outer cells are slighty larger and more eosinophilic than the adjacent basal cells.

Differential diagnoses are benign feline basal cell tumor and basal cell carcinoma, particularly those basal cell carcinomas which have cystic degeneration or slight apocrine differentiation. Ductular apocrine adenomas are distinguished from benign basal cell tumors by the presence of multiple tubular structures, the absence of a broad epidermal connection, and the absence of melanin pigment. They are distinguished from basal cell carcinomas by the absence of mitotic atypia, necrosis, melanin pigment, broad epidermal contiguity, and stromal invasion.

APOCRINE CARCINOMA
Clinical features

Malignant neoplasms of apocrine sweat glands occur uncommonly in dogs and rarely in cats. Apocrine carcinomas represented 2.2% of canine skin tumors in a large survey cited by Bevier.

Apocrine sweat gland carcinomas in dogs are usually indistinguishable clinically from their benign counterparts. Lesions are solitary, firm, circumscribed nodules 1 to 10 cm in diameter. The clinical appearance may vary, depending upon the histologic subtype. Cys-

tadenocarcinomas may have a fluctuant consistency, and compound tumors may be firmer than simple types because of the presence of cartilage. The overlying skin is frequently alopecic, and secondary ulceration may be present. Poorly differentiated tumors in dogs and cats may appear as firm, poorly circumscribed, diffusely ulcerated masses.

The reported average age of affected animals varies from 8 to 13 years. There is no known breed or site predilection.

Little information is available on the biologic behavior of apocrine sweat gland carcinomas. They are reported to have the potential for metastasis to lymph nodes and viscera, but a statement of actual metastatic incidence has not been made. Biologic behavior may be analogous to mammary gland neoplasms, in which the metastatic incidence closely correlates to histologic subtype. Retrospective studies of apocrine sweat gland carcinomas to determine the biologic behavior in relation to histomorphologic subtype are needed.

Histopathology

Apocrine cystadenocarcinoma (Figure 24-9). The cystic subtype of apocrine carcinoma is a discrete, multilocular dermal neoplasm resembling cystadenoma (see preceding discussion), but cytologic features of malignancy are present. There is patchy piling up of cells around cyst lumens, with formation of small papillary projections. Nuclei are larger and more pleomorphic

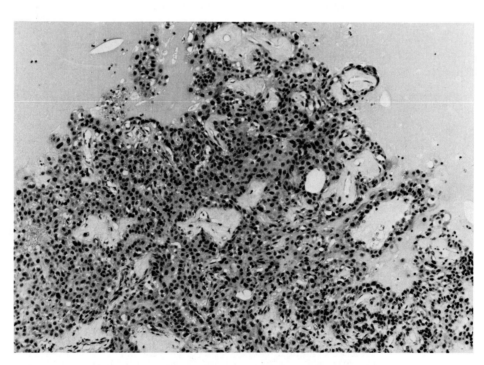

FIGURE 24-9. Apocrine cystadenocarcinoma in a dog. The epithelial cells lining this papillary structure have pleomorphic, hyperchromatic nuclei and loss of polarity. (×120.)

than in adenomas, nucleoli are prominent, and mitotic figures are easily detected. Secretory activity and apical blebbing are not obvious. Stromal invasion is rare.

Well-differentiated apocrine adenocarcinoma (Figure 24-10). This variant of sweat gland carcinoma, which is the most common in dogs, is architecturally similar to apocrine glandular adenomas with tubular or papillary patterns (see preceding discussion). The neoplastic epithelial structures are lined by one or more layers of cuboidal-to-columnar cells that have

moderately enlarged, vesicular nuclei and small nucleoli. Decapitation secretion and luminal accumulation of secretory material are common. Mitotic activity is low to moderate, and atypical mitoses are present. Secondary ulceration may be present in larger lesions. Stromal invasion is rare.

Poorly differentiated apocrine carcinoma (Figure 24-11). These are infiltrative apocrine neoplasms with ill-defined borders. They are composed of large polygonal cells arranged in acinar patterns, nests, and

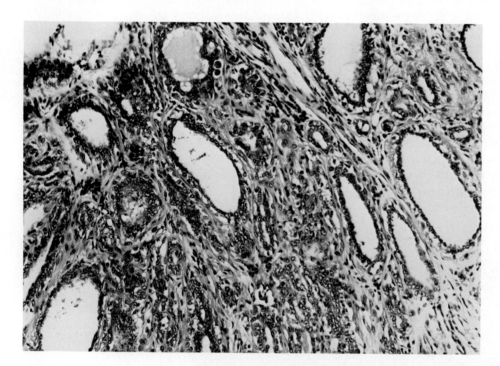

FIGURE 24-10. Well-differentiated apocrine adenocarcinoma in a dog. Epithelial cells have enlarged, vesicular nuclei and small nucleoli. Note that apocrine-type secretory activity is still evident. (×120.)

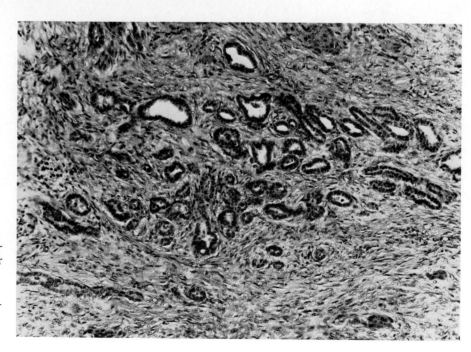

FIGURE 24-11. Apocrine adenocarcinoma in a dog. Irregular glandular structures are distributed through an abundant collagenous stroma. Note the stromal invasion by clusters of tumor cells. (×120.)

trabeculae in varying proportions. All of the poorly differentiated apocrine carcinomas have a moderate-to-abundant stroma of reactive collagenous tissue. Stromal invasion by cords and clusters of neoplastic epithelial cells is common. Ulceration is frequent and is generally a result of superficial dermal invasion.

Neoplastic cells generally have amphophilic cytoplasm and large nuclei with prominent nucleoli and moderately high mitotic activity. Mitotic atypia is frequent. Squamous metaplasia may occur. A rare variant of poorly differentiated apocrine sweat gland carcinoma is the clear-cell, or signet-ring, type. As the name implies, the cytoplasm is clear, and nuclei are usually peripherally displaced by a clear cytoplasmic secretory product, which is presumably glycogen.

Differential diagnosis of poorly differentiated apocrine sweat gland carcinoma includes other anaplastic carcinomas that may be primary or metastatic in the skin. Definitive diagnosis is likely to require immunohistochemical and ultrastructural studies. Distinction from acantholytic (pseudoglandular) squamous cell carcinoma can be difficult in lesions with squamous metaplasia. Active acantholysis, characterized by individualized keratinized cells and elongated intercellular bridges within pseudolumens, supports a diagnosis of squamous cell carcinoma.

Mixed (compound) apocrine adenocarcinoma (Figures 24-12 and 24-13). The majority of mixed apocrine carcinomas have an epithelial component of the well-differentiated type (see preceding discussion). The myoepithelial portion of the tumor usually shows myxoid or chondroid differentiation and has a benign histologic appearance, as in most compound mammary adenocarcinomas. Osseous metaplasia, however, is rare. The mesenchymal component of the tumor contains multiple nodules of small spindle and stellate cells with pale cytoplasm and bland, ovoid-to-fusiform nuclei. The mesenchymal cells are separated by a lightly basophilic mucinous stroma or are entrapped in lacunar spaces within a deeply basophilic chondroid matrix. In rare instances, when the mesenchymal cells demonstrate nuclear atypia and mitotic activity, a designation of apocrine carcinosarcoma or malignant mixed sweat gland tumor is appropriate.

Ductular apocrine adenocarcinoma (Figure 24-14). Another uncommon subtype of apocrine carcinoma resembles canine-type ductular adenoma (see preceding discussion), but is poorly circumscribed and usually lacks the multilobular configuration of its benign counterpart. Ulceration is a frequent feature, and tumor margins are infiltrative. The sparse-to-moderate stroma may have a desmoplastic appearance.

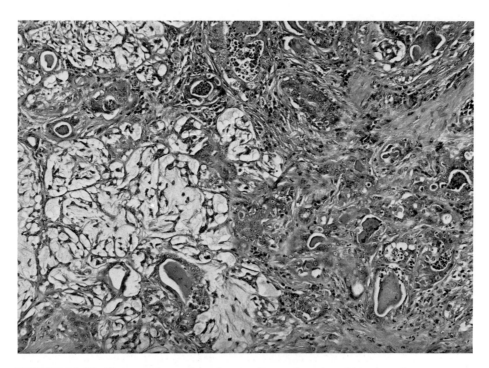

FIGURE 24-12. Compound apocrine adenocarcinoma in a dog. Irregular acinar structures containing secretory material and necrotic debris are lined by one or more layers of epithelial cells. Note the islands of myxoid myoepithelial tissue at left. (×120.)

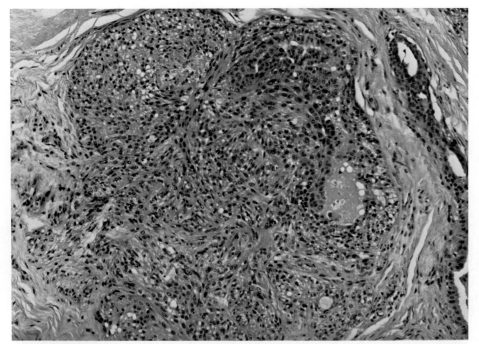

FIGURE 24-13. Compound apocrine adenocarcinoma (carcinosarcoma) in a dog. Papillary structures lined by pleomorphic epithelial cells blend into a large island of plump, spindle-shaped myoepithelial cells. Enlarged, hyperchromatic nuclei are present in both glandular and myoepithelial components. (×120.)

Solid areas and zones of squamous metaplasia may be present.

The neoplastic tubules are generally lined by a double layer of cuboidal epithelial cells, as in ductular adenoma. However, the epithelial cells are larger and more pleomorphic, and the distinction between inner and outer cell types is not apparent. The cells have moderate nuclear pleomorphism and high mitotic activity with atypia.

Differential diagnoses include acantholytic (pseudoglandular) squamous cell carcinoma and metastatic adenocarcinoma. The double layer of cells lining most of the neoplastic glandular structures is the salient feature of apocrine ductal origin.

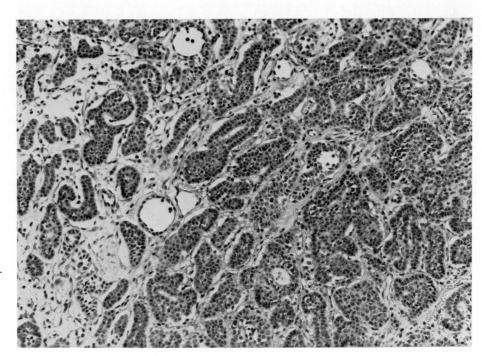

FIGURE 24-14. Ductular apocrine adenocarcinoma in a dog. The irregular glandular structures are frequently lined by a distinct double layer of plump cuboidal cells. (×150.)

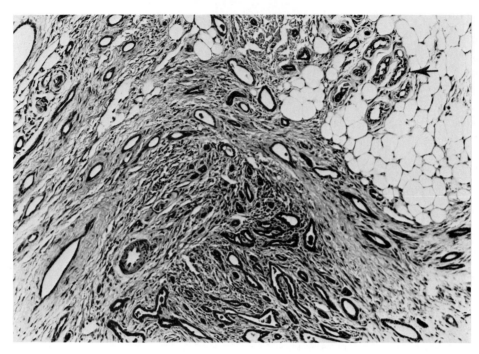

FIGURE 24-15. Eccrine carcinoma in a dog. Irregular glandular structures infiltrate the fat of the footpad. Note the residual eccrine glands at upper right *(arrow)*. (×50.)

ECCRINE CARCINOMA
Clinical features

Neoplasms of eccrine sweat glands are extremely rare in dogs and cats. This is not unexpected because eccrine glands are limited to the footpads and are few in number compared with apocrine sweat glands. In contrast, more than 15 categories of eccrine tumors exist in humans. It is unusual, however, that benign tumors of eccrine sweat glands are virtually nonexistent in animals. A single case of eccrine adenoma in a dog is mentioned by Muller, Kirk, and Scott, but there are no other known reports. The authors have occasionally observed eccrine carcinoma in the footpads of cats and dogs.

Eccrine carcinoma appears as a poorly defined swelling of the footpad and digit. Lesions may affect multiple toes in cats. The clinical appearance is indistinguishable from feline digital squamous cell carcinoma (see Chapter 25). Ulceration is common, and lysis of phalangeal bone is generally observed radiographically. Breed and age predilections have not been determined.

Eccrine carcinomas are highly aggressive neoplasms that exhibit rapid metastasis to lymph nodes and subcutaneous tissues of the affected limb. The incidence, if any, of visceral metastasis has not been determined.

Histopathology (Figures 24-15 and 24-16)

Eccrine carcinoma is a poorly circumscribed, infiltrative neoplasm involving the footpad, dermis, and phalangeal bone. Irregular tubuloacinar structures lined by one or more layers of cuboidal-to-polygonal epithelial cells are distributed through an abundant stroma of dense collagen. The neoplastic cells have amphophilic or eosinophilic cytoplasm and large, hyperchromatic nuclei. Nucleoli are usually prominent, and moderate numbers of atypical mitotic figures are present. Small foci of squamous metaplasia may be present, but orderly keratinization with keratin pearl formation is not seen. Glandular lumens often contain small numbers of necrotic cells; secretory material is sometimes observed. Bone invasion by tumor tissue is accompanied by marked desmoplasia and secondary lysis.

The differential diagnosis for eccrine carcinoma is pseudoglandular squamous cell carcinoma. Active acantholysis, characterized by individualized keratinized cells and elongated intercellular bridges within pseudotubules, supports a diagnosis of squamous cell carcinoma. The authors have employed immunohistochemical staining with carcinoembryonic antigen, which is normally present in eccrine duct and luminal cuticle, to distinguish between eccrine carcinoma and squamous cell carcinoma. The possibility of metastatic carcinoma, particularly from lung, should also be ruled out.

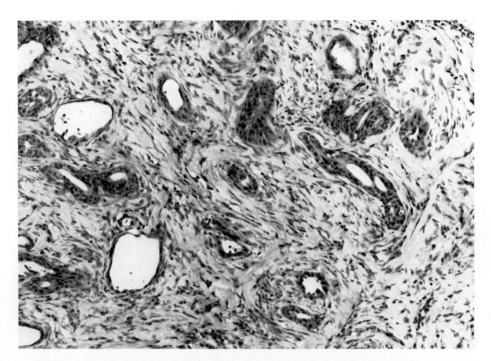

FIGURE 24-16. Eccrine carcinoma in a cat. Irregular glandular structures are lined by one or more layers of pleomorphic epithelial cells. Note the abundant cellular stroma. (×140.)

SUGGESTED READINGS

Apocrine cyst

Hashimoto K, Mehregan AH, and Kamakiri M: Tumors of skin appendages, London, 1987, Butterworth, pp 147-151.

Apocrine cystomatosis

Pulley LT and Stannard AA: Tumors of the skin and soft tissues. In Moulton J, editor: Tumors in domestic animals, ed 3, Berkeley, CA, 1990, University of California Press, p 66.

Apocrine cystadenoma

Bevier DF and Goldschmidt MH: Skin tumors in the dog. I. Epithelial tumors and tumorlike lesions, Comp Cont Ed 3:389-398, 1981.

Hashimoto K, Mehregan AH, and Kamakiri M: Tumors of skin appendages, London, 1987, Butterworth, pp 147-151.

Apocrine adenoma

Bevier DF and Goldschmidt MH: Skin tumors in the dog. I. Epithelial tumors and tumorlike lesions, Comp Cont Ed 3:389-398, 1981.

Diters RW and Walsh KM: Feline basal cell tumors: a review of 124 cases, Vet Pathol 21:51-56, 1984.

Esplin DG, Bernstein NM, and McLaughlin H: Basaloid adenoma of the mammary gland in two dogs, J Am Vet Med Assoc 184:855-857, 1984.

Hashimoto K, Mehregan AH, and Kamakiri M: Tumors of skin appendages, London, 1987, Butterworth, pp 153-157.

Hassab-El Naby HM and others: Mixed tumors of the skin: a histologic and immunochemical study, Am J Dermatopathol 11:413-428, 1989.

Weiss E and Frese K: Tumours of the skin, Bull World Health Organ 50:79-100, 1974.

Apocrine carcinoma

Bevier DF and Goldschmidt MH: Skin tumors in the dog. I. Epithelial tumors and tumorlike lesions, Comp Cont Ed 3:389-398, 1981.

Hashimoto K, Mehregan AH, and Kamakiri M: Tumors of skin appendages, London, 1987, Butterworth, pp 157-159.

Eccrine carcinoma

Hashimoto K, Mehregan AH, and Kamakiri M: Tumors of skin appendages, London, 1987, Butterworth, pp 66-79.

Muller GH, Kirk RW, and Scott DW: Small animal dermatology, ed 4, Philadelphia, 1989, WB Saunders, p 873.

Also see General References, pp 327-328.

CHAPTER 25

Nailbed epithelial tumors

Nailbed (subungual) tumors of all types are uncommon in dogs and cats. The actual incidence is difficult to estimate, since epithelial lesions other than squamous cell carcinoma are not usually described in this anatomic location in the veterinary literature. Nonneoplastic lesions, benign tumors, and malignant tumors of the nailbed have many clinical features in common because of the restrictive nature of the anatomy of distal digits and claws. Any expansile mass at this site will result in lameness, digital enlargement, replacement or lysis of the third phalanx, and, in many cases, disruption of normal nail growth.

Because of the similarity in clinical appearance of benign and malignant tumors, as well as the difficulty in obtaining adequate biopsy material by soft-tissue surgical techniques, amputational biopsy of one or more phalanges is the most accurate diagnostic technique for nailbed masses. This procedure is also curative in most cases. Parasagittal soft-tissue sections and midsagittal decalcified sections are required in almost all cases for complete evaluation of the gross architecture and histomorphology of the lesions.

NAILBED EPITHELIAL INCLUSION CYST
Clinical features

Epithelial cysts occur infrequently in a subungual location in dogs and cats. Previous onychectomy sites and dewclaws may be affected. Nailbed cysts are most likely a result of trauma leading to embedment of portions of cuticular or germinative nailbed epithelium in subjacent connective tissue; thus the term *epithelial inclusion cyst* is appropriate.

The primary presenting sign is a single swollen digit. The nail may be cracked or irregular. Radiographically, a zone of partial bone loss in the third phalanx with little periosteal response is present. The cysts are several millimeters to 1.5 cm, but size cannot usually be accurately assessed until a midsagittal section of the digit is made in preparation for histologic processing. The cysts contain semifluid, caseous material that is often pigmented. There is no known age or breed predilection.

Although epithelial inclusion cysts are nonneoplastic lesions, neoplastic transformation may occur in rare instances. The authors have observed a single case of squamous cell carcinoma arising from a nailbed epithelial inclusion cyst in a dog. A similar phenomenon occurring in human cutaneous epidermal cysts has been described by Lever.

Histopathology (Figure 25-1)

Nailbed inclusion cysts have a similar histologic appearance to follicular cysts of infundibular origin (see Chapter 22). The cyst is lined by a thick wall of archi-

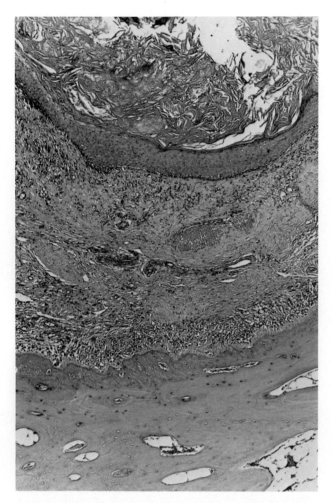

FIGURE 25-1. Nailbed epithelial inclusion cyst in a dog. A squamous epithelium-lined cyst filled with lamellar keratin is at top; phalangeal bone is at bottom. (×120.)

tecturally normal squamous epithelium, which keratinizes through a granular cell layer. The cyst lumen contains laminated keratin. The epithelium and keratinous cyst contents are often melanized in animals with dark haircoats and claws. The surrounding connective tissue often has mild infiltration by lymphocytes and plasma cells. Pressure-induced lysis and replacement of the third phalanx occur in proportion to the expanding cyst. There may be degeneration of the cyst wall accompanied by a granulomatous or pyogranulomatous inflammatory response to released keratin.

NAILBED INVERTED SQUAMOUS PAPILLOMA
Clinical features

Nailbed (subungual) inverted squamous papilloma is an uncommon benign neoplasm of dogs arising from the germinative epithelium of the claw. This lesion has not been described in a subungual location, but appears to be identical to inverted squamous papilloma arising in haired skin (see Chapter 21). The etiology of the subungual inverted squamous papilloma is unknown, but it is probable that it also is virally induced. Ultrastructural studies and immunohistochemical staining for canine papillomavirus antigen may provide further evidence in this regard.

Squamous papilloma of the nailbed appears as a single swollen digit usually with a thickened, abnormally soft claw. The nail may be broken or absent. Secondary ulceration is sometimes present. Radiographs usually show moderate-to-marked destruction of the third phalanx; periosteal proliferation of the second phalanx may also be observed.

Midsagittal section of the toe reveals a well-delineated, cup-shaped mass filled with dense keratin that usually measures less than 1 cm in diameter. In some cases, the entire nailbed has been diffusely replaced by the neoplasm. This is manifested by diffuse expansion of the nailbed, which results in a severely thickened claw without an obvious mass at its base. There is no known age or breed predisposition.

Histopathology (Figures 25-2 and 25-3)

The nailbed inverted squamous papilloma is a well-circumscribed, cup-shaped mass filled with compact keratin. The wall of the cup is a thick layer of squamous epithelial cells that form delicate conical projections extending centripetally into the keratin core. The epithelial papillae are frequently sectioned tangentially and appear as ovoid or circular structures entrapped in compact keratin. The papillae have narrow cores of bland connective tissue. In lesions in which the nailbed is diffusely replaced by neoplastic epithelium, the conical papillae have a more parallel orientation to one another, and the columns of soft keratin produced by the tumor papillae project into and partially replace the hard keratin of the claw.

The majority of the epithelial cells have moderate, pale-pink, glassy cytoplasm. Keratinization proceeds in an orderly pattern through a sparse granular cell layer. Nuclei are small and vesicular with inconspicuous nucleoli. Occasional neoplastic epithelial cells may exhibit cytoplasmic vacuolation resembling koilocytosis, which is a marker for viral induction in other papillomas (see Chapter 21). Mitotic activity is low, and mitotic figures are limited to the basal cell layer at the periphery of the mass. The third phalanx exhibits pressure-induced lysis and replacement in proportion to the size of the neoplasm. Periosteal fibrosis, periosteal bone proliferation, and secondary inflammation may be observed.

Differentiation between inverted squamous papilloma and squamous cell carcinoma of the nailbed may

FIGURE 25-2. Nailbed inverted squamous papilloma in a dog. Conical structures project into the central compact keratin core. Note the well-circumscribed tumor margin at bottom. (×50.)

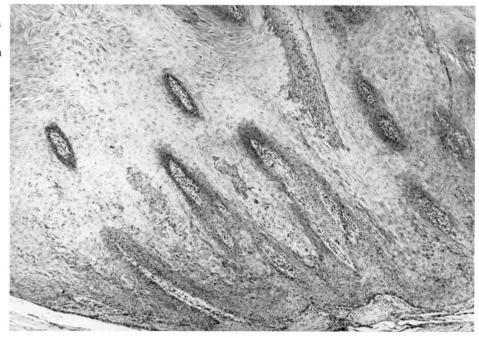

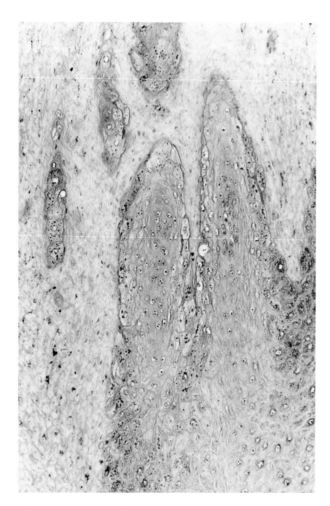

FIGURE 25-3. Nailbed inverted squamous papilloma in a dog. Note the glassy cytoplasm, sparse granular cell layer, and slight cytoplasmic vacuolation. (×160.)

be required, but the diagnosis is usually straightforward. Inverted squamous papilloma has smooth margins with no invasive tendencies. Nuclei are uniform, and mitotic figures are infrequent. The distinction between inverted squamous papilloma and subungual keratoacanthoma may be more difficult. Keratoacanthoma has islands, sheets, and peripheral trabeculae of epithelial cells in contrast to the uniform wall of cells characterizing the inverted squamous papilloma. Keratoacanthoma does not possess the central conical epithelial projections of the inverted papilloma.

NAILBED KERATOACANTHOMA
Clinical features

Nailbed (subungual) keratoacanthoma is a rare, benign neoplasm of dogs that arises from the nailbed epithelium. It is not analogous to infundibular keratinizing acanthoma, which has previously been referred to as *keratoacanthoma* in the veterinary literature (see Chapter 22). This neoplasm appears to be identical to subungual keratoacanthoma in humans, which does not undergo spontaneous involution (in contrast to human cutaneous keratoacanthoma). In a small retrospective study of 21 canine nailbed epithelial neoplasms done by one of the authors,* 9 of the tumors were biologically and histologically compatible with a diagnosis of keratoacanthoma. These data suggest that benign neoplasms may be as common as malignant neoplasms of the nailbed. Subungual keratoacanthoma

* Emily J. Walder.

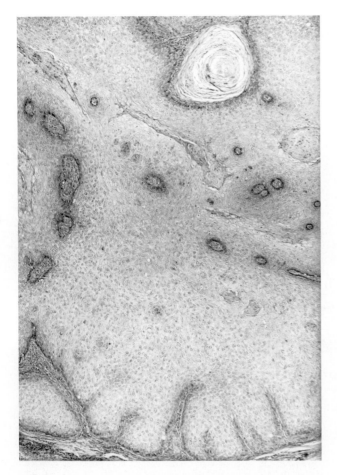

FIGURE 25-4. Nailbed keratoacanthoma in a dog. Broad sheets and trabeculae are composed of pale, glassy keratinocytes. Note the circumscribed but irregular margin of the tumor at bottom. (×50.)

in dogs was probably previously diagnosed as well-differentiated squamous cell carcinoma.

Subungual keratoacanthoma appears as a single, often severely swollen digit. Focal ulceration may be present. Almost all cases have radiographic evidence of lysis of the third phalanx. Lysis of the second phalanx and periosteal bone proliferation are observed less commonly. Affected digits may have deformed or broken claws. Midsagittal section of the toe reveals an unencapsulated mass with an irregular central zone of caseous keratin. Lesions are generally less than 1.5 cm in diameter.

There is no apparent breed or sex predilection. Affected animals in the study ranged from 6.5 to 13 years of age. Eight of nine cases were followed up for 8 months to 2 years, and no evidence of recurrence or metastasis was seen after digital amputation.

Histopathology (Figures 25-4 through 25-6)

Subungual keratoacanthomas are symmetric, circumscribed, but unencapsulated masses with a cup-shaped or inverted funnel-shaped configuration. The tumor borders are somewhat irregular or scalloped. The mass has a central core of keratin that may open onto the skin surface directly ventral or adjacent to the nail. The epithelial wall of the neoplasm is contiguous with the nailbed epithelium. The wall is composed of large squamous epithelial cells arranged in sheets, islands, and broad trabeculae. Orderly keratinization proceeds centripetally and without a granular cell layer (tricholemmal-type keratinization; see follicular cyst, Chapter 22), resulting in a central core of amorphous keratin. Many tumors have large lakes of parakeratotic

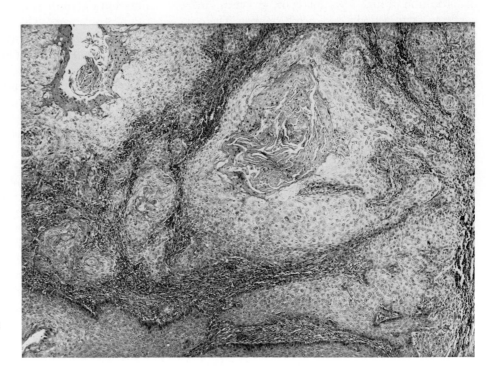

FIGURE 25-5. Nailbed keratoacanthoma in a dog shows two cores of parakeratotic cells within irregular epithelial islands. (×50.)

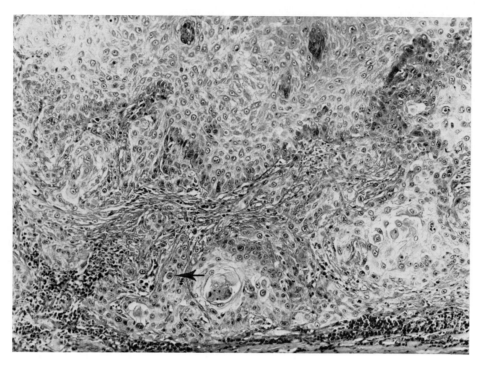

FIGURE 25-6. Higher power view of the keratoacanthoma in Figure 25-5 shows glassy cytoplasm and scattered apoptotic keratinocytes *(arrow)*. Note the mild cytologic atypia and infiltrative tendencies at the tumor margin. (×120.)

cells without nuclear atypia admixed with the amorphous keratin in the central zone.

The majority of epithelial cells have abundant, pink cytoplasm with a ground-glass appearance. This is a manifestation of high glycogen content, which can be confirmed with periodic acid–Schiff staining. There are small-to-moderate numbers of apoptotic keratinocytes, which are characterized by rounded-up, brightly eosinophilic cytoplasm and pyknotic nuclei. Occasional keratoacanthomas are composed predominantly of these apoptotic cells; the significance of this degenerative alteration is unknown. Most nuclei are moderately enlarged and vesicular with small nucleoli. Small numbers of atypical epithelial cells with amphophilic cytoplasm, enlarged nuclei, and prominent nuclei are present at the periphery of most tumors. Mitotic activity is low and is also confined to this proliferating peripheral zone.

The third phalanx exhibits pressure lysis in proportion to the size of the expansile neoplastic mass. Tumor tissue does not invade into the interstitium of the bone. Large keratoacanthomas may cause complete destruction of the third phalanx, but tumor tissue does not cross the interphalangeal joint space. The connective tissue surrounding the mass has a moderate-to-marked infiltrate of plasma cells and neutrophils. Periosteal fibrosis and bone proliferation are often present. Sec-

ondary osteomyelitis may be observed. Chronic proliferative and inflammatory changes may be present in the synovial tissue of the interphalangeal joint.

Differentiation between subungual keratoacanthoma and well-differentiated squamous cell carcinoma is often problematic. This is especially true if specimens are too small or tangential to allow adequate visualization of tumor architecture. Low-power features of a symmetric, but complex cellular wall and central keratin core are critical diagnostic features of keratoacanthoma. Soft tissue sections from the margin of a keratoacanthoma will often contain short trabeculae with atypical cells and mitotic figures, leading to an erroneous diagnosis of malignancy. Bone invasion is not observed in keratoacanthoma but is a common finding in squamous cell carcinoma. Periodic acid–Schiff reactivity has been proposed by King as an aid in distinguishing between keratoacanthoma and squamous cell carcinoma based on the high glycogen content of the former. Unfortunately, many well-differentiated subungual squamous cell carcinomas also show strong periodic acid–Schiff positivity, although the staining pattern may be irregular. Differentiation of keratoacanthoma from inverted squamous papilloma is based on the greater complexity and irregularity of the epithelial wall and on the absence of uniform, central papillary projections.

NAILBED SQUAMOUS CELL CARCINOMA

Clinical features

Squamous cell carcinoma arising from the nailbed epithelium is rare in dogs and even more rare in cats. A German survey cited by Theilen reported that approximately 60% of cutaneous squamous cell carcinomas in dogs arise in digits. However, more recent studies of nailbed squamous cell carcinomas by Liu and also Madewell indicate an incidence of 0.2% of all canine neoplasms. Subungual squamous cell carcinomas are mentioned in only one large survey on feline cutaneous tumors by Macy. In a study of bone tumors in cats by Quigley, only 1 of 25 squamous cell carcinomas involved phalangeal bone.

Nailbed squamous cell carcinoma is usually solitary but may affect multiple digits in both species. The presenting signs are similar to benign nailbed tumors and include lameness, digital swelling, deformity or loss of the nail, and radiographic evidence of phalangeal lysis. Ulceration is more common and generally more extensive than is observed with benign tumors. According to Madewell and Theilen, chronic paronychia often precedes and accompanies the development of nailbed squamous cell carcinoma. Periosteal bone proliferation is common. The appearance on midsagittal section of the digit varies considerably, depending on the degree of histologic differentiation. Tumor size varies from 0.5 to greater than 2 cm. Some lesions are well circumscribed, whereas others are diffusely infiltrative. Keratin production, manifested grossly by deposits of caseous yellow-white material, may be focal and centrally located in small, well-differentiated tumors. Larger tumors often have numerous small zones of keratinization. Poorly differentiated squamous cell carcinomas may have no gross evidence of keratin production.

In a report of multicentric subungual squamous cell carcinoma by Madewell, all of the cases were in large-breed dogs with black haircoats. Seven of twelve cases of solitary squamous cell carcinoma reviewed by one of the authors* were also in large-breed dogs, two of which were Kerry Blue Terriers. Affected animals in all studies were 7 years of age or older.

The reported metastatic incidence of these neoplasms varies markedly. Part of the inconsistency in reports of biologic behavior may be due to failure to distinguish squamous cell carcinomas involving digital skin or bone from those which truly arise from ungual epithelium. In a study of five cases by Liu, one dog had widespread nodal and visceral metastasis at the time of presentation; this is such atypical behavior for cutaneous squamous cell carcinoma that the authors suspect

that the digital neoplasm may have been a metastasis from a visceral site, such as lung. Ten dogs in Walder's survey were followed up for 9 months to 2 years; only one developed regional lymph node metastasis after digital amputation. Feline subungual squamous cell carcinomas, in contrast, are fairly aggressive neoplasms with frequent subcutaneous and nodal metastasis. However, of interest is a report by Pollack that showed several cases of multicentric feline digital carcinoma to be metastases from pulmonary epidermoid carcinoma.

Histopathology (Figures 25-7 and 25-8)

Subungual squamous cell carcinomas are unencapsulated, asymmetric neoplasms with focal or multifocal connection to nailbed epithelium. Tumor margins are irregular and infiltrative. The architecture and morphology of the neoplastic epithelial cell aggregates are identical to well-differentiated, poorly differentiated, or acantholytic variants of squamous cell carcinoma in other anatomic locations (see Chapter 21). The majority of subungual squamous cell carcinomas are of the well-differentiated type with readily identifiable foci of keratinization. All tumor types are accompanied by a desmoplastic stromal response. Infiltrates of plasma cells and neutrophils are present and may be severe in extensively ulcerated lesions.

The third phalanx shows lysis and periosteal bone proliferation, and the medullary spaces are infiltrated by aggregations of neoplastic squamous epithelial cells. Osteomyelitis may be present. The interphalangeal joint may show invasion by squamous cell carcinoma in addition to chronic synovitis. More commonly, neoplastic tissue does not violate the joint space but extends along the periosteum and infiltrates periarticular connective tissue. The second phalanx may also show lysis and periosteal proliferation, and occasional foci of neoplastic epithelial cells may be present in the distal medulla. More proximal portions of the second phalanx are rarely involved.

The primary differential diagnosis for well-differentiated nailbed squamous cell carcinoma is keratoacanthoma. Keratoacanthomas are recognizable in most cases by their symmetry, central keratin cores, and absence of bone invasion. The epithelial cells of keratoacanthoma usually contain more abundant, uniformly distributed glycogen than those of squamous cell carcinoma. The differential diagnosis for the rare acantholytic variant of subungual squamous cell carcinoma is eccrine carcinoma arising from the footpad. Serial sections to establish connection to ungual epithelium, as well as immunohistochemical stains for carcinoembryonic antigen (found in glandular neoplasms), are useful in differentiation. In cases of multicentric digital squamous cell carcinoma of any histologic subtype, a differential diagnosis of metastatic carcinoma must always be considered.

---

* Emily J. Walder.

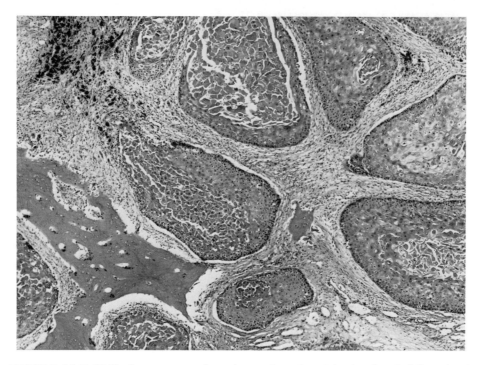

FIGURE 25-7. Nailbed squamous cell carcinoma in a dog. Islands of well-differentiated squamous epithelial cells invade phalangeal bone. Note the early acantholysis in the centers of the tumor islands. (×50.)

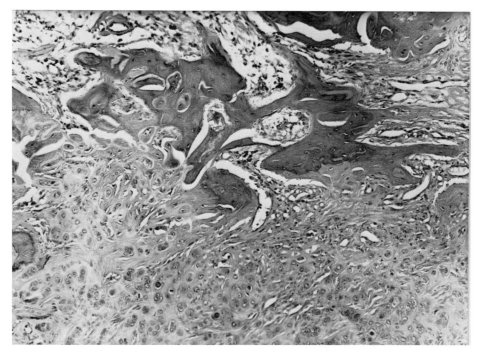

FIGURE 25-8. Poorly differentiated nailbed squamous cell carcinoma in a dog. Epithelial cells arranged individually and in clusters diffusely infiltrate phalangeal bone. (×120.)

SUGGESTED READINGS

Nailbed epithelial inclusion cyst

Lever WF and Schaumburg-Lever G: Histopathology of the skin, ed 7, Philadelphia, 1990, JB Lippincott, pp 535-536.

Nailbed inverted squamous papilloma

Campbell KL and others: Cutaneous inverted papillomas in dogs, Vet Pathol 25:67-71, 1988.

Nailbed keratoacanthoma

King DF and Barr RJ: Intraepithelial elastic fibers and intracytoplasmic glycogen: diagnostic aids in differentiating keratoacanthoma from squamous cell carcinoma, J Cutan Pathol 7:140-148, 1980.

Stoll DM and Ackerman AB: Subungual keratoacanthoma, Am J Dermatopathol 2:265-271, 1981.

Walder EJ and Barr RJ: Subungual keratoacanthoma in the dog: a clinicopathologic review of 9 cases and comparison to subungual squamous cell carcinoma. Proceedings of the Thirty-Fifth Annual Meeting of the American College of Veterinary Pathologists, Toronto, p 24, 1984.

Nailbed squamous cell carcinoma

Bevier DF and Goldschmidt MH: Skin tumors in the dog. I. Epithelial tumors and tumorlike lesions, Comp Cont Ed 3:389-398, 1981.

Liu S-K and Hohn BR: Squamous cell carcinoma of the digit of the dog, J Am Vet Med Assoc 153:411-424, 1968.

Macy DW and Reynolds HA: The incidence, characteristics and clinical management of skin tumors of cats, J Am Anim Hosp Assoc 17:1026-1034, 1981.

Madewell BR and others: Multiple subungual squamous cell carcinomas in five dogs, J Am Vet Med Assoc 180:731-734, 1982.

Pollack M, Martin RA, and Diters RW: Metastatic squamous cell carcinoma in multiple digits of a cat: a case report, J Am Anim Hosp Assoc 20:835-836, 1984.

Quigley PJ and Leedale AH: Tumors involving bone in the domestic cat: a review of fifty-eight cases, Vet Pathol 20:670-686, 1983.

Theilen GH and Madewell BR, editors: Veterinary cancer medicine, ed 2, Philadelphia, 1987, Lea & Febiger, pp 242-244.

Walder EJ and Barr RJ: Subungual keratoacanthoma in the dog: a clinicopathologic review of 9 cases and comparison to subungual squamous cell carcinoma. Proceedings of the Thirty-Fifth Annual Meeting of the American College of Veterinary Pathologists, Toronto, p 24, 1984.

See also General References, pp 327-328.

PART VI

Mesenchymal neoplasia

Fibrocytic tumors

COLLAGENOUS NEVUS
Clinical features

The concepts of *nevus* and *hamartoma* tend to be elusive and confusing in most pathology texts, but Mehregan's working definition of a nevus as a circumscribed, stable malformation of skin of presumed congenital or hereditary origin creates a category that has applications in veterinary dermatopathology. In contrast to a nevus, a hamartoma also has a presumed congenital basis but tends to deviate more from the normal histologic structure and may show more extensive growth. The terms nevus and hamartoma are used almost interchangeably and are often selected more by convention than by strict adherence to definition. Although the underlying tissue abnormality in any type of nevus or hamartoma is theoretically present at birth, lesions may not become clinically apparent until later in life. Late recognition of nevi and hamartomas is particularly common in animals, and this may be sometimes explained by the fact that thick pelage makes early small or nonelevated lesions difficult to detect. In other instances, however, nevoid and hamartomatous lesions occurring in adult animals may be acquired rather than congenital.

Collagenous nevus is a relatively common lesion in dogs characterized by a focal excess of dermal collagen. Data on the incidence are difficult to provide, since collagenous nevus was not recognized as a separate entity in dogs until it was described by Scott in 1984. Lesions in animals were probably identified previously as fibromas.

Collagenous nevus usually appears as a solitary, dome- or gumdrop-shaped, firm nodule measuring less than 1 cm in diameter. The overlying skin is intact, alopecic, and frequently hyperpigmented. Lesions occur most commonly on the head, neck, and proximal limbs.

Affected animals are middle aged or older. There is no breed predilection.

Histopathology (Figure 26-1)

Collagenous nevus is a noncircumscribed, nodular focus of redundant dermal collagen that involves primarily the superficial dermis. The collagen of the nevus has a similar fiber pattern to that of the adjacent dermis. Collagen bundles may be slightly thicker or more compact than in the normal dermis. Adnexa within the nodule are decreased in number or absent; when present, they show mild atrophy and architectural distortion. Fibroblasts are not obviously increased in size or number. Inflammation is not observed. The overlying epidermis frequently contains increased melanin pigment.

Differential diagnoses for collagenous nevus include fibroma, nodular dermatofi-

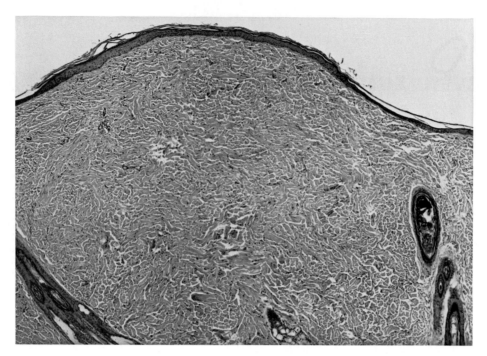

FIGURE 26-1. Collagenous nevus in a dog characterized by a dome-shaped nodule of redundant collagen within the dermis. (×50.)

brosis, and nodular scar. Fibromas in the dermis are usually larger than collagenous nevi and often encroach on the subcutis. Fibromas are slightly more cellular and have a repetitive, swirled or interlacing pattern of collagen fibers. Nodular dermatofibrosis is a multicentric condition, whereas collagenous nevus is almost always solitary. The lesions of nodular dermatofibrosis affect the full thickness of the dermis and often encroach on the subcutis. Hair follicles within the nodules of dermatofibrosis are hyperplastic rather than atrophic, and secondary inflammation is common. A nodular scar has prominently thickened, often hyalinized collagen bundles, and the overlying epidermis is hyperplastic.

NODULAR DERMATOFIBROSIS
Clinical features

This recently described rare syndrome in German Shepherd Dogs is characterized by multiple fibromatous nodules in the skin that serve as a marker for renal epithelial neoplasia. Several familial syndromes of multiple cutaneous tumors associated with specific internal malignancies exist in humans; this is the first such entity to be documented in animals. Many of the dogs in the study by Lium had a common ancestor, supporting a genetic basis for this syndrome.

The lesions of nodular dermatofibrosis appear as firm dermal and subcutaneous nodules, which are well circumscribed and vary from several millimeters to 4 cm in diameter. The overlying skin may show irregular thickening and hyperpigmentation. Larger lesions are often alopecic and ulcerated. Lesions are found primarily on limbs, head, and ears.

The average age of affected animals was 8 years in Lium's study. There was no sex predilection. The renal neoplasms are usually cystadenocarcinomas, which are often multicentric and bilateral. The metastatic rate of the renal tumors is approximately 20%.

Histopathology (Figures 26-2 and 26-3)

The dermal lesions of nodular dermatofibrosis are characterized by focal dermal thickening because of increased numbers of slightly thickened collagen bundles. There is no obvious demarcation of the lesions from the adjacent normal dermis. However, the deep margins of the dermal lesions often encroach upon and are well demarcated from the subjacent subcutaneous fat. The subcutaneous lesions are well-circumscribed nodules and plaques of mature collagen that are usually contiguous with deep dermal collagen. Fibrocytes are not increased in the dermal or subcutaneous lesions, and the collagen is ultrastructurally normal.

Adnexa within the lesions may appear essentially normal, but hair follicles are more commonly hyperplastic and hyperkeratotic. The overlying epidermis has mild-to-moderate hyperplasia. Larger lesions may have secondary folliculitis, furunculosis, and ulceration, but smaller lesions are usually noninflammatory.

The histologic appearance of this dermatosis can be subtle, and differentiation from scarring inflamma-

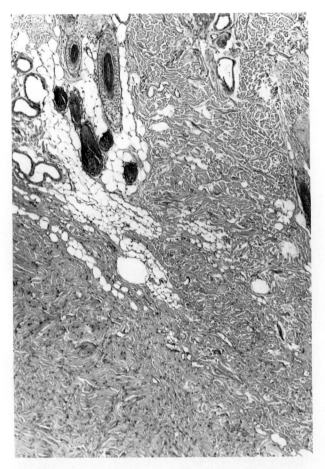

FIGURE 26-2. Nodular dermatofibrosis in a German Shepherd Dog. A poorly demarcated zone of dermal fibrosis is contiguous with a collagenous nodule in the panniculus. Note that the adnexa appear undisturbed. (×50.)

tory diseases, collagenous nevi, and fibromas may be difficult in incisional or punch biopsy specimens unless an appropriate clinical history increases the index of suspicion. Multiple excisional biopsies provide the most useful diagnostic material. Collagenous nevi are usually solitary, affect primarily the superficial dermis, and have atrophic adnexa. Fibromas are slightly more cellular than lesions of nodular dermatofibrosis and have a more complex pattern of collagen bundles.

SKIN TAG (Synonyms: skin polyp, acrochordon)
Clinical features

Skin tag is an uncommon, hyperplastic lesion of redundant epidermis and dermal collagen in dogs and cats. Skin polyps may be a proliferative response to trauma or resolving focal furunculosis.

Skin tags are solitary or multiple, polypoid or filiform masses that are usually several millimeters in diameter and less than 1 cm in length. Sternal and limb lesions may be up to 3 cm in length and 1 cm in diameter. The overlying epidermis is thickened, alopecic, and often hyperpigmented. Larger lesions may be focally eroded. Lesions are usually truncal but may also occur at pressure points on the limbs.

Affected animals are middle aged or older. There is no known breed predilection.

Histopathology (Figure 26-4)

Skin tags are composed of mature collagen resembling the meshwork pattern of normal dermis but may have slightly increased vascularity. Collagen bundles in the larger polyps may be thicker and more tightly

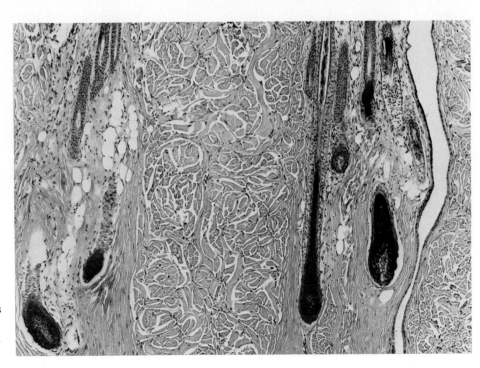

FIGURE 26-3. Higher power view of nodular dermatofibrosis shows slightly thickened collagen bundles and low cellularity. (×150.)

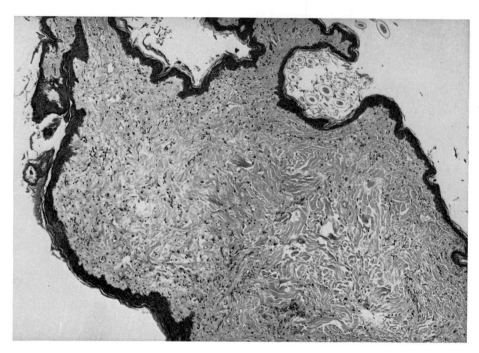

FIGURE 26-4. Skin tag in a dog. The small polypoid mass is composed of mature collagen with a sprinkling of inflammatory cells. Note the digitated configuration of overlying epithelium. (×50.)

packed than those of normal dermis. Hair follicles and adnexal glands are not present within the polyp. The overlying epidermis is acanthotic and hyperkeratotic and often has a digitated configuration. Increased epidermal melanin is frequently observed. Larger lesions often have a sprinkling of mononuclear inflammatory cells below the epidermis. Foci of erosion are accompanied by serocellular crusting and a dermal infiltrate of neutrophils and plasma cells. Hair follicles in the underlying dermis may exhibit hyperplasia, hyperkeratosis, or degeneration accompanied by trichogranuloma formation.

Differential diagnosis of a skin tag is limited because of the distinctive filiform or cylindric conformation of the lesion. Larger polypoid skin tags are differentiated from polypoid fibromas by the presence of deep and superficial inflammation, increased vascularity, and the absence of a repetitive swirled or bundled collagen fiber pattern.

DERMATOFIBROMA
Clinical features

Dermatofibroma is a rare fibrocytic tumor that occurs primarily in cats but is seen occasionally in dogs. In humans, dermatofibroma is usually included in the benign fibrohistiocytic group of tumors, but controversy exists as to whether many of the lesions in this group are reactive or neoplastic. Lever and also Enzinger state that human dermatofibromas do not undergo involution, supporting a neoplastic etiology. In contrast, Ackerman reports that human dermatofibro-

mas are a form of fibrosing dermatitis in response to trauma or arthropod bites and that the lesions slowly regress. The authors believe that dermatofibroma of dogs and cats may be a reactive proliferation of dermal fibrocytes rather than a true neoplasm, but conclusive data are not available. The natural progression of dermatofibroma in animals has not been studied, since biopsies of these lesions are invariably excisional rather than incisional.

Dermatofibromas appear as solitary, firm, circumscribed dermal nodules that are generally less than 2 cm in diameter. The overlying epidermis is alopecic and thickened. Lesions occur most often on the head, but other sites may be affected.

Affected animals are usually less than 5 years of age. There is no known breed predisposition.

Histopathology (Figures 26-5 through 26-7)

Dermatofibroma is a circumscribed, but unencapsulated dermal mass comprising spindle and stellate fibrocytic cells arranged in haphazard bundles and small whorls. The lesion extends to the dermal-epidermal junction. The tumor cells are interspersed with a moderate stroma composed of collagen fibers and bundles of varying thickness, some of which may represent preexisting dermal collagen. The whorls of fibrocytes are frequently oriented around thick collagen bundles seen in cross-section. Mineralization of collagen bundles is occasionally observed. The central portion of the nodule may have decreased cellularity as compared to the periphery, suggesting centrifugal regression. The margins of dermatofibroma often have a

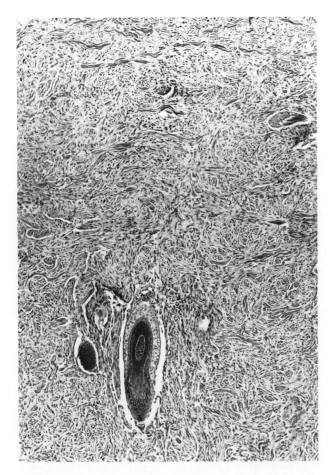

FIGURE 26-5. Dermatofibroma in a cat. Fibrocytic cells and collagen fibers are arranged in haphazard bundles and small whorls. Note the moderate cellularity. (×55.)

ragged appearance because of dissection of collagen bundles of the adjacent dermis by the fibrocytic cells.

The cells of dermatofibroma have scant, pale cytoplasm. Nuclei are fusiform and hyperchromatic. Nucleoli are inconspicuous, and mitotic figures are rare.

Differential diagnoses for dermatofibroma include fibroma, well-differentiated fibrosarcoma, and schwannoma. Fibroma has lower cellularity, a uniform collagen fiber diameter, more repetitive bundled or swirled patterning of the fibrocytic cells, and no interaction between the tumor cells and preexisting collagen bundles. The cellularity of dermatofibroma may be similar to that of well-differentiated fibrosarcoma and schwannoma (benign or malignant), but the haphazard fibrocyte arrangement mimicking normal dermal collagen, minimal mitotic activity, and entrapment of thickened collagen bundles indicate a dermatofibroma.

FIBROMA
Clinical features

Fibromas are uncommon, benign fibrocytic neoplasms of dogs and cats that arise in the dermis or subcutis. Fibromas comprise 2% to 3.5% of canine skin and subcutaneous tumors in most surveys.

Fibromas appear as solitary, firm or rubbery, circumscribed masses with an ovoid, dome-shaped or polypoid conformation. Fibromas usually range from 1 to 5 cm but are occasionally much larger. The overlying epidermis is often alopecic and atrophic. Ulceration may be present in larger lesions. Affected animals are middle aged or older. Limbs and flanks are frequently reported sites. There is no breed predilection.

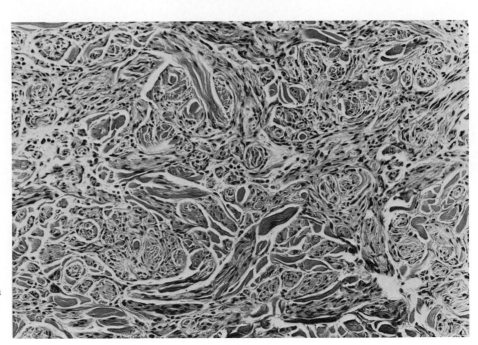

FIGURE 26-6. Higher power of the dermatofibroma in Figure 26-5 showing thick collagen bundles entrapped by whorls of proliferating fibrocytes and delicate collagen fibers. (×140.)

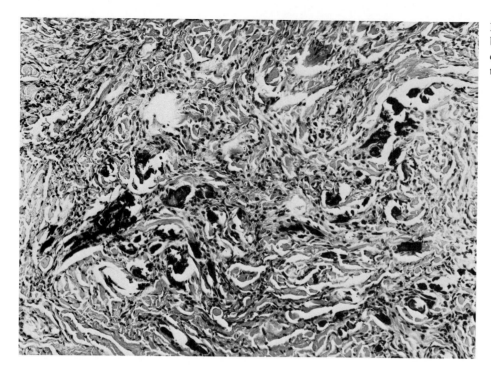

FIGURE 26-7. Dermatofibroma in a cat. Note the patchy calcification of collagen fibers at the base of the lesion. (×120.)

Histopathology (Figure 26-8)

Dermal fibromas are small and circumscribed but unencapsulated. They often blend gradually into adjacent dermal collagen. Subcutaneous fibromas are well circumscribed and usually are larger than their dermal counterparts. Fibromas are composed of collagen bundles that are generally thicker and have more repetitive patterns than those of normal dermis. The collagen of a fibroma is often arranged in interlacing bundles with a slightly undulating configuration. Broad swirls or waves of collagen may also be observed. The stroma may also contain small amounts of mucin. The overlying epidermis is generally normal or atrophic. Adnexal structures are usually completely displaced by the col-

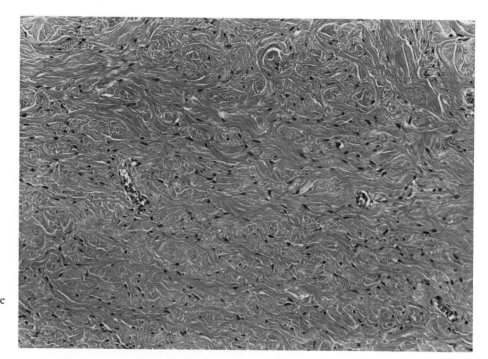

FIGURE 26-8. Fibroma in a dog. Collagen fibers and fibrocytes are arranged in a repetitive pattern of interlacing bundles and swirls. Note the low cellularity. (×120.)

lagen of dermal fibromas, but adnexal entrapment is occasionally noted.

Cellularity is low; small fibrocytic cells are distributed between the collagen bundles. The fibrocyte nuclei are slightly enlarged, fusiform, and euchromatic. Nucleoli are inconspicuous, and mitotic figures are rarely observed.

Differential diagnoses for fibroma include collagenous nevus, nodular scar, nodular dermatofibrosis, schwannoma, and skin tag. Differentiation of dermal fibroma from collagenous nevus can be problematic, particularly when adnexal entrapment is present in fibroma. Fibromas are more discrete and are often somewhat more cellular than collagenous nevi, and the collagen bundles are not arranged in a normal irregular dermal pattern, as they are in collagenous nevus. The collagen bundles of a nodular scar are thicker and more dense than those in fibroma, and there is usually some residual evidence of an inflammatory etiology, such as prominent acanthosis and hyperkeratosis or residual inflammatory cells. Differentiation of fibroma from nodular dermatofibrosis is primarily based upon the clinical history; nodular dermatofibrosis is a multicentric syndrome, whereas fibroma is almost always solitary. Fibromas are slightly more cellular than lesions of nodular dermatofibrosis and have a more repetitive pattern of collagen bundles. In comparison to schwannoma, fibroma is less cellular and lacks palisades and whorls of cells. The stromal collagen is coarser and more abundant in fibroma than in schwannoma. Larger polypoid skin tags are differentiated from polypoid fibromas by the presence of deep and superficial inflammation, increased vascularity, and the absence of a repetitive swirled or bundled collagen fiber pattern.

FIBROSARCOMA
Clinical features

Fibrosarcoma is a malignant neoplasm arising from fibroblasts in any anatomic location. Fibrosarcoma is the most common malignant mesenchymal neoplasm in cats and represented 12% to 25% of all feline skin and subcutaneous tumors in several surveys. In dogs, fibrosarcoma accounted for fewer than 6% of dermal and subcutaneous tumors in surveys from several countries. Most feline fibrosarcomas are subcutaneous, but dermal variants are not uncommon. Most canine neoplasms also arise in the subcutis; pure dermal fibrosarcomas are rare in dogs. The causal relationship between feline sarcoma virus (FeSV) and multicentric fibrosarcoma in young cats is well documented. Hendrick has recently speculated that injection site reactions may eventuate in fibrosarcomas in some cats. The etiology of canine fibrosarcoma is unknown.

Fibrosarcomas are firm, poorly circumscribed, often multilobular masses that vary from less than 1 cm to greater than 15 cm in diameter. Alopecia and ulceration are commonly observed. The majority of feline subcutaneous fibrosarcomas are on the trunk and distal limbs. Pinnae and digits seem to be preferential sites for dermal fibrosarcoma in cats. Most canine fibrosarcomas involve the trunk and proximal limbs.

The average age of animals with fibrosarcoma is 12 years in cats and 10 years in dogs. The FeSV-induced multicentric fibrosarcoma occurs in cats under 5 years of age. Fibrosarcoma is also occasionally reported in dogs under 1 year of age. There is no known breed predisposition.

In both dogs and cats, fibrosarcomas are generally of low-grade malignancy, manifested by frequent local recurrence and a fairly low incidence of distant metastasis occurring late in the course of the disease. The study by Bostock (1980) revealed a recurrence rate of 40% and a metastatic rate of 10% for canine fibrosarcomas. Tumors with a mitotic index (the total number of mitoses per 10 high-power fields) greater than 9 had a significantly higher rate of both recurrence and metastasis.

The overall recurrence rate of feline fibrosarcomas is greater than 70%, and multiple recurrences are common. The metastatic incidence is 11% to 14%, and the lung is the most common site. According to Bostock's work (1979), fibrosarcomas on the pinnae and flank of cats had a much more favorable prognosis than those on the head, thorax, or limbs; this may reflect the relative ease of wide surgical excision at those sites. A mitotic index of less than 5 was also associated with significantly longer survival times.

Histopathology (Figures 26-9 through 26-11)

Fibrosarcomas are irregular, often multilobular neoplasms involving the subcutis, dermis, or both. Some tumors are circumscribed and may be partially encapsulated; others have ill-defined, infiltrative margins. Fibrosarcomas are composed of large spindle cells arranged predominantly in interlacing bundles of varying size. The individual bundles are usually fairly broad, and the angles of intersection are highly variable. Some undulating or swirled cell groupings are often present. The classically described chevron or herringbone pattern of small bundles intersecting at consistent angles is uncommon. Cellularity varies considerably among individual tumors and often from field to field within a given tumor. The major component of the stroma is mature collagen; small amounts of mucin may be present, and small foci of chondroid metaplasia are occasionally observed. In poorly differentiated, highly cellular variants, trichrome stains may be helpful

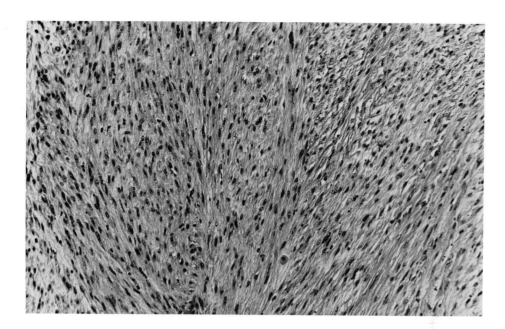

FIGURE 26-9. Fibrosarcoma in a cat. Spindle cells are arranged in broad interlacing bundles in a moderate collagenous stroma. (×140.)

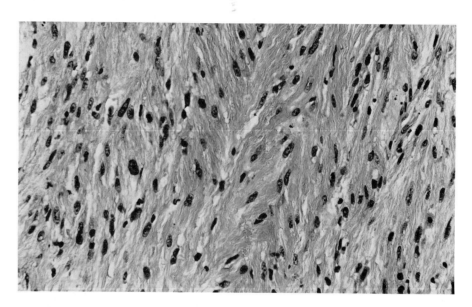

FIGURE 26-10. Higher power view of fibrosarcoma shown in Fig. 26-9 shows pleomorphic ovoid-to-fusiform nuclei, variable chromatin patterns, and prominent nucleoli. (×240.)

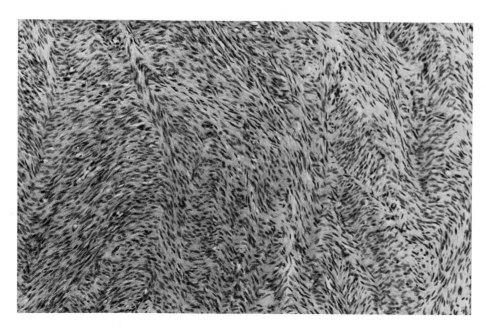

FIGURE 26-11. Fibrosarcoma in a dog. Narrow bundles of spindle cells intersecting at repetitive angles create the uncommon chevron or herringbone pattern. (×120.)

in detecting small amounts of intercellular collagen.

The tumor cells usually have pale, poorly defined, scant cytoplasm. Nuclei are usually ovoid to fusiform and vesicular and have one or more prominent nucleoli. Some neoplasms have a mixture of vesicular and hyperchromatic nuclei. Scattered multinucleated giant cells may also be present. Nuclear hyperchromatism and multinucleation are more commonly observed in feline fibrosarcomas. The mitotic rate of fibrosarcomas is highly variable, and atypical mitotic figures are present. Nuclear morphology and mitotic index do not correlate well with the degree of stromal collagen production. Fibrosarcomas with abundant, sclerotic stroma can have highly malignant cytologic features, whereas cellular neoplasms can be composed of relatively mature fibroblasts. Ulceration, necrosis, and hemorrhage are common secondary features. Lymphoplasmacytic inflammation is frequently observed around tumor margins, especially in feline fibrosarcomas. Occasional fibrosarcomas possess a diffuse inflammatory component comprising lymphocytes, plasma cells, and sometimes eosinophils.

Differential diagnoses for fibrosarcoma include malignant schwannoma, malignant fibrous histiocytoma, dermatofibroma, leiomyosarcoma, and spindle-celled squamous cell carcinoma. Malignant schwannoma usually has a more complex architecture characterized by palisades, whorls, and neuroid structures. Long, serpentine or twisted nuclei are more suggestive of a neural origin. Distinguishing features of malignant fibrous histiocytoma include radiating or cartwheel patterns in the spindle-cell component, admixtures of polygonal histiocytoid cells and multinucleated giant cells, and small amounts of intracellular lipid. Immunohistochemical markers for monocyte origin may help to confirm a diagnosis of malignant fibrous histiocytoma. The cellularity of dermatofibroma may be similar to that of fibrosarcoma, but the nonrepetitive meshwork arrangement of fibrocytes, minimal mitotic activity, and entrapment of thickened collagen bundles indicate a nonneoplastic, proliferative lesion. Leiomyosarcoma is distinguished from fibrosarcoma by the minimal collagenous stroma, abundant cytoplasm with perinuclear vacuoles, and frequent nuclear chromatin crossbars. Trichrome stains and immunohistochemical markers for smooth muscle protein are also beneficial in establishing a definitive diagnosis of leiomyosarcoma. Differentiation from spindle-celled squamous cell carcinoma is particularly important for dermal fibrosarcomas in cats. Spindle-celled squamous cell carcinoma usually shows contiguity with the epidermis and may have foci of keratinization. Immunoperoxidase staining for vimentin and keratin will allow distinction between these two neoplasms.

MYXOMA (Synonym: myxofibroma)
Clinical features

Myxoma is a rare benign neoplasm of dogs and cats arising from fibrocytes (or other primitive mesenchymal cells) that produce more mucin than collagen. The reported incidence in dogs ranges from 0.2% to 0.5%. Most tumors are subcutaneous but may involve the dermis secondarily. Purely intradermal myxomas occur occasionally.

Myxomas are soft, ill-defined masses of variable size; dermal myxomas can be smaller than 1 cm, whereas subcutaneous tumors often attain large proportions. The overlying epidermis may be partially alopecic. The cut surface of myxoma oozes clear, viscous fluid. The majority of myxomas arise on the trunk or limbs.

Affected animals are middle aged or older. There is no known breed prevalence. Myxomas may recur locally because of the difficulty in assessing tumor margins during surgery.

Histopathology (Figure 26-12)

Myxomas are unencapsulated dermal or subcutaneous neoplasms. Subcutaneous myxomas may have poorly defined margins that extend along fascial planes or interlobular septa of the panniculus. Myxomas are composed of small stellate and spindle cells scattered through an abundant stroma of acid mucopolysaccharide rich in hyaluronic acid. The mucinous matrix generally has a slightly basophilic tint with routine histologic stains. The stroma may also contain scant, wavy collagen fibers.

Overall cellularity is low. The tumor cells have discrete, eosinophilic cytoplasm and small, ovoid-to-fusiform nuclei. Nucleoli are inconspicuous, and mitotic figures are rare.

Differential diagnosis for myxoma is limited because of its distinctive stromal characteristics. Occasional variants of schwannoma, particularly neurothekeoma, have abundant stromal mucin. However, myxoid tumors of nerve sheath origin have a multilobular configuration and a tendency for arrangement in concentric whorls. Differentiation between myxoma and myxosarcoma can be problematic, since both the benign and malignant variants may have abundant stroma, low cellularity, and poor circumscription. Cytologic features of malignancy in myxosarcomas are an increased nuclear:cytoplasmic ratio, nuclear pleomorphism and hyperchromatism, and the presence of atypical mitotic figures.

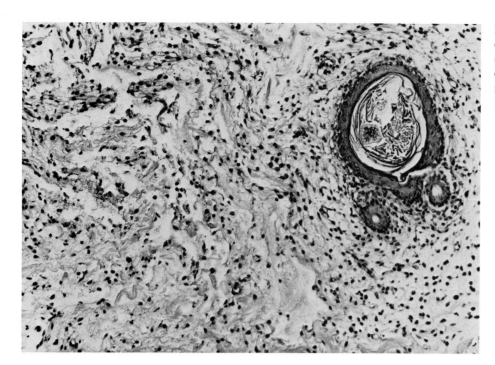

FIGURE 26-12. Myxoma in a dog. Stellate and spindle cells are scattered through an abundant stroma of mucin and small numbers of collagen fibers. (×140.)

MYXOSARCOMA (Synonym: myxofibrosarcoma)

Clinical features

Myxosarcoma is a rare malignancy of dogs and cats arising from altered fibroblasts that produce more mucin than collagen. Myxosarcomas accounted for 1% of all canine cutaneous mesenchymal tumors in a review by Goldschmidt. The clinical features are essentially the same as for myxoma (see discussion above). Secondary ulceration may be present in larger lesions. Myxosarcoma is a low-grade malignancy that exhibits frequent local recurrence and invasion, but distant metastasis is rare. The lung is reported by Pulley to be the most common metastatic site of cutaneous myxosarcoma.

Histopathology (Figures 26-13 and 26-14)

Myxosarcomas are unencapsulated, poorly circumscribed neoplasms involving the subcutis or dermis.

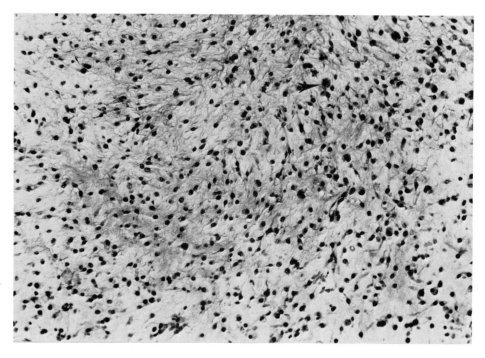

FIGURE 26-13. Myxosarcoma in a dog. Predominantly stellate cells are distributed through an abundant stroma of mucin and collagen fibers. Note that the cellularity is similar to myxoma, but there are hyperchromatic nuclei, scattered binucleated cells, and mitotic figures *(arrow)*. (×120.)

FIGURE 26-14. Myxosarcoma in a cat. Spindle cells predominate. They are arranged in broad fascicles in a moderate stroma of mucin and collagen. Note the nuclear pleomorphism, prominent nucleoli, and mitotic figures. ($\times$120.)

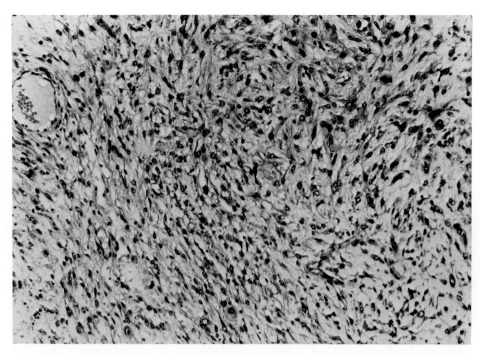

Tumor tissue frequently extends along fascial planes and interlobular septa of the panniculus. Myxosarcomas are composed of pleomorphic stellate and spindle cells distributed haphazardly through an abundant stroma of acid mucopolysaccharide. The matrix also contains small amounts of collagen. Overall cellularity is moderately low, but many tumors contain areas of increased cellularity resembling poorly differentiated fibrosarcomas. The neoplastic fibroblasts have scant, eosinophilic cytoplasm and pleomorphic nuclei that are slightly larger than those of myxoma. Nuclei are often hyperchromatic and may contain cytoplasmic invaginations. Nucleoli are inconspicuous, and mitotic activity is low. Occasional atypical mitotic figures can usually be detected. Larger neoplasms may have areas of hemorrhage, necrosis, and fibrosis. Ulceration and secondary inflammation may be present.

Differentiation between myxoma and myxosarcoma can be difficult because most benign and malignant variants have abundant stroma, low cellularity, and poor circumscription. Cytologic features of malignancy in myxosarcomas are an increased nuclear:cytoplasmic ratio, nuclear pleomorphism and hyperchromatism, and the presence of atypical mitotic figures. Myxosarcoma may be distinguished from myxoid liposarcoma by the absence of lipoblasts, well-differentiated lipocytes, and a delicate capillary meshwork.

SUGGESTED READINGS

Collagenous nevus

Mehregan AH: Pinkus' guide to dermatohistopathology, ed 4, Norwalk, Conn, 1986, Appleton-Century-Crofts, p 386.

Scott DW and others: Nevi in the dog, J Am Anim Hosp Assoc 20:505-512, 1984.

Nodular dermatofibrosis

Lium B and Moe L: Hereditary multifocal renal cystadenocarcinomas and nodular dermatofibrosis in the German Shepherd Dog: macroscopic and histopathologic changes, Vet Pathol 22:447-455, 1985.

Suter M, Lott-Stolz G, and Wild P: Generalized nodular dermatofibrosis in six Alsatians, Vet Pathol 20:632-634, 1983.

Skin tag

Lever WF and Schaumburg-Lever G: Histopathology of the skin, ed 7, Philadelphia, 1990, JB Lippincott, pp 664-665.

Mehregan AH: Pinkus' guide to dermatohistopathology, ed 4, Norwalk, Conn, 1986, Appleton-Century-Crofts, p 539.

Dermatofibroma

Ackerman AB, Niven J, and Grant-Kels JM: Differential diagnosis in dermatopathology, Philadelphia, 1982, Lea & Febiger, pp 170-173.

Enzinger FM and Weiss SE: Soft tissue tumors, ed 2, St Louis, 1988, CV Mosby, p 223.

Lever WF and Schaumburg-Lever G: Histopathology of the skin, ed 7, Philadelphia, 1990, JB Lippincott, pp 660-664.

Fibroma

Bevier DE and Goldschmidt MH: Skin tumors in the dog. II. Tumors of the soft (mesenchymal) tissues, Comp Cont Ed 3:506-514, 1981.

Enzinger FM and Weiss SE: Soft tissue tumors, ed 2, St Louis, 1988, CV Mosby, p 102.

Fibrosarcoma

Bevier DE and Goldschmidt MH: Skin tumors in the dog. II. Tumors of the soft (mesenchymal) tissues, Comp Cont Ed 3:506-514, 1981.

Bostock DE and Dye MT: Prognosis after surgical excision of canine fibrous connective tissue sarcomas, Vet Pathol 17:581-588, 1980.

Bostock DE and Dye MT: Prognosis after surgical excision of fibro-
    sarcoma in cats, J Am Vet Med Assoc 175:727-728, 1979.
Brown NO and others: Soft tissue sarcomas in the cat, J Am Vet
    Med Assoc 173:744-749, 1978.
Enzinger FM and Weiss SE: Soft tissue tumors, ed 2, St Louis,
    1988, CV Mosby, pp 201-222.

Myxoma and myxosarcoma

Bevier DE and Goldschmidt MH: Skin tumors in the dog. II. Tu-
    mors of the soft (mesenchymal) tissues, Comp Cont Ed
    3:506-514, 1981.

Goldschmidt MH: Dermal mesenchymal neoplasms of domestic an-
    imals. Proceedings of the American Academy of Veterinary
    Dermatology/American College of Veterinary Dermatology, Or-
    lando, pp 1-11, 1985.
Pulley LT and Stannard AA: Tumors of the skin and soft tissues. In
    Moulton J, editor: Tumors in domestic animals, ed 3, Berkeley,
    1990, University of California Press, pp 33-34.

See also General References, pp 327-328.

Vascular tumors

SCROTAL VASCULAR HAMARTOMA
Clinical features

Scrotal vascular hamartoma is an uncommon proliferative lesion of blood vessels in the scrotum of dogs. The lesion is believed to be a progressive vascular malformation rather than a true neoplasm; thus the designation hamartoma is appropriate (see follicular hamartoma, Chapter 22).

Scrotal vascular hamartoma begins as single or multiple, hyperpigmented macules that progress to firm plaques. Most lesions are 1 to 2 cm in diameter. The overlying epidermis becomes thickened and is frequently ulcerated because of chronic licking.

Affected animals are middle aged or older. Breeds with pigmented scrotal skin, such as Scottish Terriers and Airedale Terriers, are reported by Pulley to have a higher incidence.

Histopathology (Figures 27-1 and 27-2)

Scrotal vascular hamartoma is a poorly circumscribed dermal plaque containing multiple clusters of redundant vascular structures that surround the preexisting dermal blood vessels. Hyperplastic vessels in the center of the lesion are larger and dilated, whereas those at the periphery are capillary buds with barely discernible lumens. The vascular structures are lined by a single layer of endothelial cells with plump, dark, uniform nuclei. Mitotic figures are rare, and mitotic atypia is not present. Dermal fibrosis and proliferation of pericytes accompany the vasoformative process. The overlying epidermis shows acanthosis and increased melanin pigment. Traumatic ulceration, hemorrhage, and secondary inflammation are frequently observed.

Scrotal vascular hamartoma may be confused with hemangiosarcoma because of poor circumscription and nuclear immaturity in the peripherally developing capillaries. However, the benign and nonneoplastic nature of this lesion is manifested by the admixture of three tissue types—redundant vascular structures, increased perivascular connective tissue, and hyperplastic pericytes—and the maintenance of normal architectural relationships among them.

HEMANGIOMA
Clinical features

Hemangiomas are benign neoplasms of vascular endothelium that are common in dogs and rare in cats. The reported incidence in dogs ranges from 2% to 3% of skin and

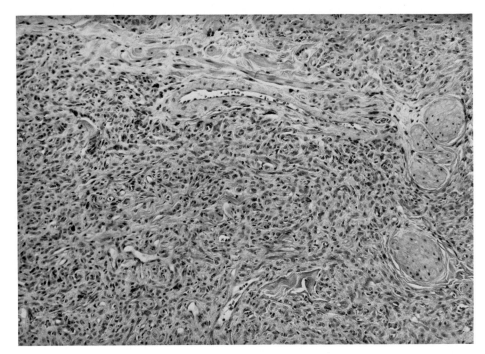

FIGURE 27-1. Scrotal vascular hamartoma in a dog. Proliferating capillaries lined by plump endothelial cells are admixed with cellular connective tissue containing pericytes and fibrocytes. Note the scrotal smooth muscle bundles at right. (×120.)

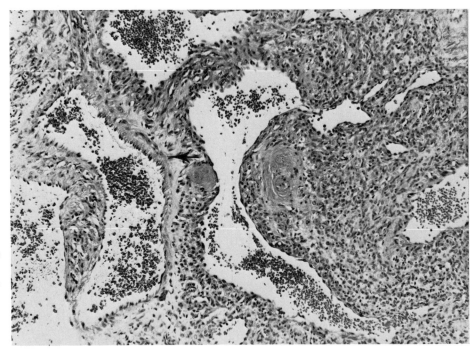

FIGURE 27-2. Scrotal vascular hamartoma in a dog. Irregular cavernous vascular structures are present in the center of the lesion. Residual scrotal blood vessels, such as the one to left of center, are recognizable by the presence of a muscularis. (×120.)

subcutaneous tumors in several surveys. The incidence in a series of 1141 canine skin and subcutaneous neoplasms by 1 of the authors* was 6%. The majority of hemangiomas arise in the subcutis, but intradermal tumors are not infrequent. The etiology of most hemangiomas is unknown, but Hargis recently reported a large group of vascular neoplasms of the ventral gla-

* Emily J. Walder.

brous skin in light-skinned breeds of dogs; chronic solar damage is considered to be of etiologic significance in the development of hemangiomas in sun-exposed sites in these animals.

Subcutaneous hemangiomas are usually solitary, well-circumscribed, meaty, ovoid or discoid masses that range from 0.5 to 4 cm in size. The overlying skin is elevated and often partially alopecic; secondary ulceration is uncommon. Subcutaneous hemangiomas have a blue or purple tint when viewed through the intact skin. Dermal hemangiomas appear as solitary or multiple, well-circumscribed, dome-shaped or polypoid masses with red or red-black coloration. They are smaller than their subcutaneous counterparts, ranging from several millimeters to 1 cm in size. The overlying epidermis is usually alopecic; ulceration and hemorrhage are frequent findings.

Dermal and subcutaneous hemangiomas can occur at any anatomic site. Hargis recently reported that dermal vascular tumors have a predilection for the ventral abdominal and inguinal skin in dogs with nonpigmented skin and short haircoats. Whippets, Bloodhounds, Salukis, and English Pointers, were found to have a higher overall incidence of cutaneous vascular tumors. In the same study, Whippets, Dalmatians, American Staffordshire Terriers, Beagles, and Bassett Hounds had a higher incidence of dermal hemangiomas and hemangiosarcomas at sun-exposed sites on the ventrum.

Females were found to be at greater risk by Hargis for the development of cutaneous vascular tumors. No sex predisposition has been reported for non-solar–associated hemangiomas. The average age of affected animals is 9 to 10 years in several surveys. The large majority of hemangiomas are benign; however, malignant transformation may occur in solar-induced dermal hemangiomas.

Angiokeratoma, a rare variant of hemangioma in dogs reported by Buyukmihci, contains both vascular and epithelial components. Angiokeratomas are small, dome-shaped or polypoid lesions that occur most often on the conjunctiva but can also arise in superficial dermis at any site. There is no known age or breed predisposition for this tumor type.

Histopathology

Cavernous hemangioma (Figure 27-3). Hemangiomas are usually well-circumscribed but unencapsulated tumors involving the dermis, the subcutis, or both. The cavernous type is by far the most common histopathologic pattern. It is characterized by a discrete mass of tightly packed, dilated vascular spaces filled with erythrocytes. Small numbers of vascular spaces may also be present beyond the main confines of the tumor within the adjacent dermis or subcutaneous fat. Each vascular structure is enclosed and lined by a single layer of normal-appearing endothelial cells. The endothelial cells are aligned on collagenous septa, which are usually thin. A small percentage of cavernous hemangiomas have broad collagenous septa, resulting in a more substantial stromal component. The septal collagen frequently shows mild infiltration by mast cells, lymphocytes, and hemosiderophages. The neoplastic endothelial cells have scant cytoplasm and flattened, dark, uniform nuclei. Nucleoli and mitotic figures are not evident.

Moderate numbers of cavernous hemangiomas

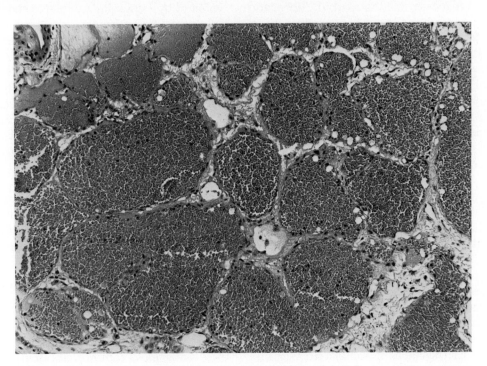

FIGURE 27-3. Cavernous hemangioma in a dog. Tightly packed, large vascular structures lined by a single layer of small, uniform endothelial cells. Note that all vascular spaces are completely enclosed.(× 120.)

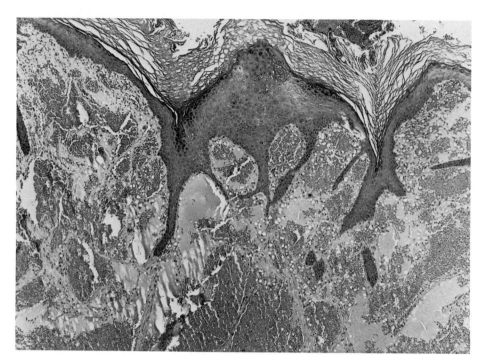

FIGURE 27-4. Angiokeratoma in a dog. The vascular component of the lesion is identical to that of cavernous hemangioma. Note that the hyperplastic epidermis forms rete pegs that appear to partially surround vascular structures in the superficial dermis. (×50.)

contain organizing thrombi that occlude one or more of the vascular structures. Thrombosis is accompanied by fibroplasia and deposition of hemoglobin breakdown pigments. The overlying epidermis of both dermal and subcutaneous hemangiomas often shows hyperplasia that varies from mild to marked. Secondary ulceration and hemorrhagic crusting are observed more often in dermal hemangiomas.

Solar-induced dermal hemangiomas of glabrous skin of lightly pigmented breeds often are less well-circumscribed than their idiopathic counterparts. Clusters and plaque-like aggregates of proliferative, nonneoplastic blood vessels may be observed in the overlying superficial dermis. Solar elastosis, as well as other features of solar dermatitis may be present. Cytologic features are identical to those of idiopathic hemangiomas.

Lymphangioma may be a differential diagnosis for hemangioma. Cavernous hemangiomas and small lymphangiomas have similar architecture and morphology, but the vascular spaces of lymphangioma contain few erythrocytes. The stroma of lymphangioma exhibits edema and lymphoplasmacytic infiltration.

Angiokeratoma (Figure 27-4). Angiokeratoma is characterized by a small, well-circumscribed mass that is elevated above the skin surface. The vascular component is essentially the same as in dermal cavernous hemangioma. The epidermis exhibits irregular hyperplasia without dysplasia, and epithelial trabeculae extend downward to separate and partially surround some of the vascular structures. Ulceration and hemorrhage are commonly present.

Capillary hemangioma (Figure 27-5). This is an uncommon histopathologic pattern of hemangioma characterized by vascular spaces of capillary caliber that are lined by a single layer of plump endothelial cells. As in cavernous hemangioma, the vascular structures are completely enclosed by their endothelial lining. A distinct collagenous supporting network is not present. Endothelial nuclei are slightly larger than in cavernous hemangioma and may protrude slightly into vessel lumens. Nucleoli are not evident, but occasional mitoses can be observed. Pure capillary hemangiomas occur only in the dermis. Subcutaneous hemangiomas may have a combination of capillary and cavernous vascular structures.

The relatively cellular appearance of capillary hemangioma may lead to confusion with hemangiosarcoma. Circumscription of tumor margins, complete enclosure of vascular spaces, nuclear uniformity, and the absence of atypical mitotic figures are important features of benign vascular neoplasms.

HEMANGIOSARCOMA (Synonyms: angiosarcoma, hemangioendothelioma)

Clinical features

Hemangiosarcomas of the skin and subcutis are uncommon malignant neoplasms of vascular endothelium. They account for slightly less than 2% of cutane-

FIGURE 27-5. Capillary hemangioma in a dog. The majority of vascular structures are of capillary caliber and are lined by a single layer of plump endothelial cells. Note that all vascular spaces are completely enclosed. (×120.)

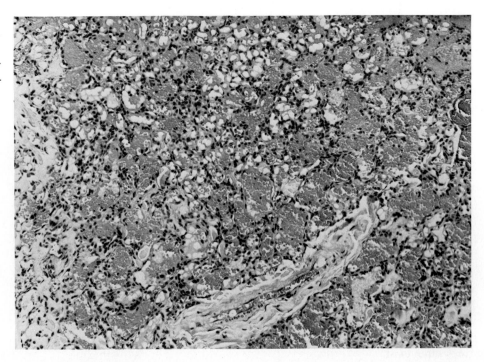

ous and subcutaneous tumors in both dogs and cats in several reports. Hemangiosarcomas occur less frequently than hemangiomas in dogs (3% to 6% incidence) but more frequently than their benign counterparts in cats. Recent work by Hargis suggests that hemangiomas and hemangiosarcomas of the skin of the ventral abdomen and inguinal region in light-skinned breeds of dogs are the result of chronic solar irradiation. Most hemangiosarcomas arise de novo, but malignant transformation within hemangiomas may occur in solar-associated lesions.

The majority of dermal hemangiosarcomas in dogs and cats appear as ill-defined, red–to–dark blue plaques or nodules that usually measure less than 2 cm in diameter. Dermal hemangiosarcomas in chronically sun-exposed anatomic sites are frequently multiple in dogs. Subcutaneous hemangiosarcomas in dogs and cats, which often involve the dermis secondarily, are poorly circumscribed, dark red or blue-black, spongy masses that can measure up to 10 cm. Lesions, particularly in cats, may resemble large ecchymoses or bruises that blanch transiently with pressure. Large subcutaneous hemangiosarcomas are generally solitary in dogs and cats. Alopecia, thickened skin, hemorrhage, and ulceration are common features regardless of dermal or subcutaneous location.

Dogs with short coats and nonpigmented skin have a higher incidence of dermal hemangiosarcomas in the glabrous skin of the caudal ventral abdomen

(solar associated). This distribution pattern is identical to those of actinic keratosis and actinic squamous cell carcinoma in dogs. Site predilection is not observed in dogs with longer coats or pigmented skin. There are also no preferential locations for subcutaneous hemangiosarcomas in dogs. Hemangiosarcomas in cats occur most frequently in the inguinal and axillary regions and on the head and ears. There is no known association at the present time between chronic solar damage and feline vascular malignancies.

Whippets, Dalmatians, Beagles, Greyhounds, American Staffordshire Terriers, and other short-haired and light-skinned breeds are at increased risk for solar-associated hemangiosarcoma. There is no reported breed predilection for non-solar–associated dermal and subcutaneous hemangiosarcomas. Female dogs, as reported by Hargis, may have a higher incidence of cutaneous vascular tumors. The average age of dogs and cats with all types of dermal and subcutaneous hemangiosarcomas in most surveys is 10 years.

Much of the published information on the metastatic rate of hemangiosarcomas in dogs fails to separate tumors by primary anatomic site, thus implying that cutaneous hemangiosarcomas have a similarly aggressive biologic behavior to their visceral counterparts. (The survey by Brown reported a 96% 1-year mortality rate.) In contrast, Culbertson's report on canine cutaneous hemangiosarcomas found metastatic lesions in only 2 of 10 animals. In the study by Hargis, it was not uncommon for dogs with solar-associated dermal or subcutaneous hemangiosarcoma to die as a result of their tumors; euthanasia as a result of recurrent or additional skin tumors was common, but the clinical course of disease was quite long (1 to 3 years). Confirmed metastasis, most commonly to the lungs, from a primary cutaneous hemangiosarcoma was occasionally observed. Accurate assessment of biologic behavior can be difficult, because it may not be possible to determine conclusively the primary site of hemangiosarcoma when multicentric lesions are present. Hemangiosarcomas in cats exhibit frequent local recurrence but have a very low incidence of metastasis.

Histopathology (Figures 27-6 through 27-10)

Hemangiosarcomas of the skin and subcutis show a continuum from well-differentiated lesions, which are difficult to distinguish from hemangiomas, to highly anaplastic tumors, which require immunohistochemistry for definitive diagnosis. When multiple tumors are present in a single animal, variable morphologic features often exist.

The majority of cutaneous hemangiosarcomas are well-differentiated neoplasms characterized by plump endothelial cells aligned on delicate collagen trabeculae or preexisting dermal collagen bundles. The trabeculae form an anastomosing meshwork of blood-filled channels of varying size. Ragged tumor margins are created by infiltration and dissection of collagen bundles by neoplastic vascular structures at the periphery. In contrast to hemangioma, the vascular spaces of hemangiosarcoma are not uniformly enclosed by endothelial cells, and blindly ending trabeculae are present. Tumor

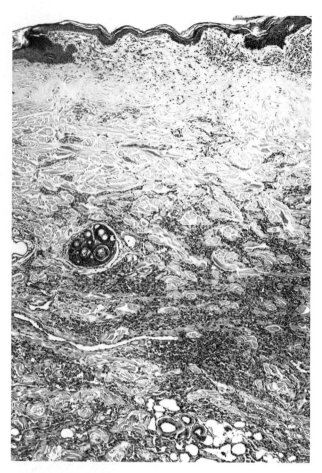

FIGURE 27-6. Hemangiosarcoma in a dog. Irregular vascular spaces dissect dermal collagen bundles, resulting in ragged tumor margins. Note the homogenization of collagen (indicative of solar elastosis) and the reactive vasoproliferation in the superficial dermis. (×120.)

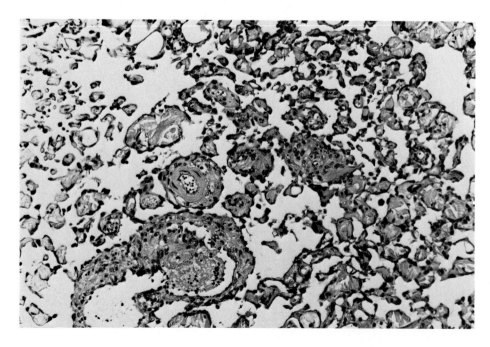

FIGURE 27-7. Hemangiosarcoma in a dog. Endothelial cell nuclei are hyperchromatic and often protrude into vascular lumens. Note the numerous blindly ending trabeculae lined by endothelial cells. (×260.)

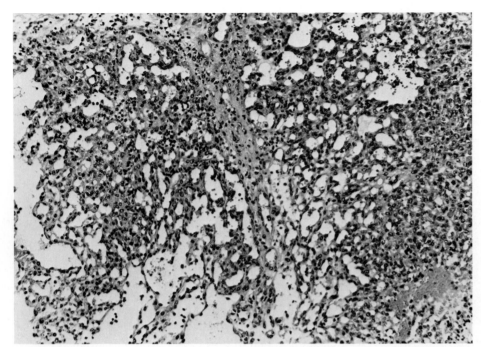

FIGURE 27-8. Hemangiosarcoma in a dog. In this less well-differentiated example, some of the vascular structures are lined by multiple layers of endothelial cells. Note the solid area of tumor cells at right. (×120.)

cells have minimal cytoplasm and slightly enlarged, hyperchromatic nuclei that bulge into the vascular lumens. Nucleoli are inconspicuous, and mitotic activity is low; atypical mitoses can usually be detected.

Piling up of tumor cells along basal laminae, nuclear pleomorphism, nucleolar prominence, an increased mitotic index, and loss of obvious vascular structures are features of hemangiosarcomas of increasing anaplasia. These histopathologic features are ob-

served more frequently in subcutaneous tumors, but dermal hemangiosarcomas may occasionally show poor differentiation. Poorly differentiated variants are highly cellular and are composed predominantly of pleomorphic spindle and polygonal cells arranged in interlacing bundles and solid sheets. Vascular differentiation may be manifested only by slit-like spaces between tumor cells that contain small numbers of erythrocytes.

Histiocytoid hemangiosarcoma, as described in

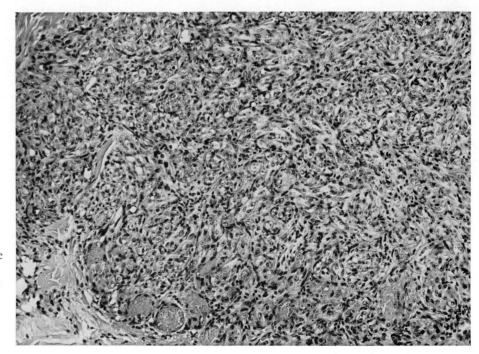

FIGURE 27-9. Histiocytoid hemangiosarcoma in a dog. The majority of the neoplasm is composed of nests of polygonal and spindle cells. Vascular differentiation is most evident at the margin of the neoplasm at lower left. (×130.)

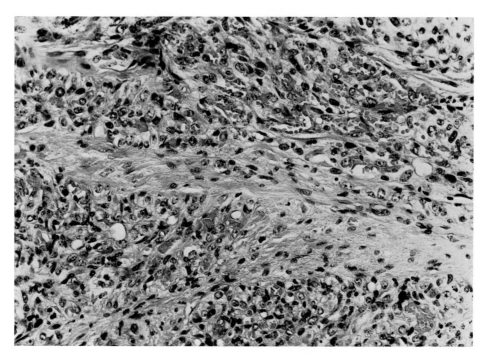

FIGURE 27-10. Higher magnification of histiocytoid hemangiosarcoma shows large polygonal cells with pleomorphic nuclei lining vascular channels containing erythrocytes. (×240.)

humans, is a rare variant in dogs that is composed predominantly of polygonal epithelioid cells with abundant, pale eosinophilic cytoplasm. Nuclei are large and vesicular and have prominent nucleoli. Mitotic activity is moderate to high. Small numbers of multinucleated tumor giant cells may be present. Vascular spaces may resemble glandular structures with luminal hemorrhage because of the epithelial appearance of the neoplastic cells. Foci of more typical endothelial differentiation can generally be found in histiocytoid hemangiosarcomas.

Most cutaneous hemangiosarcomas have mild to severe acanthosis and hyperkeratosis of the overlying epidermis. Ulceration, thrombosis, necrosis, and hemorrhage are common secondary features of larger hemangiosarcomas in dogs and cats regardless of location. Solar elastosis may be seen in the adjacent dermis of solar-associated hemangiosarcoma. Solar dermatitis, actinic keratosis and frank squamous cell carcinoma also may occur in the vicinity of hemangiosarcoma in these patients.

Differential diagnoses for hemangiosarcoma include hemangioma, fibrosarcoma, and lymphangiosarcoma. Well-differentiated hemangiosarcoma is distinguished from hemangioma by the presence of invasive tumor margins and moderate or large numbers of blindly ending, endothelium-lined trabeculae. Poorly differentiated hemangiosarcoma may be difficult to distinguish from fibrosarcoma or other spindle-cell malignancies. Clefts containing rows of erythrocytes between the neoplastic cells suggest a vascular origin. Immunohistochemical staining with factor VIII–related antigen, horse gram lectin, soybean lectin, or hairy vetch lectin may also be helpful in the definitive diagnosis of poorly differentiated hemangiosarcoma. Hemangiosarcoma and lymphangiosarcoma have similar architecture and morphology. Stromal edema and lymphoplasmacytic infiltration may be features of lymphagiosarcoma that are not observed in hemangiomas. If distinction is not possible on this basis, the more general term *angiosarcoma* may be more appropriate.

LYMPHANGIOMA
Clinical features

Lymphangiomas are benign tumors of lymphatic endothelium that are rare in both dogs and cats. Most lymphangiomas are believed to arise from a congenital failure of primitive lymphatic sacs to develop communications with the venous system. A hamartomatous etiology is supported by the prevalence of dogs less than 5 years of age in published case reports. Most lesions recur after surgical excision; one case reported by Turrel responded well to radiation therapy after multiple recurrences.

Lymphangiomas of the dermis and subcutis appear

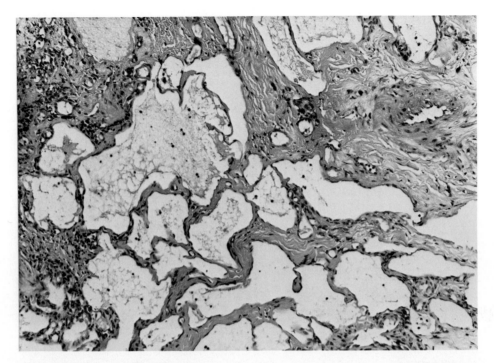

FIGURE 27-11. Lymphangioma in a dog. Cavernous, angular vascular spaces are lined by a single layer of small endothelial cells and do not contain erythrocytes. Note the lymphoplasmacytic stromal infiltrate at left. (×120.)

as fluctuant swellings up to 18 cm in size. Ulcers and tracts draining serous fluid are present in most cases. Spongiotic vesicles may be present in the overlying epidermis. There may be a predilection for intertriginous areas and limbs, based on the small number of reported cases.

There is no known breed predisposition. Affected animals range from less than 1 to 8 years of age; many have had a prolonged clinical course prior to presentation.

Histopathology (Figure 27-11)

Lymphangiomas are generally large, poorly circumscribed masses involving the dermis, subcutis, or both. Occasional small lymphangiomas occur; these are more discrete and resemble cavernous hemangiomas. Lymphangiomas are composed of angular, dilated vascular structures lined by a single layer of uniform endothelial cells. Vascular channels contain small amounts of proteinaceous fluid and mixed mononuclear cells; erythrocytes are rarely observed. The connective tissue septa supporting the vascular structures frequently have an edematous or myxomatous appearance and are infiltrated by lymphocytes, plasma cells, and small numbers of mast cells. The neoplastic cells have minimal cytoplasm, elongated hyperchromatic nuclei, inconspicuous nucleoli, and minimal mitotic activity.

The overlying epidermis shows acanthosis, spongiosis, and, in some cases, spongiotic vesiculation caused by chronic leakage of plasma proteins. Ulceration is a frequent secondary feature and may be accompanied by granulation tissue proliferation.

The majority of lymphangiomas are more extensive and diffusely organized than hemangiomas. Small lymphangiomas are architecturally similar to cavernous hemangiomas but are distinguished by the paucity of erythrocytes in the vascular spaces. Stromal edema and lymphoplasmacytic infiltration are also features that are not observed in hemangiomas.

LYMPHANGIOSARCOMA (Synonym: angiosarcoma)

Clinical features

Lymphangiosarcoma is a rare malignant neoplasm of lymphatic endothelium. Only 2 canine cases and 11 feline cases exist in recent veterinary literature. The young age of reported canine cases suggests a similar congenital basis for lymphangiosarcomas as for lymphangioma in dogs. Whether lymphangiosarcomas actually have a similar developmental origin or whether they arise from malignant transformation of lymphangioma remains to be demonstrated.

Lymphangiosarcomas appear as large, diffuse, fluc-

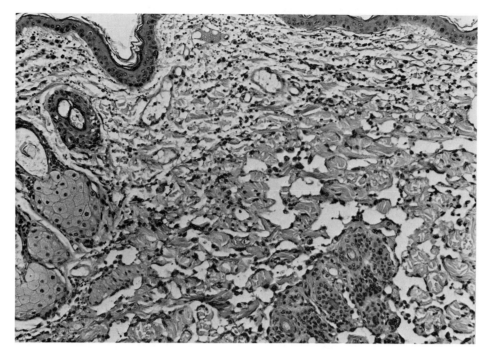

FIGURE 27-12. Lymphangiosarcoma in a cat. The dermis is diffusely infiltrated by irregular vascular spaces lined by a single layer of plump endothelial cells with hyperchromatic nuclei. Note the paucity of erythrocytes and dissection of neoplastic endothelium between dermal collagen bundles. (×120.)

tuant swellings. Ulceration and serous drainage may be present. Reported locations are the limbs, ventral neck, and ventral abdomen; this is similar to the distribution pattern of lymphangiomas (see discussion above).

The average age of cats with lymphangiosarcoma is 7 years. The two canine cases described by Kelly and Franklin were in animals less than 3 years of age. The dogs with lymphangiosarcoma had post-surgical recurrence and widespread visceral metastasis. The tumors in cats exhibited frequent local recurrence, but only one instance of confirmed distant metastasis was reported by Carpenter.

Histopathology (Figure 27-12)

Lymphangiosarcomas are ill-defined masses usually involving both the dermis and subcutis. The tumors comprise plump spindle cells aligned in one or more layers along edematous collagenous trabeculae or pre-existing dermal collagen bundles. The trabeculae form an anastomosing meshwork of large, angular vascular spaces. Blindly ending trabeculae are frequently observed. Vascular structures dissect between dermal collagen bundles, lobules of adipocytes, and fascial planes at the periphery, creating ragged tumor margins. The vascular spaces contain few erythrocytes. The sparse stromal tissue is usually infiltrated by lymphocytes,

plasma cells, and hemosiderophages. The neoplastic endothelial cells have pleomorphic, oval nuclei that bulge into the vascular lumens. Nucleoli are variable, and mitotic figures are infrequent.

It may be difficult to distinguish histopathologically between lymphangioma and lymphangiosarcoma. Peripheral dissection of collagen bundles by endothelial cells, blindly ending stromal trabeculae, and slight nuclear pleomorphism are useful indicators of malignancy. The architecture and morphology of lymphangiosarcoma also are similar to well-differentiated hemangiosarcoma. Stromal edema, lymphocytic inflammation, and the paucity of erythrocytes within vascular channels support a diagnosis of lymphangiosarcoma. If distinction is not possible on this basis, the more general term angiosarcoma may be more appropriate.

SUGGESTED READINGS

Scrotal vascular hamartoma

Pulley LT and Stannard AA: Tumors of the skin and soft tissues. In Moulton J, editor: Tumors in domestic animals, ed 3, Berkeley, Calif, 1990, University of California Press, p 46.

Hemangioma

Buyukmihci N and Stannard AA: Canine conjunctival angiokeratoma, J Am Vet Med Assoc 178:1279-1281, 1981.

Hargis AM and Ihrke PJ: Solar associated vascular tumors in dogs. Proceedings of the Fortieth Annual Meeting of the American College of Veterinary Pathologists, Baltimore, p 20, 1989.

Hemangiosarcoma

Augustin-Voss HG, Smith CA, and Lewis RM: Phenotypic characterization of normal and neoplastic canine endothelial cells by lectin histochemistry, Vet Pathol 27:103-109, 1990.

Brown NO, Patnaik AK, and MacEwen EG: Canine hemangiosarcoma: retrospective analysis of 104 cases, J Am Vet Med Assoc 186:56-58, 1985.

Culbertson MR: Hemangiosarcoma of the canine skin and tongue, Vet Pathol 19:556-558, 1982.

Hargis AM and Ihrke PJ: Solar associated vascular tumors in dogs. Proceedings of the Fortieth Annual Meeting of the American College of Veterinary Pathologists, Baltimore, p 20, 1989.

Scavelli TD and others: Hemangiosarcoma in the cat: retrospective evaluation of 31 surgical cases, J Am Vet Med Assoc 187:817-819, 1985.

Lymphangioma

Stambaugh JE, Harvey CE, and Goldschmidt MH: Lymphangioma in four dogs, J Am Vet Med Assoc 173:759-761, 1978.

Turrel JM, Lowenstine LJ, and Cowgill LD: Response to radiation therapy of recurrent lymphangioma in a dog, J Am Vet Med Assoc 193:1432-1434, 1988.

Lymphangiosarcoma

Carpenter JL, Andrew LK, and Holzworth J: Tumors and tumor-like lesions. In Holzworth J, editor: Diseases of the cat, Philadelphia, 1987, WB Saunders, pp 423, 483-486.

Franklin RT, Robertson JJ, and Thornburg LP: Lymphangiosarcoma in a dog, J Am Vet Med Assoc, 184:474-475, 1984.

Kelly WR, Wilkinson GT, and Allen PW: Canine angiosarcoma (lymphangiosarcoma): a case report, Vet Pathol 18:224-227, 1981.

Walsh KM and Abbot DP: Lymphangiosarcoma in two cats, J Comp Pathol 94:611-614, 1984.

See also General References, pp 327-328.

CHAPTER 28

Other mesenchymal tumors

LIPOMATOSIS
Clinical features

Lipomatosis refers to multicentric, neoplastic or nonneoplastic proliferations of architecturally normal adipose tissue. Several syndromes of lipomatosis occur in humans, including nevus lipomatosus superficialis, diffuse lipomatosis, pelvic lipomatosis, adiposis dolorosa (Dercum's disease), familial multiple lipomatosis, and multiple symmetric lipomatosis (Madelung's disease). Lipomatosis is rare in dogs and cats. A single case resembling multiple symmetric lipomatosis in a dog has recently been reported by Gilbert. A case of unspecified lipomatosis was described in the review of feline skin tumors by Carpenter.

The case reported by Gilbert was a 5-year-old female Dachshund with progressively enlarging, pendulous, fatty skin folds involving the neck and trunk bilaterally. The skin was atrophic, partially alopecic, and multifocally ulcerated because of trauma. The example described by Carpenter was a young cat of unspecified age that had similar fatty skin folds affecting the perineum and caudal thighs.

Histopathology

Lipomatosis in the single reported canine case was characterized by diffuse thickening of the panniculus by mature adipose tissue. The overlying epidermis and dermis were mildly atrophic. The subcutaneous fat had a normal complement of fibrous septa, blood vessels, and nerves. The interlobular septa showed mild mucin deposition. The lipocytes were cytologically normal, but small numbers of primitive mesenchymal cells and lipoblasts were present around blood vessels. The primitive mesenchymal cells were small and stellate and had dark, ovoid nuclei. The lipoblasts were stellate or polygonal and contained multiple, small, lipid vacuoles. The lipoblast nuclei were also ovoid and hyperchromatic. A detailed histopathologic description was not available for the feline case.

Differential diagnosis for lipomatosis is limited because of the unique clinical presentation. Histopathologically, differentiation of the adipose tissue in lesions of lipomatosis from that of normal subcutis may not be possible.

LIPOMA
Clinical features

Benign tumors of adipose tissue are common in dogs and uncommon in cats. Lipomas account for approximately 9% of canine skin and subcutaneous tumors.

FIGURE 28-1. Lipoma in a cat. A discrete nodule of mature lipocytes involves the dermis and subcutis. (×50.)

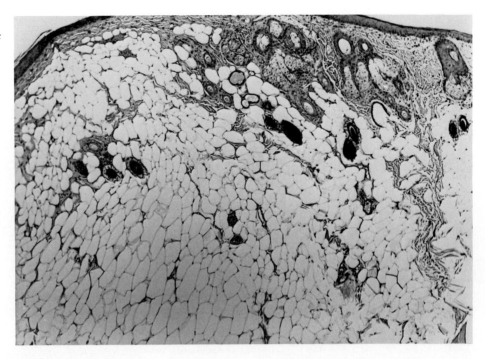

Pulley proposed that lipomas may represent foci of nodular hyperplasia or altered lipocyte metabolism rather than true neoplasms.

Lipomas appear as single or multiple, well-circumscribed, ovoid or discoid masses with a soft or rubbery consistency. The majority of lipomas are subcutaneous masses, but approximately 10% occur in a deep dermal location. Dermal lipomas are usually less than 2 cm in size, whereas subcutaneous tumors can attain sizes greater than 20 cm. The skin is freely movable over subcutaneous lipomas. Partial alopecia and epidermal atrophy may occur with larger lesions. The majority of lipomas occur on the trunk and proximal rear limbs.

The average age of affected dogs is 8 years, and females are at increased risk. Lipomas in cats occur most often in 7- to 11-year-old animals. Lipomas occur in all breeds of dogs, but Labrador Retrievers, Dachshunds, Cocker Spaniels, Poodles, and small terriers are reported to be at increased risk in studies by Bevier and also Strafuss.

Histopathology (Figures 28-1 and 28-2)

Lipomas are dermal or subcutaneous nodules composed of solid sheets of mature lipocytes that are virtually indistinguishable from their counterparts in normal fat. Most lipomas are well circumscribed but unencapsulated; some have a delicate capsule of mature fibrous tissue. Lipocytes sometimes appear larger or have more variability in size than those of adjacent normal fat. Nuclei are small, crescentic, and compressed against cell membranes by the abundant cytoplasmic stores of neutral lipid. Mitotic figures are not observed. Usually a delicate capillary vasculature is supported by thin strands of collagen.

Ischemic degenerative changes may occur in large lipomas. Lipocyte necrosis is generally accompanied by hemorrhage, fibrosis, and a mild infiltrate of macrophages. Saponification of necrotic fat may also occur.

The primary differential diagnosis for lipoma is normal adipose tissue, particularly in needle biopsy specimens. The absence of large vessels and nerve trunks is useful in distinguishing a fatty tumor from normal fat. Foci of nodular necrotizing steatitis, particularly in cats, resemble areas of ischemic degeneration in lipomas. In excisional biopsy specimens, peripheral encapsulation by mature granulation tissue indicates an inflammatory or traumatic lesion.

FIBROLIPOMA
Clinical features

Fibrolipoma is an uncommon variant of lipoma occurring in dogs and cats. Numeric incidence data are not reported. The tumors appear as solitary, well-defined, round-to-ovoid nodules involving the deep dermis or subcutis. Most lesions are 1 to 2 cm in diameter. Fibrolipomas usually occur on the trunk or limbs and are slightly firmer in consistency than lipomas. Alterations are not generally observed in the overlying skin. Age, breed, and sex predilections are probably similar to those of simple lipomas.

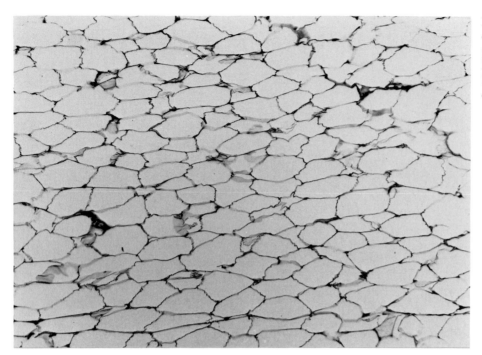

FIGURE 28-2. Lipoma in a dog. Mature lipocytes are composed almost entirely of neutral lipid. Note that nuclei are barely discernible in most of the cells. (×120.)

Histopathology (Figure 28-3)

Fibrolipoma is a well-demarcated mass, occurring in the deep dermis or subcutis, and is composed of mature lipocytes and scattered collagen bundles. A thin capsule of mature collagen is present in most tumors. The fatty component of the tumor is identical to lipoma. The fibromatous component is characterized by thick collagenous trabeculae distributed haphazardly through the mass. Cellularity is low. Fibrocyte and lipocyte nuclei are uniformly small and bland. Mitotic figures are not observed. Differential diagnoses are limited and are similar to those for simple lipoma.

INFILTRATIVE LIPOMA
Clinical features

Infiltrative lipoma is a variant of lipoma that is uncommon in dogs and rare in cats. It was first de-

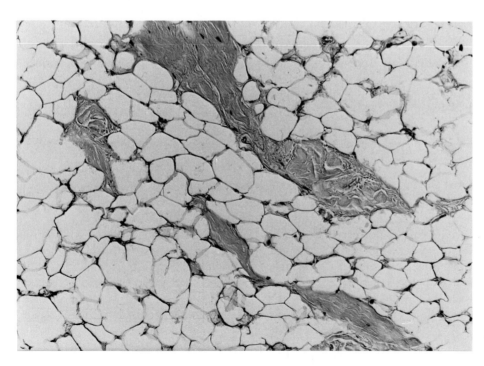

FIGURE 28-3. Fibrolipoma in a dog. Mature lipocytes are admixed with collagen bundles of low cellularity. (×120.)

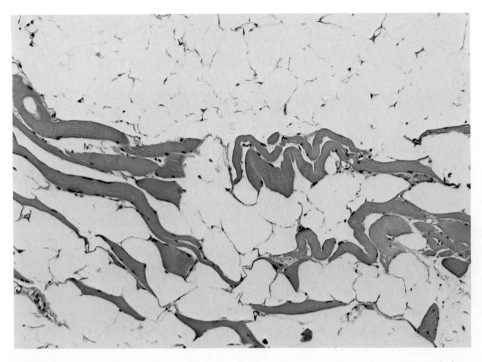

FIGURE 28-4. Infiltrative lipoma in a dog. Mature lipocytes infiltrate between muscle bundles and individual muscle fibers. (×120.)

scribed as a distinct entity in the veterinary literature in 1979 by Gleiser. Infiltrative lipomas are large, poorly defined, deep subcutaneous and intramuscular swellings that are slightly firmer than banal lipomas. Most tumors arise in the deep soft tissues of the trunk and proximal limbs. Limb lesions may produce pain or impair locomotion.

Affected animals are usually middle aged or older, but young adults occasionally develop lipomas of this type. There is no known breed or sex predilection. Although infiltrative lipomas do not undergo malignant transformation and possess no metastatic potential, they commonly require radical surgical excision to prevent local recurrence.

Histopathology (Figure 28-4)

Infiltrative lipoma is a diffusely invasive neoplasm involving the subcutis, skeletal muscle, and fascia. The tumor is unencapsulated, and margins are difficult to assess. The neoplasm is made up of sheets and trabeculae of mature lipocytes identical to those of simple lipoma. The tumor tissue spreads along fascial planes and into muscle bundles. The myofibers often become individualized and atrophic as they are entrapped by the encroaching adipose tissue. Although the adipose tissue appears poorly vascularized, degenerative changes are rarely observed.

The histopathologic appearance of infiltrative lipoma is unique in excisional biopsy specimens. Small amounts of normal fat are often present between mus-

cle bundles in obese animals, and it may be difficult to render a definitive diagnosis of infiltrative lipoma in such patients if only core needle biopsy samples are provided.

LIPOSARCOMA
Clinical features

Liposarcomas are malignant neoplasms of adipose tissue that are rare in dogs and even more rare in cats. The incidence in dogs is less than 1%. The tumors are circumscribed, soft or fleshy masses that measure 2 cm or greater in diameter. The consistency of liposarcomas varies from fatty to myxoid. Liposarcomas arise in the subcutis but frequently involve the dermis secondarily. The overlying skin is often alopecic and thickened when dermal involvement is present. Ulceration may occur in larger lesions. Most tumors involve the ventral trunk and proximal limbs.

The average age of affected animals is 10 years. In cats, however, Stephens reported that some strains of feline sarcoma virus can induce liposarcomas in kittens. Too few cases of canine or feline liposarcoma have been reported to determine breed predisposition.

Recurrence after surgical excision is common, but the incidence of distant metastasis is low. Metastatic sites reported by Theilen include lung, liver, and bone. Biologic behavior of liposarcoma in humans partially depends upon histopathologic subtype, but a similar occurrence has not been documented in animals.

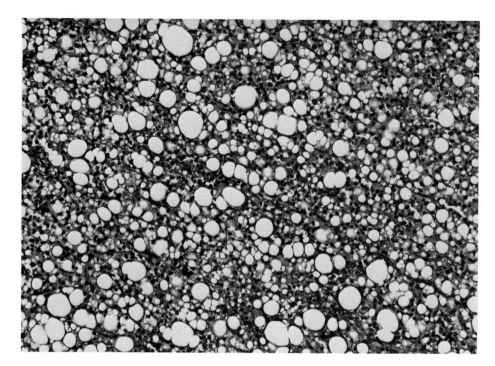

FIGURE 28-5. Well-differentiated liposarcoma in a dog. Polygonal cells are arranged in solid sheets and contain lipid vacuoles of varying size. (×120.)

Histopathology

Well-differentiated liposarcoma (Figure 28-5). This is the most common histopathologic subtype of liposarcoma. Well-differentiated liposarcomas are usually multilobular, circumscribed, but unencapsulated neoplasms comprising large polygonal cells arranged in solid sheets. Stromal collagen production is not observed. The cells have abundant cytoplasm and variable numbers of easily recognizable lipid droplets. Moderate numbers of cells have single large lipid vacuoles, resulting in peripheral nuclear displacement as in mature lipocytes. Other cells resemble lipoblasts and contain central nuclei and small numbers of delicate lipid droplets. Nuclei are large and pleomorphic and contain prominent nucleoli. Mitotic activity is low, but most of the mitoses are atypical. Hemorrhage, necrosis, fibrosis, and ulceration are secondary features that may be observed in these tumors.

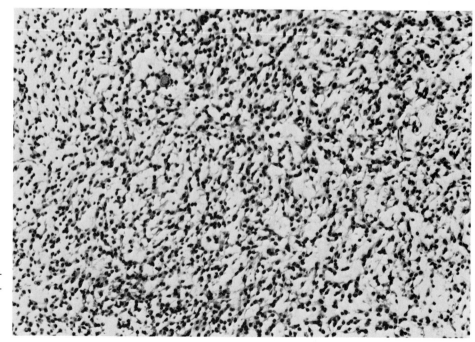

FIGURE 28-6. Myxoid liposarcoma in a dog. Spindle and stellate cells are arranged in loose bundles in a myxoid stroma. (×120.)

FIGURE 28-7. Higher power of myxoid liposarcoma shows bubbly appearance of stroma and single lipid vacuoles in many of the tumor cells. Note the mucin lake at top *(arrow).* (×240.)

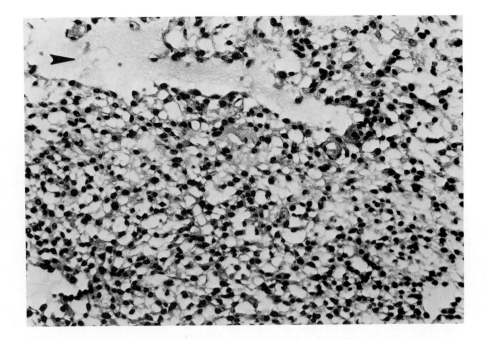

Myxoid liposarcoma (Figures 28-6 through 28-8). A less common variant is myxoid liposarcoma, which comprises predominantly small spindle cells arranged haphazardly or in interlacing bundles. Tumor margins are poorly defined. Well-differentiated lipocytes and small numbers of lipoblasts are usually scattered throughout the tumor. Nuclear features of the spindle cells resemble those of well-differentiated fibrosarcoma or myxosarcoma (see Chapter 26). The moderate stroma is composed of mucopolysaccharide ground substance and small numbers of collagen fibrils.

A delicate, anastomosing capillary vasculature is present. If cells of obvious lipocyte lineage are sparse or absent, differentiation from myxoid variants of other spindle-cell malignancies may not be possible.

Pleomorphic liposarcoma (Figure 28-9). This is a rare variant of liposarcoma. As the name implies, the tumor cells vary markedly in size and shape. Multinucleated giant cells are common. Stromal production of mucin or collagen is not observed. The cells have abundant eosinophilic cytoplasm that may appear glassy or foamy. Distinct lipid vacuoles are usually recognizable

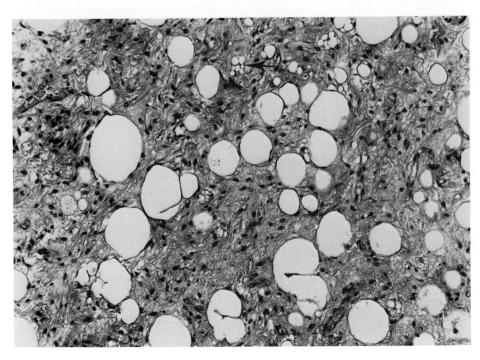

FIGURE 28-8. Myxoid liposarcoma in a dog. Spindle and stellate cells are distributed haphazardly through a stroma of mucin and collagen fibers. Note the scattered mature lipocytes with single large vacuoles and lipoblasts *(arrow)* with multiple small vacuoles. (×120.)

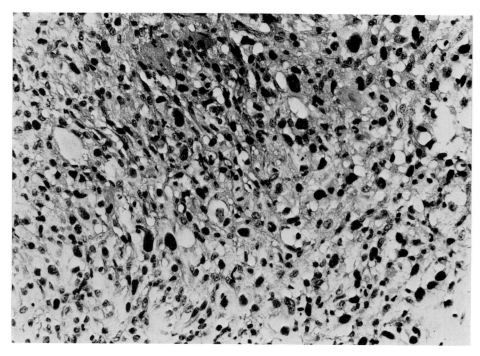

FIGURE 28-9. Pleomorphic liposarcoma in a dog. Solid sheets of highly pleomorphic polygonal cells exhibit variable lipid vacuolation. Note the markedly enlarged, hyperchromatic
nuclei. (×240.)

in small numbers of neoplastic cells. Nuclei also exhibit
marked variability in size, shape, and chromatin patterns. Nuclear hyperchromatism is a common feature.
Nucleoli are prominent, and there are many atypical
mitoses.

Pleomorphic liposarcoma may be difficult to distinguish from pleomorphic malignant fibrous histiocytoma. Intracellular lipid is present in most malignant
fibrous histiocytomas, but may be more finely dispersed or irregularly distributed than in liposarcomas.
Liposarcomas do not contain collagenous stroma or
radiating arrays of spindle cells, which are features of
malignant fibrous histiocytoma. No specific immunohistochemical markers exist for liposarcoma; positive
staining for lysozyme, alpha-1-antitrypsin and alpha-1-
antichymotrypsin may support a diagnosis of malignant fibrous histiocytoma.

HEMANGIOPERICYTOMA (Synonym:
canine hemangiopericytoma)
Clinical features

Hemangiopericytoma is a relatively common subcutaneous neoplasm reportedly arising from vascular
pericytes. Hemangiopericytomas occur exclusively in
dogs. Hemangiopericytoma accounted for 3.8% of
1141 skin and subcutaneous neoplasms in a survey by

one of the authors.* This neoplasm comprised 13.3%
of all mesenchymal neoplasms in a large review by
Goldschmidt. The pericytic origin of this neoplasm has
never been convincingly proven, despite ultrastructural
studies, and the morphology and behavior of canine
hemangiopericytoma are distinct from hemangiopericytoma in humans. Canine hemangiopericytoma has
histopathologic features in common with extracranial
meningioma and schwannoma, suggesting a possible
neural origin.

Hemangiopericytomas are solitary, multilobular,
fairly well-circumscribed masses with a firm or fatty
consistency. Approximately 20% involve the dermis as
well as the subcutis; pure dermal hemangiopericytomas
are rare. Most tumors are 5 to 10 cm in diameter, but
sizes may vary from as small as 1 cm to as large as 25
cm. The masses frequently adhere to underlying soft
tissue. Alopecia, hyperpigmentation, and ulceration are
commonly observed in the overlying skin. Hemangiopericytomas occur most frequently on the limbs; stifle
and elbow regions appear to be preferential sites.

The average age of affected animals in surveys by
Bostock, Graves, and also Postorino was 7 to 10 years.
Information on breed predisposition is variable, but
the authors concur with Postorino's data that large-

* Emily J. Walder.

breed dogs in general appear to be at greater risk. There is no obvious sex predilection.

Hemangiopericytomas exhibit frequent local recurrence with increasing invasiveness after successive surgeries. Two recent studies by Graves and Postorino reported recurrence rates of 26% and 38% respectively, and recurrence intervals of 1 to 56 months. Weiss' review article stated that necrotic hemangiopericytomas may metastasize. A case of pulmonary and regional lymph node metastasis of a hemangiopericytoma was also reported by Richardson; thus, classification of hemangiopericytoma as a low-grade malignancy seems appropriate. However, peripheral nerve sheath tumors in humans can, in rare instances, be primary in the hilus of a lymph node. These lesions are easily misinterpreted as metastatic sarcoma; therefore, it is possible that nodal schwannomas occasionally occur in dogs and may have been misinterpreted as metastatic hemangiopericytoma.

Histopathology (Figures 28-10 and 28-11)

Canine hemangiopericytomas are multilobular, unencapsulated subcutaneous or dermal masses comprising small spindle and polygonal cells. Cells are arranged

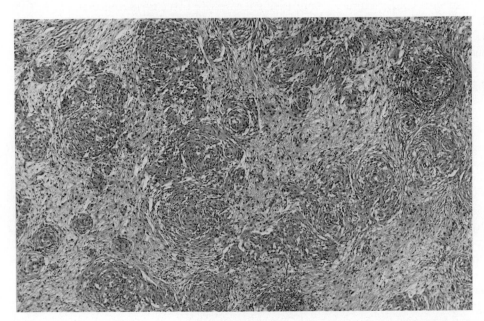

FIGURE 28-10. Canine hemangiopericytoma. Spindle cells in a whorled configuration are distributed in a stroma of collagen and mucin. (×50.)

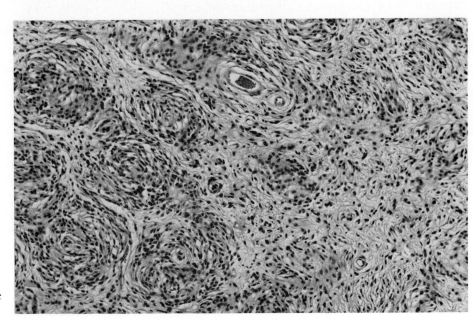

FIGURE 28-11. Canine hemangiopericytoma. The spindle and polygonal cells have uniform, ovoid nuclei. Note the capillaries at the centers of some spindle cell whorls. (×120.)

as interlacing bundles, sheets, and concentric whorls in varying proportions. Hemangiopericytomas with large numbers of whorls have the classically described "fingerprint" pattern. The whorls generally have a single capillary blood vessel at their centers, but non-perivascular whorls can also be identified. At the periphery of most hemangiopericytomas, tendrils of tumor cells extend along fascial planes, between lipocytes, and around tendon sheaths; the small caliber of these infiltrative structures makes clinical surgical assessment of tumor margins difficult. Zones of necrosis, hemorrhage, and fibrosis are common secondary features. Cellularity varies from moderately low to high, depending upon the quantity of stromal collagen and mucin. Stromal collagen is usually sparse and fibrillar. Lesions with abundant stromal mucin often appear as widely separated lobules and floating trabeculae of tumor tissue.

The tumor cells of hemangiopericytoma generally have poorly defined, pale eosinophilic or amphophilic cytoplasm. Nuclei are ovoid, pale, and uniform and have small central nucleoli. Mitotic activity is usually low. Nuclear pleomorphism and the mitotic index are often increased in recurrent lesions.

Differential diagnoses include schwannoma and the rare dermatofibrosarcoma variant of malignant fibrous histiocytoma. Differentiation of hemangiopericytoma from benign or well-differentiated malignant schwannoma can be difficult. Scattered pericapillary and noncapillary whorls are often observed in schwannomas, and the cytologic features are similar to those of hemangiopericytoma. However, schwannomas usually have a predominance of palisades and interlacing wavy bundles of cells (Antoni type A pattern). Encapsulation is also a more consistent feature of schwannomas. Predominance of fusiform and serpentine nuclei supports a diagnosis of schwannoma. The similarities between these two neoplasms often outweigh the differences, suggesting the possibility of a similiar cell of origin for both. The light microscopic and ultrastructural morphology of canine hemangiopericytoma bears a striking resemblance to that of extracranial meningioma, a rare tumor reported by Herrera in humans and one dog; these observations lend additional credence to the possibility of a neural rather than pericytic origin for canine hemangiopericytoma.

The rare dermatofibrosarcoma variant of malignant fibrous histiocytoma has similar cytoplasmic and nuclear features to hemangiopericytoma but lacks concentric whorls of spindle cells. Patterns resembling cartwheels may be observed in hemangiopericytoma but are probably formed as a result of intersection of partial whorls. Large numbers of repetitive, true storiform arrays are seen in malignant fibrous histiocytoma only.

TAIL DOCK NEUROMA
Clinical features

Tail dock neuroma is a recently described disorder that occurs rarely in dogs as a sequela to cosmetic caudectomy. Neuromas are a manifestation of traumatic or surgical nerve transection followed by disorganized proliferation of the proximal nerve stump because of poor apposition or the absence of the distal nerve segment. These tumors are reported in many species at a variety of anatomic locations.

Tail dock neuromas appear as painful, alopecic, hyperpigmented, lichenified lesions of the tail tip. The underlying connective tissue is thickened and firm, and there is focal adhesion between the connective tissue and the skin.

Affected animals are less than 4 years of age and often have a prolonged history of severe self-trauma to the tail tip. Five of six dogs in the original report were Cocker Spaniels, suggesting a possible breed predilection.

Histopathology (Figure 28-12)

Tail dock neuroma is characterized by acanthosis, compact hyperkeratosis, and diffuse dermal fibrosis. Fibrosis extends through the subcutis to the periosteum of the caudal coccygeal vertebra. The fibrous tissue is composed of thick collagen bundles with minimal cellularity, resembling scar tissue. Multiple small nerve bundles arranged individually and in clusters are distributed randomly through the connective tissue. Axons within the nerve bundles are thinly myelinated, and perineurium appears slightly thickened. The histologic appearance of tail dock neuroma is unique; there are no differential diagnoses.

SCHWANNOMA (Synonyms: peripheral nerve sheath tumor, neurofibroma, neurilemmoma)
Clinical features

Some authors in both human and veterinary disciplines have chosen to subclassify neural neoplasms based upon such features as presence or absence of encapsulation and amount and type of stroma (schwannoma, neurilemmoma, neurofibroma). Others believe that *schwannoma* is a more universal term, since all peripheral nerve sheath tumors are composed primarily of Schwann cells. In the opinion of the authors, the clinical and morphologic similarities among these proposed subclassifications outweigh the differences, and schwannoma or peripheral nerve sheath tumor is the preferred nomenclature for these neoplasms as a group.

Benign schwannomas are uncommon neoplasms in dogs and cats. This category of tumor is absent from most recent surveys. Benign schwannoma had an inci-

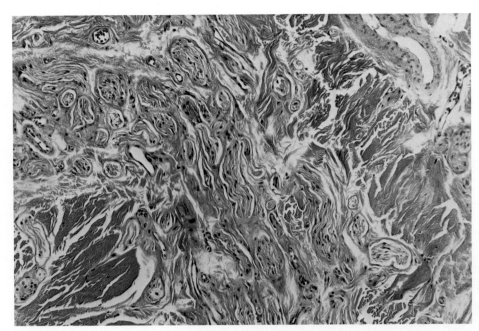

FIGURE 28-12. Tail dock neuroma in a dog. Numerous small nerve bundles are distributed haphazardly through thick collagen bundles resembling scar tissue. (×120.)

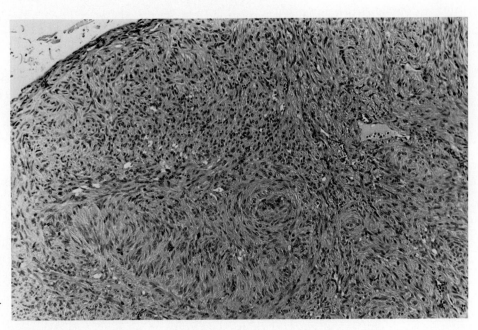

FIGURE 28-13. Schwannoma in a dog. Spindle cells are arranged in palisades and partial whorls. Note the delicate collagenous stroma. (×120.)

dence of 1% in dogs and 1.8% in cats in a survey of 1141 skin and subcutaneous neoplasms by one of the authors.* Both benign and malignant schwannomas of the dermis and subcutis in dogs and cats are probably underdiagnosed because of the histopathologic similarity to hemangiopericytoma, fibroma and fibrosarcoma, as well as the limited usage of immunohistochemical markers.

In dogs, schwannomas usually appear as circumscribed, firm or fleshy, lobulated subcutaneous masses

* Emily J. Walder.

measuring 2 to 5 cm in diameter. The overlying skin may be atrophic and alopecic. Lesions are most commonly located on the distal limbs. In cats, schwannomas are usually smaller intradermal nodules located on the head and neck. Affected animals are middle aged or older. There is no known breed predilection. Schwannomas may recur after surgical excision, but they do not metastasize.

Histopathology (Figures 28-13 through 28-15)

Classically, benign schwannomas are composed predominantly of small spindle cells arranged in wavy

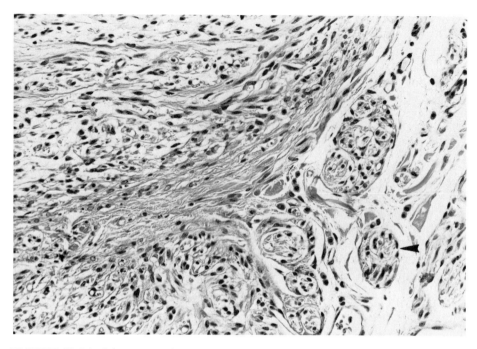

FIGURE 28-14. Schwannoma in a cat. Spindle cells are arranged in bundles and neuroid structures. Note the small nerve bundles *(arrow)* at the periphery of the tumor. (×240.)

bundles, partial whorls, and palisades. The tumors may or may not be encapsulated. Unencapsulated schwannomas in the subcutis may have delicate fingers of tumor tissue extending into adjacent fat and underlying

fascial planes. Dermal schwannomas usually extend to the dermal-epidermal junction, as in neurofibromatosis in humans. Cellularity is moderately low. There is usually a moderate collagenous stroma, but the collagen

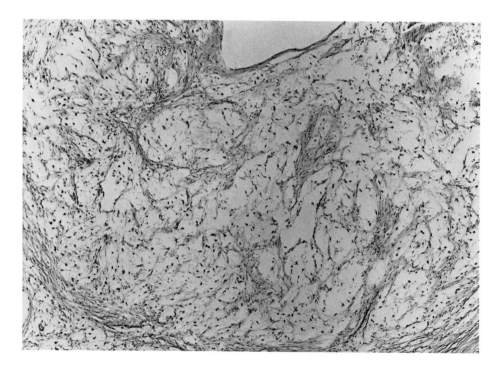

FIGURE 28-15. Myxoid schwannoma from the digit of a dog. Stellate and spindle cells tend to form loose whorls in an abundant myxoid stroma. Note the multilobular architecture created by collagen bundles. (×50.)

fibers are more delicate than in fibromatous neoplasms. The palisades of spindle cells may be oriented around small zones of sclerotic collagen. Other areas of the lesion may contain polygonal cells loosely distributed in a fibrillar and mucinous matrix.

Both spindle (Antoni type A) and polygonal (Antoni type B) cell components have ovoid, fusiform, or serpentine nuclei that are small and euchromatic. Nucleoli are inconspicuous, and mitotic figures are rare. Some schwannomas have mild nuclear hyperchromatism and pleomorphism and small numbers of mitoses. Atypical mitotic figures are not present even in the more proliferative lesions. Nerve twiglets can often be identified at the margins of schwannomas, but their presence is not requisite for the diagnosis.

An unusual variant of benign schwannoma is myxoid schwannoma (nerve sheath myxoma, neurothekeoma). One of the authors* has seen three examples in dogs, all located on a digit. Myxoid schwannomas have a multilobular configuration, with small spindle and stellate cells forming loose, concentric swirls in an abundant background of mucin. The tumor lobules are demarcated by delicate bands of collagen. These lobular structures are strongly reminiscent of pacinian corpuscles. Cytologic features are as described for typical schwannoma.

The differential diagnoses for benign schwannoma include fibroma, dermatofibroma, low-grade fibrosarcoma, hemangiopericytoma, and the dermatofibrosarcoma variant of malignant fibrous histiocytoma. Fibroma is less cellular and lacks palisades and whorls of cells. The stromal collagen is coarser and more abundant. Dermatofibroma and schwannoma have similar cellularity and architecture. Dermatofibromas can usually be distinguished by their ragged margins and entrapment of preexisting dermal collagen bundles. Fibrosarcoma usually has higher mitotic activity than schwannoma, and atypical mitoses are present. Fibrosarcomas also lack the palisaded and whorled cell arrangement found in neural tumors. Hemangiopericytoma and schwannoma are architecturally similar. The similarities between these two neoplasms often outweigh the differences, suggesting the possibility of a similar cell of origin for both. Hemangiopericytoma is often more cellular than schwannoma and pericapillary whorls are more prominent. In addition, a predominance of fusiform and serpentine nuclei is more consistent with a diagnosis of schwannoma, and nucleoli are smaller than in hemangiopericytoma. The rare dermatofibrosarcoma variant of malignant fibrous histiocytoma has cells arranged in storiform or cartwheel patterns, but these may be difficult to distinguish from the closely grouped palisades seen in schwannoma.

MALIGNANT SCHWANNOMA

(Synonyms: neurofibrosarcoma, malignant peripheral nerve sheath tumor)

Clinical features

Malignant schwannomas are generally reported to be rare malignant neoplasms of the dermis and subcutis in dogs and cats, but the authors believe these lesions to be somewhat more common in dogs. Malignant peripheral nerve sheath tumors are probably underdiagnosed because of their behavioral and histopathologic similarities to hemangiopericytoma and fibrosarcoma. In an unpublished survey of 1141 canine skin and subcutaneous neoplasms by one of the authors,* malignant schwannoma accounted for 2.8%.

Malignant schwannomas usually appear as single, lobulated, poorly circumscribed subcutaneous masses of variable consistency. Most lesions are 2 cm in diameter or larger. Primarily intradermal malignant schwannomas, which occur almost exclusively in cats, are usually smaller than 2 cm. Larger subcutaneous tumors, which are more common in dogs, usually adhere firmly to underlying soft tissue and overlying skin. The overlying skin is often alopecic, but ulceration is uncommon.

Affected animals are middle aged or older. There is no known breed predilection. Local recurrence after surgical excision is reported more commonly in cats than in dogs. There are no reports of metastasis of cutaneous or subcutaneous malignant schwannoma.

Histopathology (Figures 28-16 through 28-18)

Malignant schwannomas are unencapsulated neoplasms of the dermis or subcutis and are composed primarily of plump spindle cells arranged in interlacing bundles, palisades, and partial whorls. Palisade and whorl formation, which most likely represents an attempt to reduplicate tactile receptor structures, is generally not as prominent as in benign schwannomas. Dermal neoplasms usually extend to the dermal-epidermal junction, as in neurofibromatosis in humans. Entrapped nerve fibers, with or without infiltration by tumor, can sometimes be identified within large malignant schwannomas, and nerve twiglets may be detected at the periphery of smaller dermal neoplasms. Fingers of tumor tissue frequently invade the underlying soft tissue and along fascial planes and nerve sheaths. Small amounts of fibrous and myxoid stroma are observed and often have an irregular distribution through the neoplasm. The fibrous stroma can occasionally create a lobular or plexiform pattern. Heterologous elements— foci of cartilaginous, osseous, or epithelial metaplasia—which occur in 15% of human malignant schwan-

---

* Emily J. Walder.

* Emily J. Walder.

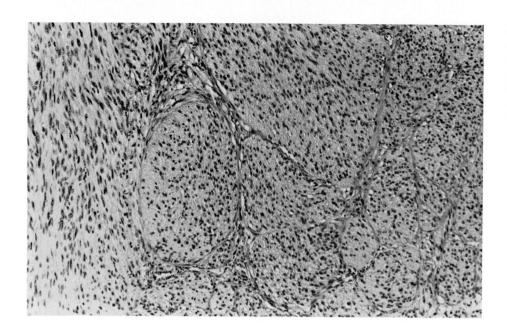

FIGURE 28-16. Malignant schwannoma in a cat. Spindle cells are arranged in bundles, partial whorls, and neuroid structures. Note the vesicular nuclei and small nucleoli. (×120.)

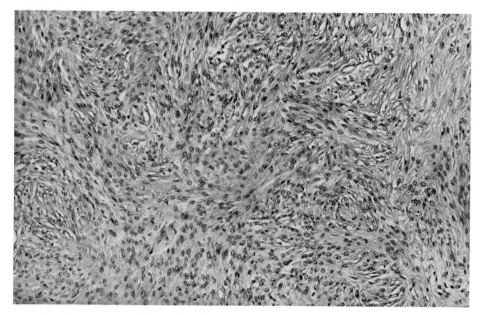

FIGURE 28-17. Malignant schwannoma in a dog. Spindle cells are arranged in palisades and partial whorls. Nuclei are ovoid and vesicular. (×120.)

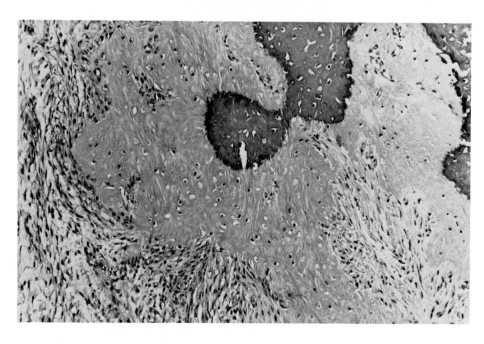

FIGURE 28-18. Same neoplasm as in Figure 28-17 shows large zone of chondro-osseous metaplasia. Spindle-cell component resembles fibrosarcoma or myxosarcoma. (×120.)

nomas, have not been previously reported in animals. Tumors with these features occur rarely, and they are easily misdiagnosed as extraskeletal chondrosarcomas or osteosarcomas.

Cellularity varies from moderate to high. The tumor cells have pale, poorly defined cytoplasm. Nuclei of the well-differentiated variants are moderately enlarged and vesicular and have fusiform, ovoid, or serpentine profiles. Nucleoli are usually small, and mitotic activity is low to moderate. Atypical mitoses are present. Patchy lymphocytic infiltrates are a fairly common feature. The less common (or less readily recognized), poorly differentiated malignant schwannomas exhibit higher cellularity and more subtle neuroid patterns. Nuclei are larger and more pleomorphic. Nucleoli are more prominent, and mitotic activity is higher.

Differential diagnoses for well-differentiated malignant schwannoma include hemangiopericytoma, fibrosarcoma, and the dermatofibrosarcoma variant of malignant fibrous histiocytoma. Well-differentiated malignant schwannomas exhibit similar cellularity and architecture to those of hemangiopericytomas. Malignant schwannomas generally have fewer and smaller whorled structures; most whorls do not contain central capillaries. Fibrosarcomas are distinguished from schwannomas by the absence of the palisaded and whorled cell arrangement characteristic of the neural tumors. Twisted and serpentine nuclei also suggest a neural origin. The rare dermatofibrosarcoma variant of malignant fibrous histiocytoma has cells arranged in storiform or cartwheel patterns, which can be difficult to distinguish from the closely grouped palisades of well-differentiated malignant schwannomas.

Separation of a poorly differentiated malignant schwannoma from fibrosarcoma or myxosarcoma may be impossible with routine histologic techniques. Immunohistochemical markers of value in identifying neural differentiation include S-100 protein, myelin basic protein, neuron-specific enolase, and neurofilament proteins. Increased application of immunohistochemical techniques should greatly enhance our ability to diagnose peripheral nerve sheath tumors and thus provide more accurate data on incidence and biologic behavior.

LEIOMYOMA
Clinical features

Leiomyomas are rare cutaneous neoplasms of dogs and cats that can arise from vascular smooth muscle, arrector pili muscle, or genital deep dermal smooth muscle. According to the review by Bevier, the reported incidence in dogs varies from 0% to 0.4%.

Leiomyomas are solitary, well-circumscribed, firm, round-to-ovoid nodules that are less than 2 cm in diameter. Cutaneous leiomyomas occur on the vulva, groin, head, and back. Interestingly, leiomyomas have not been reported in the scrotum, which contains abundant smooth muscle. Lesions do not recur after surgical excision. Age and breed predilections of affected animals have not been reported.

Histopathology (Figure 28-19)

Leiomyomas are small, circumscribed, but unencapsulated dermal nodules composed of long spindle cells arranged in interlacing fascicles. The tumor is fre-

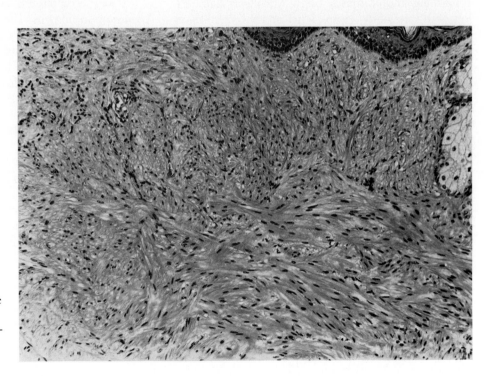

FIGURE 28-19. Leiomyoma in a dog. Long spindle cells are arranged in interlacing fascicles and exhibit perinuclear vacuolation. Note the uniform, cigar-shaped nuclei. (×120.)

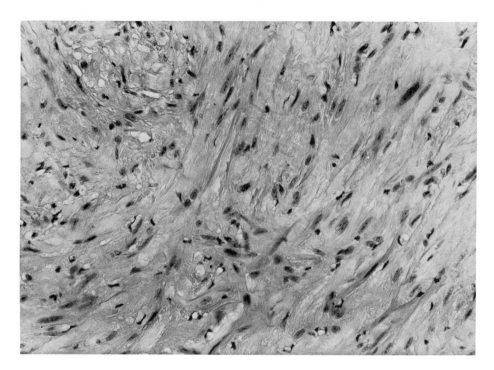

FIGURE 28-20. Leiomyosarcoma in a dog. Long spindle cells are arranged in interlacing fascicles and have patchy cytoplasmic vacuolation. Note the moderately enlarged, pleomorphic nuclei and small nucleoli. (×240.)

quently oriented around one or more hair follicles. Stromal collagen is minimal. The cells have abundant pink cytoplasm with perinuclear vacuolation. Nuclei are bland and elongate; they are blunt ended and have frequent chromatin cross-bars. Mitotic figures are not present.

The morphology of smooth muscle cells is distinctive, but leiomyomas may sometimes be confused with fibromas. Several special histologic stains are helpful in confirming smooth muscle origin: myofibers stain yellow with van Gieson's stain, whereas adjacent collagen stains red; myofibers are red with Masson's trichrome stain and often have longitudinal striations, whereas collagen stains blue; and smooth muscle cytoplasmic vacuoles contain glycogen, which can be demonstrated with a periodic acid–Schiff stain.

LEIOMYOSARCOMA
Clinical features

Cutaneous malignant smooth muscle neoplasms are rare in dogs and cats. Cutaneous smooth muscle malignancies may be underdiagnosed because of their resemblance to the far more common spindle-cell malignancies, such as fibrosarcoma and malignant schwannoma. Specific clinical information for cutaneous leiomyosarcoma is not available in the veterinary literature, but leiomyosarcomas in other anatomic locations are reported by Bevier to resemble fibrosarcomas in gross appearance and biologic behavior.

In humans, dermal smooth muscle malignancies are firm, uncircumscribed, frequently ulcerated masses that are less than 2 cm in diameter. Most lesions are located on the extremities. Subcutaneous leiomyosarcomas of humans are larger, more rapidly growing, and produce fewer changes in the overlying skin than do dermal leiomyosarcomas. The few cases of canine leiomyosarcoma observed by the authors were small, nonulcerated, predominantly dermal tumors located on the trunk.

Local recurrence of superficial leiomyosarcomas is common in humans. The metastatic rate in humans in 10% for dermal tumors and 40% for deeper lesions; metastasis is usually to the lungs but may also be to regional lymph nodes. The metastatic rate of canine leiomyosarcomas is believed to be low, but numeric data are not available.

Histopathology (Figure 28-20)

Leiomyosarcomas are usually circumscribed but unencapsulated dermal neoplasms composed of long spindle cells arranged in interlacing fascicles. They may extend secondarily into the subcutis. The overlying epidermis may show hyperplasia or ulceration. Stromal collagen is minimal. Most tumors are well differentiated, and cellularity is fairly low. The cells have abundant eosinophilic cytoplasm with variable vacuolation. Nuclei are moderately enlarged and pleomorphic, but the majority retain the typical blunt-ended, elongated configuration. Chromatin is usually stippled or marginated, and nucleoli are small. Chromatin cross-bars can usually be detected. Mitotic activity is low to moderate.

FIGURE 28-21. Benign fibrous histiocytoma in a dog. Polygonal histiocytic cells contain abundant cytoplasm with xanthomatous vacuolation. Note the scattered fibrocytic cells. (×240.)

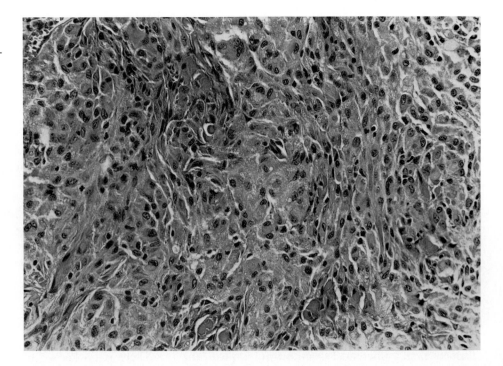

The myxoid, epithelioid, and pleomorphic variants of human leiomyosarcoma have not been reported in animals.

Diagnosis of cutaneous smooth muscle malignancies may be difficult because of their rarity and histopathologic similarities to other non–stroma producing spindle-cell malignancies, such as poorly differentiated fibrosarcoma and malignant schwannoma. The special histologic stains described for leiomyoma are potentially useful in the diagnosis of leiomyosarcoma. In addition, desmin and certain types of actin are immunohistochemical markers for smooth muscle tumors. Increased application of immunohistochemical techniques will greatly enhance the ability of the pathologist to detect the more poorly differentiated variants of leiomyosarcoma.

BENIGN FIBROUS HISTIOCYTOMA
Clinical features

The benign fibrohistiocytic tumor category in humans represents a group of tumors that have diverse etiologies but are composed of variable admixtures of fibrocytic and histiocytic cells. The fibrocytic component may exhibit storiform (cartwheel) patterning, as observed in malignant fibrous histiocytomas (see discussion below). The human entities that are usually assigned to this category include fibrous histiocytoma, dermatofibroma, eruptive histiocytoma, juvenile xanthogranuloma, and reticulohistiocytoma. The majority of these are believed to be reactive proliferations rather than true neoplasms, but the term *benign fibrohistiocytic tumor* has been retained in the literature for its descriptive and organizational value.

The authors have chosen to apply the nomenclature benign fibrous histiocytoma to a specific, uncommon cutaneous tumor occurring exclusively in dogs. These lesions are similar, but not identical, to juvenile xanthogranuloma in humans. The etiology of canine benign fibrous histiocytoma is unknown, but it may be reactive rather than neoplastic. The relationship, if any, to the common canine cutaneous histiocytoma is unknown.

Canine benign fibrous histiocytomas appear as solitary or occasionally multiple, partially alopecic, firm nodules measuring less than 1 cm in diameter. Lesions occur most often on the scrotum and legs, but other sites may be affected. Dogs with benign fibrous histiocytoma are usually 3 years of age or younger. In contrast to human juvenile xanthogranuloma, which often occurs in infants, lesions have not been observed in young puppies. There may be a breed predisposition in Golden Retrievers. Benign fibrous histiocytomas do not recur after surgical excision. It is not known if, as in juvenile xanthogranuloma of humans, spontaneous regression occurs.

Histopathology (Figure 28-21)

Benign fibrous histiocytoma is a circumscribed, but unencapsulated dermal nodule composed predominantly of histiocytic cells arranged in solid sheets. The lesion commonly has a wedge-shaped or base-narrow configuration. The cellular infiltrate usually extends to the dermal-epidermal junction, and the overlying epithelium is often hyperplastic. The infiltrate tends to spare hair follicles. Histiocytic cells in the superficial dermis may occasionally be arranged in short cords reminiscent of canine cutaneous histiocytoma. Small-to-moderate numbers of fibrocytic cells are present, but collagen production is sparse. Occasional hyalinized collagen bundles are present; these most likely represent residual dermal collagen.

The histiocytic cells are round to polygonal and have abundant, glassy, eosinophilic cytoplasm. The cytoplasm contains variable numbers of delicate vacuoles with smooth contours consistent with lipid. The nuclei are small and vary from round or oval to irregular. Nucleoli are inconspicuous, and mitotic figures are observed infrequently. Occasional multinucleated cells are present. Most benign fibrous histiocytomas have mild, patchy infiltrates of small lymphocytes. Neutrophils and eosinophils are usually present in small numbers.

The morphology of benign fibrous histiocytoma is distinctive, and differential diagnoses are limited. The histiocytes of canine cutaneous histiocytoma have sparser cytoplasm and do not exhibit lipidization. Cutaneous xanthomas associated with abnormalities of lipid metabolism are usually multiple and have much foamier cytoplasm. Granulomatous inflammation, either infectious or sterile, commonly has a pleocytic cell population with larger numbers of neutrophils, as well as a multinodular configuration.

MALIGNANT FIBROUS HISTIOCYTOMA
Clinical features

Malignant fibrous histiocytoma is a term first proposed in the human literature by Ozzello in 1963 to encompass a group of soft tissue neoplasms characterized by spindle cells in a storiform (cartwheel) growth pattern admixed with histiocytoid cells in varying proportions. These tumors were originally believed to be derived from a monocyte/macrophage cell that could undergo transition to a "facultative" fibroblast. The cell of origin of malignant fibrous histiocytoma is now considered to be more closely related to a true fibroblast. Ultrastructural studies consistently reveal mixtures of fibroblastic cells, myofibroblasts (primitive mesenchymal cells with intermediate features between fibroblasts and smooth muscle cells) and histiocytic cells in these neoplasms. Some controversy still exists as to their actual histogenesis. Nevertheless, malignant fibrous histiocytoma has been retained as an effective descriptive term for these bimorphic or pleomorphic neoplasms.

The nomenclature did not find its way into the veterinary literature until 1979 when Gleiser reviewed a small series of neoplasms in dogs and cats which were morphologically identical to malignant fibrous histiocytomas in humans. The authors concur with Gleiser that multiple subtypes of malignant fibrous histiocytoma occur in animals and are analogous to variants described in humans. Several cases were reported in the ensuing decade, and review articles by Bevier and also Macy describe these tumors. Malignant fibrous histiocytoma appears to be uncommon in cats and rare in dogs, but numeric data are not reported.

Malignant fibrous histiocytomas in animals usually appear as solitary, large, firm, poorly circumscribed, lobulated subcutaneous masses. Alopecia and ulceration are frequent features. Legs and shoulders are the most common sites.

The average age for malignant fibrous histiocytoma in both dogs and cats is 8 years, but malignant fibrous histiocytomas have been reported in cats as young as 2 years of age by Allen and also Renlund. There is no known breed predilection. Malignant fibrous histiocytomas are locally aggressive and recur frequently after surgical excision. Distant metastasis is not documented, but this may be a reflection of incomplete case follow-up. In humans, fewer than 10% of malignant fibrous histiocytomas limited to dermis and subcutis metastasize, whereas those with fascial and muscle involvement metastasize in 27% and 43% of patients, respectively.

Histopathology

Malignant fibrous histiocytoma in humans includes the low-grade malignancies of dermatofibrosarcoma protuberans and atypical fibroxanthoma, as well as a variety of histopathologic subtypes of high-grade malignancy. The variants of high-grade malignant fibrous histiocytoma designated by Enzinger are storiform-pleomorphic, myxoid, giant cell, inflammatory, and angiomatoid.

Most of these histopathologic subtypes are characterized by a bimorphic spindle and histiocytoid cell population in which the spindle cells are organized into storiform patterns. The word storiform is derived from the Latin *storea,* meaning rope mat. Individual units comprising the "mats" allegedly resemble spokes radiating from a central point. "Pinwheel" or "cartwheel" probably creates a more readily accessible word picture.

Dermatofibrosarcoma is a monomorphic neoplasm that is included by most authors in the malignant fibrous histiocytoma group because of its prominent storiform architecture; its cell of origin is still under debate. Veterinary analogs of storiform-pleomorphic type, giant cell tumor, and dermatofibrosarcoma pro-

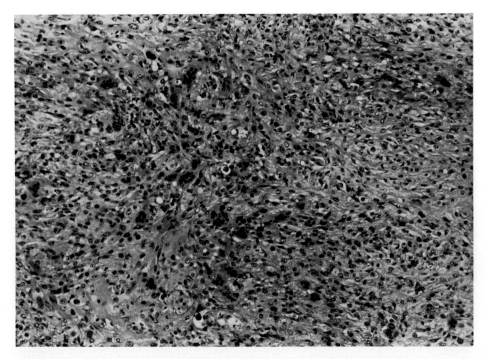

FIGURE 28-22. Malignant fibrous histiocytoma, giant cell type, in a cat. Numerous multinucleated giant cells are admixed with fibroblastic and histiocytic cells. Note the nuclear pleomorphism and variable chromatin patterns. (×120.)

tuberans have been described in the literature or observed by the authors.

Giant cell type (giant cell tumor of soft parts) (Figure 28-22). The giant cell subtype of malignant fibrous histiocytoma is the most common morphologic pattern observed in cats. These neoplasms are multilobular and are often partially encapsulated. There is a sparse-to-moderate collagenous stroma that may be hyalinized in some areas. Ulceration, necrosis, hemorrhage, and sclerosis are common secondary features. As the nomenclature indicates, these neoplasms contain large numbers of multinucleated giant cells admixed with spindle cells and mononuclear histiocytic cells. The giant cells resemble osteoclasts and have as many as 30 nuclei; however, underlying bone is not involved and the giant cells are not associated with osteoid stroma. Storiform patterns are infrequently observed in the spindle-cell population.

All three cell types of the giant cell type of malignant fibrous histiocytoma have moderate-to-abundant eosinophilic cytoplasm with variable vacuolation. Hemosiderin may be present in the histiocytic cells, indicating phagocytic capabilities. The spindle and histiocytic cells have large, pleomorphic nuclei and prominent nucleoli. Mitotic activity is fairly high, and mitotic atypia is common. Nuclei of the giant cells are usually smaller and hyperchromatic.

Differential diagnoses are fibrosarcoma and osteosarcoma. Feline fibrosarcoma may contain small or moderate numbers of multinucleated giant cells in some fields, but giant cells are never the predominant cell type, as they are in giant cell malignant fibrous histiocytoma. Both osteosarcoma and the giant cell subtype contain variable admixtures of spindle cells, polygonal cells, and multinucleated cells; multinucleated cells are more numerous in giant cell tumor, and osteoid stroma is not present.

Storiform-pleomorphic type (fibroblastic-pleomorphic type) (Figure 28-23). This subtype occurs most often in dogs but is also seen in cats. Storiform-pleomorphic malignant fibrous histiocytomas are unencapsulated, infiltrative masses composed of plump fibroblastic cells, histiocytic cells, and giant cells in varying proportions. The predominant cell type differs from case to case and from field to field within a given tumor. Reviews by Pulley, Bevier, and also Macy describe these tumors. The stroma is usually composed of delicate collagen fibers surrounding individual tumor cells. Some tumors have moderate, hyalinized stroma; patchy mucin deposition may also be seen. Ulceration, necrosis, and hemorrhage are common secondary features. The fibroblastic cells are arranged in short fascicles and storiform or cartwheel patterns; the cartwheels are frequently oriented around small blood vessels. The

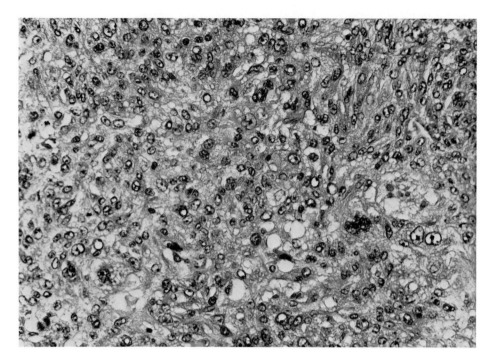

FIGURE 28-23. Malignant fibrous histiocytoma, storiform-pleomorphic type, in a dog. Pleomorphic fibroblastic and histiocytic cells are admixed with occasional multinucleated cells. Note the lipid vacuolation in moderate numbers of cells. (×240.)

pleomorphic areas have large spindle cells, polygonal cells, and giant cells arranged haphazardly.

The cytologic features are essentially as described for the giant cell type. The histiocytic cell population exhibits marked variation in cell size and shape. Nuclei have highly atypical features, including variable chromatin patterns, eccentricity, frequent cytoplasmic invaginations, and bizarre mitotic figures. Xanthoma cells (histiocytes filled with delicate lipid droplets) and lymphoplasmacytic infiltrates may also be present.

In tumors with a predominantly pleomorphic cell pattern, differential diagnoses of pleomorphic liposarcoma and even anaplastic carcinoma must be considered. Anaplastic carcinomas generally have cytoplasmic mucin, and immunohistochemistry is usually positive for cytokeratins or carcinoembryonic antigen. Intracellular lipid is present in most malignant fibrous histiocytomas, but may be more finely dispersed or irregularly distributed than in liposarcomas. Liposarcomas do not contain collagenous stroma or radiating arrays of spindle cells; however, multiple sections may be required to detect these features in this form of malignant fibrous histiocytoma. Immunohistochemical staining for lysozyme, alpha-1-antitrypsin and alpha-1-antichymotrypsin may support a diagnosis of malignant fibrous histiocytoma, but the specificity of these markers is now considered debatable.

Dermatofibrosarcoma type (dermatofibrosarcoma protuberans) (Figure 28-24). This histopathologic pattern is seen uncommonly in cats and rarely in dogs; it has not been previously described in the veterinary literature. These are unencapsulated subcutaneous neoplasms with secondary dermal involvement. In contrast, the large majority of human dermatofibrosarcomas are dermal plaque-like and nodular masses eventuating in the classic fungiform ("protuberans") appearance. Dermatofibrosarcoma is composed of a monotonous population of plump fibroblasts arranged in cartwheels and short bundles; there is no obvious perivascular orientation. The architecture resembles purely storiform areas occurring in storiform-pleomorphic malignant fibrous histiocytoma. Stromal collagen production is nominal. Necrosis is rarely observed. Cellularity is moderately high.

The spindle cells have scant, poorly defined cytoplasm and uniform, elongated nuclei. Mitotic activity is low to moderate, and there is little mitotic atypia. Giant cells, xanthoma cells, and inflammatory cells are infrequently noted.

Differential diagnoses include fibrosarcoma, hemangiopericytoma and malignant schwannoma. Differentiation between the dermatofibrosarcoma variant of malignant fibrous histiocytoma and fibrosarcoma usually is not difficult. Dermatofibrosarcoma is consis-

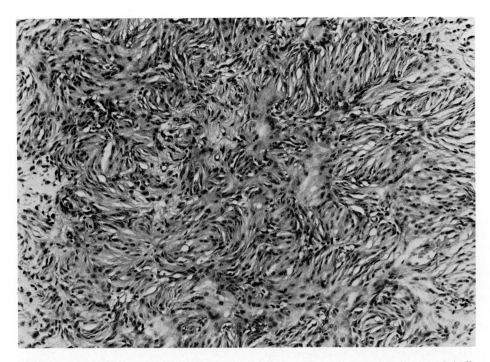

FIGURE 28-24. Malignant fibrous histiocytoma, dermatofibrosarcoma type, in a cat. Spindle cells are arranged in repetitive storiform (cartwheel) patterns. Note the relatively small, uniform nuclei. (×120.)

tently patterned, and cartwheel arrays of cells are rarely encountered in fibrosarcoma. Dermatofibrosarcoma may be confused with the more common hemangiopericytoma in dogs. Dermatofibrosarcoma lacks concentric whorls of spindle cells as seen in hemangiopericytoma. It may be difficult to distinguish dermatofibrosarcoma from malignant schwannoma; based on the close resemblance, some researchers have proposed a neural origin for dermatofibrosarcoma. Schwannian neoplasms generally have palisades and undulating bundles interspersed with whorled patterns, and foci of differentiation toward neural tactile structures are often present. Dermatofibrosarcomas also are routinely negative for S-100 protein, a common component of neural tumors.

SUGGESTED READINGS

Lipomatosis

Carpenter JL, Andrew LK, and Holzworth J: Tumors and tumor-like lesions. In Holzworth J, editor: Diseases of the cat, Philadelphia, 1987, WB Saunders, p 423.

Gilbert PA, Griffin CE, and Walder EJ: Diffuse trunkal lipomatosis in a dog, J Am Anim Hosp Assoc 26:586-588, 1990.

Lipoma

Bevier DE and Goldschmidt MH: Skin tumors in the dog. II. Tumors of the soft (mesenchymal) tissues, Comp Cont Ed 3:506-514, 1981.

Goldschmidt MH: Dermal mesenchymal neoplasms of domestic animals. Proceedings of the Annual Meeting of the American Academy of Veterinary Dermatology/American College of Veterinary Dermatology, Orlando, pp 1-11, 1985.

Pulley LT and Stannard AA: Tumors of the skin and soft tissues. In Moulton J, editor: Tumors in domestic animals, ed 3, Berkeley, Calif, 1990, University of California Press, p 31.

Strafuss AC and others: Lipomas in dogs, Proc Am Anim Hosp Assoc 9:555-556, 1973.

Fibrolipoma

Enzinger FM and Weiss SE: Soft tissue tumors, ed 2, St Louis, 1988, CV Mosby, p 305.

Pulley LT and Stannard AA: Tumors of the skin and soft tissues. In Moulton J, editor: Tumors in domestic animals, ed 3, Berkeley, Calif, 1990, University of California Press, p 31.

Infiltrative lipoma

Gleiser CA and others: Infiltrating lipomas in the dog, Vet Pathol 16:623-624, 1979.

McChesney AE and others: Infiltrative lipoma in dogs, Vet Pathol 17:316-322, 1980.

Scott DW: Feline dermatology, 1983-1985: "the secret sits," J Am Anim Hosp Assoc 23:255-274, 1986.

Liposarcoma

Bevier DE and Goldschmidt MH: Skin tumors in the dog. II. Tumors of the soft (mesenchymal) tissues, Comp Cont Ed 3:506-514, 1981.

Doster AR and others: Canine liposarcoma, Vet Pathol 23:84-87, 1986.

Enzinger FM and Weiss SE: Soft tissue tumors, ed 2, St Louis, 1988, CV Mosby, pp 346-382.

Messick JB and Radin MJ: Cytologic, histologic and ultrastructural characteristics of a canine myxoid liposarcoma, Vet Pathol 26:520-522, 1989.

Stephens LC and others: Virus-associated liposarcoma and malignant lymphoma in a kitten, J Am Vet Med Assoc 192:90-91, 1988.

Theilen GH and Madewell BR, editors: Veterinary cancer medicine, ed 2, Philadelphia, 1987, Lea & Febiger, p 292.

Hemangiopericytoma

Bevier DE and Goldschmidt MH: Skin tumors in the dog. II. Tumors of the soft (mesenchymal) tissues, Comp Cont Ed 3:506-514, 1981.

Bostock DE and Dye MT: Prognosis after surgical excision of canine fibrous connective tissue sarcomas, Vet Pathol 17:581-588, 1980.

Goldschmidt MH: Dermal mesenchymal neoplasms of domestic animals, Proceedings of the Annual Meeting of the American Academy of Veterinary Dermatology/American College of Veterinary Dermatology, Orlando, pp 1-11, 1985.

Graves G, Bjorling DE, and Mahaffey E: Canine hemangiopericytoma: 23 cases (1967-1984), J Am Vet Med Assoc 192:99-102, 1988.

Herrera GA and Mendoza A: Primary canine cutaneous meningioma, Vet Pathol 18:127-130, 1981.

Postorino NC and others: Prognostic variables for canine hemangiopericytoma: 50 cases (1979-1984), J Am Anim Hosp Assoc 24:501-509, 1988.

Richardson RC and others: Metastatic canine hemangiopericytoma, J Am Vet Med Assoc 812:705-706, 1983.

Weiss E: Tumours of the soft (mesenchymal) tissues, Bull World Health Organ 50:101-110, 1974.

Xu FN: Ultrastructure of canine hemangiopericytoma, Vet Pathol 23:643-645, 1986.

Taildock neuroma

Gross TL and Carr SH: Amputation neuroma of docked tails in dogs, Vet Pathol 27:61-62, 1990.

Schwannoma

Bevier DE and Goldschmidt MH: Skin tumors in the dog. II. Tumors of the soft (mesenchymal) tissues, Comp Cont Ed 3:506-514, 1981.

Enzinger FM and Weiss SE: Soft tissue tumors, ed 2, St Louis, 1988, CV Mosby, pp 719-780.

Goldschmidt MH: Dermal mesenchymal neoplasms of domestic animals, Proceedings of the Annual Meeting of the American Academy of Veterinary Dermatology/American College of Veterinary Dermatology, Orlando, pp 1-11, 1985.

Malignant schwannoma

Bostock DE and Dye MT: Prognosis after surgical excision of canine fibrous connective tissue sarcomas, Vet Pathol 17:581-588, 1980.

Brown NO and others: Soft tissue sarcomas in the cats, J Am Vet Med Assoc 173:744-749, 1978.

Enzinger FM and Weiss SE: Soft tissue tumors, ed 2, St Louis, 1988, CV Mosby, pp 781-815.

George E, Swanson PE, and Wick MR: Malignant peripheral nerve sheath tumors of the skin, Am J Dermatopathol 11:213-331, 1989.

Goldschmidt MH: Dermal mesenchymal neoplasms of domestic animals, Proceedings of the Annual Meeting of the American Academy of Veterinary Dermatology/American College of Veterinary Dermatology, Orlando, pp 1-11, 1985.

Leiomyoma

Bevier DE and Goldschmidt MH: Skin tumors in the dog. II. Tumors of the soft (mesenchymal) tissues, Comp Cont Ed 3:506-514, 1981.

Enzinger FM and Weiss SE: Soft tissue tumors, ed 2, St Louis, 1988, CV Mosby, p 384.

Goldschmidt MH: Dermal mesenchymal neoplasms of domestic animals, Proceedings of the Annual Meeting of the American Academy of Veterinary Dermatology/American College of Veterinary Dermatology, Orlando, pp 1-11, 1985.

Leiomyosarcoma

Bevier DE and Goldschmidt MH: Skin tumors in the dog. II. Tumors of the soft (mesenchymal) tissues, Comp Cont Ed 3:506-514, 1981.

Enzinger FM and Weiss SE: Soft tissue tumors, ed 2, St Louis, 1988, CV Mosby, pp 414-417.

Benign fibrous histiocytoma

Enzinger FM and Weiss SE: Soft tissue tumors, ed 2, St Louis, 1988, CV Mosby, pp 223-243.

Malignant fibrous histiocytoma

Allen SW and Duncan JR: Malignant fibrous histiocytoma in a cat, J Am Vet Med Assoc 192:90-91, 1988.

Bevier DE and Goldschmidt MH: Skin tumors in the dog. II. Tumors of the soft (mesenchymal) tissues, Comp Cont Ed 3:506-514, 1981.

Confer AW, Enright FM, and Beard GB: Ultrastructure of feline extraskeletal giant cell tumor (malignant fibrous histiocytoma), Vet Pathol 18:738-744, 1981.

Enzinger FM and Weiss SE: Soft tissue tumors, ed 2, St Louis, 1988, CV Mosby, pp 252-300.

Gleiser CA and others: Malignant fibrous histiocytoma in dogs and cats, Vet Pathol 16:199-208, 1979.

Macy DW and Reynolds, HA: The incidence, characteristics and clinical management of skin tumors of cats, J Am Anim Hosp Assoc 17:1026-1034, 1981.

Ozzello L, Stout AP, and Murray MR: Cultural characteristics of malignant histiocytomas and fibrous xanthomas, Cancer 16:331-344, 1963.

Pulley LT and Stannard AA: Tumors of the skin and soft tissues. In Moulton J, editor: Tumors in domestic animals, ed 3, Berkeley, Calif, 1990, University of California Press, p 27.

Renlund RC and Pritzker KPH: Malignant fibrous histiocytoma involving the digit in a cat, Vet Pathol 21:442-444, 1984.

See also General References, pp 327-328.

Melanocytic tumors

MELANOCYTOMA (Synonyms: pigmented nevus, melanocytic nevus, blue nevus, benign melanoma)

Melanocytoma is the term the authors have chosen to encompass all variants of benign neoplasms arising from melanocytes, the pigment-producing cells of epidermis, dermis, mucous membranes, and the eye. A simple, comparative classification scheme using this terminology has been proposed by Pulley. Melanocytomas are traditionally subdivided by the location of the neoplastic cells within the skin: junctional, compound, and dermal.

The nomenclature of human melanocytic tumors is fairly complex, and great confusion is engendered by the use of such terms as *congenital nevus, acquired nevus,* and *nevus cell.* The so-called nevus cells, which make up the pigmented nevi of humans, are now known to be melanocytes with slight histopathologic and biochemical alterations. Based on this fact, Magana-Garcia recently suggested that all human, noncongenital, benign proliferations of melanocytes be designated *melanocytomas.* The authors applaud this logical approach and hope that it will lead to more meaningful comparative studies. The designation *nevus* will be avoided except for comparative purposes until a congenital basis for melanocytic tumors is more adequately documented in veterinary medicine.

The term *melanoma* has been variably employed in veterinary nomenclature systems. Some classifications use the term to designate both benign and malignant neoplasms. Melanoma will be used synonymously in this text with malignant melanoma.

Clinical features

Cutaneous melanocytomas are relatively common in dogs and rare in cats. In a large series of canine cutaneous tumors reviewed by Conroy, melanocytic neoplasms accounted for 6%, and two thirds of these were benign. Melanocytic neoplasms account for fewer than 2% of tumors in all feline surveys, and the distinction often is not made between benign and malignant lesions. In reviews by Carpenter and Macy, 29% and 47%, respectively, of melanocytic feline skin tumors were histopathologically benign.

Purely junctional (intraepidermal) melanocytomas similar to human junctional pigmented nevi are not described in dogs or cats. This may be because solitary macular pigmented lesions are difficult to detect on haired skin and are unlikely to be biopsied even when present on glabrous skin. Compound melanocytomas (intraepidermal and dermal), which are similar to compound melanocytic nevi in humans, are the most common type observed in dogs. They are rare in cats. Dermal melanocytomas are also quite common in dogs; most lesions are similar to human cellular blue nevus or

common blue nevus. All of the feline benign melanocytic tumors described by Carpenter were also of this
histopathologic type. A rare variant of dermal melanocytoma is balloon-cell melanocytoma, which is analagous to human balloon-cell nevus. It has not been
previously described, but the authors have recognized
occasional cases in dogs.

Compound melanocytomas usually appear as solitary, circumscribed, brown-to-black, alopecic nodules
that are less than 1 cm in diameter. The nodules may
be smooth or slightly papillated and vary from papular
to dome shaped to pedunculated in configuration. Ulceration is uncommon. Lesions occur most often on
the trunk and head, especially on the eyelids and muzzle. Dermal melanocytomas appear as solitary, circumscribed, alopecic, fleshy, dome-shaped masses that are
0.5 to 4 cm in diameter. The lesions generally appear
blue-black when viewed through lightly pigmented
skin, but they may also appear dark brown-to-black
because of hyperpigmentation of the overlying epidermis. Dermal melanocytomas occur most often on the
trunk and occasionally on the extremities, particularly
between the digits.

The average age of dogs with melanocytomas in
the study by Bolon was 8.1 years, but dogs as young as
1.5 years were affected. Conroy reported a higher incidence of all melanocytic neoplasms in breeds with
darker pigmentation, such as Scottish and Airedale
Terriers, and male dogs. The study by Bolon reported a
higher incidence in Doberman Pinschers and Miniature
Schnauzers, but there was no sex predilection.

Malignant transformation occurs in a small percentage of benign melanocytic tumors in humans. This
phenomenon has not been well documented in animals
but Conroy has suggested that it may occur occasionally. In addition, clinical and histopathologic criteria
used to differentiate between benign and malignant
melanocytic neoplasms are not always clear-cut. In
Bostock's retrospective survey of melanocytic neoplasms in dogs, 4 of 52 dogs with apparently benign
lesions developed metastases or inoperable recurrences.
It is therefore prudent that all melanocytic neoplasms
be completely excised and clean tissue margins established by excisional biopsy.

Histopathology

Junctional melanocytomas have a predominance of
melanocytes located within the epidermis along the
dermal-epidermal junction. Clusters of melanocytes
along outer layers of follicular epithelium are also considered to be a manifestation of junctional activity.
Compound melanocytomas have tumor cells in the
dermis, as well as a dermal-epidermal or follicular component. The natural progression from junctional to
compound melanocytoma is well documented in humans and pigs but is still speculative in other species.
Dermal melanocytomas are strictly intradermal in location.

**Compound melanocytoma (Figures 29-1
through 29-3).** Compound melanocytoma is a circumscribed, but unencapsulated neoplasm composed
predominantly of small spindle and polygonal cells and

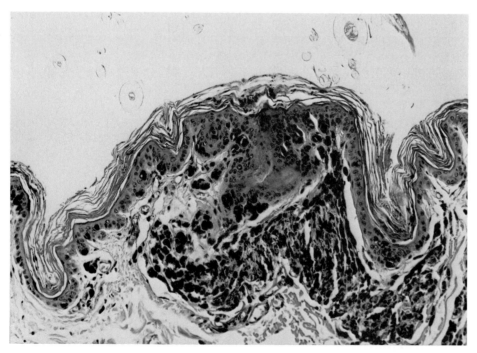

FIGURE 29-1. Compound
melanocytoma in a dog. This
small nodular neoplasm is composed of heavily pigmented,
epithelioid melanocytes arranged in nests and clusters.
Note the relative symmetry of
both dermal and epidermal
components. (×140.)

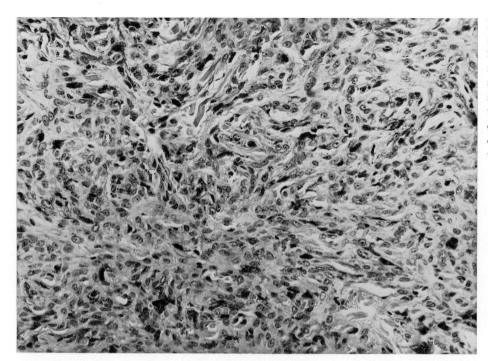

FIGURE 29-2. Compound melanocytoma in a dog. Fusiform cells in the dermal component are sparsely pigmented and are arranged in short bundles and nests. Nuclei are ovoid and uniform and have small nucleoli. Note the heavily pigmented epithelioid cells scattered through the tumor. (×240.)

large round-to-polygonal epithelioid cells. Lesions frequently have a symmetric, wedge-shaped configuration. Occasional melanocytomas are plaque-like. Focal ulceration caused by trauma may be present.

Variable numbers of nests and clusters of large epithelioid cells are distributed along the dermal-epidermal junction. Epithelioid cells may also be clustered along the outer layers of the epithelium of residual hair follicles. Some neoplasms have melanocyte nests localized to the uppermost superficial dermis and spare the epidermis; it is presumed that the cell nests have migrated downward from their previous location in the epidermis, as is observed in the life cycle of human pigmented nevi. Small spindle or polygonal

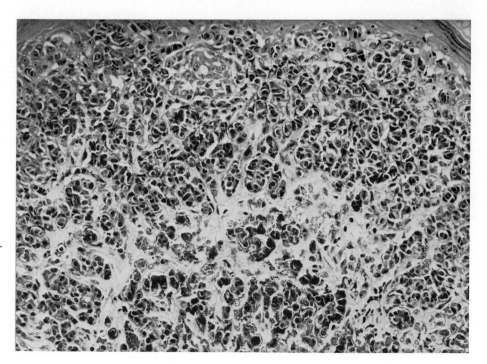

FIGURE 29-3. Compound melanocytoma in a dog. Epithelioid cells containing moderate melanin pigment are arranged in nests and clusters within the dermis and along the dermal-epidermal junction. Nuclei are relatively small and uniform. (×240.)

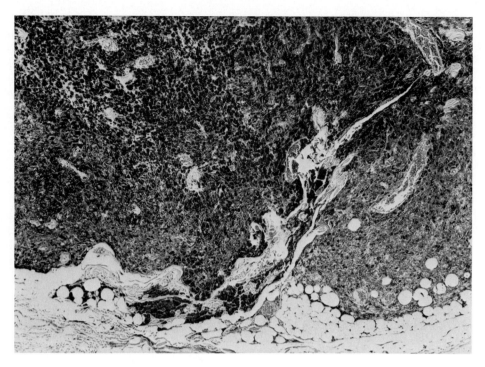

FIGURE 29-4. Dermal melanocytoma in a dog. A large, well-circumscribed mass of heavily pigmented cells encroaches on the subcutaneous fat. (×40.)

melanocytes are arranged in solid sheets, nests, and partial whorls in the dermis. The spindle-cell component in the deeper dermis is sometimes arranged in small whorls and serpentine bundles, simulating neural structures. This is not unexpected in light of the embryologic derivation of melanocytes from the neural crest.

The dermal spindle and polygonal cells usually have sparsely distributed melanin pigmentation, but some lesions are uniformly deeply pigmented. The large epithelioid cells of the dermal-epidermal junction and the outer follicular wall are heavily pigmented. The epidermis is hyperpigmented regardless of the presence of intraepidermal melanocyte clusters.

The epithelioid melanocytes have abundant melanin granules, which may obscure nuclear features. The fusiform and small polygonal melanocytes have pale, poorly defined cytoplasm with few or moderate melanin granules. Melanin granules within the neoplastic melanocytes are small and of uniform size within a given cell. All of the melanocytes have slightly enlarged, ovoid, vesicular nuclei and small or inconspicuous nucleoli. Mitotic figures are rare, and mitotic atypia is not observed. Small numbers of melanophages, sometimes accompanied by lymphocytes and plasma cells, are usually present at the base of the neoplasm. Melanophages are large, round macrophages that are distended with coarse melanin granules of varying size.

Dermal melanocytoma (Figures 29-4 through 29-7). Dermal melanocytoma is a circumscribed, but unencapsulated intradermal neoplasm with a variety of histopathologic patterns. A grenz zone is often present in the superficial dermis. Larger tumors may encroach upon subcutaneous fat. The epidermis is often hyperpigmented, and ulceration is not uncommon, especially in larger lesions.

The most common histopathologic variant is composed of plump fusiform cells arranged in whorls and nests reminiscent of nerve sheath tumors. The tumor is moderately cellular, and stromal collagen is not present. The cells have moderate numbers of fine melanin granules. Heavily pigmented melanophages are usually distributed through the tumor in small to moderate numbers. The melanophages are often grouped into small clusters. The melanocytes have ovoid, vesicular nuclei and small or prominent nucleoli. Nuclei may be quite large, but nuclear pleomorphism is minimal. Mitotic activity is low, and mitotic atypia is not observed. Small foci of necrosis may be present.

Another common variant of dermal melanocytoma is composed of large epithelioid and dendritic melanocytes with diffusely abundant, coarse melanin granules. Stromal collagen is moderate. Nuclear features are as described previously but are frequently obscured by the melanin pigment. Bleaching with permanganate or ox-

FIGURE 29-5. Dermal melanocytoma in a dog. Sparsely pigmented fusiform cells arranged in whorls and nests are interspersed with heavily pigmented epithelioid cells and melanophages. (×120.)

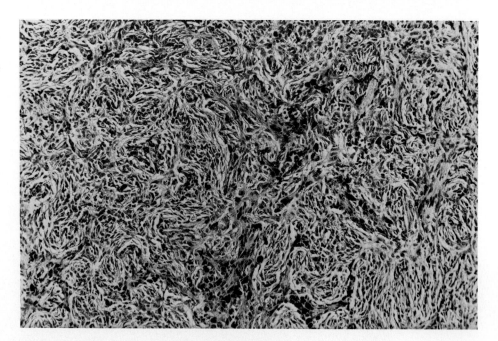

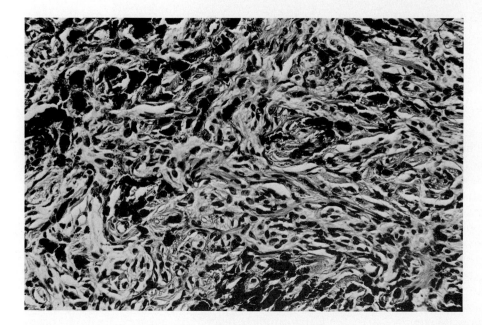

FIGURE 29-6. Higher magnification of the dermal melanocytoma in Figure 29-5 shows uniform, ovoid nuclei and inconspicuous nucleoli. Note the small bundles and nests reminiscent of neural tumors. (×240.)

FIGURE 29-7. Dermal melanocytoma in a dog. Moderately pigmented epithelioid cells are arranged in sheets and nests. Nuclei are large and vesicular but uniform. Note the coarse melanin granules in melanophages at top left. (×240.)

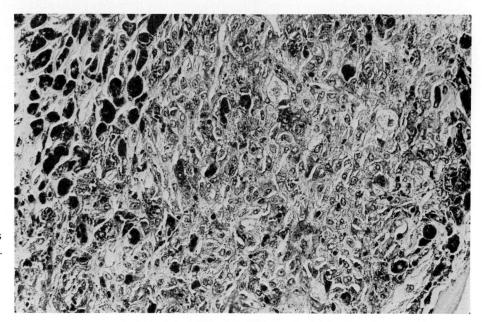

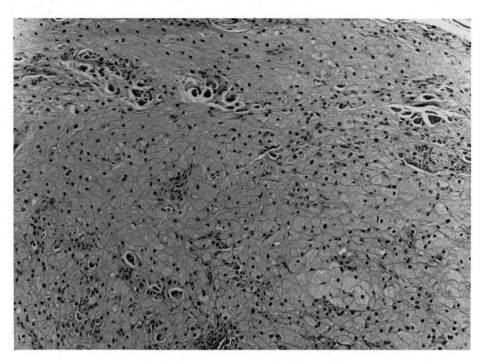

FIGURE 29-8. Balloon-cell melanocytoma in a dog. Solid sheets of large, polygonal cells have finely granular pigmentation. Nuclei are small and dark. (×120.)

alic acid is frequently helpful for accurate evaluation of nuclear morphology and mitotic index.

Balloon-cell melanocytoma (Figure 29-8). The rare balloon-cell melanocytoma is a well-circumscribed dermal nodule composed predominantly of large, epithelioid cells with abundant, pale cytoplasm. Small numbers of typical fusiform or polygonal melanocytes are often present. The cytoplasm of the balloon cells generally has a finely granular quality. Dust-like melanin granules can usually be detected in small numbers of tumor cells, but Fontana-Masson stain is often required to identify melanin pigment. Nuclei are small, uniform, and ovoid. Mitotic figures are rare.

Differentiation of melanocytoma from malignant melanoma can be problematic. Large tumor size, ulceration, and atypical nuclei can be misinterpreted in these neoplasms as features of malignancy. Architectural symmetry and well-defined tumor margins are indicators of a benign lesion regardless of size. Compound melanocytomas have nests of melanocytic cells confined to the dermal-epidermal junction; malignant melanomas may have melanocytic cells at higher levels of the epidermis. Although the nuclei of melanocytomas can be large and have prominent nucleoli, relative nuclear uniformity is observed. According to Bostock's retrospective study, the mitotic index is a significant determinant of biologic behavior of melanocytic neoplasms; a mitotic rate of fewer than 2 per 10 high-power fields indicated benign biologic behavior in most cases.

LENTIGO (Synonym: lentigo simplex)
Clinical features

A lentigo is a melanocytic proliferation that is usually confined to the epidermis. It is best interpreted as a melanocytic hyperplasia rather than a true neoplasm. Lentigines are not included in the classification systems of Pulley or Conroy and appear to be rare in animals. Lesions analogous to human lentigo simplex have been described in dogs by Muller, Kirk, and Scott and Briggs and in cats by Scott and Nash. The authors believe that the canine lesions reported as multicentric lentigo simplex (lentiginosis profusa) are more consistent with pigmented epidermal nevi than with primary melanocytic tumors (see Chapter 21). Melanocytic proliferations resembling lentigo simplex have been observed in dogs, but too few lesions have been studied to determine if the human nomenclature is applicable.

Lentigines are black, macular, or slightly raised, well-circumscribed lesions that are usually less than 1 cm in diameter. Lentigines are generally multiple and may be numerous. The lesions in cats occur predominantly on the head, often on the lips, eyelid margins, and nasal planum. Lentigines in dogs have been observed exclusively on the nipples.

Lesions in cats often first appear in animals less than 1 year of age, increase in size and number, and then become stable; this is consistent with a congenital etiology. There is no breed predilection in cats, but

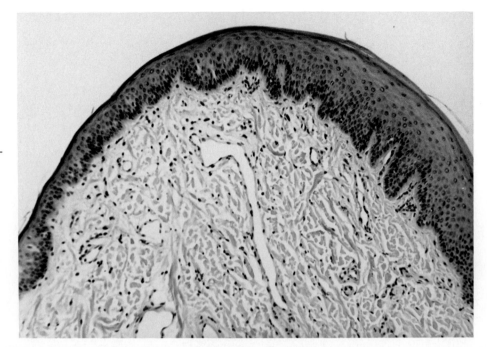

FIGURE 29-9. Lentigo in a cat. Densely pigmented melanocytes have accumulated in the basal cell layer of the lip margin. Note that epithelial hyperplasia is minimal. (×120.)

affected animals have orange, cream, red, tricolor, or silver haircoats. Lesions in dogs occur in older animals, and there is no known breed predisposition.

Histopathology (Figures 29-9 and 29-10)

Lentigines are discrete, plaque-like lesions characterized by irregular epidermal hyperplasia, hyperpigmentation, and increased numbers of deeply pigmented melanocytes. Epidermal hyperpigmentation is often severe enough to obscure the melanocytic hyperplasia in the basal layer and may extend through the epidermis into the stratum corneum. Epidermal hyperplasia is more prominent in lentigines in dogs than in cats. The melanocytes, enlarged because of engorgement with melanin, are usually distributed as single cells among the basal epithelial cells, but dermal-

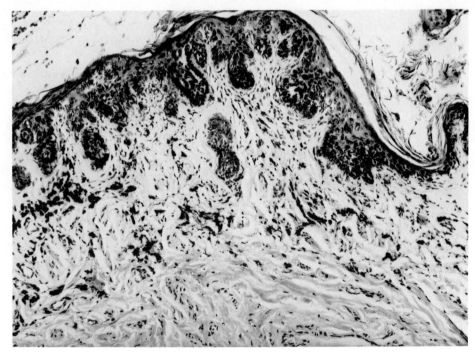

FIGURE 29-10. Lentigo in a dog. Densely pigmented melanocytes are concentrated around elongated rete ridges of the nipple. Hyperpigmentation extends into the stratum corneum. Note the stellate melanocytes in the underlying dermis. (×120.)

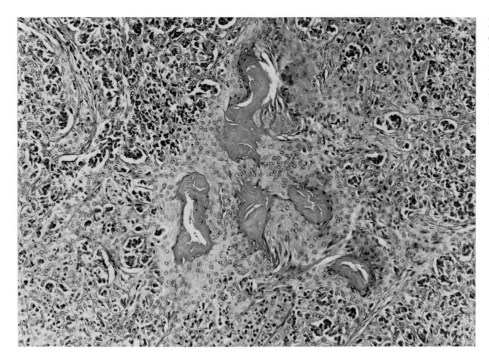

FIGURE 29-11. Melanocytoma-acanthoma in a dog. Islands of small, pale keratinocytes have central cysts filled with amorphous keratin. Clusters of small melanocytes are present in the stroma and within the epithelium. (×120.)

epidermal clusters may occasionally be present. The enlarged melanocytes may be concentrated along elongated rete ridges. Small numbers of melanophages may be present in the superficial dermis. Other than increased melanin content, the melanocytes of lentigo simplex are histologically normal.

The differential diagnosis for lentigo simplex is pigmented epidermal nevus. Simple lentigines are clinically flat or slightly elevated lesions; they do not appear papillated or scaly, as do epidermal nevi. Epidermal nevi exhibit papillomatous epidermal hyperplasia, hypergranulosis, and hyperkeratosis. Lentigines have mild or moderate epidermal hyperplasia characterized by rete ridge formation.

MELANOCYTOMA-ACANTHOMA
Clinical features

Melanocytoma-acanthoma is a rare, previously unreported neoplasm of dogs that has features of both compound melanocytoma and benign epithelial neoplasia. The epithelial component appears to show follicular differentiation, but the exact classification is unclear. The authors have chosen the general appellation *acanthoma* until the epithelial pattern can be more specifically categorized. This melanocytic neoplasm has no human analogue.*

Melanocytoma-acanthomas are solitary, circum-

scribed, pigmented, dome-shaped nodules that measure less than 1 cm in diameter. Age, breed, and site predilections are as yet undetermined.

Histopathology (Figures 29-11 and 29-12)

Melanocytoma-acanthomas are well-circumscribed, unencapsulated, ovoid dermal nodules that are focally contiguous with the epidermis. The epithelial component is characterized by anastomosing trabeculae of fairly small keratinocytes with peripheral palisading. Scattered cystic structures contain amorphous or laminated keratin. The smaller cystic structures keratinize without a granular cell layer. Occasional larger cysts demonstrate infundibular keratinization. Numerous nests and clusters of polygonal melanocytes are distributed along the peripheral layers of the epithelial trabeculae and cysts, simulating junctional activity. The keratinocytes and keratinous cyst contents show patchy melanization, often with a clumped distribution. The sparse collagenous stroma is filled with clusters of melanocytes and melanophages analogous to the dermal component of a compound melanocytoma.

The majority of keratinocytes have moderate, pale-pink cytoplasm. Nuclei are bland and ovoid, and nucleoli are inconspicuous. Mitotic activity is minimal. Scattered individual dyskeratotic cells are also noted. The melanocytes have moderate or abundant melanin granules. Nuclei are small, ovoid, and euchromatic. Nucleoli are inconspicuous, and mitotic figures are not observed.

* Barr RJ: Personal communication, 1989.

FIGURE 29-12. Higher magnification of the melanocytoma-acanthoma in Figure 29-11 shows intraepithelial nests of melanocytes with uniform, ovoid nuclei. Note the tricholemmal-type keratinization of cystic structure *(top center)* and clumps of melanin within the cyst. (×240.)

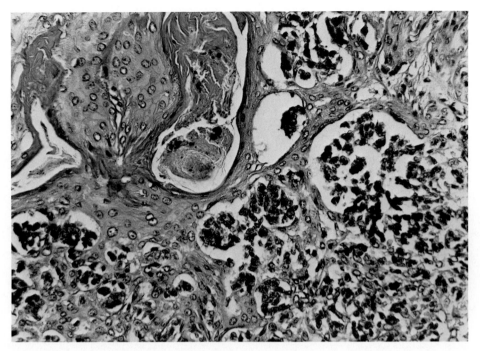

The architecture and morphology of the epithelial component of melanocytoma-acanthoma most closely resemble those of isthmus-catagen tricholemmoma but also have some features of trichoepithelioma (see Chapter 22). Although both of these follicular neoplasms may be melanized, they are readily distinguished from melanocytoma-acanthoma by the absence of aggregations of melanocytes. A "collision tumor" (two distinct neoplasms occurring at the same anatomic site) composed of compound melanocytoma and tricholemmoma or trichoepithelioma is an additional differential diagnosis. However, the consistent close interrelationship of the melanocytic and epithelial components of melanocytoma-acanthoma differentiates it from a random overlap of two neoplasms.

MALIGNANT MELANOMA
Clinical features

Malignant cutaneous neoplasms of melanocytic origin are uncommon in dogs and rare in cats. The incidence of canine malignant melanomas varies from 2% to 3% in several surveys; 33% of cutaneous melanocytic neoplasms in dogs were malignant in the survey by Conroy. Melanocytic neoplasms account for fewer than 2% of tumors in all feline surveys, but distinction often is not made between benign and malignant lesions. In reviews by Carpenter and also Macy, 71% and 53%, respectively, of melanocytic feline skin tumors were histopathologically malignant.

Malignant melanomas range in size from several millimeters to as large as 10 cm; the majority of lesions are 1 to 3 cm in diameter. Most neoplasms are sessile, but occasional melanomas are polypoid or plaque-like. Melanomas usually appear gray, brown, or black, depending upon the extent of melanin production, the presence of junctional activity, and the presence of re-active hyperpigmentation of the overlying epidermis. Ulceration is common, particularly in larger lesions.

Eyelids, digits (including nailbeds), and the trunk are the most frequent locations for cutaneous malignant melanomas in dogs. The face and digits also appear to be preferential sites in cats, based upon the small number of reported cases.

The average age of affected dogs varies from 9 to 11 years in several surveys, but malignant melanomas may develop in dogs as young as 3 years of age. The average age of cats with cutaneous melanomas was reported to be 12 years in a survey by Patnaik. Dogs with heavily pigmented skin and hair, such as Cocker Spaniels, Scottish Terriers, Boston Terriers, and Airedale Terriers, are predisposed to develop melanomas. There is no known breed predisposition in cats.

The biologic behavior of cutaneous malignant melanomas is difficult to predict, and a variety of prognostic factors have been investigated. The large majority of malignant melanomas in dogs and cats are primarily

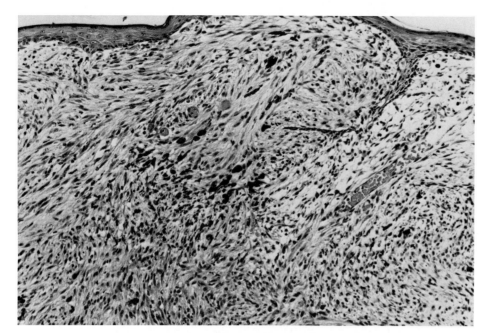

FIGURE 29-13. Malignant melanoma in a dog. A dermal nodule is composed predominantly of nonpigmented spindle cells arranged in interlacing bundles. Small numbers of heavily pigmented cells are present. Note that an intraepidermal component is not evident. (×120.)

dermal; thus the complex human classification schemes for intraepidermal melanomas and prognostic levels of dermal invasion do not apply. Mitotic activity has been shown in retrospective studies by Bostock and Bolon to be a significant predictive factor for canine melanocytic neoplasms. In Bostock's survey, a mitotic index (the total number of mitoses per 10 high-power fields) of 2 or less was associated with a 2-year mortality of 10%, whereas a mitotic index of 3 or greater was statistically linked with a 2-year mortality of 73%, independent of other histopathologic features of benignancy or malignancy. In the study by Bolon, a histo-

pathologic diagnosis of malignancy based on mitotic activity and cytologic atypia predicted recurrence or metastasis in 15 of 23 cases. A German study cited by Theilen reported large tumor size to be the only feature which correlated significantly with aggressive biologic behavior. Conversely, tumor size in Bostock's study was found not to be of prognostic value. Anatomic location, histopathologic subtype (see below), and the degree of pigmentation were not of value in predicting biologic behavior in any of the surveys.

The study by Bolon reported a 35% surgical cure rate for histopathologically malignant canine melano-

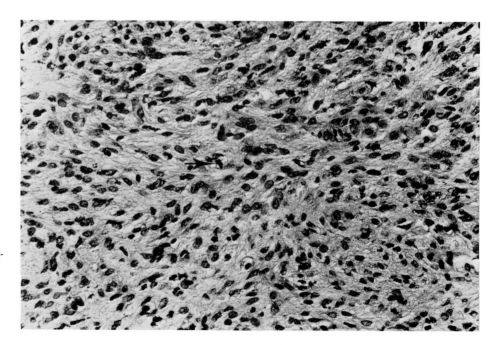

FIGURE 29-14. Higher magnification of malignant melanoma showing moderate nuclear enlargement and pleomorphism. Note the mitotic figure *(arrow)*. (×240.)

FIGURE 29-15. Malignant melanoma in a dog. Polygonal cells are arranged in sheets and nests. Note the vacuolated and granular cytoplasm. ($\times 240$.)

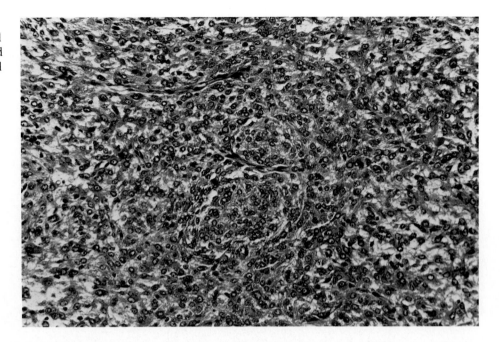

cytic tumors. The remaining 65% recurred or metastasized. Of the canine malignant melanomas in this review, 13% metastasized to regional lymph nodes and lungs. Two of five cats with cutaneous malignant melanoma in Patnaik's review had multiple recurrences, and one developed extensive visceral metastases. Satellite metastasis (the development of many small cutaneous nodules around a primary melanoma) is common in humans and has been reported in several feline cases.

Histopathology (Figures 29-13 through 29-19)

Cutaneous melanomas have a broad spectrum of histopathologic presentation. Reviews by Weiss and also Goldschmidt refer to spindle, epithelioid, epithelioid and spindle-cell, and dendritic and whorled histopathologic subtypes. However, overlaps between these categories commonly occur within a single neoplasm, and multiple retrospective studies indicate that they are not of prognostic significance. It is not unexpected that melanoma cells display such diversity of cytologic features; they share common embryologic roots with both neural and epithelial tissues.

Melanomas are usually fairly well-circumscribed, but unencapsulated neoplasms involving epidermis and dermis or dermis alone. Large tumors may encroach upon the subcutis. Purely intraepidermal melanomas,

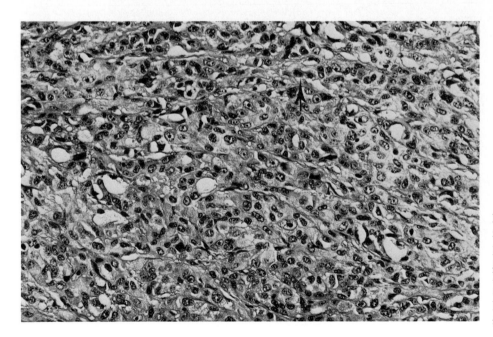

FIGURE 29-16. Malignant melanoma in a dog. Highly pleomorphic spindle and polygonal cells are arranged in nests. Nuclei are markedly enlarged and have prominent nucleoli. Note the mitotic figures *(arrow)*. ($\times 240$.)

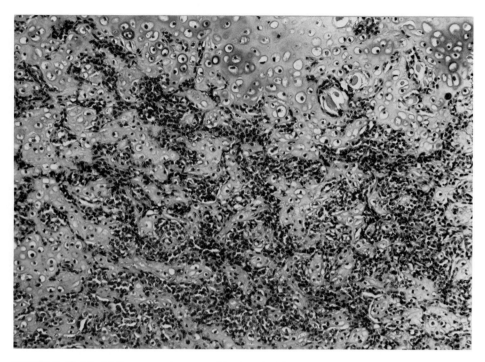

FIGURE 29-17. Malignant melanoma with chondroid metaplasia in a dog. Nests and trabeculae of darkly pigmented, polygonal melanocytes are interspersed with zones of well-differentiated cartilage. (×120.)

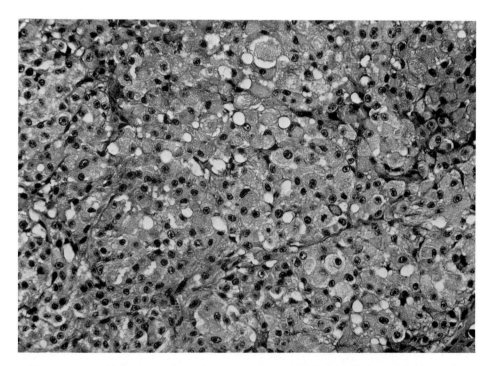

FIGURE 29-18. Malignant melanoma in a cat. Large epithelioid cells have abundant, glassy or finely granular cytoplasm. Nuclei are large and have prominent nucleoli. (×240.)

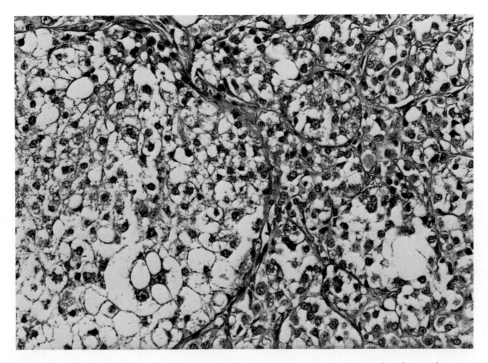

FIGURE 29-19. Balloon cell melanoma in a dog. Large cells with vacuolated cytoplasm are arranged in islands and nests. Finely granular melanin is present in small numbers of cells. Note the large nuclei with prominent nucleoli. (×240.)

such as superficial spreading melanoma or lentigo maligna in humans, are extremely rarely recognized in animals. Melanomas tend to be asymmetric, a feature most readily recognized in the epidermal component of smaller neoplasms. Ulceration and necrosis are common, particularly in larger masses. Peripheral infiltrates of lymphocytes and plasma cells may be present, and melanophages are often distributed throughout the neoplasm.

Melanomas comprise varying proportions of spindle and large polygonal cells arranged in interlacing bundles, partial whorls, solid sheets, and nests. Pure spindle-cell melanomas and pure epithelioid melanomas occur less frequently than mixed types. Giant epithelioid melanomas occur occasionally in cats. Interlacing bundles, partial whorls, and nests predominate in primarily spindle-cell melanomas; the architecture resembles fibrosarcoma or schwannoma. Sheets and nests predominate in primarily epithelioid melanomas. Many, but not all, melanomas have demonstrable "junctional activity," that is, the presence of tumor cells at the dermal-epidermal junction, as well as at higher levels of the epidermis. The intraepidermal component consists predominantly of epithelioid melanocytes that may be arranged in nests, clusters, or individually. The degree of pigmentation of melanomas varies from abundant to undetectable among individual neoplasms; no consistent degree or pattern of melanin pigmentation occurs within a given melanoma. Intraepidermal melanocytes often contain more melanin pigment than the cells of the dermal component. Most neoplasms have minimal stromal collagen. A rare feature of malignant melanomas in dogs is chondroid metaplasia of the stroma.

Melanoma cells usually have moderate-to-abundant, pale cytoplasm. The cytoplasm of amelanotic melanomas may have a gray, granular quality. The giant epithelioid melanomas of cats have a predominance of large cells with glassy, eosinophilic cytoplasm. Nuclei are enlarged and vary from ovoid to fusiform, depending upon the cytoplasmic morphology. There is moderate-to-marked nuclear pleomorphism. Chromatin patterns vary from tumor to tumor and often within a given neoplasm. Nucleoli are present and may be prominent. Mitotic activity is 3 or greater per 10 high-power fields, and mitotic atypia is present.

Balloon-cell, or clear-cell, malignant melanomas were recently described in dogs by Diters. This distinctive, rare variant has a multilobular architecture and does not possess an intraepidermal component. The cells are large and have clear or slightly eosinophilic cytoplasm. The majority of cells have an epithelioid conformation, but small zones of spindling may be detected. Most balloon-cell malignant melanomas are amelanotic or have dust-like granules similar to those of balloon-cell melanocytoma (see previous discussion). Nuclei are large and vesicular and have prominent nucleoli. Mitotic activity is relatively low.

The primary differential diagnosis for pigmented malignant melanoma is melanocytoma, particularly in smaller neoplasms. Features that support a diagnosis of malignant melanoma are a mitotic index of 3 or greater per 10 high-power fields, the presence of atypical mitoses, asymmetry, the presence of melanoma cells in the upper epidermis and at the dermal-epidermal junction, lymphoplasmacytic inflammation, and marked nuclear pleomorphism.

Differential diagnoses for amelanotic malignant melanoma include fibrosarcoma, malignant schwannoma, anaplastic carcinoma, and sebaceous carcinoma. Differentiation of predominantly spindle-cell amelanotic melanoma from fibrosarcoma or malignant schwannoma may be problematic. The majority of spindle-cell melanomas have some areas of epithelioid differentiation, and foci of junctional activity can often be identified in serial sections. Similarly, amelanotic epithelioid melanoma can be distinguished from anaplastic carcinoma by the presence of spindle-cell foci and junctional activity. Balloon-cell melanoma may be histopathologically indistinguishable from sebaceous carcinoma with routine stains if bimorphic cytologic features are absent. Fontana-Masson silver stain is helpful in identifying small amounts of melanin in largely amelanotic neoplasms of all histopathologic types. Immunoperoxidase stain for vimentin, a fibrillar protein in mesenchymal cells and melanocytes, may aid in the differentiation of epithelioid or balloon-cell melanoma from carcinoma. Unfortunately, S-100 protein, a common marker for human melanomas, is noncontributory in most canine melanomas. Specific monoclonal antibodies for melanoma in animals are currently being investigated.*

SUGGESTED READINGS

Melanocytoma

Bolon B, Calderwood Mays MB, and Hall BJ: Characterization of canine melanomas and comparison of histology and DNA ploidy to their biologic behavior, Vet Pathol 27:96-102, 1990.

Bostock DE: Prognosis after surgical excision of canine melanomas, Vet Pathol 16:32-40, 1979.

Carpenter JL, Andrew LK, and Holzworth J: Tumors and tumor-like lesions. In Holzworth J, editor: Diseases of the cat, Philadelphia, 1987, WB Saunders, pp 421, 579-583.

Conroy JD: Melanocytic tumors of domestic animals, Arch Dermatol 96:372-380, 1967.

* Naydan D: Personal communication, 1990.

Goldschmidt MH and Bevier DE: Skin tumors in the dog. III. Lymphohistiocytic and melanocytic tumors, Comp Cont Ed 3:588-594, 1981.

Macy DW and Reynolds HA: The incidence, characteristics and clinical management of skin tumors of cats, J Am Anim Hosp Assoc 17:1026-1034, 1981.

Magana-Garcia M and Ackerman AB: What are nevus cells? Am J Dermatopathol 12:93-102, 1990.

Pulley LT and Stannard AA: Tumors of the skin and soft tissues. In Moulton J, editor: Tumors in domestic animals, ed 3, Berkeley, Calif, 1990, University of California Press, pp 75-82.

Lentigo

Briggs OM: Lentiginosis profusa in the pug: three case reports, J Small Anim Pract 26:675-680, 1985.

Conroy JD: Melanocytic tumors of domestic animals, Arch Dermatol 96:372-380, 1967.

Kraft I and Frese D: Lentigo-ähnliche Proliferationen des Zitzenepithels biem Hund, Zentralbl Veterinarmed [A] 23:234-247, 1976.

Muller GH, Kirk RW, and Scott DW: Small animal dermatology, ed 4, Philadelphia, 1989, WB Saunders, pp 706-708.

Nash S and Paulsen D: Generalized lentigines in a silver cat, J Am Vet Med Assoc 196:1500-1501, 1990.

Pulley LT and Stannard AA: Tumors of the skin and soft tissues. In Moulton J, editor: Tumors in domestic animals, ed 3, Berkeley, Calif, 1990, University of California Press, pp 75-82.

Scott DW: Lentigo simplex in orange cats, Companion Anim Pract 1:23-25, 1987.

Melanocytoma-acanthoma

No references available.

Malignant melanoma

Bolon B, Calderwood Mays MB, and Hall BJ: Characterization of canine melanomas and comparison of histology and DNA ploidy to their biologic behavior, Vet Pathol 27:96-102, 1990.

Bostock DE: Prognosis after surgical excision of canine melanomas, Vet Pathol 16:32-40, 1979.

Carpenter JL, Andrew LK, and Holzworth J: Tumors and tumor-like lesions. In Holzworth J, editor: Diseases of the cat, Philadelphia, 1987, WB Saunders, pp 421, 579-583.

Conroy JD: Melanocytic tumors of domestic animals, Arch Dermatol 96:372-380, 1967.

Diters RW and Walsh KM: Canine cutaneous clear cell melanomas: a report of 3 cases, Vet Pathol 21:355-356, 1984.

Goldschmidt MH and Bevier DE: Skin tumors in the dog. III. Lymphohistiocytic and melanocytic tumors, Comp Cont Ed 3:588-594, 1981.

Howard-Martin MO and Qualls CW: Metastatic melanoma in a cat, Fel Pract 16:6-8, 1986.

Macy DW and Reynolds, HA: The incidence, characteristics and clinical management of skin tumors of cats, J Am Anim Hosp Assoc 17:1026-1034, 1981.

Patnaik AK: Feline melanoma: a comparative study of ocular, oral and dermal neoplasms, Vet Pathol 25:105-112, 1988.

Pulley LT and Stannard AA: Tumors of the skin and soft tissues. In Moulton J, editor: Tumors in domestic animals, ed 3, Berkeley, Calif, 1990, University of California Press, pp 75-82.

Theilen GH and Madewell BR, editors: Veterinary cancer medicine, ed 2, Philadelphia, 1987, Lea & Febiger, pp 315-322.

Weiss E: Tumours of the soft (mesenchymal) tissues, Bull World Health Organ 50:101-110, 1974.

See also General References, pp. 327-328.

Histiocytic and mast cell tumors

CANINE CUTANEOUS HISTIOCYTOMA

Clinical features

Histiocytoma is a common benign tumor in dogs, representing approximately 19% of all skin and subcutaneous neoplasms in a large survey by Taylor. This corresponds to a 19.6% incidence in a recent statistical review of 1141 canine skin tumors by one of the authors,* making histiocytoma the most common skin neoplasm in that survey. The etiology of histiocytoma is unknown, but it is more likely a unique proliferation or reactive hyperplasia rather than a true neoplasm. Histiocytomas are derived from cells of monocyte-macrophage lineage; this is supported by results of electron microscopy and enzyme histochemistry. It has been suspected for some time that canine histiocytomas arise from Langerhans cells—specialized monocytic-dendritic cells in the dermis and epidermis that function in antigen processing. Unfortunately, canine Langerhans cells lack Birbeck's granules, the distinctive ultrastructural markers of these cells in humans and rodents. A recent immunohistochemical study by Moore has shown that histiocytomas most likely are of Langerhans-cell origin.

Histiocytomas appear as rapidly growing, alopecic, erythematous, dome-shaped nodules that generally measure 0.5 to 1.5 cm in diameter, but can reach dimensions of up to 4 cm. Lesions may be multiple, either synchronously or sequentially. Ulceration is a frequent feature. Histiocytomas can occur anywhere on the body, but preferential sites are the muzzle, pinnae, extremities, and scrotum.

The majority of histiocytomas occur in dogs between 6 months and 3 years of age; the incidence drops markedly in older animals. Many purebred dogs may be predisposed to develop histiocytomas. Conroy reported a higher incidence in English Bulldogs, Doberman Pinschers, Schnauzers, and Scottish Terriers. Muller, Kirk, and Scott reported breed predilections in Boxers, Dachshunds, Cocker Spaniels, Great Danes, and Shetland Sheepdogs. Spontaneous regression within weeks to months is the usual natural progression of canine cutaneous histiocytoma; however, most lesions are removed before regression occurs. Occasional recurrence of histiocytoma at the previous surgical site was reported by Taylor and also Goldschmidt (1989).

Histopathology (Figures 30-1 through 30-4)

Canine cutaneous histiocytomas are circumscribed, but unencapsulated dermal neoplasms composed of round and polygonal cells arranged in cords and sheets. All

---

* Emily J. Walder.

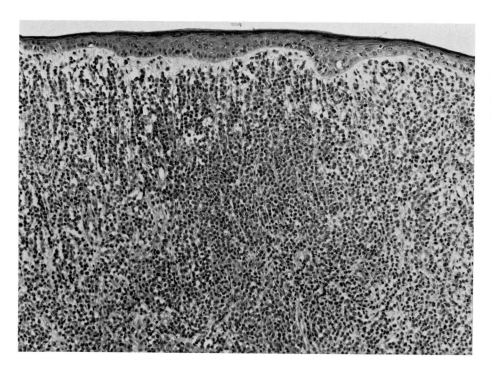

FIGURE 30-1. Histiocytoma in a dog. Cords of cells are oriented perpendicularly to the skin surface in the superficial aspect of the tumor, whereas the deep portion is composed of sheets of cells. (×120.)

histiocytomas, regardless of their stage of development, have a base-narrow or top-heavy configuration (i.e., their silhouette resembles an inverted trapezoid or wedge). Most tumors completely obliterate adnexal structures, but residual hair follicles are occasionally present. In the superficial aspects of the tumor, the cells form loose cords that stream down from the dermal-

epidermal junction. Clusters of cells may be present within the overlying epidermis. Deeper portions of the neoplasm have cells arranged in solid sheets. The youngest lesions are composed entirely of histiocytes and have an intact epidermis. Older lesions ulcerate and develop lymphocytic infiltrates starting at the base and progressing upward. Involuting histiocytomas develop

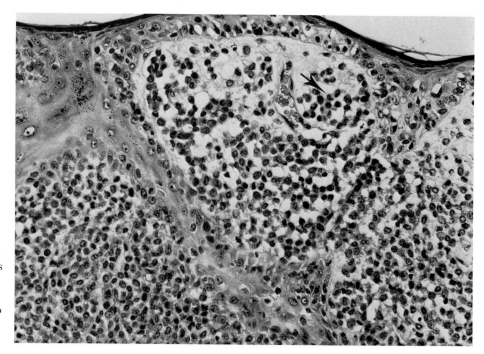

FIGURE 30-2. Higher magnification of a histiocytoma shows ovoid, reniform, and **C**-shaped *(arrow)* nuclei. Note the close approximation of tumor cells to the dermal-epidermal junction. (×240.)

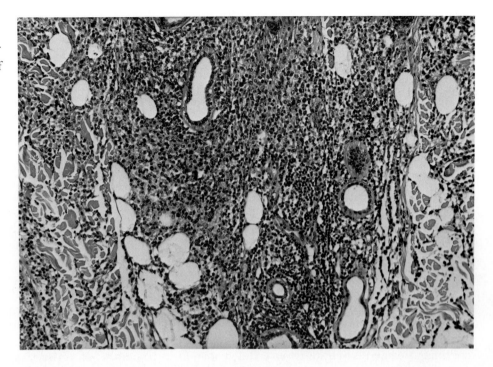

multifocal zones of necrosis that eventually coalesce. In some late-stage lesions, lymphocytes outnumber the histiocytes; diagnosis in these cases requires careful search for residual cords or clusters of histiocytic cells in the superficial dermis. Neutrophils are generally limited to the ulcerated surface unless secondary pyoderma is present in residual hair follicles. Plasma cells, mast

cells, and eosinophils are not commonly observed in histiocytomas, but may be prominent in some cases.

Superficial histiocytes have discrete cell boundaries and moderate, lightly eosinophilic, often slightly granular or vacuolated cytoplasm. Nuclei are pleomorphic; nuclear profiles vary from round to ovoid to reniform. Folded nuclei with a "coffee bean" configuration are

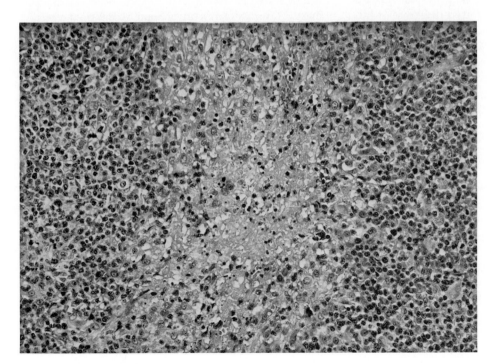

FIGURE 30-4. Histiocytoma in a dog. A zone of necrosis is surrounded by lymphocytes and histiocytes in late-stage regression. (×240.)

typical for histiocytoma. **C**-shaped nuclei are common in late or regressing histiocytomas. Regressing cells may also be individualized, rounded, and contain more intensely eosinophilic cytoplasm. These typical regressing histiocytes may be most easily observed just beneath intact epidermis. Mitotic activity in the superficial cell population is moderate to high, except in regressing histiocytomas. The deeper solid sheets of cells have abundant, poorly defined, paler cytoplasm. Nuclei are irregularly ovoid and have small nucleoli. Mitotic activity in the deep cell population is moderate, and atypical mitoses may be present.

Differential diagnoses for canine cutaneous histiocytoma are limited, especially when excisional biopsy samples are submitted. In regressing histiocytomas with marked, diffuse lymphocytic infiltration, it may be difficult to detect the typical residual histiocytes in the superficial dermis. These lesions may be difficult to distinguish from idiopathic or arthropod-induced focal lymphocytic dermatitides. The presence of plump, macrophage-like cells with **C**-shaped nuclei is helpful in confirming a diagnosis of histiocytoma. Differentiation between histiocytoma and cutaneous T-cell lymphoma in incisional or punch biopsy samples from older dogs can be problematic. Histiocytoma is usually solitary, and cutaneous lymphoma is usually multicentric, but multiple histiocytomas and solitary lymphomas may occur. Collections of histiocytes within the epidermis of a histiocytoma can mimic the epitheliotropism of mycosis fungoides. Irregular nuclear profiles are features of both cell types. Detection of superficial dermal cords of typical histiocytes and deep dermal nodular aggregates of lymphocytes supports a diagnosis of histiocytoma. Immunohistochemical studies using histiocytic and lymphocytic cell markers would also provide a definitive diagnosis, but these stains are not widely available. Finally, multicentric lesions that are histologically indistinguishable from canine cutaneous histiocytomas may be a subtype of cutaneous histiocytosis.

FELINE MAST CELL TUMOR
Clinical features

Mast cell tumors are common, usually benign, cutaneous neoplasms in cats. Older surveys cited by Pulley indicated that mast cell tumors accounted for 2% to 3% of feline skin tumors. The study by Macy reported an occurrence rate of 15%. Feline mast cell tumors had an incidence of 7.6% in a recent review by Buerger.

Feline mast cell tumors appear as discrete, firm, tan, alopecic papules and nodules, ranging from a few millimeters to 2 cm in size. Pruritus is variable. Larger lesions are often focally ulcerated. Mast cell tumors are often multicentric in the skin, both synchronously and metachronously. Buerger reported that 43% of tumors occurred on the head and neck. Another recent study by Wilcock found no site predilection. The average age of affected animals in all surveys was 10 years; the majority were greater than 4 years of age.

The biologic behavior of feline mast cell tumors has recently been re-evaluated. Scott reported in 1980 that primary cutaneous mast cell tumors were aggressive neoplasms with rapid development of nodal and visceral metastasis. In contrast, recent studies by Buerger and also Wilcock indicated recurrence rates at the original surgical site of 0% and 4% and occurrence rates of additional cutaneous tumors at other sites of 35% and 7%, respectively. Distant metastasis was not found in Buerger's report, whereas 7% of the cases in Wilcock's study had suspected, but histologically unconfirmed, metastasis to abdominal viscera. In Wilcock's report, aggressive biologic behavior, manifested by recurrence adjacent to the surgical site and suspected metastasis, correlated with poorly differentiated cell type. Morphology and biologic behavior did not appear to be related in Buerger's study, but the number of cases was quite small (14). Well-differentiated cutaneous mast cell tumors in cats would thus appear to have a reasonably good prognosis, despite their tendency to occur at additional skin sites. Visceral mastocytosis is most probably a separate neoplastic syndrome.

A histiocytic subtype of mast cell tumor, which was first described in Wilcock's study, occurs primarily in Siamese cats from 6 weeks to 4 years of age. Histiocytic mast cell tumors appear as grouped papulonodular lesions that often occur on the head. Histiocytic mast cell tumors sometimes recur as multiple crops of miliary nodules that eventually regress spontaneously.

A single case of diffuse cutaneous mastocytosis in a 1-year-old domestic short-haired cat was recently described by Brown. Generalized pruritus, lichenification, papules, and erosions were present because of dermal mastocytic infiltration. The pinnae were affected most severely. Peripheral lymph nodes were also involved.

Histopathology

Well-differentiated type (Figure 30-5). Well-differentiated feline mast cell tumors are circumscribed, but unencapsulated dermal masses composed of solid sheets and cords of uniform round cells with discrete cytoplasmic margins. Small numbers of eosinophils are scattered among the tumor cells, and nodular aggregates of lymphocytes are frequently present. A grenz zone (a narrow band of uninvolved skin) is usually present in the superficial dermis. Tumor cells sometimes extend to the dermal-epidermal junction, and Buerger reported occasional intraepithelial infiltration by mast cells. The epidermis of larger lesions is often ulcerated. The cytoplasm of the neoplastic mast cells is

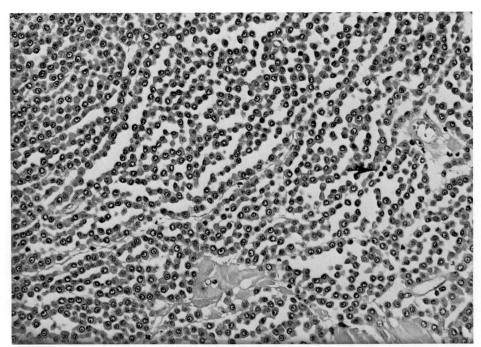

FIGURE 30-5. Well-differentiated feline mast cell tumor. Uniform round cells with centrally located nuclei are arranged in cords and sheets. Note the scattered eosinophils *(arrow)*. (×240.)

variably granular, and the nuclei are small, round, and centrally located. Nuclear pleomorphism is minimal. Nucleoli are inconspicuous, and mitotic figures are rarely observed.

Poorly differentiated type (Figure 30-6). A small percentage of feline mast cell tumors have anaplastic morphologic features. The poorly differentiated neoplasms are usually less discrete and infiltrate more

deeply than those of the well-differentiated cell type. The poorly differentiated mast cells exhibit moderate to marked pleomorphism, and partial loss of cytoplasmic granulation is evident with routine and special histologic stains. Nuclei are large, have variable chromatin patterns, and are often eccentric in location. Nucleoli are single and vary from inconspicuous to prominent. Mitotic activity is moderate to high. Tumor giant

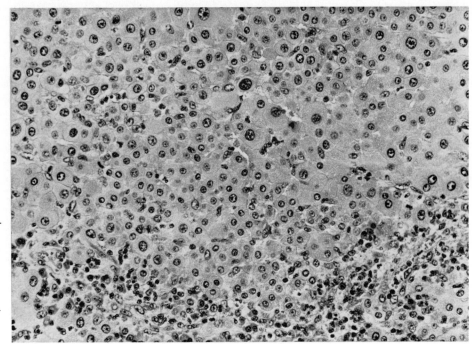

FIGURE 30-6. Poorly differentiated feline mast cell tumor. This anaplastic variant is composed of large, highly pleomorphic cells that have slightly granular cytoplasm and moderate anisokaryosis. Note the infiltrate of eosinophils and lymphocytes at bottom. (×240.)

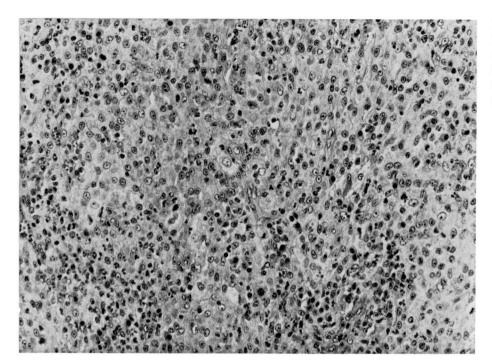

FIGURE 30-7. Histiocytic feline mast cell tumor. Polygonal cells resembling epithelioid macrophages are admixed with eosinophils, lymphocytes, and plasma cells. (×240.)

cells with single multilobate nuclei or multiple nuclei are present. The single case of diffuse cutaneous mastocytosis reported by Brown had diffuse dermal or superficial band-like infiltration by moderately pleomorphic mast cells, which often had two or three nuclei. Highly anaplastic mast cell tumors may resemble histiocytic lymphoma or epithelioid sarcoma, but Giemsa or toluidine blue stain will reveal metachromatic granulation in at least a small proportion of the tumor cells. The metachromatic granules may be so delicate that oil immersion is required for their detection.

Histiocytic type (Figure 30-7). Histiocytic mast cell tumors are small, unencapsulated, deep dermal and subcutaneous nodules composed of solid sheets of large polygonal cells admixed with moderate numbers of eosinophils and some lymphoid aggregates. The mast cells have ample, pale eosinophilic cytoplasm. Nuclei are moderately enlarged and vesicular. Nucleoli are small, and mitotic activity is low. Histiocytic mast cell tumors have a granulomatous appearance, and differential diagnoses of insect-bite granuloma and infectious granulomas must be considered. Giemsa or toluidine blue stain reveals faint to moderate metachromatic granulation, confirming the mastocytic nature of the lesions.

CANINE MAST CELL TUMOR
Clinical features

Mast cell tumors are common malignant neoplasms in dogs. Mast cell tumors accounted for 15% of all skin and subcutaneous neoplasms in a review by Conroy. A statistical survey of 1141 canine skin tumors by one of the authors* showed an incidence of 8.8%.

Mast cell tumors are generally alopecic, erythematous, edematous nodules that vary in size from several millimeters to several centimeters. Lesions on distal limbs and lips may appear as poorly defined areas of swelling. Canine mast cell tumors may be multicentric in the skin either synchronously or sequentially. Ulceration is often present in larger lesions. Mast cell tumors may develop anywhere on the body, and the subcutis as well as dermis may be involved. An increased incidence of mast cell tumors on the proximal rear limbs, perineum, and prepuce was reported by Tams.

The average age of affected animals is 8 years, but mast cell tumors are occasionally found in dogs as young as 4 months. Boxers, Boston Terriers, Bull Terriers, American Staffordshire Terriers, Fox Terriers, English Bulldogs, Dachshunds, Labrador Retrievers, and Weimaraners are reported to be predisposed.

The commonly used histopathologic grading system was developed by Patnaik in 1984 and is based primarily on nuclear morphology. The majority of canine mast cell tumors are in the grade 1, or well-differentiated, category; approximately 25% are in the grade 2 category; and poorly differentiated, or grade 3, neoplasms are uncommon. There is a strong correlation between histopathologic grade and biologic behavior; approximately 10% of dogs with grade 1

* Emily J. Walder.

FIGURE 30-8. Canine mast cell tumor, grade 1. Round cells with uniform nuclei are arranged in cords and loose sheets. Note the granular quality of cytoplasm. (×240.)

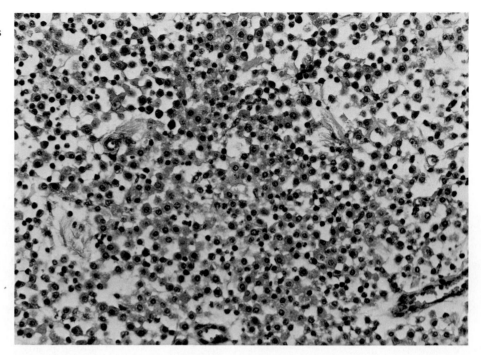

mast cell tumors die as a result of metastasis or inoperable recurrence, 45% die as a result of grade 2 mast cell tumors, and 85% die from grade 3 mast cell tumors. Complications caused by release of vasoactive amines from mast cell granules include ulceration of the gastrointestinal tract and fatal intraoperative hypotension.

Histopathology

Grade 1 (Figure 30-8). Well-differentiated mast cell tumors are usually small dermal neoplasms that are fairly well circumscribed but unencapsulated. Occasional grade 1 mast cell tumors arise in the subcutis. Neoplastic cells rarely extend to the dermal-epidermal junction, and most grade 1 mast cell tumors are nonulcerated. The tumor cells closely resemble normal mast cells and are arranged in cords and loose sheets. They have round, discrete cytoplasm with prominent, gray-blue granules as detected in most hematoxylin and eosin preparations. Nuclei are small and round-to-oval with inconspicuous nucleoli; some folded or reniform profiles may be observed. Mitotic figures are infrequent or absent. Most grade 1 mast cell tumors have moderate to large numbers of eosinophils admixed with neoplastic cells, and eosinophils outnumber mast cells in a small percentage of cases. Some tumors have scattered small foci of collagenolysis surrounded by degenerated, degranulated eosinophils ("flame figures"). There is usually a moderate stroma of hyalinized collagen bundles with variable edema. Some tumors have almost no stroma, whereas others show extensive sclerosis and low cellularity. Perivascular hyalinization is a common

feature. Tumor necrosis is uncommon, but occasional well-differentiated mast cell tumors become extensively infarcted.

Grade 2 (Figure 30-9). Dermal grade 2 mast cell tumors are usually larger, deeper, and less well-circumscribed than grade 1 tumors. Grade 2 tumors often involve the subcutis. Neoplastic cells are still arranged in cords and sheets but have a more haphazard, infiltrative pattern of growth. Ulceration and necrosis are common secondary features. The neoplastic cells are larger, slightly pleomorphic, and have less obvious cytoplasmic granules. Nuclei are moderately enlarged and pleomorphic with small nucleoli. Mitotic activity varies from low to moderate. Grade 2 mast cell tumors usually have less stroma and fewer eosinophils than the well-differentiated type, but extensive sclerosis and marked tissue eosinophilia are evident in a small percentage of lesions. Flame figures may be present.

Grade 3 (Figure 30-10). Poorly differentiated canine mast cell tumors are generally large, ulcerated, and poorly circumscribed and extend into the subcutis. Necrosis is a common secondary feature. Tumor cells are arranged primarily in solid sheets, and granules are often indiscernible without the use of Giemsa or toluidine blue stains. The cells are round to polygonal and highly pleomorphic. Cell margins are not well defined. Nuclei are usually large, round to ovoid, and vesicular. Nucleoli are often prominent. Mitotic activity is moderate to high, and many atypical mitoses are present. The eosinophilotactic effects of the mast cells continue to decrease with increasing anaplasia, but eosinophils

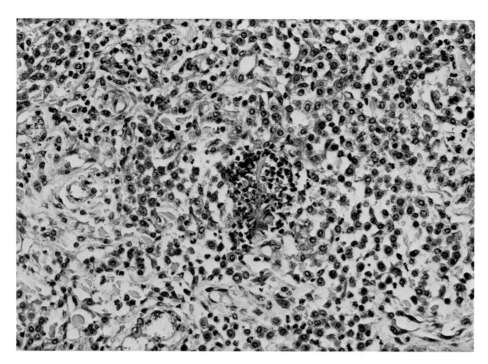

FIGURE 30-9. Canine mast cell tumor, grade 2. Nuclei are larger and slightly more pleomorphic than in the well-differentiated type. Note the central focus of eosinophilic degranulation and collagenolysis (flame figure). (×240.)

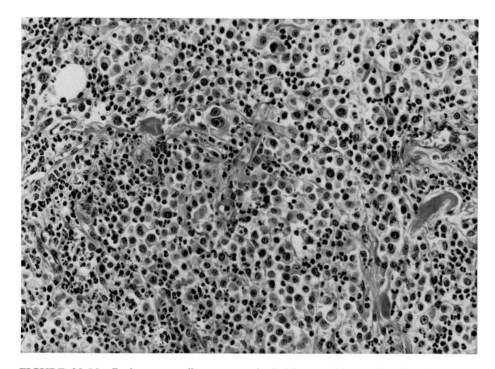

FIGURE 30-10. Canine mast cell tumor, grade 3. Pleomorphic round cells lack obvious cytoplasmic granularity. Anisokaryosis is marked, and nucleoli are often prominent. Note the atypically large population of eosinophils. (×240.)

are still detectable in small numbers in most instances and may still be abundant in rare cases. Stroma is scant to absent.

Diagnosis of grades 1 and 2 mast cell tumors is usually straightforward. Small tumors with minimal stroma may have to be differentiated from cutaneous extramedullary plasmacytomas. Giemsa or toluidine blue stain reveals moderate-to-marked metachromatic granulation of the neoplastic mast cells. Grade 3 mast cell tumors must be differentiated from other hematopoietic malignancies. Histiocytic T-cell lymphoma, poorly differentiated plasmacytoid lymphoma, and the rare cutaneous lesions of transmissible venereal tumor can have similar morphologic features, as well as eosinophilic infiltrates. Giemsa or toluidine blue stain reveals small numbers of metachromatic granules in variable proportions of tumor cells. The granules may be small, requiring the use of oil immersion for detection.

SUGGESTED READINGS

Canine cutaneous histiocytoma

Conroy JD: Canine skin tumors, J Am Anim Hosp Assoc 19:91-114, 1983.

Goldschmidt MH and Bevier DE: Skin tumors in the dog. III. Lymphohistiocytic and melanocytic tumors, Comp Cont Ed 3:588-594, 1981.

Goldschmidt MH, Shaw J, and Shofer F: Canine cutaneous histiocytoma. Proceedings of the Twenty-seventh Annual Meeting of the American Society of Dermatopathologists, San Francisco, 1989.

Moore PF and Schrenzel MD: Canine cutaneous histiocytoma represents a Langerhans cell proliferative disorder based on immunophenotypic analysis, Proceedings of the Forty-Second Annual Meeting of the American College of Veterinary Pathologists, Orlando, 1991.

Muller GH, Kirk RW, and Scott DW: Small animal dermatology, ed 4, Philadelphia, 1989, Harcourt, Brace, & Jovanovich, p 846.

Taylor DON, Dorn CR, and Luis OS: Morphologic and biologic characteristics of canine cutaneous histiocytoma, Cancer Res 29:83-92, 1969.

Feline mast cell tumor

Brown CA and Chalmers SA: Diffuse cutaneous mastocytosis in a cat, Vet Pathol 27:366-369, 1990.

Buerger RG and Scott DW: Cutaneous mast cell neoplasia in cats: 14 cases (1975-1985), J Am Vet Med Assoc 190:1440-1444, 1987.

Chastain CB, Turk MAM, and O'Brien D: Benign cutaneous mastocytomas in two litters of Siamese kittens, J Am Vet Med Assoc 193:959-960, 1988.

Macy DW and Reynolds HA: The incidence, characteristics and clinical management of skin tumors of cats, J Am Anim Hosp Assoc 17:1026-1034, 1981.

Pulley LT and Stannard AA: Tumors of the skin and soft tissues. In Moulton J, editor: Tumors in domestic animals, ed 3, Berkeley, Calif, 1990, University of California Press, p 43.

Scott DW: Feline dermatology, 1900-1978: a monograph, J Am Anim Hosp Assoc 16:331-425, 1980.

Wilcock BP, Yager JA, and Zink MC: The morphology and behavior of feline cutaneous mastocytomas, Vet Pathol 23:320-324, 1986.

Canine mast cell tumor

Bevier DE and Goldschmidt MH: Tumors in the dog. II. Tumors of the soft (mesenchymal) tissues, Comp Cont Ed 3:506-514, 1981.

Conroy JD: Canine skin tumors, J Am Anim Hosp Assoc 19:91-114, 1983.

Muller GH, Kirk RW, and Scott DW: Small animal dermatology, ed 4, Philadelphia, 1989, Harcourt, Brace, & Jovanovich, p 846.

Patnaik AK, Ehler WJ, and MacEwen EG: Canine cutaneous mast cell tumor: morphologic grading and survival time in 83 dogs, Vet Pathol 21:469-474, 1984.

Tams TR and Macy DW: Canine mast cell tumors, Comp Cont Ed 3:869-876, 1981.

See also General References, pp 327-328.

CHAPTER 31

Lymphocytic tumors

CUTANEOUS EXTRAMEDULLARY PLASMACYTOMA
(Synonym: plasma cell tumor)
Clinical features

Cutaneous extramedullary plasmacytomas are uncommon, usually benign, cutaneous neoplasms in dogs. Numeric incidence data have not been published, but these tumors accounted for 2.3% of 1141 canine skin and subcutaneous neoplasms in a statistical survey conducted by one of the authors.* Cutaneous extramedullary plasmacytomas are exceedingly rare in cats; a single case was recently reported by Carothers. Cutaneous plasmacytomas were designated in older veterinary literature as *reticulum cell sarcomas* because of their unusual morphology and have been designated more recently as *atypical histiocytomas* after their largely benign behavior was recognized. The plasma cell was confirmed as the cell of origin in reports by Rakich and also Baer in 1989, in part by demonstrating cytoplasmic immunoglobulin with immunoperoxidase staining. A similar neoplasm both clinically and histologically, but with ultrastructural features suggestive of cutaneous neuroendocrine carcinoma (Merkel cell tumor), was described by Nickoloff. The relationship between the canine Merkel cell tumor and cutaneous plasmacytoma is unclear; additional immunohistochemical studies are needed to assess epithelial properties of the proposed Merkel cell tumor. The authors suspect that both tumors may be plasmacytic in origin, based on recent evidence.†

Cutaneous extramedullary plasmacytomas are usually solitary, dome-shaped or pedunculated, alopecic nodules measuring less than 2 cm in diameter. The dermis is most commonly affected, but subcutaneous lesions occur occasionally. Tumors are occasionally multiple. Approximately one third are focally ulcerated. The most frequently affected sites are pinnae (both medial and lateral surfaces), ear canals, face, and feet. One of the authors‡ has seen two cases in dogs characterized by multiple tumors involving the pinnae and ear canals only. Extramedullary plasmacytomas also occur in the oral cavity, usually on maxillary gingiva, and the rectal submucosa. The single case of feline extramedullary plasma cell tumor involved the subcutis, lymph nodes, spleen, and liver. The average age of affected dogs is approximately 10 years. There is no apparent breed predilection.

The majority of canine cutaneous extramedullary plasmacytomas are benign; occasional lesions recur after surgical excision. Plasma cell tumors occurring in the oral

* Emily J. Walder.
† Schrenzel M: Personal communication, 1990.
‡ Thelma Lee Gross.

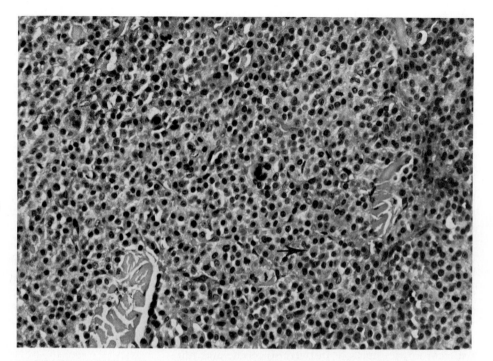

FIGURE 31-1. Plasmacytoma in a dog. Round-to-polygonal cells are arranged in tightly packed nests. Scattered cells have giant hyperchromatic nuclei. Note the smaller cells with distinct plasmacytoid features *(arrow)*. (×240.)

cavity, rectum, or subcutis are more likely to exhibit aggressive biologic behavior. There does not appear to be any correlation between behavior and the degree of differentiation of the neoplastic plasma cells. Association with systemic plasma cell dyscrasia appears to be uncommon in dogs; 2 of 75 cases in the study by Rakich had multiple myeloma. The feline case reported by Carothers had an associated monoclonal gammopathy.

Histopathology (Figures 31-1 and 31-2)

Cutaneous extramedullary plasmacytomas are circumscribed, but unencapsulated dermal nodules composed predominantly of round-to-polygonal cells arranged in tightly packed nests and cords. There is usually a narrow grenz zone (a zone of uninvolved superficial dermis between the epidermis and a dermal lesion), but tumor cells will occasionally extend to the

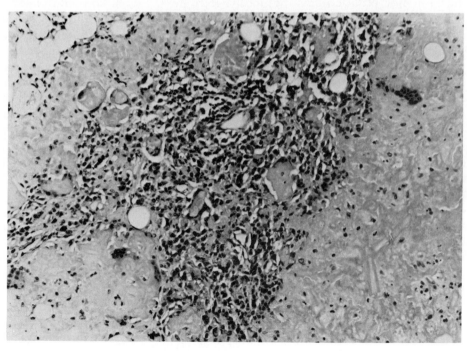

FIGURE 31-2. Plasmacytoma in a dog. Well-differentiated plasma cells with hyperchromatic nuclei are surrounded by large deposits of amyloid. Note the foreign body–type giant cells. (×240.)

dermal-epidermal junction. At the periphery of the neoplasm, the cells become smaller and less cohesive, and plasmacytoid features are more apparent. The tumor cell nests are separated by a delicate stroma of reticulin and capillary blood vessels. The reticulin fibers, which can be demonstrated with Gomori's or Wilder's silver stain, incompletely surround the plasma cell aggregates. Some cutaneous plasmacytomas have dilated vascular sinusoids, and individualized tumor cells appear to float in small lakes of erythrocytes; this may be misinterpreted as vascular invasion. Small numbers of eosinophils generally infiltrate the neoplasm; this is most likely a reflection of the eosinophilotactic properties of immunoglobulin.

The majority of tumor cells have moderate cytoplasm with a hyaline, glassy or, less commonly, granular quality. Nuclei of cutaneous plasmacytomas are quite pleomorphic and vary from round to ovoid to convoluted. Variable numbers of giant unilobulate or multilobulate nuclei are usually present. Occasional cells have multiple nuclei. Nuclei are euchromatic or hyperchromatic, nucleoli are inconspicuous, and mitotic activity is low to moderate. The smaller peripheral cells exhibit typical plasmacytoid differentiation manifested by discrete cytoplasmic margins, homogeneous or smudged-appearing amphophilic cytoplasm, and a suggestion of perinuclear halos. Nuclei of the smaller peripheral cells are usually hyperchromatic and eccentric in location. Some tumors are composed mostly of large, bizarre cells with abundant, eosinophilic, glassy cytoplasm and virtually no evidence of plasmacytoid differentiation. Ribonucleic acid can be readily demonstrated in most plasmacytomas with methyl green pyronine stain and tends to be concentrated in the more differentiated cells at the periphery. (Note that cytoplasmic ribonucleic acid stains magenta with methyl green pyronine stain, whereas mast cell granules appear orange-brown.) Cytoplasmic whole immunoglobulin or immunoglobulin light chains can also be demonstrated using immunoperoxidase techniques.

Approximately 10% of canine cutaneous extramedullary plasmacytomas show varying degrees of amyloid production. Occasional tumors are composed predominantly of amyloid and contain only scattered islands of residual plasma cells. Plasma cell tumors with amyloid production invariably are characterized by a well-differentiated cell type. Amyloid deposition is usually accompanied by a mild granulomatous inflammatory reaction that includes foreign body–type multinucleated giant cells. The single reported case of feline plasmacytoma had abundant amyloid deposition in all lesions.

Differential diagnoses for extramedullary plasma cell tumor are other round cell tumors, including histi-ocytoma, mast cell tumor, amelanotic epithelioid melanoma, and the proposed Merkel cell tumor. Plasmacytomas are distinguished from histiocytomas by the absence of cords of cells oriented perpendicularly to the skin surface, the absence of lymphocytic infiltrates, and the presence of tumor giant cells with multilobular nuclei. Plasmacytomas are usually distinguishable from mast cell tumors by the glassy as opposed to granular quality of the cytoplasm, the absence of stromal collagen, and negative Giemsa or toluidine blue stain. Amelanotic epithelioid malignant melanomas usually have paler cytoplasm with a finely granular quality as compared with plasmacytomas. Melanoma nuclei have more prominent nucleoli. Junctional activity can be detected in most malignant melanomas. Fontana-Masson stain or S-100 immunoperoxidase stain is also helpful in differentiating melanocytic neoplasms from plasma cell tumors. Detection of cytoplasmic whole immunoglobulin or immunoglobulin light chains by the use of immunoperoxidase stains confirms a diagnosis of plasmacytoma.

MALIGNANT LYMPHOMA (Synonym: lymphosarcoma)

Clinical features

Malignant lymphoma is the most common hematopoietic neoplasm of dogs and cats, but skin involvement is rare. According to a review by McKeever, primary cutaneous lymphoma accounted for 8% of all canine lymphoma cases. Only 1.7% of all feline lymphoma cases were cutaneous in a survey by Hardy. Cutaneous involvement may be primary or may occur in conjunction with disseminated lymphoma.

Cutaneous lymphomas can be divided into two major subgroups based on the absence or presence of epitheliotropism—a tendency for the tumor cells to accumulate in epidermal or adnexal epithelium. Non-epitheliotropic lymphomas are usually of presumed B-cell origin, as indicated by numerous cell marker studies in human lymphomas. Epitheliotropic lymphoma, which generally refers to mycosis fungoides and its variants, is of presumed T-cell origin. Several cases of mycosis fungoides in cats reported by Baker and also Caciolo (1983, 1984) were of proven T-cell origin. T-lymphocyte lineage is difficult to verify in dogs because of the nonspecific erythrocyte-rosetting properties of canine lymphocytes as compared to other species. Immunohistochemical markers are currently being investigated and are more likely to be of value in confirming the cell type in canine epitheliotropic lymphoma. All nine cats in Caciolo's study (1984) on cutaneous lymphoma, which included both epitheliotropic and nonepitheliotropic subtypes, were FeLV

TABLE 31-1. Comparison of classification systems for nonepitheliotropic lymphoma

Rappaport nomenclature	NCI working formulation	Grade
Well-differentiated lymphocytic	Small cell	Low
	Small cleaved B cell	Intermediate
Poorly differentiated lymphocytic	Large cell	High
Undifferentiated	Immunoblastic	High
Histiocytic	Histiocytic	High

negative using the immunofluorescent technique on blood. Nevertheless, a retroviral etiology is likely for at least some feline cutaneous nonepitheliotropic lymphomas based on extensive evidence in other forms of lymphoma, as well as in lymphoid leukemia of cats. An oncogenic virus causing canine lymphoma has not been identified.

The etiology of mycosis fungoides in dogs and cats is not yet known. In humans, the current widely supported theory is that persistence of environmental antigen and/or Langerhans cell abnormalities act as a stimulus for chronic T-cell stimulation; this may progress to neoplasia of T-helper cells. However, recent immunohistochemical studies by Moore indicate that the majority of canine mycosis fungoides cases have a predominance of T-suppressor cells.

Further histologic subtyping of lymphomas, beyond designations of epitheliotropic and nonepitheliotropic, is currently controversial because of the multiplicity of classification schemes developed over the last 10 years. Older literature generally uses the classic Rappaport nomenclature developed in 1956 and based solely on histologic criteria. A more recent classification system is the National Cancer Institute (NCI) Working Formulation, which combines the functional approach of Lukes-Parker-Collins with behavioral grading based on mitotic rate. A comparison of Rappaport and NCI nomenclature applicable to cutaneous lymphoma is provided in Table 31-1. Because functional studies, such as erythrocyte-rosetting, and fresh tissue histochemistry are rarely done on canine and feline lymphomas, a logical nomenclature primarily using histologic features is of great importance in allowing clinicians to evaluate differences in biologic behavior and response to various treatment protocols. Carter's report indicates that data support a correlation between

the biologic behavior of some canine lymphomas and the NCI grading system. The survey by Greenlee, using the Kiel classification and a similar grading system, concluded that high-grade canine lymphomas in general responded better to the chemotherapy protocol than did low-grade lymphomas. A complete discussion of B- and T-cell life cycles, morphology, and nomenclature is beyond the scope of this chapter. Readers are referred to material by Lukes, Carter, and Greenlee for additional information.

The clinical presentation of cutaneous lymphoma includes a broad spectrum of lesions that are partially determined by the cell type involved. Nonepitheliotropic lymphomas usually appear as nodular masses of varying size that may be solitary but are more often multiple. Ulceration is frequent. Pruritus is variable. Erythema, scaling, and alopecia are also common. Lesions most often occur on the trunk but may also be found on the head and extremities.

Typical clinical findings in mycosis fungoides have already been described (see Chapter 10) and correspond to the patch (premycotic, erythematous), plaque, and tumor stages of the human disease. In the rare *d'emblee* variant of mycosis fungoides, solitary or multiple tumor masses occur without preexisting patch or plaque lesions. Woringer-Kolopp disease (pagetoid reticulosis) is a rare, localized form of mycosis fungoides in humans that has minimal dermal infiltration and therefore does not progress beyond the plaque stage. A single canine case reported in 1981 by Johnson was histologically similar to human Woringer-Kolopp disease but had multicentric involvement of footpads, oral mucosa, and the nose. The authors have also observed several canine cases of focal and multicentric Woringer-Kolopp–type mycosis fungoides. Woringer-Kolopp–like disease has not been seen in cats.

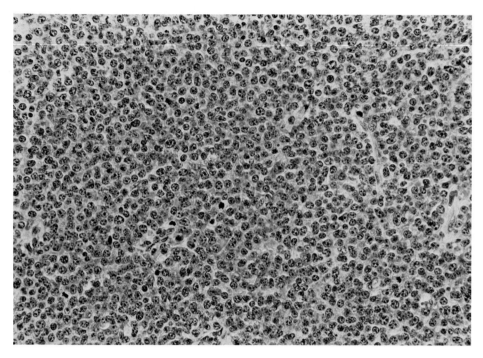

FIGURE 31-3. Malignant lymphoma in a dog, large cell type. The large, vesicular nuclei contain multiple nucleoli, which tend to have a peripheral distribution. Note the fairly high mitotic activity. ($\times$290.)

Sézary syndrome is a variant of mycosis fungoides that has typical cutaneous lesions plus a convoluted T-cell leukemia. Thrall reported a single case of Sézary syndrome in a dog with typical plaque-stage cutaneous lesions, as well as infiltration of numerous internal organs.

The average age of dogs and cats with cutaneous lymphoma is 9 to 11 years. There is no apparent breed predilection. Surgical excision of solitary tumors in dogs was curative in cases reported by Brown and also McKeever, but tumors recur rapidly after surgical excision in cats. In most cases of mycosis fungoides, with the exception of Sézary syndrome and the *d'emblee* type, lymph nodes and visceral organs are not affected until late in the course of the disease. Many animals with nonepitheliotropic lymphoma have involvement of peripheral lymph nodes and internal organs at the time of presentation.

Histopathology

Nonepitheliotropic (Figures 31-3 through 31-7). B-cell lymphomas and T-cell lymphomas that do not show affinity for epithelial structures are characterized by nodular-to-diffuse infiltration of the dermis and often the subcutis by sheets of homogeneous lymphocytes. A grenz zone is generally present in the uppermost dermis, but the cellular infiltrate may ex-

tend to the dermal-epidermal junction. Neoplastic lymphocytes are infrequently noted within epidermis. Dermal adnexa are usually effaced by tumor cells, but residual adnexal epithelium is not infiltrated. The neoplastic infiltrates have a bottom-heavy or base-wide configuration. Necrosis and ulceration may be observed in all variants but are more common in the higher grade malignancies (Table 31-1).

Because malignant lymphoma can arise from any cell type in the B or T lineage, cellular morphology is highly variable. The majority of cases of cutaneous lymphoma in dogs and cats in reviews by Brown, Caciolo (1984), and McKeever were of the large cell type (Table 31-1). Large lymphocytes are intermediate in size between small ("well-differentiated") lymphocytes and macrophages. They have scant, amphophilic cytoplasm and large, vesicular nuclei. Nuclear profiles may be predominantly round-to-ovoid (noncleaved B-cell) or mostly folded or irregular (cleaved B-cell, convoluted T-cell). One or more small nucleoli are frequently situated along the nuclear membrane. Mitotic activity is moderate to high.

Another common type of cutaneous lymphoma in dogs and cats is immunoblastic lymphoma (Table 31-1). Immunoblasts are the largest cells of the lymphocyte life cycle, and they are similar in size to macrophages. B and T immunoblasts are usually indistinguishable histologi-

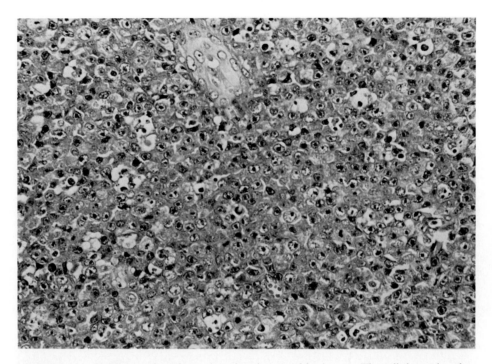

FIGURE 31-4. Malignant lymphoma in a dog, immunoblastic type. The cells have abundant amphophilic cytoplasm, large vesicular nuclei, and prominent centrally located nucleoli. Note the numerous mitotic figures. (×290.)

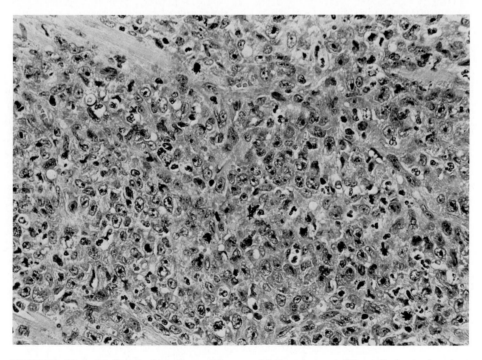

FIGURE 31-5. Malignant lymphoma in a cat, histiocytic type. The cells have abundant, poorly defined cytoplasm, large pleomorphic nuclei, and prominent nucleoli. Note the high mitotic activity. (×290.)

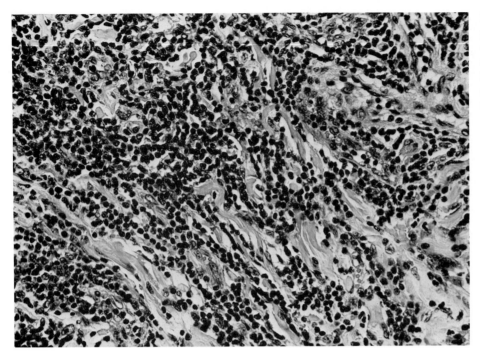

FIGURE 31-6. Malignant lymphoma in a dog, small noncleaved cell type. The cells have minimal cytoplasm and small hyperchromatic nuclei with round-to-ovoid profiles. Mitotic figures are rare. (×290.)

cally. They have moderate amphophilic or basophilic cytoplasm and large, round, vesicular nuclei. A single, prominent, centrally located nucleolus is present. Mitotic figures are numerous.

Histiocytic lymphoma is a cytologically distinct, uncommon variant that occurs more often in cats than in dogs. This cell type has many histologic features of epithelioid macrophages, but is usually of T-cell lin-

eage. "Histiocytic" lymphocytes have abundant, poorly defined, pale eosinophilic cytoplasm. Nuclei are large and highly pleomorphic with profiles varying from ovoid to reniform to convoluted. Nucleoli are usually single and large. Mitotic activity is high. Necrosis and inflammatory cell infiltrates are often more prominent than in other lymphoma variants. Eosinophils are often present in small numbers because of secretion of

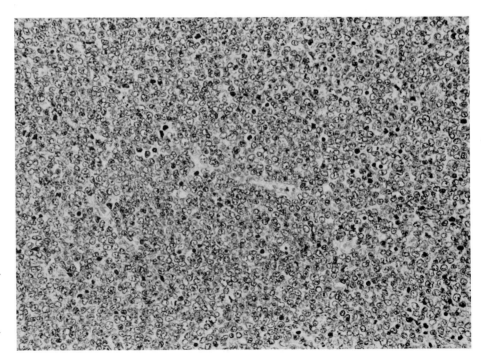

FIGURE 31-7. Malignant lymphoma in a dog, small cleaved cell type. The cells have small vesicular nucleoli with irregular or folded profiles. Mitotic activity is fairly high. (×290.)

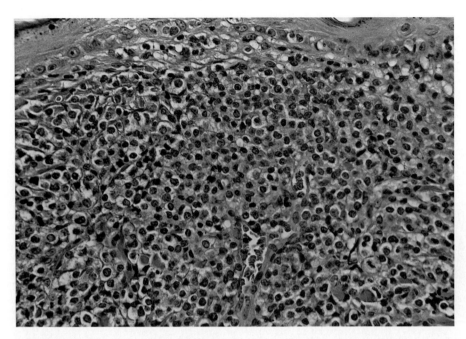

FIGURE 31-8. Mycosis fungoides (tumor stage) in a dog. Neoplastic cells are large and contain oval to irregular nuclei and moderate, pale cytoplasm. (×290.)

eosinophilotactic lymphokines. Differentiation from granulomatous inflammation can be extremely difficult, especially in punch biopsy samples. Anaplastic mast cell tumor and even anaplastic carcinoma are additional differential diagnoses that may require special stains or immunoperoxidase stains to be ruled out.

Small lymphocytic and small cleaved B-cell lymphomas are uncommon in dogs and cats. These neoplasms are composed of small cells with scant, pale cytoplasm. Nuclei have evenly dispersed chromatin and inconspicuous nucleoli. Small lymphocytes have round-to-ovoid nuclear profiles, whereas small cleaved cells have slightly larger, folded nuclei. Mitotic activity is low or moderate. Small-cell lymphomas can be difficult to distinguish from lymphocyte-predominant inflammatory lesions; fortunately, these are few in canine and feline skin. Lymphocyte-rich regressing canine cutaneous histiocytomas, insect-bite reactions, and idiopathic lymphocytic dermatitides may have a highly cellular, fairly monomorphic appearance that may mimic small-cell lymphoid neoplasia. Inflammatory processes generally have a top-heavy silhouette, a more pleocytic population, and no grenz zone, and they do not extend deeply into subcutaneous fat.

Other types of nonepitheliotropic lymphoma, such as lymphoblastic or mixed-cell types, probably occur infrequently in the skin of dogs and cats. Logical histologic classification of these uncommon lymphomas using the NCI system should be feasible in most cases by careful assessment of cell size, nuclear size and conformation, nucleolar number and prominence, and mitotic rate.

Epitheliotropic (Figures 10-37 through 10-40, 31-8, and 31-9). Cutaneous lymphomas that demonstrate affinity of tumor cells for epithelial structures are of T-cell origin and are most often, but not always, of the mycosis fungoides phenotype. The T lymphocytes are primarily attracted to Langerhans cells rather than keratinocytes, but this is manifested as progressive accumulation of neoplastic cells within epidermis and adnexal epithelium. The histologic findings in most types of mycosis fungoides were already described (see Chapter 10). The *d'emblee* variant appears identical to tumor-stage lesions of progressive mycosis fungoides. The dermis contains one or more poorly circumscribed, nodular infiltrates of homogeneous lymphoid cells that may extend into the panniculus. Ulceration is common, and the intact epidermis has diffuse or multifocal accumulations of tumor cells. Adnexa are usually obliterated by the neoplasm, but residual follicles and sweat glands show marked epitheliotropic infiltration by T lymphocytes. The residual adnexa are often demarcated only by intact glassy membranes and basement membranes. The cytologic features of the mycosis cells are scant, clear cytoplasm and large, pale nuclei. Many of the nuclei have convoluted contours. Nucleoli are inconspicuous, and mitotic activity is fairly low.

Tumors of mycosis fungoides may need to be distinguished from histiocytomas in incisional or punch biopsy specimens, since histiocytomas can demonstrate

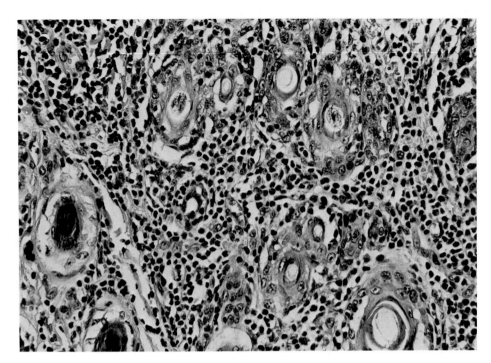

FIGURE 31-9. Mycosis fungoides in a cat. The cells have minimal cytoplasm and small hyperchromatic nuclei, resembling small noncleaved lymphocytes. Nuclear profiles often appear slightly irregular. Note infiltration of follicular epithelium by the lymphocytes. (×290.)

limited epidermotropism. Mycosis cells have paler cytoplasm, less obvious nucleoli, and lower mitotic activity than histiocytoma cells. Also, necrosis and infiltration by small lymphocytes usually are not observed in mycosis fungoides.

Woringer-Kolopp–like variants of mycosis fungoides are characterized by moderate to marked, irregular epithelial hyperplasia with variable hyperkeratosis. The lower layers of the epithelium have marked, diffuse infiltration by neoplastic cells in contrast to the mild epidermal infiltrates with cell clusters (Pautrier's microabscesses) observed in typical patch- and plaque-stage mycosis fungoides. Superficial follicular epithelium is similarly affected if haired skin is involved. The cellular infiltrate in the superficial dermis and oral submucosa is mild and predominantly lymphoplasmacytic. The intraepithelial cells of the Woringer-Kolopp–like variant generally have more abundant cytoplasm, larger nuclei, and higher mitotic activity than in other types of mycosis fungoides. Other cytologic and immunohistochemical features are identical to those of mycosis cells.

LYMPHOMATOID GRANULOMATOSIS
Clinical features

Lymphomatoid granulomatosis is an uncommon lymphohistiocytic proliferative disorder in humans that

was first described by Liebow in 1972. It is rare in dogs and has not been seen in cats. All of the canine cases reported in the literature had visceral lesions only. Two cases of lymphomatoid granulomatosis with primary cutaneous lesions have been seen by the authors, and an additional case was observed by Rosenkrantz.*

Lymphomatoid granulomatosis is an angiocentric, angiodestructive, granulomatous, systemic disease affecting primarily the lungs. Fifteen percent of the human cases progress to frank malignant lymphoma. A third of the human cases have cutaneous lesions that may precede pulmonary lesions by several months. The etiology of lymphomatoid granulomatosis is unknown but is probably related to immunoregulatory dysfunction. As in mycosis fungoides (see discussion above), T-helper cells are increased, and the lymphomas that may subsequently develop appear to be of T-cell origin, according to recent phenotypic and genetic studies.

Skin lesions of lymphomatoid granulomatosis in humans are erythematous papules, plaques, and nodules with a tendency to ulcerate. Ulceration as a primary presenting sign is rare but has been described by Wood. Canine cases have chronic histories of recurrent, punctate to crateriform ulcers that heal with scarring. The lesions involve the face, eyelids, mucocutaneous junctions, and trunk. At necropsy, in addition to multiple discrete skin ulcers, there may be nodular le-

---

* Rosenkrantz WR: Personal communication, 1990.

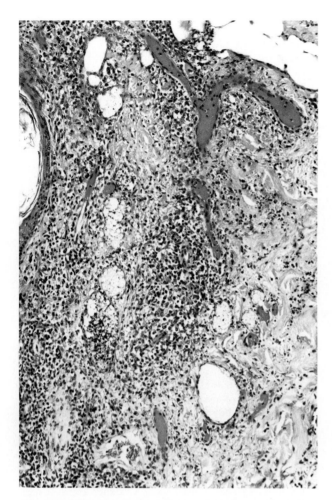

FIGURE 31-10. Lymphomatoid granulomatosis in a dog. The dermis is infiltrated by pleomorphic lymphohistiocytic cells, which tend to concentrate around blood vessels and adnexa. (×120.)

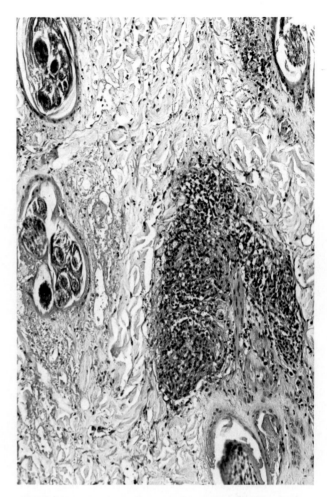

FIGURE 31-11. Lymphomatoid granulomatosis in a dog. Lymphohistiocytic infiltrate obliterates a dermal blood vessel at right. Note the granular degeneration of adjacent dermal collagen and necrosis of adnexal epithelium within the margin of a dermal infarct at left. (×120.)

sions limited to subcutaneous fat. Lungs and lymph nodes contain yellow-gray, nodular foci.

Histopathology (Figures 31-10 through 31-12)

The skin lesions of canine cases of lymphomatoid granulomatosis are similar to those of human cases and are characterized by abrupt foci of full-thickness epidermal ulceration overlying wedge-shaped zones of dermal necrosis. The surrounding intact deep dermis and hypodermal fat has moderate, periadnexal, and perivascular infiltrates of mixed lymphocytes and histiocytes with occasional neutrophils. The lymphohistiocytic cells infiltrate blood vessel walls in the panniculus, resulting in ischemic necrosis of the overlying dermis and adnexa. The infiltrate consistently has a polymorphous appearance with variable numbers of histiocytes, small lymphocytes, large lymphocytes, and plasma cells. Atypical large lymphocytes with pale cytoplasm and

hyperchromatic nuclei progressively increased in number over the course of the disease. Nuclei of the atypical lymphocytes are slightly elongated and twisted or irregular in profile. Mitotic figures are also detected with increasing frequency over time.

The lungs have patchy alveolar, perivascular, and vascular infiltration by polymorphous lymphohistiocytic cells, including atypical lymphocytes as described for the skin lesions, and atypical plasmacytoid cells with large, eccentric, hyperchromatic nuclei. Similar lesions may be present in lymph nodes, liver, and spleen.

A diagnosis of cutaneous lymphomatoid granulomatosis may be overlooked primarily because of its rarity. According to Wood, lymphomatoid granulomatosis is the only disease that shows perivascular and intravascular infiltration by a mixed population of lymphohistiocytic cells with atypical cytologic features.

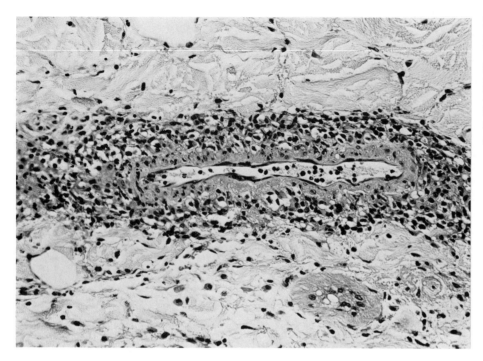

FIGURE 31-12. Lymphomatoid granulomatosis in a dog. The wall of a deep dermal arteriole is infiltrated by pleomorphic lymphohistiocytic cells. Note the elongated, hyperchromatic nuclei. (×290.) *(Case material from WS Rosenkrantz, Garden Grove, California.)*

SUGGESTED READINGS

Cutaneous extramedullary plasmacytoma

Baer KE and others: Cutaneous plasmacytomas in dogs: a morphologic and immunohistochemical study, Vet Pathol 26:216-221, 1989.

Brunnert SR and Altman NH: Identification of immunoglobulin light chains in canine extramedullary plasmacytomas by thioflavine T and immunohistochemistry, J Vet Diagn Invest 3:245-251, 1991.

Carothers MA and others: Extramedullary plasmacytoma and immunoglobulin-associated amyloidosis in a cat, J Am Vet Med Assoc 195:1593-1597, 1990.

Nickoloff BJ, Hill JR, and Weiss LM: Canine neuroendocrine carcinoma (Merkel cell tumor): a report of twenty cases, Am J Dermatopathol 7:579-586, 1985.

Rakich PM and others: Mucocutaneous plasmacytomas in dogs: 75 cases (1980-1987), J Am Vet Med Assoc 194:803-810, 1989.

Rowland PH and others: Cutaneous plasmacytomas with amyloid in six dogs, Vet Pathol 28:125-130, 1991.

Malignant lymphoma

Baker JL and Scott DW: Mycosis fungoides in two cats, J Am Anim Hosp Assoc 25:97-101, 1989.

Brown NO and others: Cutaneous lymphosarcoma in the dog: a disease with variable clinical and histologic manifestations, J Am Anim Hosp Assoc 16:565-572, 1980.

Caciolo PL and others: A case of mycosis fungoides in a cat and literature review, J Am Anim Hosp Assoc 19:505-512, 1983.

Caciolo PL and others: Cutaneous lymphosarcoma in the cat: a report of nine cases, J Am Anim Hosp Assoc 20:491-496, 1984.

Carter RF, Valli VEO, and Lumsden JH: The cytology, histology and prevalence of cell types in canine lymphoma classified according to the National Cancer Institute working formulation, Can J Vet Res 50:154-164, 1986.

Doe R and others: Canine epidermotropic cutaneous lymphoma, Am J Dermatopathol 10:80-86, 1988.

Goldschmidt MH and Bevier DE: Skin tumors in the dog. III. Lymphohistiocytic and melanocytic tumors, Comp Cont Ed 3:588-594, 1981.

Greenlee PG and others: Lymphomas in dogs, Cancer 66:480-490, 1990.

Hardy WD Jr: Hematopoietic tumors of cats, J Am Anim Hosp Assoc 17:921-940, 1981.

Johnson JA and Patterson JM: Canine epidermotropic lymphoproliferative disease resembling pagetoid reticulosis in man, Vet Pathol 18:487-493, 1981.

Lukes RJ and Parker JW: The pathology of lymphoreticular neoplasms. In Twomey JJ and Good RA, editors: The immunopathology of lymphoreticular neoplasms, New York, 1978, Plenum Publishing, pp 239-279.

McKeever PJ and others: Canine cutaneous lymphoma, J Am Vet Med Assoc 180:531-536, 1982.

Moore PF: Lymphoid neoplasia of skin and mucous membranes in the dog: a morphologic and immunophenotypic analysis. Proceedings of the Forty-First Annual Meeting of the American College of Veterinary Pathologists, Phoenix, p 22, 1990.

Thrall MA and others: Cutaneous lymphosarcoma and leukemia in a dog resembling Sézary syndrome in man, Vet Pathol 21:182-186, 1984.

Lymphomatoid granulomatosis

Fitzgerald SD, Wolf DC, and Carlton WW: Eight cases of canine lymphomatoid granulomatosis, Vet Pathol 28:241-245, 1991.

Leblanc B and others: Lymphomatoid granulomatosis in a Beagle dog, Vet Pathol 27:287-289, 1990.

Liebow AA, Carrington CRB, and Friedman PJ: Lymphomatoid granulomatosis, Hum Pathol 3:457-558, 1972.

Lucke VM and others: A lymphomatoid granulomatosis of the lungs of young dogs, Vet Pathol 16:405-412, 1979.

Postorino NC and others: Canine pulmonary lymphomatoid granulomatosis. Proceedings of Seventh Annual Conference of the Veterinary Cancer Society, Madison, Wisc, 1987.

Walder EJ and Barr RJ: A case of lymphomatoid granulomatosis with primary cutaneous manifestations in a dog. Proceedings of the Thirty-Seventh Annual Meeting of the American College of Veterinary Pathologists, New Orleans, p 62, 1986.

Wood ML and others: Cutaneous lymphomatoid granulomatosis: a rare cause of recurrent skin ulceration, Br J Dermatol 110:619-625, 1984.

See also General References, pp 327-328.

Index

A

Abscess of bite wound compared with mycobacterial infection, 170
Abyssinian cat, psychogenic alopecia in, 295
Acantholysis
  actinic keratosis and, 78, 331
  impetigo and, 12
  pemphigus erythematosus and, 19
  pemphigus foliaceus and, 18
  pemphigus vegetans and, 33
  pemphigus vulgaris and, 31
  subcorneal pustular dermatosis and, 20
Acantholytic squamous cell carcinoma, 337, 338-339
  compared with
    apocrine sweat gland carcinoma, 394
    ductular apocrine adenocarcinoma, 395
    subungual squamous cell carcinoma, 403
Acanthoma, infundibular keratinizing; *see* Infundibular keratinizing
    acanthoma
Acanthosis
  growth hormone/castration-responsive dermatosis and, 283
  hyperestrogenism and, 281
  hypothyroidism and, 274
  Sertoli cell tumor and, 278
Acanthosis nigricans of Dachshund, 79-81
Acariasis
  notoedric; *see* Notoedric acariasis
  otodectic, feline notoedric acariasis compared with, 125
  sarcoptic; *see* Sarcoptic acariasis
Acid-fast stain
  mycobacterial infection and, 170
  Nocardia and, 165
Ackerman's urticarial allergic eruption compared with angioedema
    and urticaria, 136
Acne
  actinic comedones versus, 272
  follicular destruction and
    canine, 257-258
    feline, 258-259
Acquired pattern alopecia, 306-307
  compared with
    alopecia areata, 291
    color-mutant alopecia, 299
    congenital hypotrichosis, 309
    hyperadrenocorticism, 277
Acral lick dermatitis, 71-74

Acral lick dermatitis—cont'd
  compared with
    callus and callus pyoderma, 256
    pythiosis, 184
  deep bacterial folliculitis and furunculosis and, 252, 254
Acral pruritic nodule; *see* Acral lick dermatitis
Acrochordon, 409-410, 413
Acrodermatitis
  of Bull Terrier, 106-108
  zinc-responsive dermatosis compared with, 104
Actin, smooth muscle tumors and, 445
Actinic comedones, 98
  compared with
    acne, 258
    callus and callus pyoderma, 256
  follicular destruction and, 270-272
  keratosis and, 77, 79
Actinic keratosis
  acantholytic variant of, 331
  comedones and, 270, 271
  cutaneous horn and, 331
  of dermis, 155-156
  of epidermis, 76-79, 330-331
  hemangiosarcoma and, 423, 426
  lichenoid keratosis compared with, 85
Actinic squamous cell carcinoma compared with hemangiosarcoma,
    423
Actinomyces, 163, 165
Actinomyces hordeovulnaris, 163
Actinomyces viscosus, 163
Actinomycosis
  cutaneous dirofilariasis compared with, 129
  of dermis, 163-166
Acute moist dermatitis; *see* Pyotraumatic dermatitis
Adenitis, sebaceous; *see* Sebaceous adenitis
Adenocarcinoma
  apocrine; *see* Apocrine adenocarcinoma
    ductular, 394-395
    mixed, 394, 395
    metastatic, ductular apocrine adenocarcinoma compared with,
      395
Adenoma
  apocrine; *see* Apocrine adenoma
  hepatoid gland, 381-383
  mammary gland, 390

Adenoma—cont'd
  perianal gland, 381-383
  sebaceous; see Sebaceous adenoma
Adipocytes, necrosis of, 315
Adipose tissue lipoma, 431
Adnexal atrophy, 278
Adnexal differentiation in solid basal cell carcinoma, 347
Adnexal dysplasia, focal, 358-359
Adrenal hormone synthesis, 282
Afghan Hound
  demodicosis in, 264
  hypothyroidism in, 74
  tricholemmoma in, 364
Ainu with Vogt-Koyanagi-Harada–like syndrome, 148
Airedale Terrier
  follicular dysplasia in, 304, 306
  hypothyroidism in, 74
  malignant melanoma in, 459
  melanocytic neoplasms in, 452
  scrotal vascular hamartoma in, 419
Akita
  pemphigus foliaceus in, 16
  sebaceous adenitis in, 101, 248
  Vogt-Koyanagi-Harada–like syndrome in, 148
Alaskan Malamute
  follicular dysplasia in, 304
  hypothyroidism in, 74
  post-clipping alopecia in, 285
  vitiligo in, 152
  Vogt-Koyanagi-Harada–like syndrome in, 148
  zinc-responsive dermatosis in, 103
Alcian blue, discoid lupus erythematosus and, 145
Algae
  in opportunistic cutaneous infections
    of dermis, 179-181
    versus systemic mycoses, 175
  in systemic cutaneous infections
    versus actinomycosis and nocardiosis, 165
    versus cryptococcosis, 177
Allergic contact dermatitis, 51-52; see also Hypersensitivity
  compared with
    feline psychogenic alopecia, 296
    hookworm dermatitis, 130
    hyperplastic dermatitis, 68
    irritant contact dermatitis, 54-55
  of dermis, 131-132, 133
Allergic dermatitis, 131-132, 133
  contact; see Allergic contact dermatitis
  flea; see Flea allergy dermatitis
  food and; see Food allergy
  inhalant; see Atopy
  miliary; see Allergic miliary dermatitis
Allergic eruption of Ackerman versus angioedema or urticaria, 136
Allergic miliary dermatitis, 59-61, 62, 122-123
  cheyletiellosis and, 126
  compared with
    atopy, 115
    eosinophilic plaque, 55, 215
    food allergy, 117, 119
    notoedric acariasis, 126
Alopecia
  acquired pattern; see Acquired pattern alopecia
  atopy and, 115
  cicatricial; see Cicatricial alopecia
  color-mutant; see Color-mutant alopecia
  congenital, 307-309

Alopecia—cont'd
  cyclic flank, 304
  endocrine, 274
  frictional, 282-283
  post-clipping; see Post-clipping alopecia
  post-rabies vaccination; see Post-rabies vaccination alopecia
  psychogenic; see Psychogenic alopecia, feline
  scarring; see Cicatricial alopecia
  traction; see Traction alopecia
  zinc-responsive dermatosis and, 102, 103
Alopecia areata, 291-292
  cicatricial alopecia compared with, 293
  dermatophytosis compared with, feline, 243
  mycosis fungoides compared with, 161
  post-rabies vaccination alopecia compared with, 288, 289
  traction alopecia compared with, canine, 294
Alopecic plaque, acral lick dermatitis and, 72
Alpha-1-antichymotrypsin, 448
Alpha-1-antitrypsin, 448
Amelanotic epithelioid melanoma compared with extramedullary plasma cell tumor, 476
American Staffordshire Terrier
  actinic keratosis in, 78, 330
  deep bacterial folliculitis and furunculosis in, 253
  demodicosis in, 264
  dermal hemangiomas and, 421
  hemangiosarcomas in, 421
    solar-associated, 423
  mast cell tumor in, 470
  squamous cell carcinoma in, 337
Amino acid deficiency, 104
Ampicillin, 42
Amyloid, 230
  plasmacytoma and, 476
Amyloidosis
  cutaneous, 229-232
  renal, 220
  systemic, 220, 230
ANA test; see Antinuclear antibody test
Anagen effluvium, 286
Anagen hair, telogen effluvium and, 287
Anagen hair follicle, matrical cyst and, 354
Anaplastic carcinoma
  amelanotic malignant melanoma versus, 464
  apocrine sweat gland carcinoma versus, 394
  histiocytic lymphoma versus, 481
  squamous cell carcinoma versus, 338
  storiform-pleomorphic malignant fibrous histiocytoma versus, 448
Anaplastic mast cell tumor compared with histiocytic lymphoma, 481
Ancylostoma braziliense, 130
Ancylostoma caninum, 130
Ancylostomiasis; see Hookworm dermatitis
Androgens, human, 257
Anesthesia
  for deep punch biopsy, 63
  for skin biopsy, 3, 269
  for wedge biopsy, 63, 325
Angioedema, 135
Angiokeratoma, 421, 422
Angiomatoid variant, 382
Angiosarcoma, 428; see also Hemangiosarcoma; Lymphangiosarcoma
Antibiotics, 316

Antichymotrypsin, 448
Antigen, carcinoembryonic; *see* Carcinoembryonic antigen
Antilymphocyte serum, 263
Antimelanocyte antibodies, 150
Antinuclear antibody test
    in discoid lupus erythematosus, 23
    in pemphigus erythematosus, 18, 147
    in ulcerative dermatosis of Shetland Sheepdog and Collie, 37
    in vitiligo, 152
    in Vogt-Koyanagi-Harada–like syndrome, 149
Antitrypsin, 448
Apical blebbing
    apocrine cyst and, 386, 387, 388
    apocrine cystadenocarcinoma and, 393
    mammary adenomas and, 390
Apocrine adenocarcinoma, 394-395
    poorly differentiated, 393-394
    well-differentiated, 393
Apocrine adenoma, 389-392
    ductular; *see* Ductular apocrine adenoma
Apocrine carcinoma, 392-395
    perianal gland carcinoma versus, 385
Apocrine cyst, 386, 387
Apocrine cystadenocarcinoma, 392-393
Apocrine cystadenoma, 387-388
Apocrine cystic calcinosis, 227, 228
Apocrine cystomatosis, 386-387
Apocrine decapitation-type secretory activity, 386
Apocrine differentiation in solid basal cell carcinoma, 347
Apocrine gland dilatation in atopy, 116
Apocrine gland hyperplasia
    atopy and, 116
    flea allergy dermatitis and, 122
    food allergy and, 118
Apoptosis
    discoid lupus erythematosus and, 23
    erythema multiforme and, 41, 42
    of keratinocytes in nailbed keratoacanthoma, 402
Arthritis
    hookworm dermatitis and, 130
    juvenile sterile granulomatous dermatitis and lymphadenitis and, 203
Arthropod bites
    eosinophilic furunculosis and, 269
    eosinophilic or plasma cell granuloma from, 207-209, 218
Artifact, usable
    canine familial dermatomyositis and, 36
    discoid lupus erythematosus and, 24
    hereditary lupoid dermatosis of German Shorthaired Pointer and, 28
    ulcerative dermatosis of Shetland Sheepdog and Collie and, 38
Aspergillosis, 179-181; *see also* Cutaneous infections, opportunistic fungi and algae in
Asthenia, cutaneous, 232-234
    feline skin fragility syndrome versus, 236
Atopy
    allergic contact dermatitis compared with, 52, 131-132
    chronic hyperplastic dermatitis and, 68, 69
    dermal, 114-116
    excessive grooming and, 295
    feline, 115
        eosinophilic plaque with, 55
        notoedric acariasis compared with, 125
    flea allergy dermatitis compared with, 120
        canine, 122

Atopy—cont'd
    food allergy compared with, 117
    hyperplastic dermatosis of West Highland White Terrier compared with, 81
Atrophic diseases of hair follicles, 273-297
    alopecia areata in, 291-292
    canine familial dermatomyositis in, 289-291
    canine female hyperestrogenism in, 280-281
    canine hyperadrenocorticism in, 275-278
    canine hypothyroidism in, 273-275
    canine Sertoli cell tumor in, 278-280
    canine traction alopecia in, 294-295
    cicatricial alopecia in, 292-293
    feline psychogenic alopecia in, 295-296
    growth hormone/castration-responsive dermatosis in, 281-284
    post-clipping alopecia in, 285-286
    post-rabies vaccination alopecia in, 287-289
    telogen effluvium in, 286-287
Atrophy
    adnexal, 278
    epidermal, 277
    follicular
        canine Sertoli cell tumor and, 76
        hair; *see* Atrophic diseases of hair follicles
        hypothyroidism and, 75
Atypical histiocytoma, 474
Atypical large lymphocytes, 483
Atypical mycobacteriosis; *see* Opportunistic mycobacterial infection
Autoimmune skin disease
    bullous
        epidermolysis bullosa versus, 38
        pemphigoid and, 28
    compared with
        actinic keratosis, 331
        alopecia areata and, 291
        erythema multiforme, 42
        generic dog food dermatosis, 105
        leishmaniasis, 186
        zinc-responsive dermatosis, 103
    discoid lupus erythematosus and, 22
    pemphigus foliaceus and, 16
    pemphigus vegetans and, 33
    pemphigus vulgaris and, 31
    primary seborrhea and, 89
    systemic lupus erythematosus and, 24
Autosomal recessive ichthyosis, human, 98

B

B-cell lymphoma, 481
Bacterial folliculitis
    deep; *see* Deep bacterial folliculitis and furunculosis
    erythema multiforme versus, 42
    Schnauzer comedo syndrome and, 97
    superficial; *see* Superficial bacterial folliculitis
Balloon-cell melanocytoma, 452, 456
Balloon-cell melanoma, 463, 464
    sebaceous carcinoma versus, 380
Basal cell basalioma, 341
Basal cell carcinoma
    clear-cell, 343, 348-349
    compared with
        benign feline basal cell tumor, 343
        feline ductular apocrine adenoma, 392
        sebaceous epithelioma, 378

Basal cell carcinoma—cont'd
    compared with—cont'd
        trabecular trichoblastoma, 371
    of epidermis, 343-349
    granular cells and, 371
    inner root sheath differentiation in, 348
    keratinizing; see Keratinizing basal cell carcinoma
    with sebaceous differentiation, 378
    solid, 343, 344-347
Basal cell degeneration
    bullous and vesicular diseases and, 22
    canine familial dermatomyositis and, 35
    discoid lupus erythematosus and, 23, 24, 144
    erythema multiforme and, 42
    hereditary lupoid dermatosis of German Shorthaired Pointer
        and, 28
    pemphigus erythematosus and, 147
    psoriasiform-lichenoid dermatosis of Springer Spaniel and, 85
    systemic lupus erythematosus and, 25, 26, 146
    ulcerative dermatosis of Shetland Sheepdog and Collie
        and, 38
Basal cell epithelioma; see also Basal cell carcinoma
    metastatic potential of, 343-344
    term, 341
Basal cell tumor; see also Trichoblastoma
    benign feline
        epidermal, 341-343
            solid basal cell carcinoma versus, 347
            stromal features in, 343
            trabecular trichoblastoma versus, 369-370
        garland, 367
        medusa-head, 367
        term, 341
Basal cell vacuolation
    canine familial dermatomyositis and, 35
    discoid lupus erythematosus and, 23
    erythema multiforme and, 42
    hereditary lupoid dermatosis of German Shorthaired Pointer
        and, 27, 28
    systemic lupus erythematosus and, 25
    ulcerative dermatosis of Shetland Sheepdog and Collie and,
        37, 38
Basalioma, basal cell, 341; see also Basal cell carcinoma
Basaloid apocrine adenoma, 389; see also Ductular apocrine ade-
    noma
Basaloid mammary gland adenoma, 390
Basement membrane zone
    bullous and vesicular diseases and, 22
    discoid lupus erythematosus and, 24
    epidermolysis bullosa and, 38
Basophil hypersensitivity, 119
Basophilic debris, 318
Basosquamous basal cell tumor, 343
Basosquamous carcinoma; see Keratinizing basal cell carcinoma
Bassett Hound
    actinic keratosis in, 330
    black-hair follicular dysplasia in, 301
    congenital hypotrichosis in, 308
    dermal hemangiomas and hemangiosarcomas in, 421
    primary seborrhea in, 89
Beagle
    actinic keratosis in, 78, 330
    black-hair follicular dysplasia in, 301
    congenital hypotrichosis in, 308
    dermal hemangiomas in, 421

Beagle—cont'd
    hemangiosarcomas in, 421
        solar-associated, 423
    hepatoid gland neoplasms in, 382
    sebaceous adenoma in, 377
    squamous cell carcinoma in, 337
Bearded Collie with pemphigus foliaceus, 16
Bedlington Terrier with pilomatricoma, 366
Behavior, biologic; see Biologic behavior
Belgian Sheepdog with sebaceous adenitis, 101
Belgian Tervuren
    antimelanocyte antibodies in, 150
    vitiligo in, 152
Benign basal cell tumor; see Basal cell tumor, benign
        feline
Benign fibrohistiocytic tumor, 445; see also Fibrous
        histiocytoma, benign
Benign melanoma; see Melanocytoma
Benign mixed mammary tumors compared with mixed
        apocrine adenoma, 390
Bernese Mountain Dog
    color-mutant alopecia in, 299
    dermal systemic histiocytosis in, 201-203
Bichon Frise
    congenital hypotrichosis in, 308
    post-rabies vaccination alopecia in, 288
Big head; see Juvenile sterile granulomatous dermatitis and lym-
        phadenitis
Biologic behavior
    malignant lymphoma and, 477
    malignant melanoma and, 459-460
    mast cell tumor and
        canine, 470-471
        feline, 468
    plasmacytoma and, 475
Biopsy
    punch; see Punch biopsy
    skin; see Skin biopsy
    wedge; see Wedge biopsy
Bites
    arthropod; see Arthropod bites
    opportunistic mycobacterial infection versus, 170
    spider, 185, 212-213
Black-hair follicular dysplasia, 301-302
    color-mutant alopecia versus, 299, 301
Black-widow spider bites, 212
Blastomyces dermatitidis, 174
Blastomycosis versus cryptococcosis, 178; see also Cutaneous infec-
        tions, systemic fungi and algae in
Bleaching, 454
Blebbing, apical; see Apical blebbing
Bleeding abnormalities in canine hyperadrenocorticism, 275
Bloodhounds with cutaneous vascular tumors, 421
Blue Doberman syndrome, 299
Blue dog disease; see Color-mutant alopecia
Blue line, 13
Blue nevus, 451; see also Melanocytoma
Bone invasion of nailbed squamous cell carcinoma, 403
Border Collie with flea allergy dermatitis, 120
Boston Terrier
    acquired pattern alopecia in, 307
    demodicosis in, 264
    hyperadrenocorticism in, 276
    ichthyosis in, 99
    malignant melanoma in, 459

Boston Terrier—cont'd
   mast cell tumor in, 470
   sebaceous adenoma in, 377
Botryomycosis compared with actinomycosis and nocardiosis, 166
Bowen's disease compared with actinic keratosis, 79, 331, 340-341
Boxer
   acne in, 258
   atopy in, 115
   coccidioidomycosis in, 175
   demodicosis in, 264
   follicular dysplasia in, 304, 306
   histiocytoma in, 465
   hyperadrenocorticism in, 276
   hypothyroidism in, 74
   kerion in, 261
   mast cell tumor in, 470
   sebaceous adenitis in, 101
   Sertoli cell tumor in, 76
   sterile granuloma and pyogranuloma in, 196
Brittany Spaniel; *see* English Springer Spaniel
Bronchopneumonia in Bull Terrier, 107
Brown recluse spider bites, 212
Bubble blowing, 199
Bulb-type tricholemmoma, 364-365
   clear-cell basal cell carcinoma versus, 349
Bull Terrier
   deep bacterial folliculitis and furunculosis in, 253
   lethal acrodermatitis in, 106-108
   mast cell tumor in, 470
   squamous cell carcinoma in, 337
Bulla
   in bullous and vesicular diseases, 22; *see also* Bullous and vesicular diseases of epidermis
   in bullous pemphigoid, 28, 29, 30
   cutaneous mucinosis and, 228
   in drug eruptions compared with bullous pemphigoid, 29
   in epidermolysis bullosa, 38
   hemorrhagic; *see* Hemorrhagic bulla
   in junctional epidermolysis bullosa, 38, 39
   in pemphigus vulgaris, 31
   in toxic epidermal necrolysis, 44
Bulldog
   English; *see* English Bulldog
   French; *see* French Bulldog
Bullous and vesicular diseases of epidermis, 22-40
   bullous pemphigoid in, 28-30
   canine familial dermatomyositis in, 34-36
   epidermolysis bullosa in, 38, 39
   hereditary lupoid dermatosis of German Shorthaired Pointer in, 26-28
   lupus erythematosus in
      discoid, 22-24
      systemic, 24-26
   pemphigus vegetans in, 33-34
   pemphigus vulgaris in, 31-33
   ulcerative dermatosis of Shetland Sheepdog and Collie in, 36-38
Bullous impetigo, 10, 11, 12
   pemphigus foliaceus versus, 18
Bullous pemphigoid, 28-30
   compared with
      chemical and thermal burns, 49
      epidermolysis bullosa, 38
      mucocutaneous candidiasis, 14
      mycosis fungoides, 159
      pemphigus vulgaris, 31

Bullous pemphigoid—cont'd
   compared with—cont'd
      toxic epidermal necrolysis, 44
      ulcerative dermatosis of Shetland Sheepdog and Collie, 36
Burns
   chemical and thermal, 48-50
   compared with
      erythema multiforme, 42
      feline idiopathic ulcerative dermatosis, 65
      toxic epidermal necrolysis, 46
   full or partial thickness, 48, 49

C

Cairn Terrier
   atopy in, 115
   flea allergy dermatitis in, 120
Calcification
   apocrine cystic, 227, 228
   dystrophic, 227
      calcinosis circumscripta and, 226
      calcinosis cutis and, 223
   in epithelioma; *see* Pilomatricoma
   tumoral, 226-228
Calcinosis circumscripta, 226-228
Calcinosis cutis, 223-226
   canine hyperadrenocorticism and, 275, 278
Calcium chloride, 224, 226
Callus and callus pyoderma, 255-256
   acne versus, 258
Callus dermatitis, 255-256, 258
Candida, 14, 15
Candidiasis, mucocutaneous, 14-15
Canned red tuna, 324
Capillary hemangioma, 422
Carcinoembryonic antigen, 339
   eccrine carcinoma and, 396
   malignant fibrous histiocytoma and, 448
   nailbed squamous cell carcinoma and, 403
Carcinoma
   anaplastic; *see* Anaplastic carcinoma
   apocrine; *see* Apocrine carcinoma
   basal cell; *see* Basal cell carcinoma
   basosquamous; *see* Keratinizing basal cell carcinoma
   eccrine; *see* Eccrine carcinoma
   hepatoid gland; *see* Perianal gland carcinoma
   matrical; *see* Matrical carcinoma
   metastatic; *see* Metastatic carcinoma
   nailbed squamous cell, 403, 404
   perianal gland; *see* Perianal gland carcinoma
   sebaceous; *see* Sebaceous carcinoma
   squamous cell; *see* Squamous cell carcinoma
Carcinosarcoma, 394
Carpal pad of German Shepherd Dog with sterile pedal panniculitis, 324
Caseation necrosis
   matrical carcinoma and, 371
   in solid basal cell carcinoma, 345
Castration response, 282
Cat; *see also* specific breed
   acne in, 258-259
   actinic keratosis in, 330
   allergic miliary dermatitis in; *see* Allergic miliary dermatitis
   benign basal cell tumor in; *see* Basal cell tumor
   cutaneous horn in footpad of, 331-334
   cutaneous mastocytosis in, 468

Cat; *see also* specific breed—cont'd
  cutaneous nonepitheliotropic lymphoma in, 477
  demodicosis in, 259, 262, 266
  dermatophytic mycetoma in, 172-174
    dermatophytosis and, 242
  dermatophytosis in, 172, 241-243
  diffuse cutaneous mastocytosis in, 468
  digital squamous cell carcinoma compared with eccrine carcinoma of, 396
  ductular apocrine adenoma in; *see* Ductular apocrine adenoma
  eosinophilic granuloma in; *see* Eosinophilic granuloma
  eosinophilic plaque in, 55, 56
    mosquito-bite hypersensitivity versus, 215
    prominent eosinophils or plasma cells and, 213-215
  eosinophilic ulcer in, 63-64, 117, 216
  epithelioid melanoma in, 463
  food allergy in, 117-119
  idiopathic ulcerative dermatosis in, 65-67
  indolent ulcer in, 63-64, 117, 216
  insect-bite hypersensitivity in; *see* Mosquito-bite hypersensitivity
  leprosy in; *see* Leprosy, feline
  linear granuloma in; *see* Eosinophilic granuloma
  localized demodicosis in, 264
  mast cell tumors in, 468-473
  mosquito-bite hypersensitivity in; *see* Mosquito-bite hypersensitivity
  mycosis fungoides in, 159, 161
  notoedric acariasis in, 125-127
  opportunistic mycobacterial infection in, 169
  panniculitis in, 313
  pansteatitis in, 323-324
  papillomavirus in, 334
  plasma cell pododermatitis in, 220-221
  psychogenic alopecia in; *see* Psychogenic alopecia, feline
  ribbon trichoblastoma in, 368
  ringworm in, 172, 241-243
  sebaceous adenitis in, 100
  self-induced hair loss in; *see* Psychogenic alopecia, feline
  Siamese; *see* Siamese cat
  skin fragility in, 234-236
    cutaneous asthenia versus, 233, 234
  sporotrichosis of, compared with canine sporotrichosis, 182
  ulcerative dermatosis in, 65-67
Catagen phase of hair follicle, 273
  arrested, 285
Cavernous hemangioma, 421-422
Cedar chip bedding in allergic contact dermatitis, 52
Cellulitis
  deep bacterial folliculitis and furunculosis and, 255
  juvenile; *see* Juvenile sterile granulomatous dermatitis and lymphadenitis
Ceroid pigment, 324
Chemical burns, 48-50
Chesapeake Bay Retriever with follicular dysplasia, 304
Cheyletiella, 126-128
  allergic miliary dermatitis and, 60
Cheyletiella blakei, 126
Cheyletiella parasitovorax, 126
Cheyletiella yasguri, 126
Cheyletiellosis, 126-128
  feline allergic miliary dermatitis and, 60
Chihuahua
  alopecia in
    acquired pattern, 307
    color-mutant, 299

Chihuahua—cont'd
  demodicosis in, 264
  post-rabies vaccination alopecia in, 288
Chinese Shar Pei
  atopy in, 115
  cutaneous mucinosis in, 228, 229
  demodicosis in, 264
  food allergy and, 117
  primary seborrhea in, 89
Cholesterol cleft
  cutaneous xanthoma and, 193
  feline pansteatitis and, 324
  traumatic panniculitis and, 320
Chondroid metaplasia, 462, 463
Chow Chow
  color-mutant alopecia in, 299
  growth hormone/castration-responsive dermatosis in, 283
  hypothyroidism in, 74
  pemphigus foliaceus in, 16
  sebaceous adenitis in, 101
Cicatricial alopecia, 292-293
  compared with
    alopecia areata, 291
    canine traction alopecia, 294, 295
    post-rabies vaccination alopecia, 288
Civatte bodies
  in discoid lupus erythematosus, 23
  in systemic lupus erythematosus, 25-26
Clear-cell apocrine gland carcinoma, 394
Clear-cell basal cell carcinoma, 343, 348-349
  compared with
    bulb-type tricholemmoma, 364
    sebaceous carcinoma, 380
Clear-cell malignant melanoma, 464
Clown nose, 199
Coagulation necrosis
  in chemical and thermal burns, 49
  in toxic epidermal necrolysis, 44
Coat color change in canine Sertoli cell tumor, 75
Coccidioides immitis, 174
Coccidioidomycosis, 174; *see also* Cutaneous infections, systemic fungi and algae in
Cocker Spaniel
  demodicosis in, 264
  hepatoid gland neoplasms in, 382
  histiocytoma in, 465
  lipoma in, 431
  malignant melanoma in, 459
  nodular sebaceous hyperplasia in, 374
  primary seborrhea in, 89
  sarcoptic acariasis in, 124
  sebaceous adenoma in, 377
  sebaceous carcinoma in, 380
  sebaceous epithelioma in, 378
  seborrheic dermatitis in, 91
  tail dock neuroma in, 438
  trichoblastoma in, 367
  vitamin A–responsive dermatosis in, 94
Cod liver oil supplementation, 324
Collagen
  cicatricial alopecia and, 293
  in cutaneous asthenia, 233
  eosinophilic furunculosis and, 269
  feline
    food allergy and, 119
    granuloma and; *see* Eosinophilic granuloma, feline

Collagen—cont'd
    feline—cont'd
        indolent ulcer and, 64
        skin fragility syndrome and, 235-236
    fibropruritic nodules and, 71
    laminar distribution of, 293
    sterile eosinophilic pustulosis and, 251
Collagenic granuloma, feline; *see* Eosinophilic granuloma,
        feline
Collagenolytic epidermolysis bullosa, 38
Collagenous nevus, 407-408
    compared with
        fibroma, 413
        nodular dermatofibrosis, 409
Collarette, epidermal
    erythema multiforme and, 41
    sterile eosinophilic pustulosis and, 250
    subcorneal pustular dermatosis and, 20
    superficial spreading pyoderma and, 12, 13
Collie
    Bearded, 16
    Border, 120
    bullous pemphigoid in, 29
    canine familial dermatomyositis in, 35
    cutaneous histiocytosis in, 199
    demodicosis in, 264
    discoid lupus erythematosus in, 22
    epidermolysis bullosa in, 38
    ichthyosis in, 99
    idiopathic sterile nodular panniculitis in, 321
    nose of, 22
    pemphigus erythematosus in, 18
    pyotraumatic dermatitis in, 59
    sebaceous adenitis in, 101
    systemic lupus erythematosus in, 25
    ulcerative dermatosis in, 36-38
        bullous pemphigoid versus, 29
        discoid lupus erythematosus versus, 24
        erythema multiforme versus, 43
        systemic lupus erythematosus versus, 25
    vitiligo in, 152
Collision tumor, 459
Colloid bodies
    canine familial dermatomyositis and, 35
    lupus erythematosus and
        discoid, 23
        systemic, 25-26
    ulcerative dermatosis of Shetland Sheepdog and Collie
        and, 37
Color-mutant alopecia, 298-301
    follicular dysplasia versus
        black-hair, 301, 302
        canine, 306
Comedones
    acne and, 257-258
    actinic; *see* Actinic comedones
    canine hyperadrenocorticism and, 278
    demodicosis and, 264
    feline acne and, 258-259
Comedos in Schnauzer, 96-98
Complement factor 3, 123
Compound apocrine adenocarcinoma, 394, 395
Compound apocrine adenoma, 390
Compound melanocytomas, 451, 452-453
    melanocytoma-acanthoma and, 458

Compound sebaceous adenoma
    ductular, 377, 378
    glandular, 377, 378
    nodular sebaceous hyperplasia compared with, 376
Congenital alopecia, 307-309
Congenital dermoid cysts, 355
Congenital hypotrichosis, 307-309
Congo red stain, 230
Connective tissue dermal diseases; *see* Dysplastic and depositional
        diseases of dermal connective tissue
Contact allergens, 52
Contact dermatitis
    allergic; *see* Allergic contact dermatitis
    atopy versus, 115
    irritant, 52-55
        allergic contact dermatitis versus, 51-52
        hookworm dermatitis versus, 130
        rhabditic dermatitis versus, 267
Contact irritants, 52
Cornifying epithelioma, intracutaneous; *see* Infundibular keratiniz-
        ing acanthoma
Corticosteroids
    in cutaneous histiocytosis, 199
    in sarcoptic acariasis, 124
Crusting in mucocutaneous pyoderma, 142, 143
Cryptococcosis
    dermal, 177-178
    dermatophytic mycetoma versus, 172
    feline leprosy versus, 167
    narrow-based budding in, 177
    opportunistic mycobacterial infection versus, 170
    sporotrichosis versus, 182
    systemic mycoses versus, 175
Cryptococcus neoformans, 177
Culture
    fungal; *see* Fungal infection, cultures in
    of pythiosis, 184
Curly-Coated Retriever with follicular dysplasia, 304, 306
Cushing's disease or syndrome; *see* Hyperadrenocorticism
Cutaneous horn
    defined, 331
    dilated pore and, 356
    of feline footpad, 331-334
    infundibular keratinizing acanthoma and, 361
Cutaneous infections
    leishmaniasis in
        dermal, 186-188
        sebaceous adenitis and, 101
    opportunistic fungi and algae in, 179-181
        cutaneous xanthoma versus, 194
        deep bacterial folliculitis and furunculosis versus, 254
        erythema nodosum–like panniculitis versus, 323
        idiopathic sterile nodular panniculitis versus, 321
        systemic mycoses versus, 175
        xanthoma versus, 194
    systemic fungi and algae in, 174-177
        actinomycosis and nocardiosis versus, 165
        cryptococcosis versus, 177
        cultures in, 175, 180
        deep bacterial folliculitis and furunculosis versus, 254
        erythema nodosum–like panniculitis versus, 323
        feline dermatophytic mycetoma versus, 172
        feline leprosy versus, 167
        idiopathic sterile nodular panniculitis versus, 321
        opportunistic mycobacterial infection versus, 170

Cutaneous infections—cont'd
  systemic fungi and algae in—cont'd
    sporotrichosis versus, 182, 184
Cyclic flank alopecia, 304
Cyst
  apocrine; *see* Apocrine cyst
  dermoid; *see* Dermoid cyst
  epidermal inclusion; *see* Follicular cyst
  epidermoid; *see* Follicular cyst
  follicular; *see* Follicular cyst
  hybrid; *see* Hybrid cyst
  infundibular, 351, 352-353
  isthmus-catagen, 351, 353-354
  matrical; *see* Matrical cyst
  nailbed epithelial inclusion, 398-399
  sebaceous duct, 374, 375
  solid basal cell carcinoma, 347
  tricholemmal, 351, 353-354
Cystadenocarcinoma, apocrine, 392-393
Cystadenoma, apocrine, 387-388
Cystic calcinosis, apocrine, 227, 228
Cystomatosis, apocrine, 386-387
Cytokeratins
  malignant fibrous histiocytoma and, 448
  spindle-celled squamous cell carcinoma and, 340
Cytoplasmic immunoglobulin, 474, 476
Cytoplasmic inclusion bodies, 335
Cytotoxic drugs, 263

D

Dachshund
  acanthosis nigricans in, 79-81
  alopecia in
    acquired pattern, 306, 307
    color-mutant, 299
  bullous pemphigoid in, 29
  ear margin seborrhea in, 96
  hepatoid gland neoplasms in, 382
  histiocytoma in, 465
  hyperadrenocorticism in, 276
  hypothyroidism in, 74
  idiopathic sterile nodular panniculitis in, 321
  immune-mediated vasculitis in, 138
  juvenile sterile granulomatous dermatitis in, 323
  lipoma in, 431
  Malassezia pachydermatis in, 92
  mast cell tumor in, 470
  opportunistic mycobacterial infection in, 323
  pancreatic disease in, 321
  pyogranuloma in, 196
  sebaceous adenoma in, 377
  sterile granuloma in, 196
  vitiligo in, 152
Dalmatian
  actinic keratosis in, 77, 78, 330
  atopy in, 115
  cutaneous vascular tumors in, 421
  deep bacterial folliculitis and furunculosis in, 253
  demodicosis in, 264
  dermal hemangiomas in, 421
  dermatophytosis in, 244
  hemangiosarcomas in, 421
    solar-associated, 423
  squamous cell carcinoma in, 337

Decapitation secretion
  in apocrine adenocarcinoma, 393
  in apocrine glandular adenoma, 389
Deep bacterial folliculitis and furunculosis
  acne and
    canine, 258
    feline, 259
  actinic comedones and, 271, 272
  actinic keratosis and, 78
  color-mutant alopecia and, 301
  compared with
    demodicosis, 264-265
    dermatophytosis, 245
    eosinophilic furunculosis, 270
    erythema nodosum–like panniculitis, 323
    foreign body reactions, 191, 192
    idiopathic sterile nodular panniculitis, 321
    kerion, 262
    opportunistic mycobacterial infection, 170
    pemphigus foliaceus, 247
    pyotraumatic dermatitis, 58, 59
    septic vasculitis, 140
    sporotrichosis, 182
  follicular destruction and, 252-255
  predisposing causes of, 252
Deep pyoderma; *see* Deep bacterial folliculitis and furunculosis
Degenerative diseases of epidermis, 7-110; *see also* Epidermal diseases
d'Emblee variant epitheliotropic lymphoma, 481
Demodectic mange; *see* Demodicosis
Demodicosis
  acne and
    canine, 258
    feline, 259
  adult-onset, 262, 263
  compared with
    actinic comedones, 271
    dermatophytosis, 242, 243
    familial dermatomyositis, 35
    generic dog food dermatosis, 105
    hookworm dermatitis, 130
    hyperplastic dermatosis in West Highland White Terrier, 81
    ichthyosis, 99
    juvenile sterile granulomatous dermatitis and lymphadenitis, 204
    pemphigus foliaceus, 16
    pythiosis, 184
    zinc-responsive dermatosis, 103
  deep bacterial folliculitis and furunculosis and, 252, 254, 255
  epidermal and follicular keratin in, 90
  feline, 259, 262, 266
  follicular destruction and, 262-266
  hyperadrenocorticism and, 276
  immunologic defect in, 262-263
  juvenile-onset, 262, 263
  sebaceous adenitis and, 101, 249
  septic vasculitis and, 139
  superficial bacterial folliculitis and, 239
Dendritic subtype malignant melanoma, 461
Depigmentation
  cutaneous; *see* Vogt-Koyanagi-Harada–like syndrome
  discoid lupus erythematosus and, 143
Depositional diseases of connective tissue of dermis, 223-236; *see also* Dysplastic and depositional diseases of dermal connective tissue

Dermal collagen in feline skin fragility syndrome, 235-236
Dermal diseases, 111-236
  granulomatous and pyogranulomatous
    infectious, 163-189; *see also* Infectious nodular and diffuse
      granulomatous and pyogranulomatous dermal diseases
    noninfectious, 190-206; *see also* Noninfectious nodular and
      diffuse granulomatous and pyogranulomatous dermal
      diseases
  infectious nodular, 163-189; *see also* Infectious nodular and dif-
    fuse granulomatous and pyogranulomatous dermal diseases
  lichenoid, 141-162; *see also* Lichenoid diseases of dermis
  noninfectious nodular, 190-206; *see also* Noninfectious nodular
    and diffuse granulomatous and pyogranulomatous dermal
    diseases
  perivascular, 112-134; *see also* Perivascular diseases, dermal
  vascular, 135-140
Dermal-epidermal junction
  bullous and vesicular diseases of, 22-40; *see also* Bullous and
    vesicular diseases of epidermis
  epidermolysis bullosa and, 38
  hereditary lupoid dermatosis in German Shorthaired Pointer
    and, 28
  sarcoptic acariasis and, 123
Dermal fibroma compared with fibropruritic nodules, 71
Dermal fibrosis
  acral lick dermatitis and, 72, 73
  actinic keratosis and, 155, 156
  calcinosis cutis and, 226
  fibropruritic nodules and, 70, 71
  idiopathic ulcerative idermatosis and, 65-67
Dermal melanocytomas, 451, 452, 454-456
Dermatitis
  acral lick; *see* Acral lick dermatitis
  acute moist; *see* Pyotraumatic dermatitis
  allergic contact; *see* Allergic contact dermatitis
  allergic miliary; *see* Allergic miliary dermatitis
  callus, 255-256, 258
  Cheyletiella in; *see* Cheyletiellosis
  chronic hyperplastic; *see* Hyperplastic dermatitis, chronic
  contact; *see* Contact dermatitis
  erythematous exfoliative, 158
  flea allergy; *see* Flea allergy dermatitis
  heartworm; *see* Dirofilariasis
  hookworm; *see* Hookworm dermatitis
  idiopathic periadnexal multinodular granulomatous; *see* Sterile
    granuloma and pyogranuloma
  inhalant; *see* Atopy
  interface, 141
  irritant contact, 52-55
    allergic contact dermatitis versus, 51-52
    hookworm dermatitis versus, 130
  juvenile sterile granulomatous; *see* Juvenile sterile granulomatous
    dermatitis and lymphadenitis
  lichenoid, 141; *see also* Lichenoid diseases of dermis
  lymphocytic
    histiocytoma versus, 468
    small-cell lymphoid neoplasia versus, 481
  miliary; *see* Allergic miliary dermatitis
  nasal solar, 22
  Pelodera; *see* Rhabditic dermatitis
  pyotraumatic; *see* Pyotraumatic dermatitis
  rhabditic; *see* Rhabditic dermatitis
  seborrheic; *see* Seborrheic dermatitis
  superficial necrolytic; *see* Superficial necrolytic dermatitis

Dermatofibroma, 410-411
  compared with
    benign schwannoma, 441
    fibrosarcoma, 415
Dermatofibrosarcoma
  benign schwannoma versus, 441
  hemangiopericytoma versus, 438
  malignant schwannoma versus, 443
Dermatofibrosarcoma protuberans, 446, 448-449
Dermatofibrosarcoma type malignant fibrous histiocytoma, 446,
  448-449
Dermatofibrosis, nodular; *see* Nodular dermatofibrosis
Dermatographism, 135
Dermatomyositis, familial; *see* Familial dermatomyositis
Dermatopathy, diabetic; *see* Superficial necrolytic dermatitis
Dermatophytic mycetoma
  dermal, 172-174
  dermatophytosis and, 242
Dermatophytosis
  acne and, 259
  allergic miliary dermatitis and, 60
  canine, 243-245
  compared with
    acne, 258
    cutaneous leishmaniasis, 186
    deep bacterial folliculitis and furunculosis, 255
    discoid lupus erythematosus, 23
    familial dermatomyositis, 35
    generic dog food dermatosis, 105
    ichthyosis, 99
    juvenile-onset localized demodicosis, 264
    mycosis fungoides, 159
    pemphigus foliaceus, 16
    subcorneal pustular dermatosis, 20
    superficial spreading pyoderma, 12
    zinc-responsive dermatosis, 103
  feline, 172, 241-243
  seborrhea and, 89
  seborrheic dermatitis and, 91
  superficial bacterial folliculitis and, 239
Dermatosis
  generic dog food; *see* Generic dog food dermatosis
  in German Shorthaired Pointer with hereditary lupoid, 26-28
    versus discoid lupus erythematosus, 24
    versus familial dermatomyositis, 36
    versus systemic lupus erythematosus, 26
  growth hormone/castration-responsive; *see* Growth
    hormone/castration-responsive dermatosis
  idiopathic ulcerative, pyotraumatic dermatitis versus, 59
  nutrient-responsive, 102
  psoriasiform-lichenoid, 83-85, 156-157
    lichenoid keratosis compared with, 85
  subcorneal pustular; *see* Subcorneal pustule
  ulcerative; *see* Ulcerative dermatosis
  vitamin A–responsive; *see* Vitamin A–responsive dermatosis
  in West Highland White Terrier, 81-83
    versus hyperplastic ichthyosis, 99
  zinc-responsive; *see* Zinc-responsive dermatosis
Dermatosparaxis, 232-234, 236
Dermoid cyst
  follicular, 355
  trichofolliculoma compared with, 359
Dermoid sinus; *see* Dermoid cyst
Desmin, 445

Diabetes mellitus
dermatopathy in; *see* Superficial necrolytic dermatitis
skin fragility syndrome and, 234
vitiligo and, 152
Diarrhea in Bull Terrier, 107
Differential diagnosis; *see* specific disease
Dilated pore
cutaneous horn in, 331
follicular tumors and, 356-357
Dipetalonema reconditum, 128
Dirofilaria immitis, 128
Dirofilariasis, 128-130
rhabditic dermatitis compared with, 267
Discoid lupus erythematosus, 22-24, 143-145
actinic keratosis and, 78
compared with
erythema multiforme, 43, 153
familial dermatomyositis, 35
hereditary lupoid dermatosis of German Shorthaired Pointer, 28
mucocutaneous pyoderma, 141, 143
mycosis fungoides, 159
pemphigus erythematosus, 18
psoriasiform-lichenoid dermatosis of Springer Spaniel, 157
systemic lupus erythematosus, 25, 146
ulcerative dermatosis of Shetland Sheepdog and Collie, 38
vitiligo, 152, 153
Vogt-Koyanagi-Harada–like syndrome, 149, 150
Disease
Bowen's, 79, 331, 340-341
Cushing's; *see* Hyperadrenocorticism
Voygt-Koyanagi-Harada–like, pemphigus erythematosus compared with, 18
Woringer-Kolopp, 477
Dissociative anesthesia, 3
Doberman Pinscher
acne in, 258
acral lick dermatitis in, 72
bullous pemphigoid in, 29
coccidioidomycosis in, 175
color-mutant alopecia in, 299
deep bacterial folliculitis and furunculosis in, 253
demodicosis in, 264
histiocytoma in, 465
hypothyroidism in, 74
ichthyosis in, 99
melanocytic neoplasms in, 452
pemphigus foliaceus in, 16
sarcoptic acariasis in, 124
seborrhea in, 89
sporotrichosis in, 182
vitiligo in, 152
zinc-responsive dermatosis in, 103
Dog; *see also* specific breed
callus and callus pyoderma in
acne compared with, 258
follicular destruction and, 255-256
collagenolytic granuloma in; *see* Eosinophilic granuloma
cutaneous histiocytoma in; *see* Histiocytoma
demodicosis in; *see* Demodicosis
dermatophytosis in, 243-245
dirofilariasis in, 128-130, 267
ductular apocrine adenoma in, 390-391
ear margin seborrhea in, 95-96, 97
eosinophilic granuloma in, 218-220

Dog; *see also* specific breed—cont'd
familial dermatomyositis in; *see* Familial dermatomyositis
female hyperestrogenism in, 280-281
flea allergy dermatitis in; *see* Flea allergy dermatitis
follicular destruction and acne in, 257-258
follicular dysplasia in; *see* Follicular dysplasia
hemangiopericytoma in; *see* Hemangiopericytoma
hereditary black-hair follicular dysplasia in, 299, 301-302
hyperadrenocorticism in, 275-278
telogen effluvium versus, 287
hypothyroidism in; *see* Hypothyroidism
mast cell tumors in, 465-468, 470-473
opportunistic mycobacterial infection in, 169
panniculitis in, 313
papillomavirus in, 334
ringworm in; *see* Dermatophytosis
sarcoptic acariasis in; *see* Sarcoptic acariasis
scabies in; *see* Sarcoptic acariasis
Sertoli cell tumor in, 75-76, 278-280
sporotrichosis in, 182
traction alopecia in; *see* Traction alopecia
Dog food dermatosis; *see* Generic dog food dermatosis
Drug eruption
erythema multiforme and, 41
pemphigus vulgaris versus, 33
septal panniculitis and, 323
superficial necrolytic dermatitis versus, 47
toxic epidermal necrolysis and, 44
Ductular adenoma, compound sebaceous, 377, 378
Ductular apocrine adenocarcinoma, 394-395
Ductular apocrine adenoma, 389
canine, 390-391
feline, 391-392
solid basal cell carcinoma compared with, 347
Dudley nose, 150, 152
Dyskeratosis
acrodermatitis of Bull Terrier and, 108
actinic keratosis and, 78
erythema multiforme and, 42
generic dog food dermatosis and, 106
Dyslipoproteinemia, 193
Dysplasia; *see also* Inflammatory, dysplastic, and degenerative diseases
adnexal, focal, 358-359
black-hair follicular; *see* Black-hair follicular dysplasia
epidermal
actinic keratosis and, 78
hyperplastic dermatosis of West Highland White Terrier and, 82
follicular; *see* Follicular dysplasia
hyperplastic, 68-87; *see also* Hyperplasia
Dysplastic and depositional diseases of dermal connective tissue, 223-236
calcinosis circumscripta in, 226-228
calcinosis cutis in, 223-226
cutaneous amyloidosis in, 229-232
cutaneous asthenia in, 232-234
cutaneous mucinosis or myxedema in, 228-229
skin fragility syndrome in, 234-236
Dysplastic hair follicle, 298-309
acquired pattern alopecia in, 306-307
black-hair, 301-302
color-mutant alopecia in, 298-301
congenital hypotrichosis in, 307-309
follicular dysplasia in, 302-306

Dystrophic calcification
  calcinosis circumscripta and, 226
  calcinosis cutis and, 223
Dystrophic cutaneous calcification, 227
Dystrophic epidermolysis bullosa, 38

E
Ear cropping, 226
Ear-margin seborrhea, 307
Eccrine carcinoma, 396, 397
  subungual squamous carcinoma compared with, 403
Ehler-Danlos syndrome, 232
Ehrlichiosis, 139
Elastosis, solar
  actinic keratosis and, 155
  hemangioma and, 422
Electromyography, 36
Elizabethan collar, 295
Elliptical wedge biopsy, 2
Endocrine alopecia, 274
Endocrine tumor, pancreatic, 46
Endocrinopathy
  acquired pattern alopecia and, 307
  congenital hypotrichosis and, 308
  primary seborrhea and, 89
English Bulldog
  acne in, 258
  demodicosis in, 264
  female hyperestrogenism and, 281
  follicular dysplasia in, 304, 306
  hepatoid gland neoplasms in, 382
  histiocytoma in, 465
  hypothyroidism in, 74
  mast cell tumor in, 470
  sterile granuloma and pyogranuloma in, 196
English Pointer with cutaneous vascular tumors, 421
English Setter with atopy, 115
English Springer Spaniel
  follicular dysplasia in, 304
  hypothyroidism in, 74
  primary seborrhea in, 89
  psoriasiform-lichenoid dermatosis in, 83-85, 156-157
  sebaceous adenitis in, 101
Eosinophilia, peripheral, 250
Eosinophilic exocytosis, 55, 56
Eosinophilic folliculitis
  allergic miliary dermatitis and, 123
  mosquito-bite hypersensitivity versus, 211
Eosinophilic furunculosis
  allergic miliary dermatitis and, 123
  follicular destruction and, 269-270
  granuloma versus, 219
  sterile eosinophilic pustulosis and, 251
Eosinophilic granuloma
  canine, prominent eosinophils or plasma cells in, 218-220
  feline
    indolent ulcer and, 63-64, 216
    mosquito-bite hypersensitivity versus, 211
    oral, 216
    prominent eosinophils or plasma cells and, 215-217
    specific pathogen–free cats in, 215
Eosinophilic plaque, 55, 56
  compared with
    allergic miliary dermatitis, 61, 123

Eosinophilic plaque—cont'd
  compared with—cont'd
    idiopathic ulcerative dermatosis, 67
    indolent ulcer, 64
    mosquito-bite hypersensitivity, 211
  food allergy and, 117
  idiopathic ulcerative dermatosis compared with, 67
  prominent eosinophils or plasma cells in, 213-215
Eosinophilic pustulation, spongiotic, 18
Eosinophilic pustulosis, sterile, 12, 239, 241
Eosinophilic ulcer; see Indolent ulcer
Eosinophils
  food allergy and, 119
  nodular and diffuse diseases with prominent; see Nodular and diffuse dermal diseases with prominent eosinophils or plasma cells
Epidermal atrophy, 277
Epidermal collarette; see Collarette, epidermal
Epidermal contiguity
  benign basal cell tumor and, 342
  carcinoma and
    clear-cell, 349
    keratinizing basal cell, 347-348, 361
    matrical, 371
    sebaceous, 380
    solid basal cell, 344, 345
    squamous cell, 385
  ductular apocrine adenoma and, 391
  fibrosarcoma and, 415
  isthmus-catagen tricholemmoma and, 365
  melanocytoma-acanthoma and, 458
  sebaceous epithelioma and, 378
  trichoepithelioma and, 360
Epidermal diseases, 10-111
  bullous and vesicular, 22-40; see also Bullous and vesicular diseases of epidermis
  exudative and ulcerative, 58-67; see also Exudative and ulcerative diseases of epidermis
  hyperkeratotic, 88-110; see also Hyperkeratotic diseases of epidermis
  hyperplastic, 68-87; see also Hyperplastic diseases of epidermis
  necrotizing, 41-50; see also Necrosis
  spongiotic, 51-57
  superficial pustular, 10-21; see also Superficial pustular diseases, epidermal
Epidermal dysplasia; see also Hyperplastic dermatosis of West Highland White Terrier
  actinic keratosis and, 78
  generic dog food dermatosis and, 106
  hyperplastic dermatosis of West Highland White Terrier and, 82
Epidermal hyperplasia compared with acral lick dermatitis, 73
Epidermal inclusion cyst; see Follicular cyst
Epidermal necrolysis
  generic dog food dermatosis and, 106
  toxic; see Toxic epidermal necrolysis
Epidermal nevus
  linear, human, 331
  pigmented; see Pigmented epidermal nevus
Epidermal pustules, superficial, 12
Epidermal tumors, 330-350
  actinic keratosis in, 330-331
  basal cell carcinoma in, 343-349
  benign feline basal cell tumor in, 341-343
  cutaneous horn of feline footpad in, 331-334
  pigmented epidermal nevus in, 331

Epidermal tumors—cont'd
  squamous cell carcinoma in, 336-340
    in situ, 340-341
  squamous papilloma in
    idiopathic, 336
    viral, 334-335
Epidermoid cyst; *see* Follicular cyst
Epidermolysis bullosa, 38, 39
  bullous pemphigoid compared with, 30
Epidermolytic epidermolysis bullosa, 38
Epidermolytic hyperkeratosis
  human, 98
  pigmented epidermal nevus and, 331
Epinephrine, 3
Epithelial inclusion cyst, nailbed, 398-399
Epithelial tumors
  epidermal tumors and, 330-350; *see also* Epidermal tumors
  follicular tumors and, 351-373; *see also* Follicular tumors
  nailbed, 398-405; *see also* Nailbed epithelial tumors
  neoplastic diseases and, 329-405
  renal, fibromatous nodules and, 408
  sebaceous tumors and, 374-385; *see also* Sebaceous tumors
  sweat gland tumors and, 386-397; *see also* Sweat gland tumors
Epithelioid melanoma, 461
  amelanotic, extramedullary plasma cell tumor versus, 476
  feline, 463
Epithelioid sarcoma, 469
Epithelioma
  basal cell, 341; *see also* Basal cell carcinoma
  calcifying; *see* Pilomatricoma
  intracutaneous cornifying; *see* Infundibular keratinizing acanthoma
  meibomian, 378
  perianal gland, 384
  sebaceous; *see* Sebaceous epithelioma
Epitheliotropic lymphoma, 476, 481-482
  d'emblee variant of, 481
  malignant; *see* Mycosis fungoides
  mucocutaneous candidiasis versus, 14
Erysipelothrix rhusiopathiae, 139
Erythema, necrolytic migratory, 46; *see also* Superficial necrolytic dermatitis
Erythema multiforme, 41-44
  compared with
    bullous pemphigoid, 29
    chemical and thermal burns, 49
    discoid lupus erythematosus, 24
    hereditary lupoid dermatosis of German Shorthaired Pointer, 28
    mucocutaneous candidiasis, 14
    pemphigus vulgaris, 31
    systemic lupus erythematosus, 26
    toxic epidermal necrolysis, 44, 46
    ulcerative dermatosis of Shetland Sheepdog and Collie, 36, 38
    urticaria and angioedema, 136
  of dermis, 153, 154
  older dogs with, 41, 42
  superficial necrolytic dermatitis compared with, 47
Erythema nodosum–like panniculitis, 323
  immune-mediated vasculitis versus, 138, 333
Erythematous exfoliative dermatitis, 158
Estrogen, 280
Estrous cycles, 281
Exclamation-mark hairs, 291
Exfoliative erythroderma, 158

Exocytosis, eosinophilic plaque and, 55, 56
Exophytic papilloma, 334-335
Exophytic warts, 334
Extramedullary plasmacytoma, 230, 474-475
  mast cell tumors versus, 473
Exudate in opportunistic mycobacterial infection, 170
Exudative and ulcerative diseases of epidermis, 58-67
  allergic miliary dermatitis in, 59-61, 62
  idiopathic ulcerative dermatosis in, 65-67
  indolent ulcer in, 63-64
  pyotraumatic dermatitis in, 58-59

F
FAD; *see* Flea allergy dermatitis
Familial dermatomyositis, 34-36, 289-291
  compared with
    alopecia areata, 292
    cicatricial, 293
    discoid lupus erythematosus, 24
    hereditary lupoid dermatosis of German Shorthaired Pointer, 28
    juvenile-onset localized demodicosis, 264
    post-rabies vaccination alopecia, 289
    ulcerative dermatosis of Shetland Sheepdog and Collie and, 36
Fat, infiltrative lipoma and, 433
Fat necrosis
  pansteatitis and, 324
  traumatic panniculitis and, 319
Fatty acids, unsaturated, 324
Fecal flotation
  cheyletiellosis and, 127
  sarcoptic acariasis and, 124
Feline leprosy; *see* Leprosy, feline
Feline leukemia virus, 331; *see also* Cat
  cutaneous horn of footpads and, 331
  epitheliotropic and nonepitheliotropic subtypes of lymphoma and, 477-478
Feline sarcoma virus, 413
  liposarcoma and, 433
Female hyperestrogenism in dog, 280-281
Female variant perianal gland adenoma, 382
Feminization in Sertoli cell tumors, 75
Fibrocytic tumors, 407-418
  collagenous nevus in, 407-408
  dermatofibroma in, 410-411
  fibroma in, 411-413
  fibrosarcoma in, 413-415
  myxoma in, 415, 416
  myxosarcoma in, 416-417
  nodular dermatofibrosis in, 408-409
  skin tag in, 409-410
Fibrohistiocytic tumors, benign, 445
Fibrolipoma, 431-432
Fibroma, 411-413
  compared with
    benign schwannoma, 441
    collagenous nevus, 407-408
    dermatofibroma, 411
    nodular dermatofibrosis, 409
    skin tags, 410
  schwannoma and, 439
Fibropapilloma, 336
Fibropruritic nodules, 70-71
  flea allergy dermatitis and, canine, 120, 122

Fibrosarcoma, 413-415
    compared with
        amelanotic malignant melanoma, 464
        benign schwannoma, 441
        cutaneous smooth muscle malignancies, 445
        dermatofibroma, 411
        hemangiosarcoma, 426
        malignant fibrous histiocytoma, 447, 448-449
        spindle-celled squamous cell carcinoma, 340
    malignant schwannoma and, 439, 441, 443
    post-rabies vaccination and, 318
Fibrosing steatitis compared with traumatic panniculitis, 320
Fibrosis
    dermal
        acral lick dermatitis and, 72, 73
        actinic keratosis and, 155, 156
        calcinosis cutis and, 226
        fibropruritic nodules and, 70, 71
    perifollicular, 241
    ulcerative dermatosis with linear subepidermal; see Idiopathic ulcerative dermatosis
Fibrous histiocytoma; see also Histiocytoma
    benign, 445-446
        dermatofibroma and, 410
        histopathologic variants of, 194
    malignant, 446-449
        fibrosarcoma compared with, 415
        pleomorphic liposarcoma compared with, 435
Fish-scale disease; see Ichthyosis
Fite-Faraco modification of acid-fast stain, 165, 170
Flame figures
    canine
        eosinophilic granuloma versus, 219
        mast cell tumors and, 471
    feline, mosquito-bite hypersensitivity versus, 211
Flame follicles
    in atrophic diseases, 273
    female hyperestrogenism and, 281
    follicular dysplasia and, 305
    growth hormone/castration-responsive dermatosis and, 283
    hyperadrenocorticism and, 278
    hypothyroidism and, 274
    post-clipping alopecia and, 285
    Sertoli cell tumor and, 278
Flank alopecia, cyclic, 304
    atopy versus, 115, 116
Flea allergy dermatitis, 63
    canine, 119-122
        food allergy versus, 119
        hookworm dermatitis versus, 131
        hyperplastic dermatosis of West Highland White Terrier versus, 81
        sarcoptic acariasis versus, 124, 125
    chronic hyperplastic dermatitis and, 68, 69
    excessive grooming and, 295
    experimentally induced, 121
    feline
        allergic miliary dermatitis and, 59-60
        eosinophilic plaque and, 55
        fibropruritic nodules and, 70, 71
        food allergy versus, 117, 119
        impetigo versus, 10
        pyotraumatic dermatitis and, 59
        superficial spreading pyoderma versus, 12
Flea and tick dip in chemical burn, 48

Flea-bite hypersensitivity; see Flea allergy dermatitis
Follicle nevus, 357-358
Follicles
    acne in destruction of, 258-259
    dysplasia of; see Follicular dysplasia
    flame; see Flame follicles
    hair; see Hair follicle
    inferior segment of, 351
        matrical cyst and, 354
    pustular and nodular diseases of
        destruction in; see Pustular and nodular diseases with follicular destruction
        no destruction in; see Pustular and nodular diseases without follicular destruction
Follicular atrophy
    familial dermatomyositis and, 36
    hypothyroidism and, 75
    panniculitis and, 314
    Sertoli cell-tumor and, 76
Follicular casts
    ear margin seborrhea and, 96
    sebaceous adenitis and, 101
    vitamin A–responsive dermatosis and, 94
Follicular cyst, 351-355
    callus and callus pyoderma and, 256
    inner root sheath differentiation in hybrid, 348
Follicular dysplasia, 302-306; see also Dysplastic hair follicle
    black-hair; see Black-hair follicular dysplasia
    compared with
        alopecia areata, 115, 116
        color-mutant alopecia, 299
        growth hormone/castration-responsive dermatosis, 283, 284
        hyperadrenocorticism, 277
        hypothyroidism, 74
        post-rabies vaccination alopecia, 288
    congenital hypotrichosis and, 308
Follicular epaulets, 91
Follicular fronds
    ear margin seborrhea and, 96
    sebaceous adenitis and, 101
    vitamin A–responsive dermatosis and, 94
Follicular hamartoma, 357-358
Follicular keratosis
    ear margin seborrhea and, 97
    ichthyosis and, 100
    seborrhea versus, 91
    vitamin A–responsive dermatosis and, 94
Follicular melanocytes compared with alopecia areata, 291
Follicular papilla compared with ribbon-type trichoblastoma, 367
Follicular root sheath mineralization, 278
Follicular telogen arrest, 241
Follicular tumors, 351-373
    adnexal dysplasia in, 358-359
    congenital etiology of, 351
    cyst in, 351-355
    dilated pore in, 356-357
    hamartoma in, 357-358
    infundibular keratinizing acanthoma in, 361-363
    matrical carcinoma in, 371-372
    pilomatricoma in, 365-367
    trichoblastoma in, 367-371
    trichoepithelioma in, 360-361
    trichofolliculoma in, 359-360
    tricholemmoma in, 364-365

Folliculitis
  allergic miliary dermatitis and, 60
  bacterial
    deep; *see* Deep bacterial folliculitis and furunculosis
    erythema multiforme versus, 42
    Schnauzer comedo syndrome and, 97
    superficial; *see* Superficial bacterial folliculitis
  dermatophytosis and
    canine, 245
    feline, 242
  eosinophilic; *see* Eosinophilic folliculitis
  generic dog food dermatosis and, 106
  superficial perforating, 239, 240
Fontana-Masson stain
  balloon-cell melanocytoma and, 455
  malignant melanoma and, 464
  melanin pigment and, 380
  plasmacytoma and, 476
Food allergy, 117-119
  compared with
    allergic contact dermatitis, 52
    allergic miliary dermatitis, 59, 123
    atopy, 115
    chronic hyperplastic dermatitis, 68
    eosinophilic granuloma, 217
    eosinophilic plaque, 55
    flea allergy dermatitis, 120, 122
    hookworm dermatitis, 131
    mosquito-bite hypersensitivity, 210, 211
    notoedric acariasis, 125, 126
  excessive grooming and, 295
  hyperplastic dermatosis of West Highland White Terrier and, 81
  indolent ulcer and, 63, 64
Footpads
  in acrodermatitis of Bull Terrier, 106
  in calcinosis circumscripta, 227
  cutaneous horn of feline, 331-334
  eccrine carcinoma of, 396
  eosinophilic granuloma of, 216
  hookworm dermatitis of, 131
  ichthyosis of, 99
  irritant contact dermatitis of, 53
  pemphigus foliaceus of, 16
  pemphigus vulgaris of, 31
  sterile pedal panniculitis of German Shepherd Dog and, 324
  superficial necrolytic dermatitis of, 46, 47
  systemic lupus erythematosus of, 25
  toxic epidermal necrolysis of, 44
  vitiligo of, 150
  zinc-responsive dermatosis of, 103
Foreign body granuloma; *see* Foreign body reactions
Foreign body reactions
  actinomycosis and, 163
    nocardiosis compared with, 166
  compared with
    arthropod-bite granuloma, 208
    cutaneous infections of systemic fungi and algae, 180
    eosinophilic granuloma, 216, 218
    opportunistic mycobacterial infection, 170
    spider bites, 213
    sporotrichosis, 182, 184
    sterile pedal panniculitis, 325
    traumatic panniculitis, 319
  of dermis, 190-192
Formalin, neutral phosphate-buffered, 3-4

Fox Terrier with mast cell tumor, 470
Foxtail, reaction to, 120
French Bulldog
  female hyperestrogenism in, 281
  follicular dysplasia in, 304
Frictional alopecia, 282-283
Frozen sections, 170
Fungal infection
  compared with
    acral lick dermatitis, 72
    pythiosis, 185
    sterile granuloma and pyogranuloma, 198
  cultures in
    actinomycosis and nocardiosis and, 165
    cutaneous cryptococcosis and, 177
    cutaneous infections of systemic fungi and algae and, 175, 180
    sporotrichosis and, 182
  opportunistic; *see* Cutaneous infections, opportunistic fungi and algae in
  systemic; *see* Cutaneous infections, systemic fungi and algae in
Furunculosis
  deep bacterial; *see* Deep bacterial folliculitis and furunculosis
  eosinophilic; *see* Eosinophilic furunculosis
  self-trauma and, 72

G

Gammopathy, monoclonal, 230
Garland basal cell tumor, 367
Gastrointestinal mucosa in toxic epidermal necrolysis, 44
General anesthesia
  in punch biopsy, 63
  in skin biopsy, 3, 269
  in wedge biopsy, 63, 325
Generic dog food dermatosis, 104-106
  compared with
    acrodermatitis of Bull Terrier, 108
    erythema multiforme, 42
    superficial necrolytic dermatitis, 47, 48
    zinc-responsive dermatosis, 103, 104
German Shepherd Dog
  deep bacterial folliculitis and furunculosis in, 253
  demodicosis in, 264
  dermatitis in
    acral lick, 72
    allergic contact, 51
    pyotraumatic, 59
  discoid lupus erythematosus in, 22
  familial dermatomyositis in, 35
  fibropruritic nodules in, 70
  hepatoid gland neoplasms in, 382
  mucocutaneous pyoderma in, 141
  nodular dermatofibrosis in, 408
  opportunistic fungal and algae infections in, 180
  pemphigus erythematosus in, 18
  pythiosis in, 184
  seborrhea in, 89
  sterile pedal panniculitis of, 324-325
  systemic lupus erythematosus in, 25
  vitiligo in, 152
German Shorthaired Pointer
  acne in, 258
  follicular dysplasia in, 304, 306
  hereditary lupoid dermatosis in, 26-28
    discoid lupus erythematosus versus, 24
    familial dermatomyositis versus, 26-28

German Shorthaired Pointer—cont'd
  hereditary lupoid dermatosis in—cont'd
    ulcerative dermatosis of Shetland Sheepdog and Collie versus, 38
German Wirehaired Pointer
  follicular dysplasia in, 304, 306
  oral eosinophilic granuloma and, 218
Giant cell malignant fibrous histiocytoma, 446, 447
Giant cell pansteatitis, 324
Giant cell tumor of soft parts, 446, 447
Giant epithelioid melanoma, 463
Giemsa stain
  leishmaniasis and, 188
  mast cell tumors and, 469, 470, 471
  plasmacytoma and, 476
Glandular adenoma
  apocrine, 389-390
  compound sebaceous, 377, 378
Glandular neoplasms compared with acantholytic squamous cell carcinoma, 339
Glomerulonephritis, 123, 220
Glucocorticoids
  actinic comedones and, 271
  demodicosis and, 263
  in oral eosinophilic granuloma, 219
  in sterile granulomatous or pyogranulomatous syndrome, 196
Golden Retriever
  atopy in, 115
  benign fibrous histiocytomas in, 445
  deep bacterial folliculitis and furunculosis in, 253
  food allergy and, 117
  hypothyroidism in, 74
  kerion in, 261
  pyotraumatic dermatitis in, 59
  seborrhea in, 89
  sterile granuloma and pyogranuloma in, 196
  vitiligo in, 152
Gomori's stain
  plasmacytoma and, 476
  pythiosis and, 185
Gonadal hormones, 384
Grading system of mast cell tumor, 470
Graft-versus-host disease, 42
Grains, actinomycosis and, 164, 165
Gram-positive cocci
  impetigo and, 11
  pyotraumatic dermatitis and, 59
  superficial spreading pyoderma and, 12-13
Granular cell basal cell carcinoma compared with trabecular trichoblastoma, 371
Granular cell trichoblastoma, 370-371
  bulb-type tricholemmoma compared with, 364-365
Granules in Splendore-Hoeppli reaction, 173
Granuloma
  collagenic; *see* Eosinophilic granuloma
  collagenolytic; *see* Eosinophilic granuloma
  eosinophilic; *see* Eosinophilic granuloma
  foreign body; *see* Foreign body reactions
  fungal, acral lick dermatitis compared with, 72
  histiocytic mast cell tumors versus, 470
  insect-bite
    arthropod, 207-209, 218
    histiocytic mast cell tumors compared with, 470
  lick; *see* Acral lick dermatitis
  linear; *see* Eosinophilic granuloma

Granuloma—cont'd
  opportunistic mycobacterial; *see* Opportunistic mycobacterial infection
  palisading, 219
  pressure-point; *see* Callus and callus pyoderma
  sterile; *see* Sterile granuloma and pyogranuloma
Granuloma annulare, human, 218
  canine eosinophilic granuloma compared with, 219
Granulomatosis, lymphomatoid; *see* Lymphomatoid granulomatosis
Granulomatous dermal diseases
  infectious nodular and diffuse; *see* Infectious nodular and diffuse granulomatous and pyogranulomatous dermal diseases
Granulomatous dermatitis; *see* Sterile granuloma and pyogranuloma
  juvenile; *see* Juvenile sterile granulomatous dermatitis and lymphadenitis
Granulomatous diseases of dermis
  noninfectious nodular and diffuse; *see* Noninfectious nodular and diffuse granulomatous and pyogranulomatous dermal diseases
Granulomatous inflammation
  benign fibrous histiocytoma versus, 44
  histiocytic lymphoma versus, 481
Granulomatous sebaceous adenitis, 264, 265
Grass awns
  actinomycosis and, 163, 164
  reaction to, 120
Great Dane
  acne in, 258
  acral lick dermatitis in, 72
  color-mutant alopecia in, 299
  deep bacterial folliculitis and furunculosis in, 253
  demodicosis in, 264
  histiocytoma in, 465
  hypothyroidism in, 74
  sterile granuloma and pyogranuloma in, 196
  zinc-responsive dermatosis in, 103
Greyhound
  Italian; *see* Italian Greyhound, alopecia in
  solar-associated hemangiosarcoma in, 423
Growth hormone, response to, 282
Growth hormone/castration-responsive alopecia compared with follicular dysplasia, 305, 306
Growth hormone/castration-responsive dermatosis, 281-284
  compared with
    follicular dysplasia, 304
    post-clipping alopecia, 285
Gynecomastia
  female hyperestrogenism and, 281
  Sertoli cell tumor in, 75

H

Hair
  acquired pattern alopecia and, 307
  foreign bodies and, eosinophilic granuloma and feline, 216
  post-clipping alopecia and, 285
  self-induced psychogenic loss of; *see* Psychogenic alopecia, feline
Hair bulb, 351
  pilomatricoma and, 365, 366
Hair follicle, 237-309; *see also* Follicles
  anagen phase of
    inferior segment of, 354
    telogen effluvium and, 287
  atrophy in, 273-297; *see also* Atrophic diseases of hair follicles
  calcinosis cutis and, 226
  dysplastic diseases of; *see* Dysplastic hair follicle

Hair follicle—cont'd
    matrical cyst and, 354
    mineralization of external root sheaths of, 226
    pustular and nodular diseases of
        follicular destruction in, 252-272
        no follicular destruction in, 238-251
Hair follicle nevus, 357-358
Hair growth cycle arrest, 274
    female hyperestrogenism and, 281
    growth hormone/castration-responsive dermatosis and, 283
    hyperadrenocorticism and, 278
    post-clipping alopecia and, 285
    Sertoli cell tumor and, 278
Haircoat, salivary staining of, 115
Hamartoma
    defined, 357, 407
    follicular, 357-358
    human
        focal adnexal dysplasia and, 358
        trichofolliculoma and, 359
    lymphangioma etiology and, 426
    scrotal vascular, 419, 420
Hand lens for cicatricial alopecia, 292
Head mange; *see* Notoedric acariasis
Heartworm dermatitis, 128-130
Helper T cells in mycosis fungoides, 158
Hemangioendothelioma; *see* Hemangiosarcoma
Hemangioma
    actinic keratosis and, 78
    capillary, 422
    cavernous, 421-422
    compared with
        hemangiosarcoma, 426
        lymphangioma, 427
    solar-induced, 422
    vascular, 419-422
Hemangiopericytoma, 436-438
    compared with
        benign schwannoma, 441
        dermatofibrosarcoma type malignant fibrous histiocytoma,
           448-449
        malignant schwannoma, 439, 441, 443
    neural origin of, 436, 438
Hemangiosarcoma
    compared with
        hemangioma, 422
        lymphangiosarcoma, 428
        scrotal vascular hamartoma, 419
    poorly differentiated, 425
    vascular, 422-426
    well-differentiated, 424
Hemorrhagic bulla
    deep bacterial folliculitis and furunculosis and, 255
    demodicosis and, 264
    immune-mediated vasculitis and, 138
    septic vasculitis and, 139
Hepatic lipidosis, 234
Hepatocutaneous syndrome; *see* Superficial necrolytic dermatitis
Hepatoid glands
    adenoma of, 381-383
    anatomic distribution of, 381
    carcinoma of; *see* Perianal gland carcinoma
    hyperplasia of, 381-383
Hepatopathy, vacuolar, 46
Hereditary black-hair follicular dysplasia, 299, 301-302

Hereditary hyperchylomicronemia, 193
Hereditary hyperlipoproteinemia, 193
Hereditary lupoid dermatosis of German Shorthaired Pointer,
    26-28
    compared with
        discoid lupus erythematosus, 24
        familial dermatomyositis, 36
        systemic lupus erythematosus, 26
        ulcerative dermatosis of Shetland Sheepdog and Collie, 38
Hidradenitis suppurativa, 36
Histiocytic and mast cell tumors, 465-473
    anaplastic, histiocytic lymphoma versus, 481
    canine, 470-473
        cutaneous histiocytoma in, 465-468
    extramedullary plasma cell tumor versus, 476
    feline, 468-470
    histiocytic, 468
    poorly differentiated, 468, 469-470
    well-differentiated, 468-469
Histiocytic lymphoma, 480-481
    mast cell tumors versus, 469, 473
Histiocytoid hemangiosarcoma, 425-426
Histiocytoma, 199, 465-468
    atypical, 474
    compared with
        benign fibrous histiocytoma, 44
        extramedullary plasma cell tumor, 476
        histiocytosis, 199
        mycosis fungoides, 481-482
        small-cell lymphoid neoplasia, 481
    fibrous; *see* Fibrous histiocytoma
    spontaneous regression of, 465
    small-cell lymphoid neoplasia versus, 481
Histiocytosis, 198-201
    of Bernese Mountain Dog, 202
    compared with
        cryptococcosis, 177
        histiocytoma, 468
        sebaceous glands, 249
        sterile granuloma and pyogranuloma syndrome, 195-196, 198
        systemic mycoses, 175
    systemic
        Bernese Mountain Dog with, 201-203
        cutaneous versus, 202
        fungi and algae infections compared with, 180
Histiocytosis X, human, 201
Histoplasma capsulatum, 174; *see also* Cutaneous infections, systemic
    fungi and algae in
Hives, 135; *see* Urticaria
Hookworm dermatitis, 130-131
    compared with
        flea allergy dermatitis, 122
        rhabditic dermatitis, 267
Hordeum, 120
Hormones, gonadal, 384
Horn, cutaneous; *see* Cutaneous horn
Hot spots; *see* Pyotraumatic dermatitis
Hound
    Afghan; *see* Afghan Hound
    Bassett; *see* Bassett Hound
Hybrid cyst, 351, 354-355
    follicular
        inner root sheath differentiation in, 348
        matrical carcinoma versus, 372
21-Hydroxylase deficiency, 282

Hyperadrenocorticism, 98, 275-278
    telogen effluvium compared with, 287
Hyperchylomicronemia, 193
Hyperestrogenism, 280-281
    Sertoli cell tumors and, 75
Hyperglucocorticoidism, 10; *see also* Hyperadrenocorticism
    actinic comedones versus, 271, 272
    calcinosis cutis and, 223
    iatrogenic, 98, 275
    skin fragility syndrome and, 234
Hyperhidrosis
    apocrine gland and, 116
    atopy and, 115
Hyperkeratosis
    demodicosis and, 264
    dermatophytosis and, 243
    epidermolytic
        human, 98
        pigmented epidermal nevus and, 331
    hypothyroidism and, 274
Hyperkeratotic diseases of epidermis, 88-110
    acrodermatitis of Bull Terrier in, 106-108
    ear margin seborrhea in, 95-96, 97
    generic dog food dermatosis in, 104-106
    ichthyosis in, 98-99, 100
    Schnauzer comedo syndrome in, 96-98
    sebaceous adenitis in, 100-102
    seborrhea in, 88-90
    seborrheic dermatitis in, 90-92
        Malassezia pachydermatis and, 92-94
    vitamin A–responsive dermatosis in, 94
    zinc-responsive dermatosis in, 102-104
Hyperlipoproteinemia, hereditary, 193
Hypermelanosis, Sertoli cell-tumor and, 77
Hyperplasia
    apocrine gland
        flea allergy dermatitis and, 122
        food allergy and, 118
    hepatoid gland, 381-383
    mucocutaneous pyoderma and, 142
    perianal gland, 381-383
    pseudoepitheliomatous, acral lick dermatitis versus, 72
    psoriasiform, lichenoid keratosis and, 85
    sebaceous gland
        atopy and, 115
        flea allergy dermatitis and, 122
        food allergy and, 118
        nodular, 374-376, 377
        senile, 374-376, 377
Hyperplastic dermatitis, chronic, 14, 68-70
    allergic contact dermatitis and, 54-55
    atopy and, 115
    compared with
        acanthosis nigricans of Dachshund, 81
        flea allergy dermatitis, 122
        superficial spreading pyoderma, 112
    food allergy and, 118
    hypothyroidism and, 75
    Sertoli cell-tumor and, 76
Hyperplastic dermatosis of West Highland White Terrier, 81-83
    ichthyosis versus, 99
Hyperplastic diseases of epidermis, 68-87
    acanthosis nigricans of Dachshund in, 79-81
    acral lick dermatitis in, 71-74
    actinic keratosis in, 76-79

Hyperplastic diseases of epidermis — cont'd
    dermatitis in, 68-70
    dermatosis of West Highland White Terrier in, 81-83
    fibropruritic nodules in, 70-71
    hypothyroidism in, 74-75
    lichenoid keratosis in, 85-86
    psoriasiform-lichenoid dermatosis of Springer Spaniel in, 83-85
    Sertoli cell tumor in, 75-76
Hypersensitivity; *see also* Allergic contact dermatitis
    arthropod-bite granuloma and, 207
    basophil, 119
    delayed, 51
        flea allergy dermatitis and, 119
    drug; *see* Drug eruption
    experimentally induced flea-bite, 121
    flea allergy dermatitis and, 119, 121
    food allergy and, 117
    immune-mediated vasculitis and, 138
    mosquito-bite; *see* Mosquito-bite hypersensitivity
    tick-bite, 207, 269
    Vogt-Koyanagi-Harada syndrome and, 148
Hypertrophic osteodystrophy, 227
Hypoaminoacidemia, 46
Hyposomatotropism; *see* Growth hormone/castration-responsive dermatosis
Hypothyroidism, 74-75
    compared with
        color-mutant alopecia, 299
        female hyperestrogenism, 281
        post-clipping alopecia, 285
        Sertoli cell tumor, 76, 280
        telogen effluvium, 287
    myxedema and, 228
    seborrhea and, 89
Hypotrichosis, congenital, 307-309

I
Iatrogenic hyperglucocorticoidism, 98, 275
Ichthyosis
    epidermal, 98-99, 100
    hereditary lupoid dermatosis of German Shorthaired Pointer versus, 26
    human, 98
Ichthyosis vulgaris, 98
Idiopathic calcinosis cutis, 224
Idiopathic leukoderma; *see* Vitiligo
Idiopathic lobular panniculitis, 321
Idiopathic lymphocytic dermatitis, 481
Idiopathic nodular xanthoma, 193-194
Idiopathic periadnexal multinodular granulomatous dermatitis; *see* Sterile granuloma and pyogranuloma
Idiopathic squamous papilloma of epidermis, 336
Idiopathic sterile nodular panniculitis
    erythema nodosum–like panniculitis versus, 323
    systemic lupus erythematosus versus, 25
Idiopathic ulcerative dermatosis
    feline, 65-67
    pyotraumatic dermatitis compared with, 59
IgE; *see* Immunoglobulin E
IgG; *see* Immunoglobulin G
IgM; *see* Immunoglobulin M
Immune-mediated glomerulonephritis, 123, 220
Immune-mediated vasculitis, 138, 139
    compared with
        septic vasculitis, 140

Immune-mediated vasculitis—cont'd
  compared with—cont'd
    spider bites, 213
Immunoblastic lymphoma, 478-480
Immunofluorescence
  in bullous pemphigoid, 30
  in discoid lupus erythematosus, 24
  in epidermolysis bullosa, 38
  in pemphigus erythematosus, 18, 19, 147
  in pemphigus foliaceus, 17, 18
  in pemphigus vulgaris, 32
  post-rabies vaccination alopecia and, 316
  rabies-specific, 288, 289
  specimen selection for, 2, 3
  in subcorneal pustular dermatosis, 20
  in systemic lupus erythematosus, 25
  in ulcerative dermatosis of Shetland Sheepdog and Collie,
      37, 38
Immunoglobulin
  cytoplasmic, plasmacytoma and, 474, 476
  septal panniculitis and, 315
Immunoglobulin E
  atopy and, 114
  flea allergy dermatitis and, 119
  sarcoptic acariasis and, 123
Immunoglobulin G
  atopy and, 114
  in bullous pemphigoid, 30
  in discoid lupus erythematosus, 24
  in pemphigus erythematosus, 20
  in pemphigus foliaceus, 18
  in pemphigus vulgaris, 32
Immunoglobulin M
  in bullous pemphigoid, 30
  in discoid lupus erythematosus, 24
  in pemphigus erythematosus, 20
  in pemphigus foliaceus, 18
  in sarcoptic acariasis, 123
Immunohistochemistry
  in bullous pemphigoid, 30
  in discoid lupus erythematosus, 24
  in epidermolysis bullosa, 38
  in pemphigus erythematosus, 18, 19, 147
  in pemphigus foliaceus, 17, 18
  in pemphigus vulgaris, 32
  specimen selection for, 2
  in subcorneal pustular dermatosis, 20
  in systemic lupus erythematosus, 25
  in ulcerative dermatosis of Shetland Sheepdog and Collie,
      37, 38
Immunostains
  in fibrosarcoma, 415
  in hemangiosarcoma, 426
  in leiomyoma, 445
  in malignant fibrous histiocytoma, 448
  in malignant schwannoma, 443
  in spindle-celled squamous cell carcinoma, 340
Immunosuppression
  cutaneous cryptococcosis and, 177
  demodicosis and, 262-263
  dermatophytosis and, 241, 244
Impetiginization
  superficial spreading pyoderma versus, 13
  term, 70
Impetigo, 10-12
  bullous, 10, 11, 12

Impetigo—cont'd
  compared with
    pemphigus erythematosus, 20
    superficial bacterial folliculitis, 239
    superficial spreading pyoderma, 13
  hyperadrenocorticism and, 276
Inclusion cyst, nailbed epithelial, 398-399
Indolent ulcer
  feline, 63-64, 216
  food allergy and, 117
Infection
  cutaneous; see Cutaneous infections
  erythema nodosum—like panniculitis and, 323
  opportunistic mycobacterial; see Opportunistic mycobacterial in-
      fection
Infectious nodular and diffuse granulomatous and pyogranuloma-
      tous dermal diseases, 163-189; see also Granuloma; Pyogran-
      uloma
  actinomycosis in, 163-166
  algae in, 179-181
  cryptococcosis in, 177-178
  dermatophytic mycetoma in feline, 172-174
  leishmaniasis in, 186-188
  leprosy in, 166-169
  mycobacteria in, 169-171
  nocardiosis in, 163-166
  opportunistic, 169-171, 179-181
    biopsy site for, 180
    clinical features of, 179-180
    fungi and algae in, 179-181, 194
    histopathology of, 180-181
    mycobacterial infection in, 169-171, 179-181
  pythiosis in, 184-186
  sporotrichosis in, 181-184
Infiltrative lipoma, 432-433
Inflammation
  canine traction alopecia and, 295
  granulomatous; see Granulomatous inflammation
  lichenoid; see Lichenoid inflammation
  lymphocytic, feline psychogenic alopecia and, 296
Inflammatory, dysplastic, and degenerative diseases, 7-110
  of dermis, 111-236; see also Dermal diseases
  of epidermis, 10-111; see also Epidermal diseases
  inflammatory diseases in, 7-67
    bullous and vesicular, 22-40; see also Bullous and vesicular dis-
        eases of epidermis
    exudative and ulcerative, 58-67; see also Exudative and ulcer-
        ative diseases of epidermis
    necrotizing, 41-50; see also Necrosis
    scarring, nodular dermatofibrosis compared with, 408-409
    spongiotic, 51-57
    superficial pustular, 10-21; see also Superficial pustular diseases,
        epidermal
Infundibular cyst, 351, 352-353
Infundibular keratinization
  in basal cell carcinoma, 348
  melanocytoma-acanthoma and, 458
Infundibular keratinizing acanthoma
  compared with
    inverted papilloma, 335
    isthmus-catagen tricholemmoma, 365
    proliferating isthmus-catagen cyst, 354
  cutaneous horn in, 331
  of follicle, 361-363
  nailbed keratoacanthoma and, 400
  stromal features in, 363

Infundibulum
    dilated pore and, 357
    follicular cysts and, 353
    hair follicle and, 351
    keratinizing acanthoma and, 363
    matrical carcinoma and, 371
    trichoepithelioma and, 360
    trichofolliculoma and, 359
Inhalant dermatitis, allergic; see Atopy
Inherited disease
    black-hair follicular dysplasia in, 299, 301-302
    hereditary lupoid dermatosis of German Shorthaired Pointer in;
        see Hereditary lupoid dermatosis of German Shorthaired
        Pointer
    hyperchylomicronemia in, 193
Injection site reactions in feline fibrosarcomas, 413
Inner root sheath, 351
    hybrid cysts and, 355
    matrical carcinoma and, 371
        keratinization in, 348
    pilomatricoma and, 366
Insect-bite reactions
    arthropod, 207-209, 218
    compared with
        histiocytic mast cell tumors, 470
        small-cell lymphoid neoplasia, 481
    mosquito; see Mosquito-bite hypersensitivity,
    urticaria and angioedema and, 136
Interdigital pyoderma, 191
Interface dermatitis, 141; see also Lichenoid diseases of dermis
Intertrigo, 143
Intracutaneous cornifying epithelioma; see Infundibular keratinizing
    acanthoma
Intragranular pustule, 17
Intranuclear inclusions, 335
Irish Setter
    atopy in, 115
    color-mutant alopecia in, 299
    deep bacterial folliculitis and furunculosis in, 253
    dermatitis in
        acral lick, 72
        flea allergy, 120
    hypothyroidism in, 74
    ichthyosis in, 99
    seborrhea in, 89
Irish Water Spaniel with follicular dysplasia, 304, 306
Irish Wolfhound with hypothyroidism, 74
Irradiation in hemangiosarcoma etiology, 423
Irritant contact dermatitis, 52-55
    compared with
        allergic contact dermatitis, 51-52
        hookworm dermatitis, 130
    irritants in, 52
Ischemia
    in lymphomatoid granulomatosis, 483
    post-rabies vaccination alopecia and, 289
    traumatic panniculitis and, 319
Isthmus of hair follicle, 351
    trichoepithelioma and, 360
    tricholemmoma and, 364, 365
Isthmus-catagen cyst, 351, 353
    proliferating, 353-354
Isthmus-catagen tricholemmoma, 365
    compared with
        melanocytoma-acanthoma, 459
        trabecular trichoblastoma, 370

Isthmus-type keratinization in basal cell carcinoma, 348
Italian Greyhound, alopecia in
    acquired pattern, 307
    color-mutant, 299

J
Jack Russell Terrier with ichthyosis, 99
Jadassohn, nevus sebaceus of, 376
Junctional activity
    in melanocytoma-acanthoma, 458
    in melanomas, 463
Junctional epidermolysis bullosa, 38, 39
Junctional melanocytoma, 451, 452
Juvenile cellulitis; see Juvenile sterile granulomatous dermatitis and
    lymphadenitis
Juvenile pyoderma; see Juvenile sterile granulomatous dermatitis
    and lymphadenitis
Juvenile sterile granulomatous dermatitis and lymphadenitis,
    203-205
    compared with
        acne, 258
        sterile nodular panniculitis, 323

K
Keeshond with growth hormone/castration-responsive dermatosis,
    283
Keratinization
    acne and, 259
    in basal cell carcinoma; see Keratinizing basal cell carcinoma
    ductular apocrine adenoma and, 390
    fibrosarcoma and, 415
    in hyperkeratotic diseases of epidermis, 88; see also Hyperkera-
        totic diseases of epidermis
    in infundibular acanthoma; see Infundibular keratinizing acanth-
        oma
    Malassezia pachydermatis in, 92
    matrical; see Matrical keratinization
    melanocytoma-acanthoma and, 458
    in Schnauzer Comedo syndrome, 96
    tricholemmal; see Tricholemmal keratinization
    vitamin A–responsive dermatosis and, 94, 95
Keratinizing basal cell carcinoma, 343, 347-348
    compared with
        matrical carcinoma, 372
        pilomatricoma, 367
        trichoepithelioma, 361
    stromal features in, 348
Keratinocyte necrosis, erythema multiforme and, 42, 43, 153
Keratoacanthoma
    nailbed, 400-402
        squamous cell carcinoma compared with, 403
    subungual, 400-402
Keratosis
    actinic; see Actinic keratosis
    follicular; see Follicular keratosis
    lichenoid; see Lichenoid keratosis
Kerion
    compared with
        acral lick dermatitis, 72
        arthropod-bite granuloma, 207
        deep bacterial folliculitis and furunculosis, 255
        follicular destruction and, 261-262
Kerry Blue Terrier with pilomatricoma, 366
Ketoconazole, 92
Koilocytosis
    nailbed inverted squamous papilloma and, 399

Koilocytosis—cont'd
papillomavirus and, 334
Kunkers of pythiosis, 185
Kuvaszok, familial dermatomyositis and, 35

L

Labrador Retriever
congenital hypotrichosis in, 308
dermatitis in
acral lick, 72
allergic contact, 51
pyotraumatic, 59
ichthyosis in, 99
lipoma in, 431
mast cell tumor in, 470
sarcoptic acariasis in, 124
vitiligo in, 152
Lamellar ichthyosis, human, 98
Laminar distribution of collagen, 293
Langerhans cells
alopecia areata and, 291
histiocytomas and, 465
Latrodectus mactans, 212
Leiomyoma, 443-444
Leiomyosarcoma, 444-445
fibrosarcoma versus, 415
Leishmania, 188
Leishmania chagasi, 186
Leishmania donovani, 186
Leishmaniasis
dermal, 186-188
epidermal and follicular keratin and, 90
geographic restriction of, 186
sebaceous adenitis and, 101
Lentiginosis profusa, 456
Lentigo, 456-458
pigmented epidermal nevus and, 331
Lentigo simplex, 456
Leprosy, feline, 166-169
compared with
cutaneous cryptococcosis, 177
cutaneous xanthoma, 194
sporotrichosis, 182
systemic fungi and algae infections, 180, 181
systemic mycoses, 175
Lesion, primary or secondary, 2
Lethal acrodermatitis
of Bull Terrier, 106-108
zinc-responsive dermatosis versus, 104
Leukemia cutis compared with immune-mediated vasculitis, 138
Leukemia virus, feline; *see* Feline leukemia virus
Leukocytoclastic vasculitis
immune-mediated vasculitis and, 138
urticaria and, 136-137
Leukoderma, 148
Leukotrichia, 148
Lhasa Apso
atopy in, 115
flea allergy dermatitis in, 120
sebaceous adenitis in, 101
Lichenoid dermatitis, 141
Lichenoid diseases of dermis, 141-162
actinic keratosis in, 155-156
discoid lupus erythematosus in, 143-145
erythema multiforme in, 153, 154

Lichenoid diseases of dermis—cont'd
keratosis in, 157, 158
mucocutaneous pyoderma in, 141-143
mycosis fungoides in, 158-161
pemphigus erythematosus in, 147
psoriasiform-lichenoid dermatosis of Springer Spaniel in, 83-85, 156-157
systemic lupus erythematosus in, 145-146
vitiligo in, 150-153
Vogt-Koyanagi-Harada-like syndrome in, 148-150
Lichenoid inflammation
actinic keratosis and, 79
dermatophytosis and, 245
pemphigus foliaceus and, 18
Lichenoid keratosis, 85-86
actinic keratosis versus, 79, 156
dermal, 157, 158
psoriasiform-lichenoid dermatosis of Springer Spaniel and, 83-85, 156-157
Lick dermatitis, acral; *see* Acral lick dermatitis
Lick granuloma; *see* Acral lick dermatitis
Lidocaine, 3
Linear epidermal nevus, human, 331
Linear preputial erythema, Sertoli cell tumor and, 75-76
Lip-fold pyoderma, 141
Lipidosis, hepatic, 234
Lipoblasts in myxoid liposarcoma, 435
Lipoma, 430-431
infiltrative, 432-433
Lipomatosis, 430
Liposarcoma, 433-436
compared with
myxosarcoma, 417
sebaceous carcinoma, 380
storiform-pleomorphic malignant fibrous histiocytoma, 448
well-differentiated, 434
Liquefying panniculitis, 313
Lobular panniculitis, 314
idiopathic, 321
sterile nodular panniculitis and, 322
pansteatitis and, 324
Local anesthesia, 3
Long-haired breeds
basal cell tumor in, 343
demodicosis in, 264
Loxosceles reclusus, 212
Lupoid dermatosis of German Shorthaired Pointer, 24, 26-28
Lupus erythematosus
compared with
familial dermatomyositis, 36
hereditary lupoid dermatosis of German Shorthaired Pointer, 28
pemphigus foliaceus, 16
discoid; *see* Discoid lupus erythematosus
pemphigus erythematosus and, 18
systemic; *see* Systemic lupus erythematosus
Lupus panniculitis
compared with
erythema nodosum–like panniculitis, 323
idiopathic sterile nodular panniculitis, 321
Lutzomyia, 186
Lymphadenitis, juvenile sterile granulomatous; *see* Juvenile sterile granulomatous dermatitis and lymphadenitis

Lymphadenopathy
  acariasis and
    notoedric, 125
    sarcoptic, 124
  actinomycosis and nocardiosis and, 165
  cryptococcosis and, 177
  demodicosis and, 264
  generic dog food dermatosis and, 104
  ichthyosis and, 99
  kerion and, 261
  leishmaniasis and, 186
  leprosy and, 166
  mosquito-bite hypersensitivity and, 210
  mycosis fungoides and, 159
  seborrhea and, 89
  sterile eosinophilic pustulosis and, 250
  sterile pedal panniculitis of German Shepherd Dog and, 324
  superficial bacterial folliculitis and, 239
  systemic histiocytosis of Bernese Mountain Dog and, 201
Lymphangioma
  compared with
    hemangioma, 422
    lymphangiosarcoma, 428
  vascular, 426-427
Lymphangiosarcoma
  developmental origin of, 427
  hemangiosarcoma versus, 426
  vascular, 427-428
Lymphocytes in lymphomatoid granulomatosis, 483
Lymphocytic dermatitis
  dense accumulation of lymphocytes in, 292
  histiocytoma versus, 468
  in psychogenic alopecia, 296
  small-cell lymphoid neoplasia versus, 481
Lymphocytic lymphoma, 481
Lymphocytic thyroiditis, 74
Lymphocytic tumors, 474-484
  cutaneous extramedullary plasmacytoma in, 474-475
  lymphomatoid granulomatosis in, 482-483
  malignant lymphoma in, 476-482
Lymphoma
  B-cell, small cleaved, 481
  cell type of, 478
  epitheliotropic, 476, 481-482
    d'emblee variant of, 481
    mucocutaneous candidiasis versus, 14
  histiocytic, 480-481
    mast cell tumors versus, 469, 473
  histiocytosis versus, 199
  immunoblastic, 478-480
  lymphocytic, 481
  malignant, 476-482
    epitheliotropic; see Mycosis fungoides
    histiocytosis versus, 200
    lymphomatoid granulomatosis and human, 482
    systemic histiocytosis of Bernese Mountain Dog versus, 201
  nonepitheliotropic, 476, 477, 478-481
  plasmacytoid, grade 3 mast cell tumors versus, 473
  T-cell; see T-cell lymphoma
Lymphomatoid granulomatosis, 482-483, 484
  immune-mediated vasculitis versus, 138
Lymphosarcoma; see Lymphoma, malignant
Lysozyme, 448

M
Major basic protein, 215, 218
Malassezia
  acne and, 259
  seborrheic dermatitis and, 92-94
  West Highland White Terrier and, 81-83
Malassezia pachydermatis
  seborrheic dermatitis and, 92-94
  in West Highland White Terrier, 81-83
Malignant fibrous histiocytoma; see Fibrous histiocytoma, malignant
Malignant histiocytosis, 201
Malignant lymphoma; see Lymphoma, malignant
Malignant melanoma, 459-464
  melanocytoma compared with, 455
Malignant peripheral nerve sheath tumor; see Schwannoma, malignant
Malignant pilomatricoma; see Matrical carcinoma
Malignant schwannoma; see Schwannoma, malignant
Maltese, traction alopecia in, 294
Mammary gland adenoma
  apocrine glandular adenoma versus, 389-390
  basaloid, 390
Mammary tumors, benign mixed, 390
Manchester Terrier, acquired pattern alopecia in, 307
Mange
  demodectic; see Demodicosis
  notoedric, 125-127
  sarcoptic; see Sarcoptic acariasis
Masson's trichrome stain, 444
Mast cell tumors; see Histiocytic and mast cell tumors
Mast cells, food allergy and, 118
Mastocytosis
  diffuse cutaneous, 468
  visceral, 468
Matrical carcinoma
  compared with
    keratinizing basal cell carcinoma, 348
    pilomatricoma, 367
  follicular, 371-372
  stromal features in, 371
Matrical cyst, 351, 354
  pilomatricoma and, 367
Matrical keratinization
  basal cell carcinoma and, 348
  carcinoma and, 348, 371
  pilomatricoma and, 366
  trichoepithelioma and, 360
Mechanobullous disease, 38
Medusa-head basal cell tumor, 367
Megaesophagus, 35
Megestrol acetate–induced diabetes mellitus, 193
Meibomian gland adenoma, 377
Meibomian gland epithelioma, 378
Melanin pigmentation
  black-hair follicular dysplasia and, 302
  color-mutant alopecia and, 301
  Sertoli cell-tumor and, 76
  in solid basal cell carcinoma, 347
Melanocytes, follicular, 291
Melanocytic nevus; see Melanocytoma
Melanocytic tumors, 451-464
  lentigo in, 456-458
  malignant melanoma in, 459-464
  melanocytoma-acanthoma in, 458-459
  melanocytoma in, 451-456

Melanocytoma, 451-456
  pigmented malignant melanoma compared with, 464
Melanocytoma-acanthoma, 458-459
Melanoma
  benign; *see* Melanocytoma
  compared with
    extramedullary plasma cell tumor, 476
    sebaceous carcinoma, 380
  epithelioid, 463
  malignant; *see* Malignant melanoma
Melanophages
  compound melanocytoma and, 454
  dermal melanocytoma and, 454
Merkel cell tumor, 474
  extramedullary plasma cell tumor versus, 476
Mesenchymal neoplasia, 406-484
  benign fibrous histiocytoma and, 445-446
  fibrocytic tumors and, 407-418; *see also* Fibrocytic tumors
  fibrolipoma and, 431-432
  hemangiopericytoma and, 436-438
  histiocytic and mast cell tumors and, 465-473; *see also* Histiocytic
    and mast cell tumors
  infiltrative lipoma and, 432-433
  leiomyoma and, 443-444
  leiomyosarcoma and, 445
  lipoma and, 430-431
  lipomatosis and, 430
  liposarcoma and, 433-436
  lymphocytic tumors and, 474-484; *see also* Lymphocytic
    tumors
  malignant fibrous histiocytoma and, 446-449
  malignant schwannoma and, 441-443
  melanocytic tumors and, 451-464; *see also* Melanocytic tumors
  schwannoma and, 438-441
  tail dock neuroma and, 438
  vascular tumors and, 419-429; *see also* Vascular tumors
Metaplasia, chondroid, 462, 463
Metaplastic bone, calcinosis cutis and, 226
Metastasis
  of basal cell epithelioma, 343-344
  of eccrine carcinoma, 396
  of fibrosarcoma, 413
  of fibrous histiocytoma, 446
  of hemangiopericytoma, 437
  of hemangiosarcoma, 423
  of leiomyoma, 444
  of mast cell tumor, 468
  of matrical carcinoma, 371
  of melanocytic neoplasms, 452
  of myxosarcoma, 416
  of renal tumors, 408
  of schwannoma, 441
  of squamous cell carcinoma, 337
Metastatic carcinoma
  compared with
    ductular apocrine adenocarcinoma, 395
    sebaceous carcinoma, 380
  eccrine carcinoma and, 396
  squamous cell carcinoma and, 403
Methyl green pyronine stain, 476
Michel's fixative and transport media, 3, 4
Microabscess of Pautrier, 160
Microfilaria, 130
Microsporum canis
  canine, 243

Microsporum canis—cont'd
  feline
    dermatophytic mycetoma and, 172
    dermatophytosis and, 241
Microsporum gypseum
  dermatophytosis and, 243, 244
  kerion and, 261
Miliary dermatitis; *see* Allergic miliary dermatitis
Mineralization of external follicular root sheath in hyperadrenocorticism, 278
Minerals
  calcinosis circumscripta and, 227
  calcinosis cutis and, 225
Miniature Pinscher with color-mutant alopecia, 299
Miniature Poodle
  growth hormone/castration-responsive dermatosis in, 283
  idiopathic sterile nodular panniculitis in, 321
Miniature Schnauzer; *see also* Schnauzer
  atopy in, 115
  dermatosis in
    subcorneal pustular, 20
    vitamin A–responsive, 94
  follicular dysplasia in, 304
  food allergy and, 117
  hypothyroidism in, 74
  melanocytic neoplasms in, 452
Mites
  demodicosis and, 265, 266
  sarcoptic acariasis and, 124
Mitotic index
  fibrosarcoma and, 413
  malignant melanoma and, 460
  melanocytic neoplasms and, 455
Mixed apocrine adenocarcinoma, 394, 395
Mixed apocrine adenoma, 390
Mixed mammary tumors, apocrine adenoma compared with, 390
Moist dermatitis, acute; *see* Pyotraumatic dermatitis
Monoclonal gammopathy, 230
Mosquito-bite hypersensitivity
  allergic miliary dermatitis and, 123
  compared with
    eosinophilic furunculosis, 269
    eosinophilic granuloma, 217
    eosinophilic plaque, 55
    food allergy, 117, 119
    indolent ulcer, 64
  prominent eosinophils or plasma cells and, 210-211
Mott cells, 220
Mucicarmine stain, 178
Mucin
  discoid lupus erythematosus and, 145
  skin disease and, 229
Mucinosis, 228-229
  eosinophilic plaque compared with, 55
  papular, 228
Mucocutaneous candidiasis, 14-15
  superficial necrolytic dermatitis versus, 48
  superficial spreading, 14
Mucocutaneous junctions
  acrodermatitis of Bull Terrier and, 106, 107
  bullous pemphigoid and, 29
  erythema multiforme and, 41
  generic dog food dermatosis and, 105
  juvenile sterile granulomatous dermatitis and lymphadenitis and,
    203

Mucocutaneous junctions—cont'd
  mucocutaneous candidiasis and, 14
  pemphigus vulgaris and, 31
  superficial necrolytic dermatitis and, 46
  systemic lupus erythematosus and, 25
  toxic epidermal necrolysis and, 44
  ulcerative dermatosis of Shetland Sheepdog and Collie and, 36
  Vogt-Koyanagi-Harada–like syndrome and, 148
  zinc-responsive dermatosis and, 103
Mucocutaneous pyoderma, 141-143
  compared with
    discoid lupus erythematosus, 145
    psoriasiform-lichenoid dermatosis of Springer Spaniel, 157
Mucosa
  nasal, 199, 200
  oral; see Oral mucosa
  toxic epidermal necrolysis and gastrointestinal, 44
Multicentric squamous cell carcinoma in situ, 340-341; see also Actinic keratosis
Multiple myeloma, 230
Munro's microabscess, 85
Muscle atrophy, familial dermatomyositis and, 34-35
Mycetoma, 179-181; see also Cutaneous infections, opportunistic fungi and algae in
  dermatophytic, 172-174, 242
  granule formation and, 173
Mycobacterial infection; see Opportunistic mycobacterial infection
Mycobacteriosis, atypical; see Opportunistic mycobacterial infection
Mycobacterium avium
  leprosy versus, 168
  opportunistic mycobacterial infection versus, 170
Mycobacterium avium-intracellulare, 169
Mycobacterium chelonei, 169
Mycobacterium fortuitum, 169
Mycobacterium lepraemurium, 166
Mycoses, systemic, 174-175
Mycosis fungoides; see also Epitheliotropic lymphoma
  clinical findings of, 477
  compared with
    cutaneous leishmaniasis, 186
    histiocytoma, 468
    pemphigus erythematosus, 18
    pemphigus foliaceus, 16
    pemphigus vulgaris, 31
  d'emblee variant of, 477
  dermal, 158-161
  epitheliotropic lymphoma and, 476, 481
  etiology of, 477
  feline, 159, 161
  Woringer-Kolopp–like variants of, 482
Myeloma, multiple, 230
Myocutaneous junctions, 159
Myoepithelium
  apocrine adenomas and, 390
  mixed apocrine carcinoma and, 394
Myositis
  familial dermatomyositis and, 36
  ulcerative dermatosis of Shetland Sheepdog and Collie and, 36
Myxedema, cutaneous, 228-229
Myxofibroma; see Myxoma
Myxofibrosarcoma; see Myxosarcoma
Myxoid liposarcoma, 434, 435
  myxosarcoma compared with, 417
Myxoid schwannoma, 441

Myxoma, 415, 416
  myxosarcoma compared with, 417
  nerve sheath, 441
Myxosarcoma, 416-417
  myxoma versus, 415

N
Nail deformation, hookworm dermatitis and, 130
Nailbed epithelial tumors, 398-405
  inclusion cyst in, 398-399
  inverted squamous papilloma in, 399-400
  keratoacanthoma in, 400-402
  squamous cell carcinoma in, 403, 404
    inverted squamous papilloma versus, 399-400
Nasal mucosa, 199, 200
Nasal pyoderma, discoid lupus erythematosus versus, 23
Nasal solar dermatitis, 22
Necrolysis, toxic epidermal; see Toxic epidermal necrolysis
Necrolytic dermatitis, superficial; see Superficial necrolytic dermatitis
Necrolytic migratory erythema, human, 46; see also Superficial necrolytic dermatitis
Necrosis
  adipocyte, lobular panniculitis and, 315
  caseation
    matrical carcinoma and, 371
    solid basal cell carcinoma and, 345
  epidermal, 41-50
    chemical and thermal burns in, 48-50
    erythema multiforme in, 41-44
    superficial necrolytic dermatitis in, 46-48
    toxic epidermal necrolysis in, 44-46
  fat; see Fat necrosis
  keratinocyte
    erythema multiforme and, 42
    hereditary lupoid dermatosis of German Shorthaired Pointer and, 28
    ulcerative dermatosis of Shetland Sheepdog and Collie and, 37
  lymphomatoid granulomatosis and, 483
  in thermal burns, 49, 50
Necrotoxins, Loxosceles and, 212
Neomycin, 132
Neoplasia, 327-484
  compared with
    acantholytic squamous cell carcinoma, 339
    acral lick dermatitis, 72
    arthropod-bite granuloma, 208
    calcinosis circumscripta, 227
    cutaneous cryptococcosis, 177
    cutaneous infections from systemic fungi and algae, 180
    deep bacterial folliculitis and furunculosis, 254
    dermatophytic mycetoma, 172
    eosinophilic granuloma, 216, 218
    eosinophilic plaque, 55
    erythema multiforme, 41
    erythema nodosum–like panniculitis, 323
    fibropruritic nodules, 70
    idiopathic sterile nodular panniculitis, 321
    indolent ulcer, 63
    kerion, 261
    panniculitis, 313, 318
    post-injection panniculitis, 318
    pyotraumatic dermatitis, 59
    pythiosis, 184

Neoplasia—cont'd
  compared with—cont'd
    seborrhea, 89
    sporotrichosis, 182
    systemic mycoses, 175
    toxic epidermal necrolysis, 44
    traumatic panniculitis, 319
  epithelial tumors as, 329-405; *see also* Epithelial tumors
  mesenchymal, 406-484; *see also* Mesenchymal neoplasia
  in nailbed epithelial inclusion cyst, 398
  renal epithelial, fibromatous nodules and, 408
Nerve sheath tumor
  malignant peripheral, 437; *see also* Schwannoma, malignant
  myxoma as, 441
Neurilemmoma; *see* Schwannoma
Neurofibroma; *see* Schwannoma
Neurofibrosarcoma; *see* Schwannoma, malignant
Neuroma, tail dock, 438
Neurothekeoma, 441
  myxoma compared with, 415
Neurotoxins, *Latrodectus* and, 212
Nevus
  blue; *see* Melanocytoma
  collagenous; *see* Collagenous nevus
  defined, 331, 407
  hair follicle, 357-358
  human, linear epidermal, 331
  melanocytic, 451-456
  pigmented, 451-456
    epidermal, 331, 458
    lentigo simplex and, 458
  sebaceous, 376
  term, 357, 451
Nevus comedonicus, 96
Nevus sebaceus of Jadassohn, 376
Newfoundland
  hypothyroidism in, 74
  pemphigus foliaceus in, 16
Nikolsky's sign
  pemphigus vulgaris and, 31
  toxic epidermal necrolysis and, 44
Nocardia, 163, 165
Nocardia asteroides, 163, 164
Nocardia brasiliensis, 163, 164
Nocardia caviae, 163
Nocardiosis, 163-166
  compared with
    dirofilariasis, 129
    opportunistic mycobacterial infection, 170
Nodular and diffuse dermal diseases with prominent eosinophils or
    plasma cells, 207-222
  arthropod-bite granuloma in, 207-209
  eosinophilic granuloma in
    canine, 218-220
    feline, 215-217
  eosinophilic plaque in, 213-215
  mosquito-bite hypersensitivity in, 210-211
  plasma cell pododermatitis in, 220-221
  spider bites in, 212-213
Nodular and diffuse granulomatous diseases of dermis
  infectious; *see* Infectious nodular and diffuse granulomatous and
    pyogranulomatous dermal diseases
  noninfectious; *see* Noninfectious nodular and diffuse granuloma-
    tous and pyogranulomatous dermal diseases
Nodular cutaneous amyloidosis, 230

Nodular dermatofibrosis, 408-409
  compared with
    collagenous nevus, 407-408
    fibroma, 413
Nodular diseases
  with follicular destruction; *see* Pustular and nodular diseases with
    follicular destruction
  without follicular destruction; *see* Pustular and nodular diseases
    without follicular destruction
Nodular necrotizing steatitis versus lipoma, 431
Nodular panniculitis, sterile idiopathic, 204
  opportunistic mycobacterial infection compared with, 170
Nodular perianal gland hyperplasia and perianal gland adenoma,
    381-383
Nodular scar
  collagenous nevus versus, 407-408
  fibroma versus, 413
Nodular sebaceous hyperplasia, 374-376
  compared with
    compound sebaceous adenoma, 377
    sebaceous nevus, 376
    simple sebaceous adenoma, 377
Nodular stage in mycosis fungoides, 160
Nodular xanthoma, solitary, 193
Nodules, fibropruritic, 70-71
Nonepitheliotropic lymphoma, 476, 477, 478-481
  feline, 477
Noninfectious nodular and diffuse granulomatous and pyogranulo-
    matous dermal diseases, 190-206
  foreign body reactions in, 190-192
  histiocytosis in, 198-201
  juvenile sterile granulomatous dermatitis in, 203-205
  lymphadenitis in, 203-205
  pyogranuloma syndrome in, 194-198
  sterile granuloma in, 194-198
  systemic histiocytosis of Bernese Mountain Dog in, 201-203
  xanthoma in, 193-194, 195
Nontuberculous mycobacterial infection; *see* Opportunistic myco-
    bacterial infection
Norwegian Elkhound with infundibular keratinizing acanthoma,
    362
Norwegian scabies, 123, 124, 125
Notoedres cati, 125
Notoedric acariasis, 125-127
  compared with
    cheyletiellosis, 128
    food allergy, 117, 119
Notoedric mange, 125-127
Nutrient-responsive dermatosis, 102

O

Oil-red-O stain, 193
Old English Sheepdog
  demodicosis in, 264
  sebaceous adenitis in, 101
  vitiligo in, 152
Onychomycosis, 242
Oomycosis; *see* Pythiosis
Opportunistic algae in cutaneous infections, 179-181
  systemic mycoses compared with, 175
Opportunistic fungal infections, 179-181; *see also* Cutaneous infec-
    tions, opportunistic fungi and algae in
  compared with
    feline leprosy, 167
    idiopathic sterile nodular panniculitis, 321

Opportunistic fungal infections—cont'd
    compared with—cont'd
        pythiosis, 185
        systemic mycoses, 175
        xanthoma, 194
Opportunistic mycobacterial granulomas; *see* Opportunistic myco-
        bacterial infection
Opportunistic mycobacterial infection, 169-171
    compared with
        actinomycosis and nocardiosis, 165, 166
        deep bacterial folliculitis and furunculosis, 254
        erythema nodosum–like panniculitis, 323
        idiopathic sterile nodular panniculitis, 321
        leprosy, 168
        pyogranulomatous type of sterile granuloma and pyogranu-
            loma, 198
        sterile nodular panniculitis, 323
        systemic fungi and algae, 180
        systemic mycoses, 175
    facial form of, 170
Oral mucosa
    bullous pemphigoid and, 29
    discoid lupus erythematosus and, 22
    erythema multiforme and, 41
    foreign body reactions and, 191
    immune-mediated vasculitis and, 138
    mucocutaneous candidiasis and, 14
    mycosis fungoides and, 158
    pemphigus vulgaris and, 31
    systemic lupus erythematosus and, 25
    toxic epidermal necrolysis and, 44
    vitiligo and, 150
Osseous metaplasia, calcinosis circumscripta and, 228
Osteosarcoma compared with giant cell malignant fibrous
        histiocytoma, 447
Otodectic acariasis compared with notoedric acariasis,
        125
Outer root sheath of hair follicle, 351, 352
    matrical carcinoma and, 371
    tricholemmoma and, 364
Ovarian imbalance type I, 75, 280-281
Oxalic acid, 455

P

Paecilomycosis, 179-181; *see also* Cutaneous infections, opportunis-
        tic fungi and algae in
Pagetoid reticulosis, 477
Palisading, peripheral
    clear-cell basal cell carcinoma and, 348-349
    melanocytoma-acanthoma and, 458
    solid basal cell carcinoma and, 345
    trabecular trichoblastoma and, 343, 369, 370
    trichoblastoma and, 367
    trichoepithelioma and, 360
    tricholemmoma and, 364
Palisading granulomas, 219
Pancreatic disease
    endocrine tumor and, 46
    idiopathic sterile nodular panniculitis in, 321
Panfollicular cyst, 355
Panniculitis, 312-315
    diffuse
        idiopathic sterile nodular panniculitis and, 322
        pansteatitis and, 324
        sterile pedal, of German Shepherd Dog, 325

Panniculitis—cont'd
    erythema nodosum–like, 323
        immune-mediated vasculitis compared with, 138, 333
    idiopathic sterile nodular, 321-323
        systemic lupus erythematosus versus, 25
    juvenile sterile granulomatous dermatitis and lymphadenitis and,
        204
    lobular; *see* Lobular panniculitis
    lupus, 146
        idiopathic sterile nodular panniculitis compared with, 321
    post-injection, 316-319
    post-rabies vaccination alopecia and, 289
    septal, 315, 323
    sequela to, 313
    sterile nodular, opportunistic mycobacterial infection compared
        with, 170
    sterile pedal
        fistulation in, 325
        German Shepherd Dog and, 324-325
    systemic lupus erythematosus and, 25
    traumatic, 319-320; *see* Traumatic panniculitis
Panniculus diseases, 311-326
    panniculitis in; *see* Panniculitis
    pansteatitis in, 323-324
    post-rabies vaccination alopecia in, 316, 317
Pansteatitis, 323-324
Papilloma
    cutaneous horn in, 331
    exophytic, 334-335
    idiopathic squamous, 376
    inverted, 335
    squamous
        nailbed inverted, 399-400
        subungual inverted, 399-400
        viral, 334-335
Papillomatous hyperplasia, pemphigus vegetans and, 34
Papillomavirus
    verruca plana and, 334
    viral squamous papilloma and, 334
Papular mucinosis, 228
Papules
    allergic contact dermatitis and, 51, 52
    allergic miliary dermatitis and, 60-61
Paronychia
    acrodermatitis of Bull Terrier and, 106
    hookworm dermatitis and, 130
    nailbed squamous cell carcinoma and, 403
Patch tests in allergic contact dermatitis, 51, 52
Pattern analysis in skin biopsy, 4-5
Pattern baldness; *see* Acquired pattern alopecia
Pautrier's microabscess, 160
Pedal panniculitis of German Shepherd Dog, 324-325
Pelodera dermatitis, 130, 266-268
Pelodera strongyloides, 266
Pemphigus erythematosus, 18-20, 147
    pemphigus foliaceus versus, 18
Pemphigus foliaceus, 16-18, 245-247
    compared with
        actinic keratosis, 78
        allergic miliary dermatitis, 61
        dermatophytosis, 242, 244
        discoid lupus erythematosus, 23
        mosquito-bite hypersensitivity, 210
        notoedric acariasis, 125
        pemphigus vegetans, 33, 34

Pemphigus foliaceus—cont'd
  compared with—cont'd
    subcorneal pustular dermatosis, 20
    superficial bacterial folliculitis, 239
    superficial necrolytic dermatitis, 47
    superficial spreading pyoderma, 12
   facial, 16
    pemphigus erythematosus and, 18
   impetigo and, 12
   pemphigus erythematosus and, 18, 20, 147
Pemphigus vegetans, 33-34
  compared with
   pemphigus foliaceus, 247
   pemphigus vulgaris, 33
Pemphigus vulgaris, 31-33
  compared with
   bullous pemphigoid, 29
   chemical and thermal burns, 49
   mucocutaneous candidiasis, 14
   mycosis fungoides, 159
   pemphigus vegetans, 33
   toxic epidermal necrolysis, 44
   ulcerative dermatosis of Shetland Sheepdog and Collie, 36
Perforating folliculitis, superficial, 239, 240
Periadnexal multinodular granulomatous dermatitis, idiopathic; see
    Sterile granuloma and pyogranuloma
Periadnexal pyogranuloma, 204
Perianal gland adenoma, 381-383
Perianal gland carcinoma, 384-385
  poorly differentiated variants of, 384
  sebaceous carcinoma compared with, 380
  well-differentiated, 384
Perianal gland epithelioma, 384
Perianal gland hyperplasia and perianal gland adenoma, nodular,
    381-383
Perifollicular fibrosis, 241
Periodic acid–Schiff stain
  leiomyoma and, 444
  nailbed keratoacanthoma and, 402
Peripheral nerve sheath tumor, 437; see also Schwannoma
Peripheral palisading; see Palisading, peripheral
Perivascular diseases, dermal, 112-134
  acariasis in
   notoedric, 125-127
   sarcoptic, 123-125
  allergic contact dermatitis in, 131-132, 133
  allergic miliary dermatitis in, 122-123
  atopy in, 114-116
  cheyletiellosis in, 126-128
  cutaneous dirofilariasis in, 128-130
  flea allergy dermatitis in, 119-122
  food allergy in, 117-119
  hookworm dermatitis in, 130-131
  superficial spreading pyoderma in, 112-113, 114
Permanganate, 454-455
Persian cat
  dermatophytic mycetomas in, 172
  dermatophytosis in, 242
Phaeohyphomycosis, 179-181; see also Cutaneous infections, oppor-
    tunistic fungi and algae in
Phlebectasia, 275, 276
Phlebotomus, 186
Phosphate-buffered formalin, 3-4
Photo-aggravation
  familial dermatomyositis and, 34

Photo-aggravation—cont'd
  lupus erythematosus and
   discoid, 22
   systemic, 25
  pemphigus erythematosus and, 18
  Vogt-Koyanagi-Harada–like syndrome and, 148
Phrynoderma, 94
Phycomycosis; see Pythiosis
Pigmentary incontinence
  acanthosis nigricans of Dachshund and, 80-81
  discoid lupus erythematosus and, 24, 145
  hereditary lupoid dermatosis of German Shorthaired Pointer and,
    28
  post-rabies vaccination alopecia and, 289
  psoriasiform-lichenoid dermatosis of Springer Spaniel and, 157
Pigmentation, melanin; see Melanin pigmentation
Pigmented epidermal nevus, 331
  lentigo simplex and, 458
Pigmented nevus; see Melanocytoma
Pigmented tumors, 378
Pilomatricoma, 365-367
  compared with
   matrical carcinoma, 372
   proliferating matrical cyst, 354
   trichoepithelioma, 361
  malignant; see Matrical carcinoma
Pilomatrixoma; see Pilomatricoma
Pink, white, and blue sandwich, 48
Pit Bull Terrier with ichthyosis, 99
Pityrosporum canis, 92
Plant foreign body reaction, 191
Planum nasale
  discoid lupus erythematosus and, 22, 23
  histiocytosis and, 199
  leishmaniasis and, 186
  mosquito-bite hypersensitivity and, 210
  pemphigus erythematosus and, 18
  systemic histiocytosis of Bernese Mountain Dog and, 201
  systemic mycoses and, 175
Plaque
  acral lick dermatitis and, 72
  eosinophilic; see Eosinophilic plaque
  in mycosis fungoides, 160
Plasma cell pododermatitis
  eosinophilic granuloma versus, 216
  prominent eosinophils or plasma cells in, 220-221
Plasma cell stomatitis, 220
Plasma cell tumor, 230
Plasma cells, nodular and diffuse diseases with prominent, dermal;
    see Nodular and diffuse dermal diseases with prominent
    eosinophils or plasma cells
Plasmacytoid lymphoma, 473
Plasmacytoma
  extramedullary, 230
Pleomorphic liposarcoma, fibrous histiocytoma compared with,
    448
Pluripotentiality of basal cell carcinoma, 343
Pododemodicosis, 264
Pododermatitis
  plasma cell
   eosinophilic granuloma versus, 216
   prominent eosinophils or plasma cells in, 220-221
Pointer
  English, 421
  German Shorthaired; see German Shorthaired Pointer

Pointer—cont'd
    German Wirehaired; *see* German Wirehaired Pointer
Polyp, skin; *see* Skin tag
Polypoid fibromas, skin tags versus, 410
Pomeranian with growth hormone/castration-responsive dermato-
        sis, 282, 283
Poodle
    alopecia in
        post-rabies vaccination, 288
        traction, 294
    congenital hypotrichosis in, 308
    dermatophytosis in, 244
    hyperadrenocorticism in, 276
    hypothyroidism in, 74
    lipoma in, 431
    nodular sebaceous hyperplasia in, 374
    pilomatricoma in, 366
    sebaceous adenoma in, 377
    sebaceous epithelioma in, 378
    Standard; *see* Standard Poodle
    systemic lupus erythematosus in, 25
    Toy; *see* Toy Poodle
    trichoblastoma in, 367
Pores, dilated, 331, 356-357
Portuguese Water Dog with follicular dysplasia, 304, 306
Post-clipping alopecia, 285-286
    growth hormone/castration-responsive dermatosis and, 283, 284
Post-injection panniculitis, 316-319
Post-rabies vaccination alopecia, 287-289, 316, 317
    compared with
        alopecia areata, 291, 292
        cicatricial alopecia, 293
        post-injection panniculitis, 319
Preauricular xanthogranuloma, 196, 197-198
    compared with
        cutaneous xanthoma, 194
        leprosy, 168
Preputial erythema, Sertoli cell tumor and, 75-76
Pressure-point granuloma, 255-256, 258
Primary lesion, 2
Progestational compounds, 234
Proliferating cyst
    infundibular keratinizing acanthoma and, 363
    isthmus-catagen, 353-354
        infundibular keratinizing acanthoma and, 363
    matrical, 354
Protein, major basic, 215, 218
Prototheca, 181
Protothecosis, 179-181; *see also* Cutaneous infections, opportunistic
        fungi and algae in
Pruritus
    atopy versus, 115
    food allergy and, 117
Pseudoepitheliomatous hyperplasia, 72
Pseudoglandular squamous cell carcinoma, 338-339; *see also* Acan-
        tholytic squamous cell carcinoma
    eccrine carcinoma compared with, 396
Psoriasiform hyperplasia
    human, 84
    lichenoid keratosis and, 85
    psoriasiform-lichenoid dermatosis of Springer Spaniel and, 156
Psoriasiform-lichenoid dermatosis
    compared with
        actinic keratosis, 156
        lichenoid keratosis, 85

Psoriasiform-lichenoid dermatosis—cont'd
    of Springer Spaniel, 83-85, 156-157
Psychogenic alopecia, feline, 295-296
    compared with
        atopy, 115
        dermatophytosis, 242
Psychogenic hair loss, self-induced; *see* Psychogenic alopecia, feline
Public hazard in sporotrichosis, 181-182
Pug
    atopy in, 115
    demodicosis in, 264
    pigmented epidermal nevus in, 331
Punch biopsy, 2-3
    acne and
        canine, 258
        feline, 259
    in acral lick dermatitis, 72
    in alopecia areata, 291
    in amyloidosis, 230
    in calcinosis cutis, 225
    in eosinophilic granuloma, 216
    in idiopathic sterile nodular panniculitis, 322
    in indolent ulcer, 63
    in juvenile sterile granulomatous dermatitis and lymphadenitis,
        203
    in mosquito-bite hypersensitivity, 210
    in mucocutaneous pyoderma, 142
    in panniculitis, 313
    in sporotrichosis, 182
    in xanthoma, 193
Puppy pyoderma; *see* Impetigo
Puppy strangles; *see* Juvenile sterile granulomatous dermatitis and
        lymphadenitis
Purpura
    cutaneous amyloidosis and, 230
    immune-mediated vasculitis and, 138
    septic vasculitis and, 139
Pustular and nodular diseases with follicular destruction, 252-272
    acne in
        canine, 257-258
        feline, 258-259
    actinic comedones in, 270-272
    callus and callus pyoderma in, 255-256
    deep bacterial folliculitis and furunculosis in, 252-255
    demodicosis in, 262-266
    eosinophilic furunculosis of face in, 269-270
    kerion in, 261-262
    rhabditic dermatitis in, 266-268
Pustular and nodular diseases without follicular destruction,
        238-251
    dermatophytosis in
        canine, 243-245
        feline, 241-243
    pemphigus foliaceus in, 245-247
    sebaceous adenitis in, 247-249
    sterile eosinophilic pustulosis in, 250-251
    superficial bacterial folliculitis in, 238-241
Pustular dermatosis, subcorneal; *see* Subcorneal pustule
Pustular diseases, superficial; *see* Superficial pustular diseases, epi-
        dermal
Pustulation, spongiotic eosinophilic, 18
Pustule
    intraepidermal, psoriasiform-lichenoid dermatosis of Springer
        Spaniel versus, 85
    intragranular, pemphigus foliaceus and, 17

Pustule—cont'd
  subcorneal; *see* Subcorneal pustule
Pustules
  superficial epidermal, 12
  suprabasilar
    pemphigus vegetans and, 33, 34
Pustulosis, sterile eosinophilic; *see* Sterile eosinophilic pustulosis
Pyoderma
  callus, 255-256, 258
  compared with
    familial dermatomyositis, 35
    generic dog food dermatosis, 105
    nasal discoid lupus erythematosus, 23
    zinc-responsive dermatosis, 103
  deep; *see* Deep bacterial folliculitis and furunculosis
  juvenile; *see* Juvenile sterile granulomatous dermatitis and lymphadenitis
  lip-fold, mucocutaneous pyoderma and, 141
  mucocutaneous, 141-143
    discoid lupus erythematosus versus, 145
    psoriasiform-lichenoid dermatosis of Springer Spaniel versus, 157
  pruritic superficial, atopy versus, 115
  puppy; *see* Impetigo; Superficial spreading pyoderma
  seborrhea and, 89
  seborrheic dermatitis and, 91, 92
  secondary, 299; *see also* Deep bacterial folliculitis and furunculosis; Superficial bacterial folliculitis
    black-hair follicular dysplasia and, 301
  superficial; *see* Superficial bacterial folliculitis
  superficial spreading; *see* Superficial spreading pyoderma
Pyogranuloma
  with central clear zones, opportunistic mycobacterial infection and, 170
  compared with
    cryptococcosis, 177
    cutaneous infections of systemic fungi and algae, 180
    leishmaniasis, 188
    leprosy, 167
    sebaceous adenitis, 248-249
  periadnexal, juvenile sterile granulomatous dermatitis and lymphadenitis and, 204
  sterile, systemic mycoses versus, 175
Pyogranulomatous diseases of dermis; *see* Infectious nodular and diffuse granulomatous and pyogranulomatous dermal diseases; Noninfectious nodular and diffuse granulomatous and pyogranulomatous dermal diseases
Pyogranulomatous inflammation, acne and, 259
Pyogranulomatous sterile granuloma and pyogranuloma, 197
Pyotraumatic dermatitis, 58-61; *see also* Deep bacterial folliculitis and furunculosis
  deep bacterial folliculitis and furunculosis and, 253, 254
  idiopathic ulcerative dermatosis compared with, 67
Pythiosis, 184-186
  compared with
    deep bacterial folliculitis and furunculosis, 254
    spider bites, 213
Pythium, 184
  morphologic features of, 185

R

Rabies
  post-injection panniculitis and vaccination for, 316-317
  rabies-specific immunofluorescence and, 288, 289
Rats in *Mycobacterium lepraemurium* transmission, 166

Regional anesthesia, 3
Renal amyloidosis, 220
Renal epithelial neoplasia, 408
Reticulum cell sarcoma, 474
Retriever
  Chesapeake Bay, 304
  Curly-Coated, 304, 306
  Golden; *see* Golden Retriever
  Labrador; *see* Labrador Retriever
Rhabditic dermatitis
  follicular destruction and, 266-268
  hookworm dermatitis versus, 130
Rhodesian Ridgeback with dermoid cysts, 355, 359
Ribbon trichoblastoma, 367-368
Ridgeback, Rhodesian, dermoid cysts in, 355, 359
Ring block in skin biopsy, 3
Ringworm
  canine, 243-245
  feline, 172, 241-243
Rocky Mountain spotted fever, 139
Rodent ulcer, 63-64, 216
Root sheath
  inner; *see* Inner root sheath
  outer; *see* Outer root sheath of hair follicle
Rottweiler
  congenital hypotrichosis in, 308
  immune-mediated vasculitis in, 138
  vitiligo in, 152
Runyon group IV mycobacteria, 169
Rupture
  of infundibular cyst, 353
  of pilomatricoma, 367
Russell body, 220

S

S-100 protein
  dermatofibrosarcomas and, 449
  malignant melanoma and, 464
Saint Bernard with pyotraumatic dermatitis, 59
Salivary staining of haircoat, 115
Salukis with cutaneous vascular tumors, 421
Samoyed
  hepatoid gland neoplasms in, 382
  post-clipping alopecia in, 285
  sebaceous adenitis in, 101, 248
  Vogt-Koyanagi-Harada–like syndrome in, 148
Sandfly, 186
Sarcoidosis, cutaneous, 195, 198
Sarcoma, reticulum cell, 474
Sarcoma virus, feline, 413
  liposarcoma and, 433
Sarcoptes scabiei, 104
  variant *canis*, 123, 125
  variant *hominis*, 123
Sarcoptic acariasis, 104, 123-127
  canine, 123-125
  compared with
    cheyletiellosis, 128
    dirofilariasis, 129
    flea allergy dermatitis, 122
    food allergy, 117, 119
    hookworm dermatitis, 130, 131
    rhabditic dermatitis, 267
  ear margin seborrhea and, 96
  feline, 125-127

Sarcoptic acariasis—cont'd
  Norwegian, 123, 124, 125
Sarcoptic mange; *see* Sarcoptic acariasis
Satellitosis
  erythema cultiforme and, 153
  term, 42
Scabies; *see* Sarcoptic acariasis
Scar
  in alopecia; *see* Cicatricial alopecia
  compared with
    collagenous nevus, 407-408
    nodular dermatofibrosis, 408-409
Schipperke
  color-mutant alopecia in, 299
  pemphigus foliaceus in, 16
Schnauzer
  comedo syndrome in, 96-98
    acne versus, 258
    actinic comedones versus, 272
  histiocytoma in, 465
  miniature; *see* Miniature Schnauzer
  pigmented epidermal nevus in, 331
  pilomatricoma in, 366
  Standard, 421
Schwannoma, 438-441
  compared with
    dermatofibroma, 411
    fibroma, 413
    hemangiopericytoma, 438
    myxoma, 415
  malignant, 441-443
    amelanotic malignant melanoma versus, 464
    cutaneous smooth muscle malignancies versus, 445
    dermatofibrosarcoma type malignant fibrous histiocytoma versus, 448-449
    fibrosarcoma versus, 415
    heterologous elements in, 441-443
Scottish Terrier
  atopy in, 115
  flea allergy dermatitis in, 120
  histiocytoma in, 465
  malignant melanoma in, 459
  melanocytic neoplasms in, 452
  scrotal vascular hamartoma in, 419
Scrotal vascular hamartoma, 419, 420
Sebaceoma, 377
Sebaceous adenitis, 90, 247-249
  compared with
    demodicosis, 264, 265, 266
    hereditary lupoid dermatosis of German Shorthaired Pointer, 26
    ichthyosis, 99
    leishmaniasis, 188
    pemphigus foliaceus, 16
    periadnexal type of sterile granuloma and pyogranuloma, 198
    vitamin A–responsive dermatosis, 94
  epidermal and follicular keratin and, 100-102
  feline, 100
Sebaceous adenoma, 376-377
  compound ductular, 377, 378
  compound glandular, 377, 378
  nodular sebaceous hyperplasia versus, 375
  simple; *see* Simple sebaceous adenoma

Sebaceous carcinoma, 380-381
  compared with
    amelanotic malignant melanoma, 464
    basal cell carcinoma, 347, 349, 378
    perianal gland carcinoma, 385
    poorly differentiated perianal gland carcinoma versus, 385
Sebaceous duct cyst, 374, 375
Sebaceous epithelioma, 377-380
  solid basal cell carcinoma versus, 347
Sebaceous gland
  absence of, 248
  atrophy of, sebaceous adenitis and, 102
  carcinoma of; *see* Sebaceous carcinoma
  hyperplasia of
    atopy and, 115
    dermatosis of West Highland White Terrier and, 82
    flea allergy dermatitis and, 122
    food allergy and, 118
    nodular, 374-376, 377
    senile, 374-376, 377
  squamous metaplasia of, atopy and, 116
Sebaceous nevus, 376
Sebaceous tumors, 374-385
  adenoma in; *see* Sebaceous adenoma
  carcinoma in; *see* Sebaceous carcinoma
  cyst in, 374, 375
  epithelioma in, 347, 377-380
  hyperplasia in; *see* Sebaceous gland, hyperplasia of
  nevus in, 376
  nodular perianal gland hyperplasia and perianal gland adenoma in, 381-383
  perianal gland carcinoma in, 384-385
Seborrhea
  ear-margin, 95-96, 97, 307
  primary, 88-90
    cheyletiellosis and, 127
    ear margin seborrhea versus, 96
    follicular keratosis versus, 91
    hereditary lupoid dermatosis of German Shorthaired Pointer versus, 26
    hypothyroidism versus, 74
    ichthyosis versus, 99
    psoriasiform-lichenoid dermatosis of Springer Spaniel and, 85
    Schnauzer comedo syndrome and, 98
    sebaceous adenitis versus, 102
    seborrheic dermatitis and, 92
    vitamin A–responsive dermatosis and, 94
    Westie and, 81-83, 89, 99
  secondary, 88
  vitamin A–responsive dermatosis versus, 94
Seborrhea oleosa, 88, 91
Seborrhea sicca, 88
Seborrheic dermatitis, 90-92
  compared with
    dermatophytosis, 244
    hyperplastic dermatosis of West Highland White Terrier, 82-83
    Malassezia pachydermatis infection, 92-94
    primary seborrhea, 90
    vitamin A–responsive dermatosis, 94
  hyperkeratotic diseases and, 88, 89
Secondary lesion, 2
Self-induced psychogenic feline hair loss; *see* Psychogenic alopecia, feline

Self-trauma, atopy and, 114, 115
Senile sebaceous hyperplasia, 374-376, 377
Septal panniculitis, 315, 323
Septic vasculitis, 139-140
   immune-mediated vasculitis versus, 138
Serocellular crusting, allergic miliary dermatitis and, 61
Sertoli cell tumors
   canine, 75-76, 278-280
   hypothyroidism and, 75, 275
   malignant, 76
Setaria, 120
Sézary syndrome, 478
Shadow cells, 352
   matrical carcinoma and, 371
Shar Pei, Chinese
   atopy in, 115
   food allergy and, 117
   primary seborrhea in, 89
Shetland Sheepdog
   color-mutant alopecia in, 299
   cutaneous histiocytosis in, 199
   discoid lupus erythematosus in, 22
   familial dermatomyositis in, 35
   histiocytoma in, 465
   Sertoli cell tumor in, 76
   systemic lupus erythematosus in, 25
   ulcerative dermatosis in, 36-38
      bullous pemphigoid versus, 29
      discoid lupus erythematosus versus, 24
      erythema multiforme versus, 43
      systemic lupus erythematosus versus, 26
Shih Tzu
   post-rabies vaccination alopecia in, 288
   traction alopecia in, 294
Siamese cat
   basal cell tumor in, 343
   histiocytic subtype of mast cell tumor in, 468
   psychogenic alopecia and, 295
   systemic lupus erythematosus in, 25
   vitiligo in, 152
   xanthomas in, 193
Siberian Husky
   discoid lupus erythematosus in, 22
   follicular dysplasia in, 304, 305
      growth hormone/castration-responsive dermatosis versus, 284
   oral eosinophilic granuloma and, 218
   post-clipping alopecia in, 285
   vitiligo in, 152
   Vogt-Koyanagi-Harada–like syndrome in, 148
   zinc-responsive dermatosis in, 103
Sign, Nikolsky's
   pemphigus vulgaris and, 31
   toxic epidermal necrolysis and, 44
Signet-ring apocrine sweat gland carcinoma, 394
Silvery scales in leishmaniasis, 186
S-100 immunoperoxidase stain, 476
Simple sebaceous adenoma, 377
   nodular sebaceous hyperplasia versus, 375
Skin biopsy, 1-5; *see also* specific pathology
   in acanthosis nigricans of Dachshund, 80
   in acrodermatitis of Bull Terrier, 107
   in actinic comedones, 271
   alopecia and
      acquired pattern, 307
      cicatricial, 293

Skin biopsy—cont'd
   alopecia and—cont'd
      color-mutant, 299
      post-clipping, 285
      post-rabies vaccination, 288, 316
      psychogenic, 295
      sharply defined areas of, 291
      traction, 294
   in asthenia, 233
   in atopy, 115
   in bullous pemphigoid, 29
   in chemical and thermal burns, 49
   in cheyletiellosis, 127
   in congenital hypotrichosis, 308
   in deep bacterial folliculitis and furunculosis, 254
   in demodicosis, 264
   dermatitis and
      allergic contact, 52, 131
      allergic miliary, 61, 122
      chronic hyperplastic, 69
      flea allergy, 120
      hookworm, 131
      irritant contact, 54
      pyotraumatic, 59
      rhabditic, 267
      seborrheic, 91, 92
      superficial necrolytic, 47
   in dermatophytic mycetoma, 172
   in dermatophytosis, 242, 244
   dermatosis and
      generic dog food, 105
      growth hormone/castration-responsive, 283
      hereditary lupoid, of German Shorthaired Pointer, 27
      hyperplastic, of West Highland White Terrier, 82
      psoriasiform-lichenoid, in Springer Spaniel, 84, 156
      subcorneal, 20
      vitamin A–responsive, 94
      zinc-responsive, 103
   in dirofilariasis, 129
   in discoid lupus erythematosus, 23
   in eosinophilic furunculosis, 269
   in eosinophilic plaque, 55, 213
   in erythema multiforme, 42, 153
   in familial dermatomyositis, 35, 290
   in feline skin fragility syndrome, 234-235
   in female hyperestrogenism, 281
   follicular dysplasia and, 304-305
      black-hair, 302
   in food allergy, 117-118
   granuloma and
      arthropod-bite, 208
      eosinophilic, 218-219
      sterile, and pyogranuloma, 196
   handling of, 3-4
   in histiocytosis, 199
   histopathology of, 4-5
   in hyperadrenocorticism, 277
   in hypothyroidism, 75, 274
   in ichthyosis, 99
   in impetigo, 10
   indications for, 1
   instrumentation for, 3
   keratosis and
      actinic, 78, 155
      lichenoid, 85

Skin biopsy—cont'd
    in kerion, 261
    in leishmaniasis, 187
    methods of, 2
    in mucocutaneous candidiasis, 14
    mycoses and
        mycosis fungoides in, 159
        systemic, 175
    pattern analysis in, 4-5
    in pemphigus erythematosus, 19, 147
    in pemphigus foliaceus, 17, 245-246
    in post-injection panniculitis, 318
    in sarcoptic acariasis, 124
    in Schnauzer comedo syndrome, 97
    in sebaceous adenitis, 101, 247
    seborrhea and
        ear margin, 96
        primary, 89
    in Sertoli cell tumor, 76, 278
    specimen for, 2-3
    in sterile eosinophilic pustulosis, 250
    submission of, 4
    in superficial bacterial folliculitis, 239
    in superficial spreading pyoderma, 12, 112
    systemic fungi and algae and, 180
    in systemic histiocytosis of Bernese Mountain Dog, 202
    in systemic lupus erythematosus, 25, 145-146
    technique for, 3
    in telogen effluvium, 287
    in toxic epidermal necrolysis, 44
    in urticaria and angioedema, 136
    in vitiligo, 152
    in xanthoma, 193
Skin disease
    autoimmune; see Autoimmune skin disease
    patterns of, 5
Skin-fold pyoderma, 143
Skin fragility syndrome in cat, 234-236
    cutaneous asthenia versus, 233, 234
Skin polyp; see Skin tag
Skin scrapings
    in acariasis, 124, 125
    in cheyletiellosis, 127
Skin tag, 409-410
    fibroma compared with, 413
Sled-dog breeds with post-clipping alopecia, 285
Smears of exudate in mycobacterial infection, 170
Smooth muscle markers, 415
SND; see Superficial necrolytic dermatitis
Soap bubble appearance in cryptococcosis, 178
Solar damage; see also Solar elastosis
    hemangiomas and, 420, 422
    hemangiosarcoma and, 423
    nasal dermatitis and, 22
    vascular malignancy and, 423
Solar dermatitis, nasal, 22
Solar elastosis; see also Solar damage
    actinic comedones and, 272
    actinic keratosis and, 76, 77, 155; see also Actinic keratosis
    hemangioma and, 422
    hemangiosarcoma and, 426
Solar keratosis; see Actinic keratosis
Solid basal cell carcinoma; see Basal cell carcinoma, solid
Spaniel
    Cocker; see Cocker Spaniel

Spaniel—cont'd
    English Springer; see English Springer Spaniel
    Irish Water, 304, 306
    Springer; see English Springer Spaniel
Spider bites
    prominent eosinophils or plasma cells in, 212-213
    pythiosis versus, 185
Spindle-cell malignancy
    liposarcoma and myxoid variant of, 435
    malignant melanoma and, 461
    squamous cell carcinoma and, 339-340
        fibrosarcoma versus, 415
Spitz with systemic lupus erythematosus, 25
Splendore-Hoeppli reaction, 165
    dermatophytic mycetoma and, 173
Spongiosis
    eosinophilic pustulation and, 18
    epidermal, 51-57
        allergic contact dermatitis in, 51-52
        eosinophilic plaque in, 55, 56
        irritant contact dermatitis in, 52-55
Sporothrix schenckii, 181
    morphologic features of, 184
Sporotrichosis, 181-184
    canine versus feline, 182
    compared with
        cryptococcosis, 177
        dermatophytic mycetoma, 172
        leprosy, 167
        systemic mycoses, 175
Springer Spaniel; see English Springer Spaniel
Squamous cell carcinoma
    acantholytic; see Acantholytic squamous cell carcinoma
    actinic; see also Actinic keratosis
        comedones and, 270
        hemangiosarcoma versus, 423
        keratosis and, 330, 331
    compared with
        hemangiosarcoma, 426
        perianal gland carcinoma, 385
    early, 341
    epidermal, 336-340
    in situ, 340-341; see also Actinic keratosis
    multicentric, 79, 331, 340-341
    nailbed, 403-404
    poorly differentiated, 338
    pseudoglandular, 338-339, 396
    sebaceous gland, atopy and, 116
    solid basal cell carcinoma and, 347
    spindle-celled, 339-340
        fibrosarcoma versus, 415
    well-differentiated, 337
        subungual keratoacanthoma versus, 402
Squamous papilloma
    idiopathic, 336
    inverted
        keratoacanthoma versus, 402
        nailbed or subungual, 399-400
    viral, 334-335
Staffordshire Terrier, American; see American Staffordshire Terrier
Stain
    Congo red, 230
    Fite-Faraco modification of acid-fast, 165, 170
    Fontana-Masson; see Fontana-Masson stain
    Giemsa; see Giemsa stain

Stain—cont'd
    Gomori's, 185, 476
    Masson's trichrome, 444
    methyl green pyronine, 476
    mucicarmine, 178
    oil-red-O, 193
    periodic acid–Schiff, 402, 444
    pH requirements of mucin, 145
    S-100 immunoperoxidase, 476
    thioflavine T, 230
    toluidine blue; *see* Toluidine blue stain
    trichrome, 413, 415, 444
    van Gieson's, 444
    von Kossa, 226
    Wilder's silver, 476
Standard Poodle
    color-mutant alopecia in, 299
    sebaceous adenitis in, 101, 248
Standard Schnauzer with cutaneous vascular tumor, 421
Staphylococci in seborrheic dermatitis, 91
Staphylococcus intermedius
    in deep bacterial folliculitis and furunculosis, 252
    in impetigo, 10
    in superficial bacterial folliculitis, 238
    in superficial spreading pyoderma, 12
Steatitis
    fibrosing, traumatic panniculitis and, 320
    vitamin E deficiency, 323-324
Sterile eosinophilic pustulosis
    eosinophilic furunculosis versus, 270
    superficial bacterial folliculitis versus, 239, 241
    superficial spreading pyoderma versus, 12
Sterile granuloma and pyogranuloma, 194-198
    compared with
        cryptococcosis, 177
        histiocytosis, 199, 201
        juvenile sterile granulomatous dermatitis and lymphadenitis, 204
        leishmaniasis, 188
        leprosy, 167
        sebaceous adenitis, 248-249
        systemic fungi and algae, 180
        systemic histiocytosis, 202
        systemic mycoses, 175
    syndromes similar to, 195-196
Sterile granulomatous dermatitis and lymphadenitis, juvenile, 203-205
    compared with
        acne, 258
        sterile nodular panniculitis, 323
Sterile nodular panniculitis
    idiopathic, 25, 323
    juvenile sterile granulomatous dermatitis and lymphadenitis versus, 204
    opportunistic mycobacterial infection versus, 170
Sterile pedal panniculitis of German Shepherd Dog, 324-325
Stipa, 120
Stomatitis
    plasma cell, 220
    uremic, mucocutaneous candidiasis versus, 14
Storea, 446
Storiform-pleomorphic malignant fibrous histiocytoma, 446, 447-448
Strangles, puppy; *see* Juvenile sterile granulomatous dermatitis and lymphadenitis

Styling devices, traction alopecia from, 294
Subcorneal pustule, 20
    compared with
        impetigo, 11
        pemphigus erythematosus, 19
        pemphigus foliaceus, 17
        superficial bacterial folliculitis, 239
        superficial spreading pyoderma, 12
Subcutis, lipomatosis of, 430
Subungual inverted squamous papilloma, 399-400
Subungual keratoacanthoma, 400-402
    inverted squamous papilloma versus, 400
Sulfur granules, actinomycosis and, 164
Sun-damaged skin, squamous cell carcinoma and, 336
Sunbathing, actinic keratosis and, 78
Superficial bacterial folliculitis, 238-241
    coexistent diseases or syndromes with, 238
    compared with
        acral lick dermatitis, 72
        acrodermatitis of Bull Terrier, 106
        atopy, 115
        color-mutant alopecia, 301
        dermatophytosis, 244
        pemphigus erythematosus, 20
        pemphigus foliaceus, 16
        sarcoptic acariasis, 124
        sterile eosinophilic pustulosis, 250, 251
        subcorneal pustular dermatosis, 20
        superficial spreading pyoderma, 12
        urticaria and angioedema, 136
Superficial epidermal pustules, 12
Superficial necrolytic dermatitis, 46-48
    compared with
        acrodermatitis of Bull Terrier, 108
        candidiasis, 14, 15
        erythema multiforme, 42
        generic dog food dermatosis, 105, 106
        zinc-responsive dermatosis, 103, 104
Superficial perforating folliculitis, 239, 240
Superficial pustular diseases, epidermal, 10-21
    impetigo in, 10-12
    mucocutaneous candidiasis in, 14-15
    pemphigus erythematosus in, 18-20
    pemphigus foliaceus in, 16-18
    subcorneal pustular dermatosis in, 20
    superficial spreading pyoderma in, 12-14
Superficial pyoderma; *see also* Superficial bacterial folliculitis
Superficial spreading pyoderma, 12-14, 112-113, 114, 239
    compared with
        acanthosis nigricans of Dachshund, 80
        atopy, 116
        erythema multiforme, 42
        flea allergy dermatitis, 120
        mucocutaneous candidiasis, 15
        sterile eosinophilic pustulosis, 250
        superficial bacterial folliculitis, 241
        urticaria, 136
Suppurative arthritis, 203
Suprabasilar cleft
    pemphigus vegetans and, 33
    pemphigus vulgaris and, 31, 32, 34
Swarm of bees lymphocytic inflammation, 292
Sweat gland tumors, 386-397
    apocrine
        adenoma in, 389-392

Sweat gland tumors—cont'd
  apocrine—cont'd
    carcinoma in, 392-395
    cyst in, 386, 387
    cystadenoma in, 387-388
    cystomatosis in, 386-387
  eccrine, 396, 397
Syndrome
  Cushing's; *see* Hyperadrenocorticism
  Ehlers-Danlos, 232-234, 236
  Schnauzer comedo, 96-98, 258, 272
  Sézary, 478
  Vogt-Koyanagi-Harada–like; *see* Vogt-Koyanagi-Harada–like
    syndrome
Systemic amyloidosis of skin compared with multiple myeloma,
  230
Systemic fungal infection
  idiopathic sterile nodular panniculitis versus, 321
  morphologic features in, 175
Systemic lupus erythematosus, 24-26
  compared with
    discoid lupus erythematosus, 23, 24, 145
    erythema multiforme, 42, 43
    hereditary lupoid dermatosis of German Shorthaired Pointer,
      28
    mucocutaneous candidiasis, 14
    panniculitis, 313
    pemphigus vulgaris, 31
    superficial necrolytic dermatitis, 47
    toxic epidermal necrolysis, 44
    ulcerative dermatosis of Shetland Sheepdog and Collie, 36, 38
    vitiligo, 152
    Vogt-Koyanagi-Harada–like syndrome, 149
  dermal, 145-146

T

T-cell lymphoma; *see also* Mycosis fungoides
  epitheliotropic, 476
  histiocytic, mast cell tumors versus, 473
  histiocytoma versus, 468
  lymphomatoid granulomatosis and, 482
T-suppressor cells, 477
Tag, skin, 409-410, 413
Tail dock neuroma, 438
Tarsal pad in sterile pedal panniculitis, 324
Telogen defluxion; *see* Telogen effluvium
Telogen effluvium, 286-287
  compared with
    hyperadrenocorticism, 278
    hypothyroidism, 275
  inducers of, 286
Telogen phase of hair follicle, 273
TEN; *see* Toxic epidermal necrolysis
Terrier
  Airedale; *see* Airedale Terrier
  American Staffordshire; *see* American Staffordshire Terrier
  Boston; *see* Boston Terrier
  Bull; *see* Bull Terrier
  Cairn; *see* Cairn Terrier
  hyperplastic dermatosis of West Highland White, ichthyosis ver-
    sus, 99
  Jack Russell, 99
  lipoma in, 431
  Manchester, 307
  Pit Bull, 99

Terrier—cont'd
  Scottish; *see* Scottish Terrier
  West Highland White; *see* West Highland White Terrier
  Yorkshire; *see* Yorkshire Terrier, alopecia in
Thermal injury, 48-50
  squamous cell carcinoma and, 336
Thioflavine T stain in amyloid, 230
Thrombosis, pythiosis and, 185
Thyroid gland
  disorders of, 74
Tick-bite hypersensitivity
  arthropod-bite granuloma and, 207
  eosinophilic furunculosis versus, 269
Toluidine blue stain
  mast cell tumors and, 469, 470, 471
  plasmacytoma and, 476
Tombstone cells, 32
Toxic epidermal necrolysis, 44-46
  compared with
    bullous pemphigoid, 29
    chemical and thermal burns, 49, 50
    erythema multiforme, 42, 43
    pemphigus vulgaris, 31
Toy Poodle
  epidermolysis bullosa in, 38
  sebaceous adenitis in, 101
Trabecular trichoblastoma, 369-370
  compared with
    benign basal cell tumor, 343
    isthmus-catagen tricholemmoma, 365
    solid basal cell carcinoma, 347
    stromal features in, 369
Traction alopecia, 294-295
  compared with
    alopecia areata, 291
    cicatricial alopecia, 293
Tranquilization in skin biopsy, 3
Traumatic panniculitis, 319-320
  compared with
    pansteatitis, 324
    post-injection panniculitis, 319
Trichoblastoma; *see also* Basal cell tumor
  ductular apocrine adenoma versus, 390-391
  follicular, 367-371
  granular cell, bulb-type tricholemmoma versus, 364-365
  trabecular; *see* Trabecular trichoblastoma
  trichogenic, 367
Trichoepithelioma, 360-361
  compared with
    ductular apocrine adenoma, 390-391
    keratinizing basal cell carcinoma, 348
    melanocytoma-acanthoma, 459
    pilomatricoma, 367
    proliferating matrical cyst, 354
    inner root sheath differentiation in, 348
Trichofolliculoma, 359-360
  compared with
    dermoid cyst, 355
    matrical carcinoma, 372
Trichogranuloma
  callus and callus pyoderma and, 256
  deep bacterial folliculitis and furunculosis and, 255
Trichohyalin
  hair follicle and, 352
  hybrid cysts and, 355

Trichohyalin—cont'd
  matrical carcinoma and, 371
Tricholemmal cyst; see Isthmus-catagen cyst
Tricholemmal keratinization
  bulb-type tricholemmoma and, 364
  follicular cyst and, 351
  hair follicle and, 352
  isthmus-catagen cyst and, 353
  isthmus-catagen tricholemmoma and, 365
  keratinizing basal cell carcinoma and, 348
  melanocytoma-acanthoma and, 458
  nailbed keratoacanthoma and, 401
  ribbon-type trichoblastoma and, 368
  trabecular trichoblastoma and, 370
Tricholemmoma, 364-365
  bulb-type; see Bulb-type tricholemmoma
  isthmus-catagen, 365
    melanocytoma-acanthoma compared with, 459
Trichophyton mentagrophytes in dermatophytosis
  in cat, 241
  in dog, 243, 244
Trichrome stain
  in fibrosarcoma, 413, 415
  in leiomyoma, 444
Trimethoprim-sulfa reactions, 42
Tumor
  basal cell; see Basal cell tumor
  benign fibrohistiocytic, 445
  benign mixed mammary, mixed apocrine adenoma versus, 390
  collision, 459
  epidermal; see Epidermal tumors
  epithelial; see Epithelial tumors
  fibrocytic; see Fibrocytic tumors
  follicular; see Follicular tumors
  lymphocytic; see Lymphocytic tumors
  malignant peripheral nerve sheath; see Schwannoma, malignant
  mast cell; see Histiocytic and mast cell tumors
  melanocytic; see Melanocytic tumors
  Merkel cell, 474
  nailbed epithelial; see Nailbed epithelial tumors
  pancreatic endocrine, 46
  peripheral nerve sheath, 437
  pigmented, 378
  plasma cell, 230
  sebaceous; see Sebaceous tumors
  Sertoli cell; see Sertoli cell tumors
  stage in mycosis fungoides, 160
  sweat gland; see Sweat gland tumors
  transmissible venereal, mast cell tumors versus, 473
  vascular; see Vascular tumors
Tumoral calcinosis, 226-228
Tuna, canned red, 324

U
Ulcer
  discoid lupus erythematosus and, 143
  feline
    eosinophilic, 63-64, 216
    indolent, 63-64, 216
  food allergy and, 117
  immune-mediated vasculitis and, 138
  indolent
    eosinophilic granuloma versus, 216
    food allergy and, 117
  rodent, 63-64, 216

Ulcer—cont'd
  septic vasculitis and, 139, 140
Ulcerative dermatosis
  idiopathic, 65-67
    pyotraumatic dermatitis versus, 59
    linear subepidermal fibrosis and, 65-67
    Shetland Sheepdog and Collie and, 36-38
      bullous pemphigoid versus, 29
      discoid lupus erythematosus versus, 24
      erythema multiforme versus, 43
      hereditary lupoid dermatosis of German Shorthaired Pointer versus, 28
      systemic lupus erythematosus versus, 26
Ulcerative diseases of epidermis; see Exudative and ulcerative diseases of epidermis
Ultraviolet radiation, 330; see also Solar damage
Umbilical fold, flea allergy dermatitis in, 120
Uncinariasis; see Hookworm dermatitis
Unsaturated fatty acids in pansteatitis, 324
Uremic stomatitis compared with mucocutaneous candidiasis, 14
Urticaria, 135-137
  in Ackerman's allergic eruption compared with angioedema, 136
  erythema multiforme compared with, 42
  immunologic and nonimmunologic causes of, 135
Uveitis; see Vogt-Koyanagi-Harada–like syndrome

V
Vaccination reaction
  idiopathic ulcerative dermatosis versus, 65
  rabies
    alopecia in; see Post-rabies vaccination alopecia
    post-injection panniculitis and, 316-317
Vacuolar degeneration
  in familial dermatomyositis, 290
  in liver with superficial necrolytic dermatitis, 46
  in post-rabies vaccination alopecia, 289
van Gieson's stain, 444
Vascular diseases, dermal, 135-140
  angioedema in, 135-137
  pythiosis and, 185
  systemic histiocytosis and, 202
  urticaria in, 135-137
  vasculitis in; see Vasculitis
Vascular tumors, 419-429
  hemangioma in, 419-422
  hemangiosarcoma in, 422-426
  lymphangioma in, 426-427
  lymphangiosarcoma in, 427-428
  scrotal hamartoma in, 419, 420
Vasculitis
  compared with
    canine ear margin seborrhea, 96
    chemical and thermal burns, 49, 50
    erythema multiforme, 42
    erythema nodosum–like panniculitis, 323
    post-rabies vaccination alopecia, 316
    septal panniculitis, 315
    spider bites, 213
    systemic lupus erythematosus, 25
    toxic epidermal necrolysis, 44
    urticaria and angioedema, 136
  immune-mediated, 138, 139
    septic vasculitis versus, 140
    spider bites versus, 213

Vasculitis—cont'd
  leukocytoclastic
    immune-mediated vasculitis and, 138
    urticaria and, 136-137
  nonleukocytoclastic, 138
  septic, 139-140
    immune-mediated vasculitis versus, 138
Vasoactive amines, 471
Vellus hairs, acquired pattern alopecia and, 307
Venereal tumor compared with mast cell tumors, 473
Verruca, 336
Verruca plana, 334, 335
Verrucous nevus, human, 331
Vesicle
  in bullous and vesicular diseases, 22; see also Bullous and vesicu-
    lar diseases of epidermis
  in bullous pemphigoid, 28, 29
  dermatitis and
    allergic contact, 51, 52, 132
    feline allergic miliary, 61
    irritant contact, 54
  in epidermal diseases; see Bullous and vesicular diseases of epider-
    mis
  in epidermolysis bullosa, 38
  in familial dermatomyositis, 34, 36
  in junctional epidermolysis bullosa, 38
  in mucinosis, 228
  in pemphigus vulgaris, 31
Vimentin
  in fibrosarcoma, 415
  in malignant melanoma, 464
  in squamous cell carcinoma, 340
Viral disease
  in feline leukemia
    versus cutaneous horn of footpads, 331
    with epitheliotropic and nonepitheliotropic lymphoma,
      477-478
  in feline sarcoma; see Feline sarcoma virus
  in squamous papilloma of epidermis, 334-335
Visceral disease, 174
  in mastocytosis, 468
Vitamin A–responsive dermatosis, 94
  primary, 102
  primary seborrhea compared with, 90
Vitamin E deficiency, 323-324
Vitiligo
  of dermis, 150-153
  Vogt-Koyanagi-Harada–like syndrome compared with, 149
Vitreous sheath tricholemmoma, 364
Vizslas
  cutaneous vascular tumors in, 421
  sebaceous adenitis in, 101, 248
    leishmaniasis versus, 188
VKH; see Vogt-Koyanagi-Harada–like syndrome
Vogt-Koyanagi-Harada–like syndrome, 148-150
  compared with
    discoid lupus erythematosus, 23, 145
    mycosis fungoides, 159
    pemphigus erythematosus, 18
    vitiligo, 152
von Kossa stain, 226

W
Wart, 324-325, 336
  exophytic, 334

Wedge biopsy
  in actinomycosis and nocardiosis, 165
  in amyloidosis, 230
  in calcinosis circumscripta, 227
  in calcinosis cutis, 225
  in canine callus and callus pyoderma, 256
  in cryptococcosis, 177
  elliptical, 2
  in eosinophilic granuloma, 219
  in epidermolysis bullosa, 38
  in erythema nodosum–like panniculitis, 323
  in fibropruritic nodules, 70
  foreign body reactions and, 191
  in immune-mediated vasculitis, 138
  in indolent ulcer, 63
  in leprosy, 167
  in mucinosis, 229
  in opportunistic mycobacterial infection, 170
  in pansteatitis, 324
  in pemphigus vegetans, 33
  in pemphigus vulgaris, 31
  in plasma cell pododermatitis, 220
  in pythiosis, 184
  in septic vasculitis, 140
  in spider bites, 213
  in sporotrichosis, 182
  in sterile pedal panniculitis of German Shepherd Dog, 325
  in traumatic panniculitis, 319
  in ulcerative dermatosis, 65
  in ulcerative dermatosis of Shetland Sheepdog and Collie, 37
  in xanthoma, 193
Wedge-shaped necrosis in arthropod-bite granuloma, 208
Weimaraner with mast cell tumor, 470
West Highland White Terrier
  atopy in, 115
  flea allergy dermatitis in, 120
  food allergy and, 117
  hyperplastic dermatosis of, 81-83
    ichthyosis versus, 99
  Malassezia pachydermatis infection in, 93
  primary seborrhea in, 81-83, 89, 99
Westie; see West Highland White Terrier
Wheals
  food allergy and, 117
  urticaria and angioedema and, 135, 136
Whippet
  actinic keratosis in, 78
  alopecia in
    acquired pattern, 307
    color-mutant, 299
  cutaneous vascular tumors in, 421
  hemangiosarcomas in
    dermal hemangiomas versus, 421
    solar-associated, 423
White cats with squamous cell carcinoma, 337
White-faced cat with actinic keratosis, 330
Wilder's silver stain, 476
Winer, dilated pore of, 331, 356-357
Wirehaired Fox Terrier with atopy, 115
Woringer-Kolopp disease, 477
Woringer-Kolopp–like variants of mycosis fungoides, 482

X
X-linked ichthyosis, human, 98
Xanthogranuloma, preauricular; see Preauricular xanthogranuloma